Walter Finnegan, M.D.

HUP — Ortho.

Please return to 110 Maloney.

THE SPINE

Volume II

Edited by

RICHARD H. ROTHMAN, M.D., Ph.D.

Associate Professor of Orthopaedic Surgery,
The University of Pennsylvania School of Medicine;
Chief of Orthopaedic Surgery,
The Pennsylvania Hospital, Philadelphia

and

FREDERICK A. SIMEONE, M.D.

Associate Professor of Neurosurgery,
The University of Pennsylvania School of Medicine;
Chief of Neurosurgery,
The Pennsylvania Hospital;
Director of Neurosurgery,
Elliott Neurological Center of Pennsylvania Hospital, Philadelphia

1975

W. B. SAUNDERS COMPANY

Philadelphia • London • Toronto

W. B. Saunders Company: West Washington Square
Philadelphia, PA 19105

12 Dyott Street
London, WC1A 1DB

833 Oxford Street
Toronto, Ontario M8Z 5T9, Canada

The Spine — *Volume II*

ISBN 0-7216-7717-7

Last digit is the print number: 9   8   7   6   5   4   3   2   1

CONTRIBUTORS

ROBERT W. BAILEY, M.D.

Professor of Surgery, University of Michigan Medical School; Active Staff in Orthopedic Surgery, St. Joseph Mercy Hospital, Ann Arbor, Michigan.

Surgical Considerations in Arthritis of the Spine

M. VALLO BENJAMIN, M.D.

Associate Professor of Clinical Neurosurgery, New York University School of Medicine; Attending Physician, University Hospital; Associate Director, University Hospital; Visiting Attending Physician, Bellevue Hospital; Consultant Physician, Veterans Hospital, New York, New York.

Thoracic Disc Disease

DIETRICH BLUMER, M.D.

Associate Professor of Psychiatry, Harvard Medical School; Associate Psychiatrist, McLean Hospital, Belmont, Massachusetts.

Psychiatric Aspects of Spinal Pain

DAVID S. BRADFORD, M.D.

Associate Professor of Orthopedic Surgery, University of Michigan; Associate Professor of Orthopedic Surgery, Fairview Hospital Spine Service, Gillette Children's Hospital, Minneapolis, Minnesota.

Scoliosis

HOWARD DUNCAN, M.B., B.S.(Syd), M.S., M.R.C.P., F.A.C.P.

Staff Rheumatologist, Co-Director, Calcified Tissue Laboratory, Henry Ford Hospital, Detroit, Michigan.

Metabolic Bone Disease Affecting the Spine

KENNETH C. FRANCIS, B.A., M.S., M.D.

Professor of Clinical Orthopedic Surgery, New York University School of Medicine; Attending Orthopedic Surgeon, University

Hospital, New York University Medical Center, New York, New York.

Tumors of the Spine

FREDIE P. GARGANO, M.D.

Professor of Radiology, Neurology, and Neurological Surgery, University of Miami School of Medicine; Chief of Diagnostic Radiology, Jackson Memorial Hospital; Consultant in Neuroradiology, Veterans Administration Hospital, Miami, Variety Children's Hospital, Miami, and Boward General Hospital, Fort Lauderdale, Florida.

Transverse Axial Tomography of the Lumbar Spine

RICHARD N. HARNER, M.D.

Associate Professor of Neurology, University of Pennsylvania School of Medicine; Chief, Department of Neurology, Graduate Hospital of The University of Pennsylvania; Associate Professor of Neurology, Hospital of The University of Pennsylvania; Neurologist, Presbyterian-University of Pennsylvania Medical Center; Consultant in Neurology, Pennsylvania Hospital and Children's Hospital, Philadelphia, Pennsylvania.

Differential Diagnosis of Spinal Disorders

ROBERT N. HENSINGER, M.D.

Assistant Professor of Surgery, Section of Orthopedics, University of Michigan. University Hospital, Ann Arbor; Wayne County Hospital, Detroit, Michigan.

Congenital Anomalies of the Spine

A. R. HODGSON, O.B.E., F.R.C.S.E., F.A.C.S., F.R.A.C.S.

Professor of Orthopaedic Surgery, University of Hong Kong Faculty of Medicine; Chief of Orthopaedic Surgery, Duchess of Kent Children's Orthopaedic Hospital, Hong Kong; Consultant Orthopaedic Surgeon to H. M. Forces in Hong Kong.

Infectious Disease of the Spine

JOHN H. HUBBARD, M.D.

Assistant Professor of Surgery (Neurosurgery), University of Pennsylvania School of Medicine; Staff Neurosurgeon, Hospital of The University of Pennsylvania; Chief, Division of Neurosurgery, Veterans Administration Hospital; Consultant Neurosurgeon, Philadelphia General Hospital, Philadelphia, Pennsylvania.

Management of Chronic Pain of Spinal Origin

ROLLIN M. JOHNSON, M.D.

Assistant Professor of Orthopedic Surgery, Yale University School of Medicine; Chief, Rehabilitation Medicine, West Haven Veterans Administration Hospital, New Haven, Connecticut.

Surgical Approaches to the Spine

THOMAS A. KELLEY, JR., M.D.

Medical Director, Adjunct Professor of Medicine; Medical Director, Institute of Physical Medicine and Rehabilitation, University of Louisville School of Medicine, Louisville, Kentucky.

Rehabilitation of the Spinal Cord Injured Patient

G. DEAN MACEWEN, M.D.

Associate Professor, Thomas Jefferson University School of Medicine, Philadelphia, Pennsylvania; Medical Director and Surgeon-in-Chief, Alfred I. Dupont Institute, Wilmington, Delaware.

Congenital Anomalies of the Spine

PAUL E. MCMASTER, M.D.

Clinical Professor of Orthopedic Surgery, University of California at Los Angeles Medical School, Los Angeles; Senior Consultant, Orthopaedic Surgery, Veterans Administration Hospital, West Los Angeles; Senior Attending, St. John's Hospital, Santa Monica; Orthopaedic Hospital, Los Angeles; Hollywood Presbyterian Hospital, Los Angeles, California.

Osteotomy of the Spine for Fixed Flexion Deformity

IAN MACNAB, F.R.C.S.(Eng), F.R.C.S.(Can)

Associate Professor of Surgery, University of Toronto; Chief of Division of Orthopaedic Surgery, Wellesley Hospital, Toronto, Ontario, Canada.

Acceleration Extension Injuries of the Cervical Spine

JOHN H. MOE, M.D.

Emeritus Professor of Orthopedic Surgery, University of Minnesota. Former Chairman and Professor, Department of Orthopedic Surgery, University of Minnesota; Director, Twin City Scoliosis Center, Fairview Hospital, Minneapolis, Minnesota.

Scoliosis

HORACE A. NORRELL, M.D.

Former Professor and Chairman, Division of Neurological Surgery, University of Kentucky; Staff, Sarasota Memorial Hospital, Sarasota Florida.

Fractures and Dislocations of the Spine

ALWYN M. PARFITT, B.A., M.B., B.Chir., F.R.C.P., F.A.C.P.

Clinical Associate Professor, University of Michigan Medical School; Director of Mineral Metabolism Research Laboratory; Physician, Fifth Medical Division, Henry Ford Hospital, Detroit, Michigan.

Metabolic Bone Disease Affecting the Spine

WESLEY WILKIN PARKE, Ph.D.

Professor of Anatomy, Southern Illinois University School of Medicine, Carbondale, Illinois.

Development of the Spine
Applied Anatomy of the Spine

JOSEPH RANSOHOFF, M.D.

Professor and Chairman, Department of Neurosurgery, New York University School of Medicine; Director Neurological Service, University Hospital; Director Neurological Service, Veterans Administration Hospital; Attending, St. Vincent's Hospital and Medical Center, New York, New York.

Thoracic Disc Disease

RICHARD H. ROTHMAN, M.D., Ph.D.

Chief of Orthopaedic Surgery, The Pennsylvania Hospital; Associate Professor of Orthopaedic Surgery, The University of Pennsylvania School of Medicine, Philadelphia, Pennsylvania.

Cervical Disc Disease
Lumbar Disc Disease

FREDERICK A. SIMEONE, M.D.

Chief of Neurosurgery, The Pennsylvania Hospital; Associate Professor of Neurosurgery, The University of Pennsylvania School of Medicine, Philadelphia, Pennsylvania.

Cervical Disc Disease
Lumbar Disc Disease
Intraspinal Neoplasms

NATHAN M. SMUKLER, M.D.

Professor of Medicine, Thomas Jefferson University School of Medicine; Attending Physician, Thomas Jefferson University Hospital, Philadelphia, Pennsylvania.

Arthritic Disorders of the Spine

WAYNE O. SOUTHWICK, M.D.

Professor of Orthopaedic Surgery, Yale University School of Medicine, New Haven, Connecticut.

Surgical Approaches to the Spine

MICHAEL A. WIENIR, M.D.

Assistant Instructor of Neurology, University of Pennsylvania School of Medicine; Resident in Neurology, Hospital of The University of Pennsylvania, Philadelphia, Pennsylvania.

Differential Diagnosis of Spinal Disorders

ROBERT B. WINTER, M.D.

Associate Professor, University of Minnesota; Director of Medical Education, Gillette Children's Hospital, St. Paul; Director, Orthopaedic Education, Fairview Hospital and St. Mary's Hospital, Minneapolis, Minnesota.

Scoliosis

CONTENTS

CONTENTS

CHAPTER 9

Lumbar Disc Disease

RICHARD H. ROTHMAN, M.D., Ph.D.

FREDERICK A. SIMEONE, M.D.
Pennsylvania Hospital and the University of Pennsylvania

INTRODUCTION

Back pain has plagued man for many thousands of years. Descriptions of lumbago and sciatica are found in the Bible and in the writings of Hippocrates. Despite the long history of awareness of this problem, a reasonable and scientific explanation of the source of low back and leg pain did not emerge until 1934 with the publication of the classic paper by Mixter and Barr.[78] These investigators for the first time delineated prolapse of the intervertebral disc as the etiologic agent in the production of these symptoms. It is commonly acknowledged today that derangements of the intervertebral disc represent the great majority of cases of back pain and sciatica.

Human disease assumes importance as a cause of either death or disability. Degenerative disease of the spine, for all intents and purposes, is a nonlethal entity, and its priority must rest on a determination of its prevalence in the population and its impact on this population in terms of pain and disability.

INCIDENCE

In Sweden, each member of the National Health Insurance, in order to receive compensation, reports his or her illness by telephone to a central bureau. Thus, excellent statistics are readily available in terms of population analysis. Back pain has been reported in 53 per cent of light workers and 64 per cent of those engaged in heavy labor.[60] An extensive investigation by Horal showed that low back pain of a significant degree begins in the younger age groups, with a mean age of onset of 35 years.[58] Of the individuals complaining of low back pain, only 35 per cent will develop sciatica. After subsidence of the original attack of low back pain, 90 per cent have a future recurrence. The recurrent attacks tend to be more prolonged than the original episode. It is of interest that 50 per cent of individuals in this study of the population with low back pain also had cervical spine discomfort but that the age of onset was, on the average, 6 years later. Twenty per cent also had pain in the thoracic spine. It would appear that at least half of the adult population at some time in their lives is incapacitated with low back pain secondary to degenerative disc disease.

A clinical and radiographic survey of the British town of Leigh revealed that in males between the ages of 55 and 64 years, 83 per cent showed evidence of significant lumbar disc degeneration.

Several excellent reviews on the impact of spine disease on industrial disability are found in the medical literature. The Department of Labor and Industry of the State of Washington carefully analyzed its experience in 1965 and was able to come to the following conclusions: 24 per cent of days lost from work were due to low back disorders. Of those individuals who were out of work for greater than six months, only 50 per cent ultimately returned to work. Of those off work for longer than one year, only 25 per cent ultimately returned to work. Although the average industrial claim was 25.7 days, the average days lost per back claim were 123. The implication of these figures is obvious and has been repeated in every major analysis of industrial back disease.

NATURAL HISTORY

Intelligent treatment of lumbar disc degeneration must be predicated on a thorough knowledge of the natural history of this disorder. If this information is not available to the treating physician and to the patient, they will be unable to honestly and effectively make the decisions necessary in the management of this disorder. All too often, decisions either for or against surgical intervention are based on distorted concepts of disc disease. A group of 583 patients were studied at the Karolinska Institute after their first attack of sciatica. Surgery was undertaken in 28 per cent of the group, and both the operative and nonoperative patients were followed for an average of seven years.[46] The results of this study indicated that the acute episodes of sciatica ran a relatively brief course in most cases, regardless of whether the treatment was conservative or surgical. However, the subacute or chronic symptoms secondary to disc degeneration, although less dramatic, were prolonged and had a profound effect on the patient's life. At the end of the follow-up period approximately 15 per cent of the conservatively treated group continued to have a reduced working capacity, a restriction in leisure activities and regular sleep disturbances. Twenty per cent of the conservatively treated group continued to have pronounced residual sciatica. Colonna studied a group of 28 patients with radiographically proved disc herniations for a period of up to eight years.[15] Fifty-seven per cent of the patients had intermittent disability for five years or longer. Pearce has reported a group of 91 patients with a diagnosis of lumbar disc protrusion who were followed conservatively.[83] At the time of follow-up evaluation eight years later, 26.5 per cent were free of pain, 41 per cent were troubled by mild pain and 32.4 per cent were having minor to severe pain.

Disability from lumbar disc disease must be considered in terms of back and leg pain with its attendant limitation of function. Neurologic deficits including motor weakness, although helpful diagnostically, are not necessarily compelling surgical factors, since residual weakness is not markedly different in patients treated operatively or conservatively.[46] Bowel and bladder dysfunction affects a relatively small percentage of patients but assumes greater significance in terms of surgical urgency.

With this background, the treating physician and his patient must take their decision for the role of surgery. If, after careful diagnostic evaluation, a firm diagnosis can be established, and a concerted course of conservative treatment has failed, and the treating surgeon feels that his operative intervention would with certainty shorten the disease process, then surgery can be recommended.

PATHOLOGY OF THE LUMBAR INTERVERTEBRAL DISC

The biochemical, autoimmune and genetic factors in disc degeneration have been discussed in detail in Chapter 7, and the reader is referred to that section for a discussion of those aspects of lumbar disc disease. The lumbar intervertebral disc undergoes a type of degeneration which is different in many respects from the pattern found in the cervical spine. Chronic cervical disc degeneration is the major cause of neck pain and radiculitis. Herniations of soft nuclear material are the exception rather than the rule. In the lumbar spine herniations of soft disc material are frequent and, indeed, are the most common cause of acute sciatica in conjunction with low back pain. This is not to say that acute disc herniations do not occur in the cervical area or that chronic disc degeneration cannot produce sciatica, but that it is not the usual case.

In both the cervical and lumbar areas, disc degeneration is not usually due to one major traumatic insult. Approximately 25 per cent of patients presenting with back pain and sciatica will give a history of trauma. Injury will most often play a precipitating role in what is truly a chronic degenerative process.

Ballooned Disc

Ballooning of the intervertebral disc is characteristically seen in association with diseases which weaken the body of the vertebra. Classically, osteoporosis, more accurately termed osteopenia, will sufficiently weaken the vertebral body to allow expansion of the intervertebral disc into the upper and lower plates of the body. For this to occur the disc must still have its elastic gelatinous nucleus.[17] If the disc has lost its integrity, collapse and wedging of the vertebral body will occur rather than ballooning of the disc. Malignant processes such as multiple myeloma will produce sufficient weakness of the vertebral body to allow this ballooning to take place (Fig. 9–1).

Intra-Spongy Nuclear Herniations

(Schmorl's Node)

It has been noted for over 100 years that the intervertebral disc can herniate through the cartilaginous end plate into the cancellous bone of the vertebral body. This herniation of disc material takes place through a defect in the cartilaginous plate which may represent

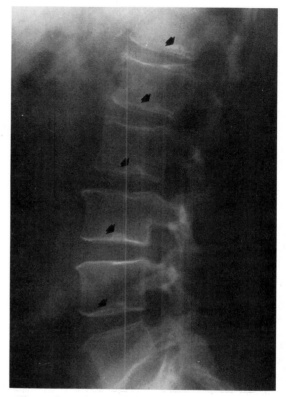

Figure 9–2. X-ray of the lumbar spine illustrating multiple intra-spongy nuclear herniations into the central portion of the adjacent end plate of the vertebral body.

the point of passage of blood vessels from the body of the vertebra to the disc during early life. These herniations are irregular in size and shape, and ultimately will be surrounded by a rim of bony sclerosis. These defects are seen throughout all adult life. The adjacent disc space frequently exhibits thinning (Fig. 9–2).

Osteophyte Formation

Peripheral osteophyte formations, anteriorly and laterally and to a lesser extent posteriorly, are often found in the bodies of lumbar vertebrae associated with disc degeneration. These osteophytes represent pathologic stimulation of new bone formation at the attachment of the longitudinal ligaments of the annulus to the bodies. This stimulation may be due to hypermobility of the vertebral body or abnormal distribution of stresses on the annulus and ligaments associated with degeneration of the intervertebral disc. MacNab has

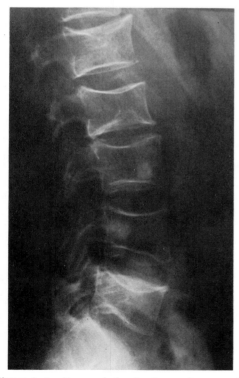

Figure 9–1. X-ray of the lumbar spine revealing severe osteoporosis with ballooning of multiple discs into the softened adjacent vertebral body.

differentiated the traction spur from other osteophytes.[72] It is horizontally directed and arises two millimeters away from the discal border of the anterior and lateral surfaces of the vertebral body. MacNab feels that it denotes segmental instability. The decreased incidence of posterior osteophytes as compared to those in the anterior and lateral position may be explained by the absence of a strong attachment of the posterior longitudinal ligament to bone. This osteophyte formation in association with disc degeneration has often been termed lumbar spondylosis, which has its counterpart in cervical spondylosis.

Thinned Discs

Three distinct situations are present which may be associated with thinning of the disc space. The first situation occurs in the presence of a transitional fifth lumbar vertebra (Fig. 9–3). Between the transitional vertebra and the sacrum, a vestigial disc is often found which is devoid of a nucleus pulposus.[48] This loss of height and disc space is not usually the product of degenerative changes. When the transverse process of this transitional vertebra is incompletely sacralized on one side and normal on the other it is possible that the caudal intervertebral disc may be degenerated. More often there is a broad sacralization of the transverse processes, either unilaterally or bilaterally. In these situations one should look for disc degeneration above this transitional vertebra rather than below it.

A second group of thinned intervertebral discs is associated with the degeneration of the nucleus pulposus, with or without herniation. This mechanical loss of disc material is often associated with invasion of granulation tissue through rents in the annulus. Progressive dehydration will contribute markedly to the diminished volume of the disc.

Disc thinning may also occur subsequent to infection of the disc space, and is more completely discussed in Chapter 12, Infections of the Spine.

Disc Protrusion

The process of nuclear herniation and annular protrusion is caused by a combination of biochemical factors previously discussed, chronic degenerative structural changes and superimposed mechanical stress. The pathologic cycle has been described in detail by Armstrong.[6] Prior to actual displacement of disc material, the nucleus and annulus undergo certain well-defined structural changes. Radiating cracks in the annulus fibrosus develop in the most centrally situated lamellae and extend outward toward the periphery.[53] These radiating clefts in the annulus weaken its resistance to nuclear herniation. If they are

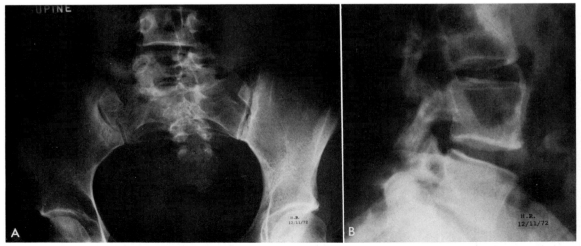

Figure 9–3. A, Anterior posterior X-ray of the lumbar spine reveals a transitional fifth lumbar vertebra. B, Lateral view of the same patient reveals loss of height of the disc space between the transitional vertebra and the sacrum. This is not due to disc degeneration but rather to the congenital variation of the transitional vertebra.

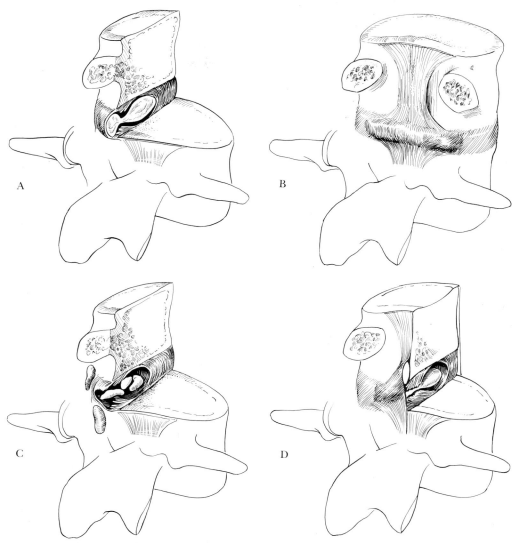

Figure 9–4. *A,* Herniation of a lumbar disc beneath the posterior longitudinal ligament in the common lateral position. *B,* Herniation of a lumbar disc in the less frequent central position beneath the strong portion of the posterior longitudinal ligament. *C,* Complete herniation of a lumbar disc through a rupture in the annulus and the posterior longitudinal ligament, with free fragments in the neural canal. These fragments may migrate cranially, caudally or into the intervertebral foramen. *D,* Herniation of a lumbar disc, with upward migration of the disc fragments, beneath the posterior longitudinal ligaments. These fragments may go unnoticed unless specific exploration in these areas is undertaken. (From DePalma, A. F., and Rothman, R. H.: The Intervertebral Disc. Philadelphia, W. B. Saunders Co., 1970.)

subject to persistent mechanical pressure by a turgid nucleus, herniation may ensue. Herniation is a much greater threat in the younger individual, between the ages of 30 and 50, having good turgor in the nucleus, than in the elderly, in whom the nucleus is desiccated and fibrotic. In the older individual the degenerated, thinned disc will often develop without any of the signs and symptoms of acute nerve root compression. This may explain the pre-

dominance of acute disc syndromes in the middle-aged population and their rarity in the elderly.

Posterior displacement of the nucleus pulposus may occur in a variety of ways (Fig. 9–4). In an extreme circumstance, there may be a massive nuclear retropulsion, in which a large volume of disc material is suddenly thrust into the spinal canal, producing a profound neurologic catastrophe. More commonly, the extrusion is a gradual and intermittent process. The nucleus progressively bulges through the rent in the annulus, being retained in position by the posterior longitudinal ligament. This ligament, which may be stretched and detached by the herniating nuclear material as it forces its way relentlessly backward to the spinal canal, may rupture, with the formation of a free sequestrum into the spinal canal. This disc fragment may then migrate cephalad or caudad or laterally into the intervertebral foramen. It is not only the size of the nuclear herniation which determines its clinical significance but also the direction in which this herniation takes place. In addition, the shape of the spinal canal is shown to be of great importance. Failure to recognize the variety of types of disc pathology having significant spatial relationships will lead to inadequate surgical treatment of these problems. It should also be pointed out that posterior protrusion of disc material may often occur at some site other than that of an obviously thin disc.[16]

Subsequent to the loss of the integrity of the annulus fibrosus, there may be invasion of the disc by granulation material, either through rents in the annulus or through cracks in the cartilaginous end plate. The role of this granulation tissue in regard to the production of pain is as yet unclear.

It should be emphasized that, as the process of disc herniation occurs, biochemical as well as mechanical irritation of the nerve root must be considered. The clinical symptoms which are produced are in all likelihood closely related to biochemical irritation of the nearby nerve root by degradation products of the degenerating disc. It has been dramatically demonstrated by Falconer that myelographic defects are unchanged after successful conservative treatment of sciatica.[32] Thus, mechanical factors alone are insufficient explanations for nerve root symptomatology.

Variations in the Shape of the Spinal Canal

Verbiest has highlighted the importance of the narrow spinal canal in the production of nerve root compression in the cauda equina.[119, 120] It is not only the absolute dimensions of the spinal canal which are of importance but also the configuration (Fig. 9–5). The trefoil canal, with narrow lateral recesses, presents a configuration in which the nerve roots are particularly vulnerable to compression.

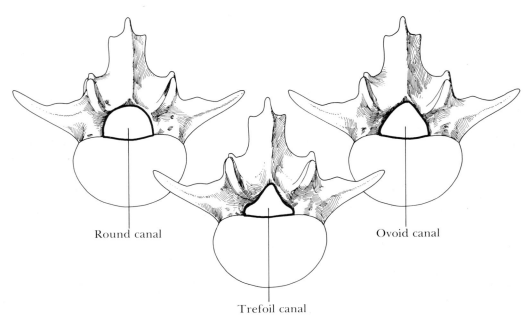

Round canal   Ovoid canal   Trefoil canal

Figure 9–5. The three variations of the spinal canal: round, ovoid and trefoil. The lateral recesses of the trefoil canal render the lumbar roots particularly vulnerable to compression by extruded disc material. (From DePalma, A. F., and Rothman, R. H.: The Intervertebral Disc. Philadelphia, W. B. Saunders Co., 1970.)

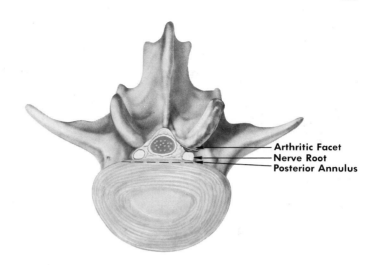

Figure 9–6. This drawing illustrates entrapment of a lumbar nerve root in a lateral narrow recess secondary to degenerative changes. Note how posterior buckling of the annulus and arthritic changes in the facet joints can compromise the nerve root in the anterior-posterior direction. Failure to decompress this recess will result in persistent sciatica after surgery.

The anterior-posterior diameter of the canal is the most critical dimension and can be measured precisely only during surgery. Myelography will suggest this diagnostic entity when there is anterior-posterior compromise of the dye column. Plain radiograms will only imply this diagnosis. A "canal to body ratio" developed by Jones is felt to be helpful in substantiating this diagnosis.[64]

It is of interest that this problem is seen most often in males and most frequently at the L4 level. This is, of course, the most narrow area in the lumbar canal.

Patients with congenitally small lumbar spinal canals, and particularly those with a narrow lateral recess, will be susceptible to degenerative changes of the intervertebral disc in terms of nerve root compression. Often a small nuclear herniation of only one to two millimeters in height will cause marked nerve root compression under these circumstances. If the canal were round in configuration this type of herniation would undoubtedly cause little difficulty. In addition to nuclear herniations, posterior osteophytes and/or degenerative changes in the apophyseal joints can produce nerve root compression in this lateral recess. If this type of pathology is unrecognized, failure to adequately decompress these recesses may result in failure to relieve symptoms after back surgery (Fig. 9–6).

A great variety of clinical manifestations may be produced by these structural abnormalities. Unilateral or bilateral sciatica may result, with both motor and sensory disturbance. So-called "cauda equina claudication" can also occur, with bilateral leg pain accentu-ated by walking and relieved by rest. It may be that the symptoms are produced by relative ischemia of the cauda equina during exercise.

Foraminal Encroachment

It should be recalled that the lumbar nerve root rests well up at the most cranial part of the intervertebral foramen, a relatively protected position. Soft disc protrusions will only infrequently compress nerve root exiting at the same level. However, as disc degeneration progresses the dimensions of the intervertebral foramen may decrease owing to loss of height of the disc space, formation of posterior-lateral osteophytes and osteoarthritis of the apophyseal joints. As the disc space narrows the superior articular facet of the inferior vertebra will tend to sublux in a superior direction and may impinge the nerve root. These considerations make it mandatory that in all nerve root decompression, the root be followed well out beyond the foramen, and the surgeon must be completely satisfied that there is no compression in this area (Fig. 9–7).

Pedicle Migration

It has been lucidly shown by MacNab that as disc degeneration occurs, with subsequent loss of height of the disc space, the pedicles will migrate in a caudal direction relative to the nerve root and may tether the root during its descent.[72, 73] This may produce an intractable radiculitis and, again, if unrecog-

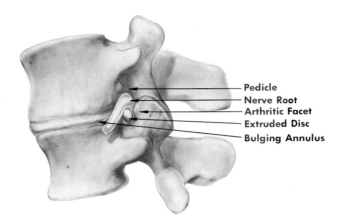

Pedicle
Nerve Root
Arthritic Facet
Extruded Disc
Bulging Annulus

Figure 9–7. Foraminal encroachment secondary to chronic disc degeneration. The nerve root exiting the foramen will be compressed by the arthritic facet joint posteriorly, the relative descent of the pedicle superiorly and the posterior bulge of the annulus or disc extrusion anteriorly. The surgeon must satisfy himself that the nerve root is entirely free throughout the entire course of the foramen when the nerve root is decompressed.

nized, will lead to failure of nerve root decompression. This entity is most often seen in the elderly individual (Fig. 9–8).

CLINICAL SYNDROME OF LUMBAR DISC DISEASE

Lumbar disc disease represents the most common cause of back and leg pain. It is a multifaceted syndrome and must be recognized as such if a diagnosis is to be correct and the treatment effective. One sees with disturbing regularity missed diagnoses of herniated lumbar discs that present in an atypical fashion, unfamiliar to the practitioner. It is equally precarious, however, to polarize one's thinking at the opposite extreme and attribute all cases of back and leg pain to abnormalities of the intervertebral disc. A wide variety of vascular, infectious and space-occupying lesions can mimic the herniated lumbar disc. An

attempt will be made in this section to outline the classic picture of the lumbar disc syndrome as well as the more common variants.

History

BACK PAIN

The majority of patients with degenerative disc disease in the lumbar spine have low back pain as the earliest symptom. The onset is most often in the third decade of life and is insidious in nature. The patient recalls that after periods of prolonged physical activity or working in a position that stresses the spine, pain appears in the lumbosacral area. These early episodes of low back pain are usually not accompanied by sciatica. The pain may last a few days and usually subsides with limitation of activity and bedrest. The pain pattern at this time is mechanical in nature, in the sense

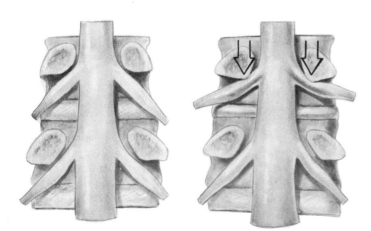

Figure 9–8. These drawings illustrate the relative caudal migration of the pedicles during disc degeneration which may tether the nerve roots. During exploration of a nerve root it must be ascertained that the root is free not only of compression but also of tension as well. If the root is tethered about the pedicle, excision of the offending pedicle must be undertaken.

that it is made worse by standing and lifting and is relieved by rest. It is the authors' feeling that the pain at this stage is due to early degeneration of the annulus fibrosus. The nucleus pulposus is beginning to desiccate, and no longer functions as a perfect gel, so that forces are transmitted in an asymmetrical fashion (Fig. 9–9). This results in areas of excessive tension on the outer layers of the annulus, which are known to contain pain fibers. It should be pointed out that at this early stage, disc disease cannot be clearly differentiated from certain other common causes of low back pain, such as neural arch defects, postural strain, and an unstable lumbosacral mechanism.

With the passage of time, these episodes may become more frequent and more intense and lead to more disability. Between acute episodes of back pain the patient usually describes a sense of stiffness, weakness or instability that is present at a low but noticeable level. Discogenic pain usually has the definite mechanical quality of being accentuated with prolonged standing or sitting. Pain that is accentuated while the patient is in bed at night is more suggestive of a neoplastic process. An intermittent character of the pain is also characteristic of disc disease, and one should be wary when the patient states that from the onset the pain has been unrelenting and progressive.

Injury is frequently noted by the patient at some time during the clinical course, but in most instances spine pain to a greater or lesser degree was present prior to the injury. Our current concepts of the pathophysiology of disc disease show trauma to be a precipitating rather than a causative event. Excessive stress applied to a young, healthy spine will fracture the osseous elements of the vertebra before the disc is ruptured. Often trivial accidents, such as bending forward to shave, coughing, or stooping to pick up an object from the floor will precipitate a severe attack. It is interesting that these usually occur during the early hours of the day when the turgor of the nucleus pulposus is at its maximum.

REFERRED PAIN

When certain of the mesodermal structures, such as the ligaments, periosteum, joint capsules, and the annulus, are subjected to such abnormal stimuli as excessive stretching or injection with hypertonic saline, a deep ill-defined, dull, aching discomfort is noted that may be referred into the area of the sacroiliac joints, the buttocks or the posterior thighs. The pattern of referral is to the area that has

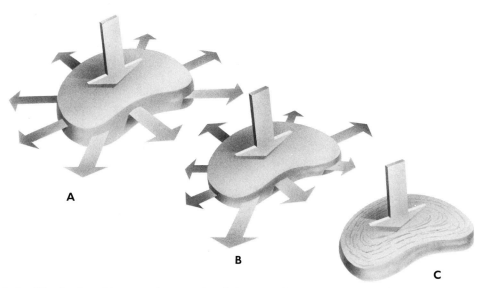

Figure 9–9. Distribution of forces in the normal and abnormal disc. *A,* When the disc functions normally, as in the early decades of life, the nucleus distributes the forces of compression and tension equally to all parts of the annulus. *B,* With degeneration, the nucleus no longer functions as a perfect gel and the forces transmitted to the annulus are unequal. *C,* With advanced degeneration of the nucleus, the distribution of forces to the annulus from within is completely lost since the nucleus now acts as a solid rather than a liquid. For this reason, disc herniation is unusual in the elderly.

the same embryonic origin as the mesodermal tissues stimulated. This is designated the sclerotome. Pain of this type is often present concurrently with radicular pain from nerve root compression, and the two may be easily confused. It should be emphasized that all pain referred from the back into the lower extremities is not caused by nerve root compression.

RADICULAR SYMPTOMS

Compression of an inflamed nerve root by a disc fragment or bulging annulus may produce pain and motor and sensory symptoms in the lower extremities. It is a well recognized fact that a normal nerve root can be retracted with production of only minimal symptoms, whereas an inflamed nerve root is exquisitely sensitive. Thus, not only is mechanical stimulation necessary but also a concurrent inflammatory reaction.

PAIN

Patients note a sharp, lancinating pain, usually starting at the proximal portion of the leg and ultimately progressing distally in a pattern typical of a dermatome. The L5 and S1 nerve roots are most frequently involved. The onset of the leg pain may be insidious or extremely rapid and dramatic and associated with a tearing or snapping sensation in the spine. The latter events may be caused by sudden rupture of the annulus, with extrusion of a fragment of disc against a nerve root. At the time of onset of the sciatica, the back pain may suddenly abate. The explanation for this is that once the annulus has ruptured, it no longer is placed under tension, and there is no longer a stimulus for pain in the low back. When the sciatic pain is acute, the patient or family of the patient may note that he is listing, usually away from the side of the sciatica. Occasionally, if the disc herniation is axillary or central in position, the patient may list toward the side of his sciatica. The pain is made worse by any maneuver that increases intraspinal pressure, such as a Valsalva maneuver, coughing, sneezing or bearing down during defecation. The patient may be aware of marked limitation of motion in his spine and he often states that his back is "locked." In extreme cases the pain may prevent any stress from being placed on the leg or back, and the patient may lie helpless on the floor or in bed

with the feeling that he is "paralyzed," while in reality the limiting factor is pain. In certain instances the patient may simply state that he is unable to tolerate any weight whatsoever on the painful leg, without being able to localize his difficulty to the lumbar spine. In high disc lesions affecting the fourth lumbar nerve root the pain may be isolated to the area of the knee, and the patient may protest vigorously that the difficulty is confined only to the knee joint and discourage any examination of his lumbar spine. If this has progressed to motor weakness involving quadriceps muscle, he may complain of buckling in his knee in addition to the knee pain, and make the situation still more confusing.

MOTOR SYMPTOMS

Occasionally a patient may present with weakness in his lower extremities as the outstanding symptoms. This is particularly true in lesions affecting the fourth and fifth nerve roots. If the fifth nerve root is compressed the patient may note weakness on dorsiflexion of the foot and toes and occasionally a complete foot drop. He may be able to relate a slapping sensation of his foot when he walks, and a space-taking lesion of the cord itself should be carefully considered.

DISC SYNDROMES

SCIATIC PAIN ALONE. It is not uncommon with the acute extrusion of a fragment of nuclear material against a nerve root to have the sudden onset of sciatica without concomitant back pain. The diagnosis of discogenic disease is suggested by accentuation of this leg pain by the Valsalva maneuver. This, of course, would not be present in leg pain caused by affections of the joints of the lower extremities or lesions of the sciatic nerve itself. Although the patient may be free of back pain, he may have a marked list, muscle spasm and limitation of motion in the lumbar spine. The specific sensory, reflex and motor change noted will vary with the nerve root compressed.

It should be pointed out that in certain individuals, isolated areas of pain in the lower extremities are noted by the patient rather than the typical pattern of dermatome involvement. The prime complaint may be pain of the knee, calf, ankle or heel in these individuals (Fig. 9–10). The unwary examiner who fails to

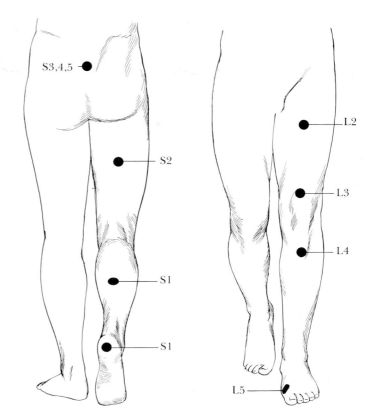

Figure 9–10. Pain may radiate to small, isolated, specific areas along the course of a dermatome.

completely undress the patient and perform a meticulously thorough examination can obviously be led astray in these instances.

BACK PAIN ALONE. It has been pointed out that most patients with discogenic pain have intermittent episodes of back pain at the onset of the clinical course. Many of these individuals may proceed through the entire natural course of their disease and never experience sciatica. During acute exacerbation pain will be accentuated by the Valsalva maneuver, and they will have the typical findings in the lumbar area noted with disc disease. It is in this group of patients that great judgment must be utilized before surgical intervention is elected. It is far too easy to place patients with lumbar pain into this category without careful diagnostic evaluation. The treating physician must discipline himself to rule out all other causes of back pain, such as tumor, infection and intraabdominal disease, before this diagnostic category is utilized.

INTERMITTENT CLAUDICATION

In a small group of patients, symptoms are suggestive of vascular insufficiency. These patients complain of pain in the posterior aspect of their thighs and calves, made worse with exertion and walking. There are subjective complaints similar to those noted with occlusive arteriosclerosis of the aortic and femoral vessels. Physical examination, however, reveals normal peripheral pulses and skin temperature. The symptoms are produced by a stenotic configuration of the spinal canal, which may be further compromised by acute or chronic disc protrusion. A complete block is often noted on myelography, particularly at the L3–L4 or L4–L5 level. In cases in which the diagnosis is unclear arteriography may be indicated.

THE CAUDA EQUINA SYNDROME

Occasionally, a large midline disc herniation may compress several roots of the cauda equina. If the lesion reaches a large size, it may mimic an intraspinal tumor, particularly if it has been slowly progressive. Often back or perianal pain will predominate, and radicular symptoms may be masked. Difficulty with urination, consisting of frequency or overflow incontinence may develop relatively early. In males a history of recent impotence may be elicited by the probing examiner. If leg pains develop they may be followed by numbness of the feet and difficulty in walking. The large midline disc lesions, which ordinarily produce a complete myelographic block when associated with these symptoms, compress several nerve roots. The centrally placed sacral fibers to the lower abdominal viscera, when compressed, produce symptoms which characterize a cauda equina compression. Perianal numbness and the loss of the "anal wink" reflex characterize an advanced cauda equina syndrome.

The significance of this entity is that it must be considered a reason for prompt surgical intervention. If incontinence is present, only prompt surgery can offer a chance to prevent the hazards of a permanent indwelling bladder catheter. True surgical emergency is indicated by the inability to walk. When these symptoms are florid, a careful myelogram with the insertion of only a small amount of contrast material (because a complete block is anticipated) should be planned (Fig. 9–11).

BLADDER SYMPTOMS

It has been recently recognized that disc protrusions may present as an abnormality of bowel or bladder function in patients with minimal or absent back pain and sciatica. It has been well documented, by Emmett and Love and by Ross and Jackson, that disc disease should be ruled out in young or middle-aged patients who develop problems of urinary retention, vesical irritability or incontinence.[31, 90] This is particularly true in the absence of infection or other pelvic abnormalities. Four syndromes have been described in regard to bladder abnormalities caused by disc derangements: total urinary retention, chronic longstanding partial retention, vesical irritability and loss of desire to void associated with unawareness of the necessity to void. This last syndrome is often associated with difficulty in initiating micturition. If these symptoms, particularly in their more subtle forms, are not specifically sought out they will often be overlooked.

Cystoscopy and a cystometrogram, in

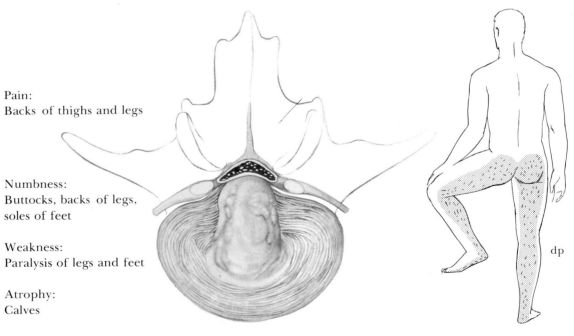

Pain:
Backs of thighs and legs

Numbness:
Buttocks, backs of legs, soles of feet

Weakness:
Paralysis of legs and feet

Atrophy:
Calves

Paralysis:
Bladder and bowel

Figure 9–11. Massive herniation at the level of the third, fourth or fifth disc may cause severe compression of the cauda equina. Pain is confined chiefly to the buttocks and the back of the thighs and legs. Numbness is widespread from the buttocks to the soles of the feet. Motor weakness or loss is present in the legs and feet with loss of muscle mass in the calves. The bladder and bowels are paralyzed. (From DePalma, A. F., and Rothman, R. H.: The Intervertebral Disc. Philadelphia, W. B. Saunders Co., 1970.)

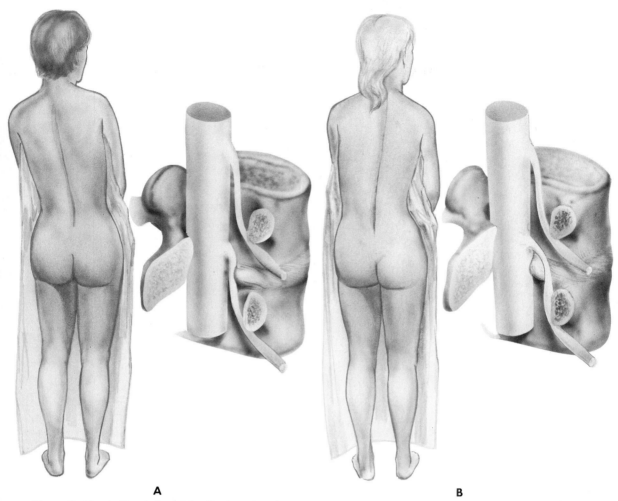

A   **B**

Figure 9–12. *A,* Herniation of the disc lateral to the nerve root. This will usually produce a sciatic list away from the side of the irritated nerve root. *B,* Herniation of the disc medial to the nerve root and in an axillary position. This will usually produce a sciatic list toward the side of the irritated nerve root.

conjunction with a myelogram, are most helpful in obtaining a definitive diagnosis.

These clinical syndromes are often seen with high disc lesions and in lesions with a large central protrusion. Single nerve root lesions are unlikely to cause bladder dysfunction.

Physical Examination

INSPECTION

Limitation of motion is usually noted during this symptomatic phase of disc disease. The range of motion should be noted not only in flexion and extension but also in rotation. The examiner must not equate flexion of the hips with flexion of the lumbar spine, and at-

tention should be directed to whether reversal of the normal lumbar lordosis occurs. It has been previously noted that even in patients who have only sciatica, marked restriction of motion may be present in the lumbar spine.

When acute sciatica is present, the patient usually lists away from the side of his sciatica, producing a "sciatic scoliosis" (Fig. 9–12). When the disc herniation is lateral to the nerve root, the patient will incline away from the side of the irritated nerve root in an attempt to draw the nerve root away from the disc fragment. In a contrary fashion, when the herniation is in an axillary position medial to the nerve root, the patient will list toward the side of the lesion, also in an effort to decompress the nerve root.

The gait and stance of patients with acute disc syndrome are also characteristic. The patient usually holds the painful leg in a flexed position and is reluctant to place his foot completely flat on the floor. Presumably, flexion of the leg relaxes the sciatic nerve roots and is an involuntary effort at decompression of the root. When walking, the patient has an antalgic gait, putting as little weight on the extremity as possible and quickly transferring his weight to the unaffected side.

Loss of normal lumbar lordosis and paravertebral muscle spasm are also usually seen during the acute phase of the disease. These abnormalities are readily seen and easily palpable. The boardlike tightness of the muscles in extreme cases is striking. Occasionally, in less acute situations, the muscle spasm can be elicited only when the patient is stressed by prolonged standing or forward flexion of the spine. In less marked cases of paravertebral muscle spasm, palpation should not be directed over the muscle belly but should start in the midline, with pressure exerted laterally in order to appreciate more subtle differences in tone. Muscle spasm may on occasion be unilateral.

PALPATION AND PERCUSSION

Palpation of the lumbar spine in the midline usually elicits pain at the level of the deranged disc. It is not unusual to find tenderness laterally along the iliac crest and the iliolumbar ligament, and over the sacroiliac joint. In many instances this tenderness does not reflect disease in these lateral areas but rather hyperesthesia from nerve root irritation. Occasionally, no tenderness is elicited with palpation of the lumbar spine in the erect position, and it will be necessary to have the patient flex his spine, to apply pressure in the midline, and then to direct him to extend his spine. This may produce marked pain in certain instances. Percussion of the lumbar spine may either elicit local pain or, more significantly, reproduce sciatica when nerve root compression is present. As with many of the previously noted findings, it is suggestive but not pathognomonic of a herniated disc.

Palpation should also be performed in the sciatic notch and along the course of the sciatic nerve itself. Hyperesthesia along the nerve is often found; in addition, local tumors of the nerve may be discovered in this manner. Occasionally, calf tenderness is found, which

again is a reflection of hyperesthesia of the sciatic nerve and has often been misinterpreted as thrombophlebitis.

NEUROLOGIC EXAMINATION

A meticulous neurologic examination will yield objective evidence of nerve root compression. It will suggest the level of disc herniation, but it is not conclusive in this regard. The two most common levels of disc herniation are L4–L5 and L5–S1. The L3–L4 disc level is the next most common. A herniated disc at L5–S1 will most often compress the first sacral nerve root. A herniated disc at L4–L5 will most often compress the fifth lumbar nerve root, and a herniated disc at L3–L4 will most often compress the fourth lumbar nerve root (see Table 9–1). However, owing to variation in root configuration and in the position of the herniation itself, disc herniation at L4–L5 can affect not only the fifth lumbar nerve root but also the first sacral nerve root, or both. For this reason it is the authors' feeling that, even though the neurologic picture is well defined, myelography should be performed to further localize the level of the lesion when surgery is indicated. If myelography is not performed, exploration of both the L4–L5 and L5–S1 disc spaces is mandatory. This is particularly important in view of the fact that there may be a disc abnormality at more than

---

TABLE 9–1. NERVE ROOT PATTERNS

L4 Nerve root
1. *Pain and numbness*—L4 dermatome, posterolateral aspect of thigh, across patella, anteromedial aspect of leg
2. *Weakness and atrophy*—weak extension of knee, and quadriceps muscle atrophy
3. *Reflex*—depression of patellar reflex

L5 Nerve root
1. *Pain and numbness*—L5 dermatome, posterior aspect of thigh, anterolateral aspect of leg, medial aspect of foot and great toe
2. *Weakness and atrophy*—weak dorsiflexion of foot and toes and atrophy of anterior compartment of leg
3. *Reflex*—none, or absent posterior tibial tendon reflex

S1 Nerve root
1. *Pain and numbness*—S1 dermatome, posterior aspect of thigh, posterior aspect of leg, posterolateral aspect of foot, lateral toes
2. *Weakness and atrophy*—weak plantar flexion of foot and toes and atrophy of posterior compartment of leg
3. *Reflex*—depression of Achilles reflex

one level. The incidence of these double herniations has, in the authors' experience, been approximately 10 per cent.

MOTOR FINDINGS

Compression of the motor fibers of the nerve root results in weakness or paralysis of the muscle group, associated with loss of tone and loss of mass of the muscle belly. Usually a group of muscles rather than a particular muscle is involved. The patient may not be aware of this weakness unless the loss is rather profound. With compression of the first sacral nerve root little motor involvement is noted other than occasional weakness in flexion of the foot and great toe. With compression of the fifth lumbar nerve root, weakness of the toe extensors and dorsiflexors of the foot is noted, with atrophy at the anterior and lateral compartment of the leg. With compression of the fourth lumbar nerve root the quadriceps muscle is affected, and the patient may note a weakness of extension of the knee and, more often, instability of the knee. Atrophy is usually prominent.

SENSORY CHANGES

The pattern of sensory involvement when nerve root compression is present usually follows the dermatome of the affected nerve root. The sensory pattern in the thigh and buttock is less specific than in the leg and foot. With compression of the fourth lumbar nerve root, loss of sensation may be noted in the anteromedial aspect of the leg. With compression of the fifth lumbar nerve root, loss of sensation will be noted in the anterior lateral portion of the leg and along the medial aspect of the foot to the great toe. With S1 nerve root compression, sensation is affected on the posterior aspect of the calf and the lateral aspect of the foot.

REFLEX CHANGES

The deep tendon reflexes are frequently altered in nerve root compression. The Achilles reflex is diminished or absent with compression of the first sciatic nerve root. Compression of the fifth lumbar nerve root most commonly causes no reflex change, but occasionally results in a loss of the posterior tibial reflex. The absence of this reflex must be asymmetrical to have clinical significance. Involvement of the fourth lumbar nerve root results in a decrease or absence of the patellar reflex. The reader should again be reminded that many etiologic agents other than disc herniation can produce abnormalities of the deep tendon reflex. Indeed, on a statistical basis, absence of the Achilles reflex is most often a concomitant of advanced age.

STRAIGHT LEG RAISING TEST AND ITS VARIANTS

There are several maneuvers that tighten the sciatic nerve and, in doing so, further compress an inflamed nerve root against a herniated lumbar disc. An excellent comprehensive view of the so-called tension signs in lumbar disc prolapse has been presented by Scham and Taylor.[95] With the straight leg raising maneuver the L5 and S1 nerve roots move two to six millimeters at the level of the foramen. The L4 nerve root moves a lesser distance, and the more proximal roots show little motion. Thus the straight leg raising test is of most importance and value in lesions of the fifth lumbar and first sciatic nerve root. Their value is also greatest in younger individuals.[108] In a review of 2000 patients with operatively proved lumbar disc herniation the straight leg raising sign was positive in 97 per cent. Young patients were shown to have a marked propensity for a positive straight leg raising test although the test itself is not pathognomonic. However, a negative test excludes with great probability the presence of a herniated disc. After the age of 30 the negative straight leg raising test no longer excludes this diagnosis (Fig. 9–13).

The straight leg raising test is performed with the patient supine and the head flat or on a low pillow. One hand is placed on the ilium to stabilize the pelvis, and the other hand slowly elevates the leg by the heel with the knee straight. The patient should be questioned as to whether this reproduces his leg pain. Only when leg pain or radicular symptoms are reproduced is this test considered positive. Back pain alone is not a positive finding in this maneuver.

Many variations of this test have been described. The knee may first be flexed to 90 degrees and the hip then flexed to 90 degrees. Next, the knee is gradually extended. If this maneuver reproduces leg pain, the test is considered positive. Both this test and the straight leg raising test have been attributed to La-

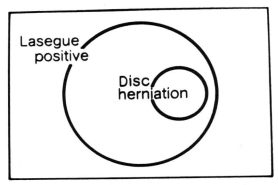

Age: under 30 years

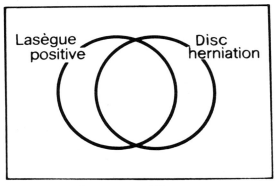

Age: over 30 years

Figure 9–13. These ven diagrams illustrate the marked propensity for a positive Lasegue test with disc herniation in the young. Over the age of 30 the propensity decreases, although the specificity increases for this test in disc herniation. (From Spangfort, 1971.)

segue. Fajersztan described a variation to the straight leg raising test in which the foot is dorsiflexed. This not only may produce an exacerbation of the pain in a straight leg raising test but also could reproduce radicular pain when the conventional straight leg raising test was negative. The sitting root test is yet another variation on this theme. With the patient sitting and his cervical spine flexed, the knee is extended while the hip remains flexed to 90 degrees. The patient may complain of leg pain or may attempt to extend his hip, indicating again nerve root compression.

The contralateral straight leg raising test is performed in the same manner as the straight leg raising test except that the non-painful leg is raised. If this reproduces the patient's sciatica in the opposite extremity, the test is considered positive. This is very

suggestive of a herniated disc and also is an indication of the location of the extrusion. The prolapse will often be large but not in the usual lateral position. At surgery the disc will be noted medial to the nerve root in the axilla (Fig. 9–14).

It should be noted that when the roots of the femoral nerve are involved, they are tensed not by the straight leg raising test but by the reverse straight leg raising test; i.e., by hip extension and knee flexion.

PERIPHERAL VASCULAR EXAMINATION

No examination of a patient with back or leg pain can be considered complete without evaluation of the peripheral circulation. Examination of the posterior tibial and dorsalis pedis arteries should be performed, as well as examination of the skin temperature and inspection for the presence of the trophic changes seen with ischemic disease.

ABDOMINAL AND RECTAL EXAMINATION

Many intra-abdominal and retroperitoneal abnormalities can result in back and leg pain. Careful palpation of the abdomen together with rectal examination will disclose many of these lesions and lead to a correct diagnosis.

Radiographic Examination and Special Tests

ROUTINE RADIOGRAPHY

Radiographic examination of the lumbar spine is considered an integral part of the evaluation of a patient with low back pain. It should be emphasized, however, that the radiographic examination is only one facet of the total picture, and that the treating physician should not allow his judgment to be superseded by the x-ray. It is well known that advanced radiographic changes of disc degeneration may be present with complete absence of symptomatology. Conversely, a marked disc prolapse with incapacitating pain may be present in the face of a completely normal x-ray. It is thus obvious that the specific radiographic findings can be of use only to reinforce the clinical diagnosis of a lumbar disc abnormality.

The radiograph must be of excellent quality, and should be taken with great attention to

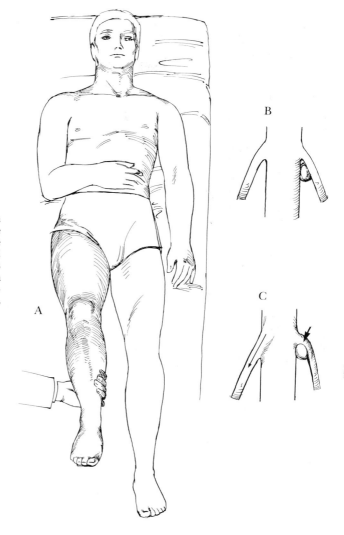

Figure 9–14. Movement of nerve roots when the leg on the opposite side is raised. *A,* When the leg is raised on the unaffected side the roots on the opposite side slide slightly downward and toward the midline. *B,* In the presence of a disc lesion, this movement increases the root tension. (From DePalma, A. F., and Rothman, R. H.: The Intervertebral Disc. Philadelphia, W. B. Saunders Co., 1970.)

detail. It should routinely include anterior-posterior, lateral and oblique views. Special views will be necessary if visualization of the sacroiliac joints is indicated.

Thinning or loss of height of the disc space is frequently seen in disc degeneration. DePalma and Rothman found that in operatively proven disc degeneration at L5 there was radiographic evidence of disc space narrowing in 41 per cent, and in disc degeneration at L4, radiographic evidence of disc space narrowing in 19 per cent.[26] It should be emphasized that thinning of the disc space, while an indication of disc degeneration, may be noted at levels other than that producing the symptomatology, and may not be present at all. It should also be recalled that narrowing of the disc space is not unique to disc degeneration but may also occur in metabolic and infectious disease of the intervertebral disc. It is also frequently seen below a transitional lumbosacral vertebra.

Sclerosis of the subchondral bone and formation of peripheral osteophytes are frequently seen in chronic disc degeneration. Again, bone spurs are not pathognomonic of disc degeneration but must be differentiated from other conditions such as Reiter's disease and ankylosing spondylitis.[30] Osteophytes are usually more prominent anteriorly than posteriorly, and this phenomenon is in all likelihood related to the nature of the ligamentous attachment to the bodies of the vertebrae above and below the disc space. MacNab has described a unique horizontal osteophyte found two to three millimeters distant from the disc space which he terms the traction spur, thought to arise from stress at the site of the ligamentous insertion during the hypermobile phase of disc degeneration. The sclerosis seen adjacent to the end plate of the vertebra may be a thin, diffuse zone or it may be localized anteriorly or posteriorly. Occasionally, a considerable portion of the vertebra will be involved and this can simulate a neoplastic process (Figs. 9–15 and 9–16).

Disc herniations may occur directly into the body of the vertebra (Schmorl's nodes), and are most commonly seen in the upper lumbar and lower thoracic areas. They most often occur in the central portion of the body just posterior to the mid position. The herniation in all likelihood follows the vascular channel but pierces the cartilaginous vertebral end plates. A sclerotic ring of bone surrounds these herniations. There is no correlation between this type of pathology and posterior herniations causing nerve root compression.

During the course of disc degeneration derangements may occur in the alignment of the vertebrae and their motion. A particular motor unit, i.e., the disc and its two adjacent vertebrae will often go through a hypermobile phase early in the course of disc degeneration, and at a later stage achieve a hypomobile phase, with focal suppression of mobility. There is a wide variation in this tendency. It is common to see posterior displacement of the vertebral body above a degenerated disc relative to the body below the degenerated disc. This is termed pseudoretrospondylolisthesis. Less often, anterior displacement of the superior vertebral body will be noted, and this is termed pseudospondylolisthesis (Fig. 9–17). These changes in alignment may produce significant symptoms in a congenitally narrow spinal canal, and if this occurs at the L3–L4 level one not uncommonly will see a complete myelographic block due to this phenomenon (Fig. 9–18).

Encroachment of the intervertebral foramina often occurs but it should be realized

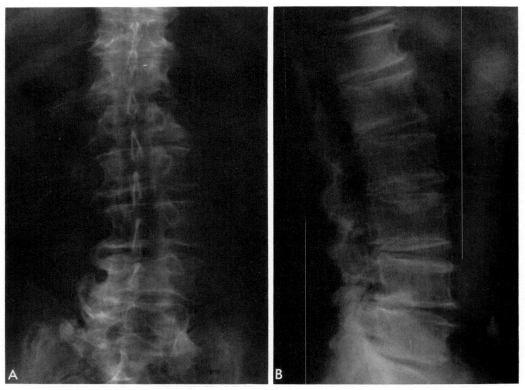

Figure 9–15. X-rays of the lumbar spine illustrate advanced multilevel disc degeneration with loss of height of the disc space, marked osteophyte formation and sclerosis of the end plates. Foraminal encroachment is present.

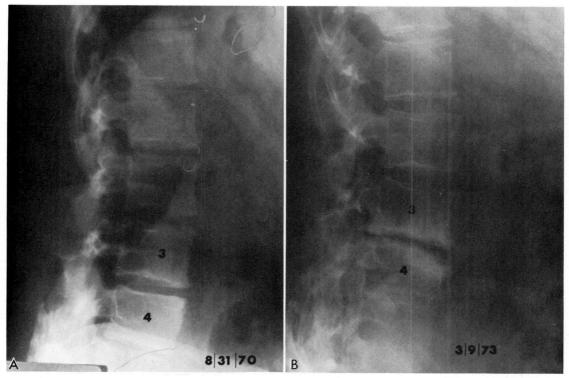

Figure 9–16. X-rays illustrate the development of disc degeneration at the L3-L4 disc space over a period of three years. Note the loss of height of the disc space, osteophyte formation and sclerosis of the end plates. In this instance the radiographic appearance was suggestive of infection, and biopsy was performed but revealed only evidence of chronic disc degeneration. At times the sclerosis can be so marked as to simulate a neoplasm of the vertebral body.

that the spatial relations are such that more leeway is present for the nerve root in the lumbar foramen than in the cervical area. Posterior osteophytes, hypertrophy, subluxation of the facets and narrowing of the disc space with approximation of the pedicle may be seen in the presence of disc degeneration. The nerve root rests in the uppermost portion of the foramen, usually well above the disc space. The tip of the superior articular facet may impinge the nerve root as it subluxes in a cranial direction.

Calcification of the nucleus does not occur often in lumbar disc degeneration but may be noted in the annulus fibrosus. Ratheke, in a postmortem study of human spines, found this type of calcification present in 71 per cent of spines examined. Magnuson first called attention to the so-called vacuum phenomenon as a sign of disc degeneration. This presence of a gas shadow in the area of the nucleus may be due to release of dissolved gases from nuclear material during extension

stress on the spine which tends to separate the vertebrae (Fig. 9–19).

As previously noted, these stigmata of disc degeneration are seen in a very large percentage of the population, many of whom have no symptoms referable to their lumbar spine. For this reason, significance should be attached to their presence only when symptoms are present, and they should be carefully correlated with the history and physical examination.

OIL MYELOGRAPHY

A carefully performed myelogram is an invaluable aid in the surgical treatment of lumbar disc disease. It is the authors' feeling, at the present time, that myelography should be performed in most instances before surgical intervention is undertaken. The rationale for performing myelography is that it will yield the following advantages.

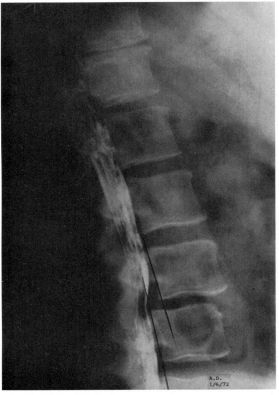

Figure 9–17. Flexion view of the lumbar spine reveals marked anterior migration of L3 on L4 secondary to disc degeneration. This is termed pseudospondylolisthesis.

Tumors of the spinal canal that may clinically mimic disc disease will be revealed. Several striking examples have been seen in which the history and neurologic findings were characteristic of a herniated lumbar disc at the L4 or L5 level and yet, to the surprise of the treating surgeon, a myelogram revealed a tumor of the lower thoracic or upper lumbar spine. Tragic errors of this nature can be easily avoided. Examples have also been seen of double pathology in which a herniated disc was found in the lower lumbar spine with a coincident tumor in the upper lumbar area. These in all likelihood would have been missed had it not been for the performance of a myelogram.

A second advantage of routine myelography is the more exact localization of disc herniation and nerve root compression. It has been stated that a careful neurologic examination will accurately localize the level of the disc pathology. While this is true in a great number of cases, it is also true that variation in

the nerve root configuration and in the location of the extrusion can lead to erroneous decisions if neurologic deficit alone is considered. An axillary or central protrusion at the L4 level may well cause an S1 nerve root syndrome usually characteristic of an L5 protrusion. Double disc herniations, i.e., more than one level, can also cloud the neurologic picture and are not uncommon occurrences.

Many complications of myelography have been described including meningitis, herniation of disc material, epidermoid formation, venous intravasation, pulmonary embolism, transection of a nerve filament and adhesive arachnoiditis. Despite this ominous list of potential problems, the incidence of these complications is small and the value of the procedure great. This is not to imply that a myelogram enjoys 100 per cent accuracy, for this is not the case. The accuracy will depend on the contrast medium utilized and the care and accuracy with which the various views are obtained. Despite great care, both false posi-

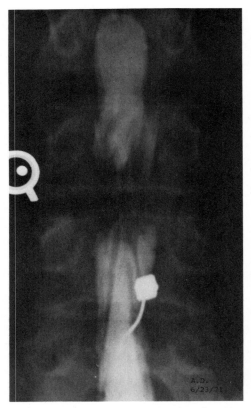

Figure 9–18. Myelogram reveals a complete block at the level of L3-L4 secondary to the pseudospondylolisthesis seen in Figure 9–17.

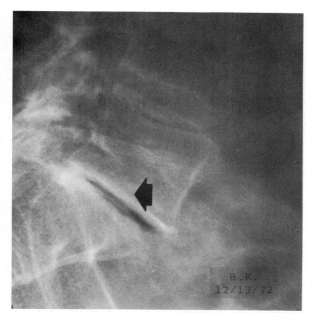

Figure 9–19. X-ray illustrates the vacuum phenomena at the L5-S1 disc space due to release of dissolved gas during extension stress on the spine.

tive and false negative myelograms will occur. False negative studies most often are found with a disc protrusion at the L5 level when a large space is present between the disc and the dural sac. There is a great variation in configuration at this level. In some individuals, the sac may lie directly against the disc while in others, 3 to 4 millimeters may separate them. False positive studies are more often noted at the L4–L5 level.

It should be emphasized that exposures should be made in the anterior-posterior, oblique and lateral planes, with the patient standing and prone. Flexion and extension views will increase the yield of this study.

ABNORMAL PATTERNS OF MYELOGRAPHY

Various patterns of myelographic abnormalities are noted, depending on the size and location of the protrusion. Soft disc herniations will yield a much different pattern than the defects noted with chronic disc degeneration and osteophyte formation.

LATERAL DISC HERNIATIONS. The defects most often noted with lateral disc herniations are incomplete filling or elevation of the root sleeve, lateral indentation of the dural sac

and a double density of the sac noted in the lateral view. A large lateral herniation may also produce a complete myelographic block at the level of the disc space. Elevation of a root sleeve may be the only abnormality noted in a lateral disc protrusion, but it is the least reliable of the findings. This is particularly true in oil myelography, since the viscid material may on occasion fail to completely fill a normal root sleeve. Indentation of the dural sac seen in the anterior posterior or oblique view and the double density seen in the lateral view are more convincing findings (Fig. 9–20).

CENTRAL HERNIATIONS. Large central disc herniations will often produce a characteristic complete myelographic block. The block will occur at the level of the disc space and in the anterior-posterior view will show an irregular sawtooth or paint-brush appearance. The lateral view will show the anterior portion of the dural sac being compressed and elevated, owing to ventral pressure from the disc herniation (Fig. 9–21). Waisting defects are commonly noted with smaller central discs, as the rootlets are forced into the lateral recess, preventing dye from filling this area.

FREE FRAGMENTS. Free fragments of disc material may migrate in either a caudal or cranial direction, and will be seen as well circumscribed masses of varying diameters at a distance from the disc space (Fig. 9–22).

CHRONIC DISC DEGENERATION. Chronic disc degeneration will often produce myelographic defects due to a diffuse posterior bulging of the annulus and osteophyte formation. In the anterior-posterior views a symmetrical waisting of the dye column will be noted owing to obliteration of the lateral recess. In the lateral views the indentation of the dye column at the level of the disc space will be noted. If no osteophytes are present this will usually be two to three millimeters in height, or if osteophytes are present they are easily seen and coincide with the defect in the dye column (Fig. 9–23).

ARTIFACTS

Many artifacts present in myelography can create defects not truly representative of disc degeneration. The defect created by the spinal needle can vary tremendously in size, and occasionally is so dramatic as to mimic a space-taking lesion. For this reason the spinal puncture should be performed at a level well away from the expected site of disc herniation.

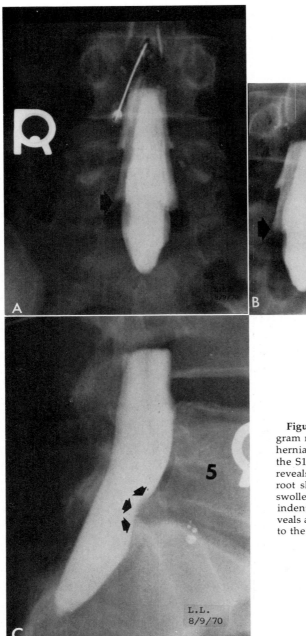

Figure 9–20. *A,* A-P view of a lumbar myelogram reveals the typical defect from a lateral disc herniation. There is shortening and elevation of the S1 nerve root on the right. *B,* Oblique view reveals again shortening and elevation of the S1 root sleeve, with displacement of dye along the swollen and edematous nerve root. There is also indentation of the dural sac. *C,* Lateral view reveals a ventral indentation of the dye column due to the disc herniation.

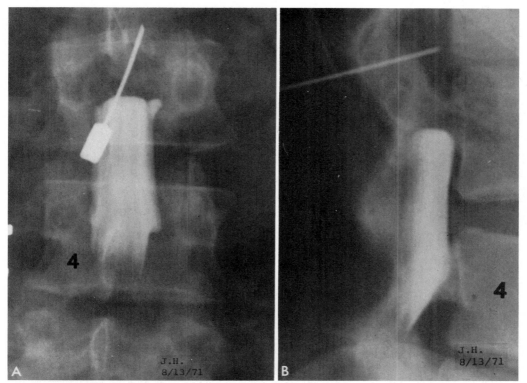

Figure 9–21. *A*, This myelographic pattern was produced by a large central disc herniation. The anterior-posterior view reveals a complete block at the level of L4-L5, with an irregular sawtooth or paint-brush appearance characteristic of the block defect produced by disc herniations. *B*, Lateral view of the same patient reveals characteristic block pattern due to disc herniation with ventral pressure on the dye column producing a complete block at the level of the large central disc herniation.

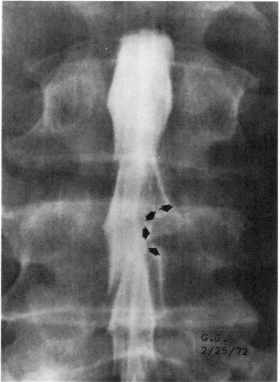

Figure 9–22. Free fragments of disc material produce a myelographic defect characterized by smooth, well-circumscribed indentations in the dye column. They may be at the level of the disc space or migrate at a distance. They may be difficult to differentiate from neurofibromata.

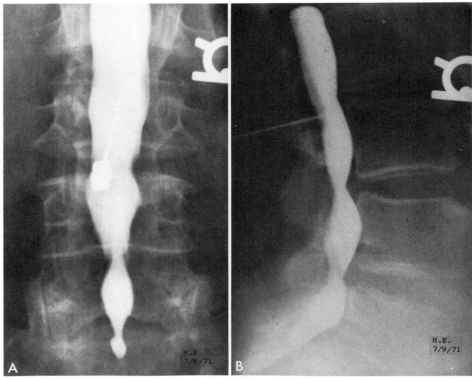

Figure 9–23. Myelograms show the characteristic appearance of chronic disc degeneration with diffuse posterior bulging of the annulus, and osteophyte formation. There is symmetrical wasting of the dye column in the AP view. The lateral view will show indentation of the dye column by the annulus anteriorly and the buckled ligamentum flavum posteriorly.

The usual site of election is the L2–L3 level unless a high lumbar disc is suspected. Artifacts are also commonly seen with previous spinal puncture, with extradural hematomas and, notoriously, in the presence of previous surgery (Figs. 9–24 and 9–25).

In conclusion, although it is appreciated that the myelogram is only 80 to 90 per cent accurate, with both false positive and false negative results, it still remains an extremely helpful and essential diagnostic tool in the preoperative evaluation of the patient with a suspected herniated disc. It should not be used in patients who are not surgical candidates in order to substantiate or disprove legal claims. Nor should it be used as the primary deciding factor as to whether or not a particular patient should undergo surgical intervention. A patient with a classic history of a disc herniation, with a clear-cut neurologic deficit and a positive straight leg raising test who has not responded to conservative treatment should not be denied surgery simply on the basis of an equivocal or negative myelogram.

RADICULOGRAPHY (MYELOGRAPHY) WITH WATER-SOLUBLE CONTRAST MEDIUM

Radiopaque water soluble contrast media have been used extensively in arteriography and intravenous pyelography, and in a variety of radiologic tests in order to visualize internal organs. These substances, when injected into the subarachnoid space, are absorbed in a few hours.[42] Because arachnoiditis and other disturbing complications are sometimes seen following myelography with the usual oil-based contrast media, an effort was made to develop a safe water-soluble agent to reduce the incidence of these disasters. A variety of water-soluble media were used during the 1940's and 1950's; all were too toxic for human investigations. Contact with the spinal cord or nerve roots induced permanent damage, and extreme pain was associated with their use.

In 1969, Ahlgren reported the use of meglumine iothalamate (Conray) for lumbar radiculography. (The term "radiculography" is used here to indicate the visualization of the subarachnoid space below the termination of the spinal cord, since all water-soluble contrast media are still considered toxic to the spinal cord.)[2] This agent was considered safe in contact with lumbar nerve roots and, in comparison with other water-soluble contrast materials, was sufficiently nonirritating. Then, in 1970, Ahlgren and Baumgartner reported on the use of meglumine iocarmate—the synthesized dimer of meglumine iothalamate—an agent developed to avoid the use of spinal anesthesia (previously required for water-soluble contrast agents) in lumbar radiculography.[3, 10] This substance was produced in order to achieve a less toxic agent by the conjunction of two molecules of meglumine iothalamate. In 1971, Skalpe indicated that no serious complications were observed in a series of 100 lumbar radiculograms.[104] He indicated that, although 8 per cent of this series had clonic spasms of the lower extremities after radiculography, the spasms were less severe though not less frequent than those seen with meglumine iothalamate. The quality of radiographs was adequate for interpretation of most lesions for which lumbar myelography is ordi-

narily performed. Although the density of the contrast is less, the water-soluble contrast material seems to extend farther along the nerve root sleeves.

A water-soluble positive contrast radiculogram is performed somewhat differently than is an ordinary lumbar myelogram. After spinal puncture with a 20 gauge needle, 5 ml. of contrast medium is mixed with 5 ml. of spinal fluid and reinjected. Care is taken to make certain that contrast material is not allowed to pass above the first lumbar vertebra. After the examination the patient must stay in bed with torso and head elevated about 30 degrees for six to eight hours. The incidence of headache and nausea is relatively high, but these symptoms are transient.

Because of the relatively recent use of meglumine iocarmate (Dimer X), it is too early to determine whether the incidence of late sequelae is reduced when compared to ordinary oily-medium myelography. In 1972, Ahlgren, Autio, and Halaburt and Lester observed radiologic signs of arachnoiditis following radiculography with these water-soluble contrast media.[4, 7, 47]

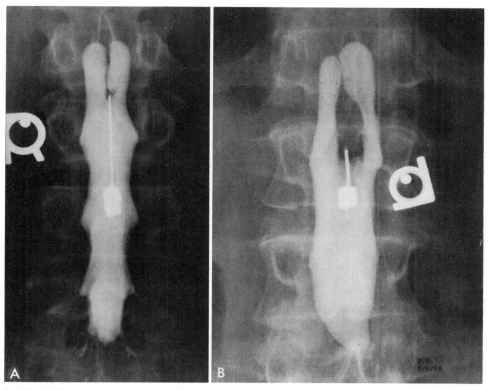

Figure 9–24. A, The myelographic defect from the spinal needle itself. In this case it is small and symmetrical. B, A more dramatic needle defect which is larger and less symmetrical.

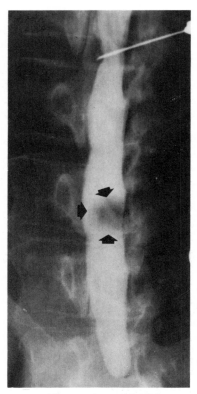

Figure 9–25. This myelographic defect represents a small extradural hematoma produced from a previous puncture.

It is obvious that a better water-soluble contrast agent must be developed for myelography. This agent should be nontoxic to the spinal cord and relatively painless, and should induce no adverse late pathological changes.

AIR LUMBAR MYELOGRAPHY

With the elucidation of the "ideal" characteristics of a contrast agent for lumbar myelography, one might indicate that air, or some other safe gaseous medium, would offer an obvious alternative. Although air is, in fact, safe and relatively quickly absorbed, the quality of radiographs of an air-filled lumbar theca leaves much to be desired. In addition, a relatively large amount of spinal fluid must be exchanged so that the injected air will float to the top of the spinal fluid column when the patient is in a marked head-down angulation. Some experienced clinicians still prefer the safety of this technique and indicate that its interpretation improves with experience. Nonetheless, lumbar myelography with air is rarely done in the United States.

DISCOGRAPHY

Discography has not proved to be essential or reliable in our experience and that of others.[27, 57] Discography is performed by placing a fine gauge spinal needle into a disc space under image intensification. Radiopaque dye is then injected into the interspace and information recorded as to the amount of dye accepted, the pressure necessary to inject the material, the configuration of the opaque media and reproduction of the patient's pain. A normal discogram may be helpful in ruling out disc degeneration but abnormalities are so common that little significance can be placed on the presence of an abnormal discogram in terms of localizing the source of a patient's pain. Three instances have been recorded in which the puncture of an intervertebral disc after a diagnostic study has led to spontaneous fusion of that disc space. It is our feeling that in most cases the study is not essential and not without hazard. For these reasons, we do not perform this as a routine study.

INTRAOSSEOUS VENOGRAPHY

It is possible, by the insertion of a large gauge needle into the marrow of a lumbar spinous process with the subsequent injection of angiographic contrast material, to visualize the epidural venous plexus. Schobinger, Krueger, and Sobel (1961) were thereby able to demonstrate intervertebral disc herniations and certain intraspinal tumors. Intervertebral disc herniations can produce displacement of the epidural venous plexus and even a complete obstruction to the flow of contrast substance. Because the veins are laterally placed, evidence of disc herniation which may not appear on routine myelography can be suggested.

Unfortunately, the procedure is both painful and difficult to interpret. The variations in anatomy of the lumbosacral intraspinal venous plexus are great: furthermore, deviation of these veins does not necessarily imply nerve root compression, since the intraspinal neural structures are not visualized. This procedure, although rarely used, may have occasional indications in difficult cases for which further evidence of suspected disc herniation may affect a borderline decision for future treatment. As such, its use requires considerations similar to those involved in the selection of lumbar discography as a diagnostic procedure.

TRANSVERSE AXIAL TOMOGRAPHY OF THE LUMBAR SPINE

FREDIE P. GARGANO, M.D.*

Transverse axial tomography of the spine is a radiographic technique which portrays any level of the spine in cross section in the living patient. The examination provides a non-distorted, magnified axial view of a preselected area of the spine. The Toshiba Tomographic Unit (Fig. 9–26) was adopted for examination of the spine. With our equipment the magnification factor is 1.33. The thickness of the tomographic cuts is 2 to 3 millimeters. The technique of examination has been described in a previous publication.[39a]

The description of the axial anatomy of the lumbar spine has been limited to the study of axial radiographs or photographs of single vertebral bodies. In the articulated spine it is evident that the lumbar spine canal at each vertebral level can be divided into two segments, an intraosseous and an articular segment (Fig. 9–27). The intraosseous segment is formed by the vertebral bodies ventrally, the pedicles laterally, the pars intra-articular posterolaterally, and the laminae and neural spine posteriorly. The articular segment is formed by the posterior aspects of the vertebral body and intervertebral disc ventrally,

*Professor of Radiology, Neurology, and Neurosurgery, University of Miami School of Medicine, Chief, Division of Diagnostic Radiology and Head, Section of Neuroradiology.

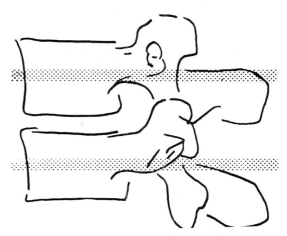

Figure 9–27. The dotted area represents the intraosseous segment of the vertebral body and canal. The segment between the dotted areas is the junctional or articular segment of the vertebral canal.

the articular processes laterally and posterolaterally, and the laminae and neural spine posteriorly. The articular segment is the most important clinically and pathologically because it contains the components of the "lumbar disc syndrome," spondylosis and lumbar stenosis. A series of normal segments from L4 to S1 is diagrammatically shown in Figure 9–28. The concept that the spinal canal is a uniform tubular shape is seen not to be tenable. The spinal canal is a constantly changing geometric space with repetitive intraosseous and articular segments.

Clinically, the indications for lumbar axial tomography are: 1) back pain with radicular symptoms; 2) suspected lumbar stenosis; 3) laminectomy and fusion failure; and 4) lumbar spondylosis.

Radiologically, we can demonstrate lumbar stenosis (Fig. 9–29), unilateral facet hypertrophy (Fig. 9–30), lumbar spondylosis (Fig. 9–31), pseudospondylolisthesis (Fig. 9–32), lateral recess syndrome (Fig. 9–33), fusion overgrowth (Fig. 9–34), spondylolisthesis (Fig. 9–35), laminectomy (Fig. 9–36) and congenital defects (Fig. 9–37).

STENOSIS. In lumbar stenosis, the pathological change is articular process hypertrophy primarily involving the inferior facets, particularly of L4. The medial overgrowth of the articular processes leads to transverse and anteroposterior narrowing of the canal. The normally biconvex configuration of the canal becomes biconcave. Laminar hypertrophy and a constricted dorsal arch may contribute to the stenosis. The pedicles were

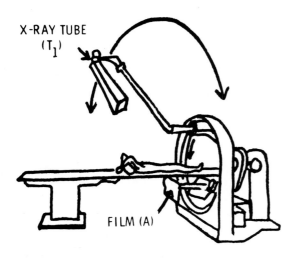

X-RAY TUBE
(T$_1$)

FILM (A)

Figure 9–26. Toshiba transverse axial tomographic unit.

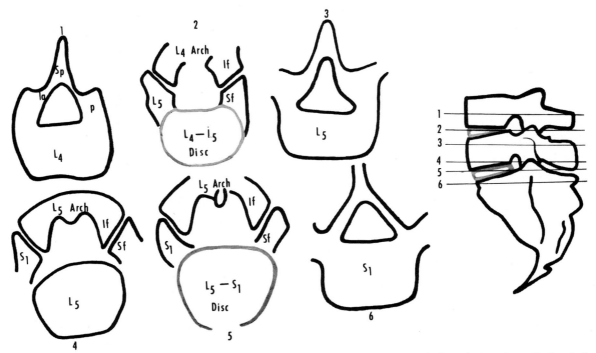

Figure 9–28. Line drawings of a series of normal lumbosacral axial tomograms. The lateral view shows the level of the tomographic cuts. It is noted that various components of adjacent vertebrae contribute to the axial tomogram at any level. The inferior articular processes of the superior vertebra are always dorsal and medial to the subadjacent superior articular processes. Sp, la, p, if and sf represent spinous process, lamina, pedicle, inferior and superior articulating processes, respectively.

rarely involved in our series. Verbiest[120a] was the first to recognize and describe stenosis secondary to posterolateral encroachment in the canal by hypertrophied articular processes. Our work has confirmed his findings. Most of our cases of stenosis have been due to spondylosis. A few patients have had developmental stenosis. One case of generalized stenosis was secondary to hyperphosphatemic bone changes.

Unilateral facet hypertrophy may be on a developmental basis or secondary to spondylosis. The end result is unilateral narrowing of the spinal canal and, usually, encroachment on the lateral recess.

SPONDYLOSIS. Lumbar spondylosis may be manifested by osteophytes, facetal arthritis, articular process hypertrophy, increased bony density and pseudospondylolisthesis. The osteophytes may mimic herniated disc disease. Facetal arthritis may so deform the articular processes that lumbar stenosis or unilateral facet hypertrophy can result. Pseudospondylolisthesis may be a prime factor in causing secondary lumbar stenosis. As a result of the slipping of the facets secondary to degenerative disc disease, the inferior facets slide anterior to the superior facets. The result is stenosis or lateral recess encroachment, or both. The facets become vertically oriented, and present a characteristic picture on the axial tomogram.

LATERAL RECESS SYNDROME. Epstein et al. have described constriction of the normal lateral recess by articular process overgrowth, primarily due to superior facet hypertrophy.[31a] The normal lateral recess is medial to the pedicles and ventral to the superior facet. Any encroachment on this recess will compress the spinal nerve lying within it. Inferior process hypertrophy, anterior migration of the inferior facets (pseudospondylolisthesis), pediculate or superior facet hypertrophy, and osteophytes may encroach on the lateral recess. It can be seen that the lateral recess is an area vulnerable to pathological change. Occasionally, the lateral recess may appear to be enlarged transversely because of inferior process hypertrophy that reaches the roof of the lateral recess. This is actually an osteoarthritic gutter adjacent to the true lateral recess.

SPONDYLOLISTHESIS. Spondylolisthesis can occur at any level but most often at L5.

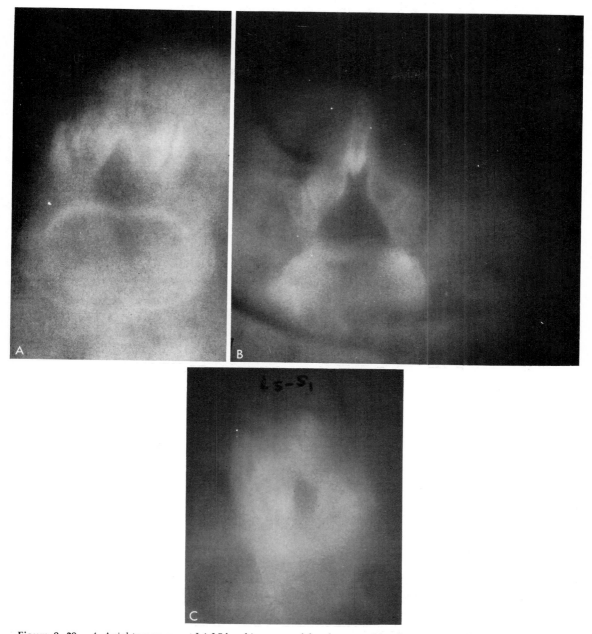

Figure 9–29. *A,* Axial tomogram at L4-L5 level in a case of developmental lumbar stenosis. The canal is narrowed in all diameters but especially at the level of the articular processes. The processes are sclerotic, and bulge convex medially to narrow the vertebral canal. *B,* Axial tomogram at L4-L5 level in a case of developmental lumbar stenosis. The inferior articular processes bulge medially at the waist of the canal, forming a posterior recess. *C,* Axial tomogram through articular segment of L5-S1. There is severe stenosis secondary to spondylosis. There is hypertrophy of the inferior articulating processes of L5 and marked facetal deformity.

The change in the axial tomogram depends on the degree of subluxation. Typically, the canal has a figure-8 configuration. The anteroposterior diameter of the canal is elongated, and there is a constriction of the lateral margins. The inferior articular processes superior to the level of subluxation are hypertrophied and sclerotic. The spondylitic defect can be demonstrated on the axial tomogram. The constrictive effect is much less with spondylolisthesis than with pseudospondylolisthesis.

VENTRAL OVERGROWTH OF SPINAL

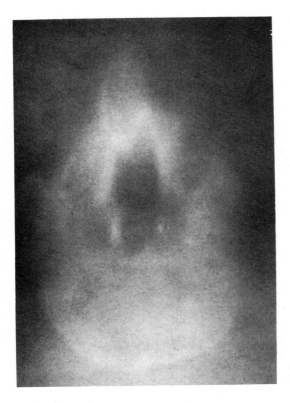

Figure 9–30. Axial tomogram at the level of the intraosseous segment of L4-L5. The right inferior articulating process is hypertrophic, constricting the canal unilaterally.

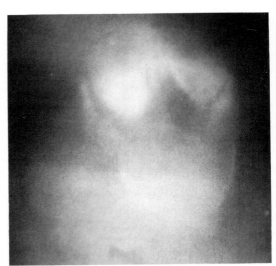

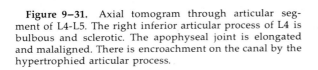

Figure 9–31. Axial tomogram through articular segment of L4-L5. The right inferior articular process of L4 is bulbous and sclerotic. The apophyseal joint is elongated and malaligned. There is encroachment on the canal by the hypertrophied articular process.

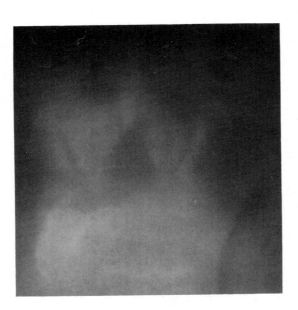

Figure 9–32. Axial tomogram through articular segment of L4-L5 in a case of pseudospondylolisthesis. The orientation of the apophyseal joints is vertical. The inferior articular processes have migrated ventrally, producing a stenotic canal. The degenerative changes are well demonstrated in the apophyseal joints.

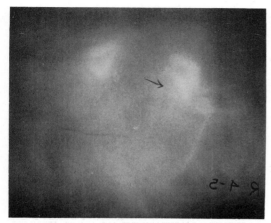

Figure 9–33. The lateral recess (arrow) is obliterated by hypertrophy of the inferior articulating process extending anteriorly.

FUSIONS. MacNab and Doll reported that over 20% of their patients subjected to posterior lumbar fusions required subsequent decompression for stenosis.[74a] Ventral overgrowth of posterior lumbar fusions into the lumbar canal, with encasement of multiple lumbosacral roots, has been recognized by other clinicians. Some patients subjected to bony fusion have had preexisting unrecognized spinal stenosis. In these patients the transverse axial tomograms reveal a typical stenotic canal with the bony fusion mass posterior in a dorsal and dorsolateral location.

Another group of patients develop lumbar canal narrowing secondary to encroachment by the fusion mass. The axial tomograms in these patients show loss of normal outline of the spinal canal. The fusion mass intrudes into the canal, causing varying degrees of constriction. On occasion, there is complete obliteration of the spinal canal by the bony overgrowth.

LAMINECTOMY AND CONGENITAL DEFECTS. Postoperative laminectomy defects, spina bifida, transitional vertebrae, malformed non-constrictive dorsal arches, and a variety of other abnormalities can be demonstrated on the transverse axial tomogram. All but the malformed dorsal arches can be demonstrated by routine radiography of the lumbar spine.

SUMMARY. Transverse axial tomography is a simple technique to view the spinal canal in cross section. It gives information unobtainable by any other radiographic technique. It clarifies the underlying pathologic change responsible for symptoms in lumbar stenosis, spondylosis, pseudospondylolisthesis, the lateral recess syndromes, and fusion overgrowths. The dorsal arch and articular process hypertrophy is demonstrated as the primary location and source of encroachment on the spinal canal, as advocated by Verbiest.

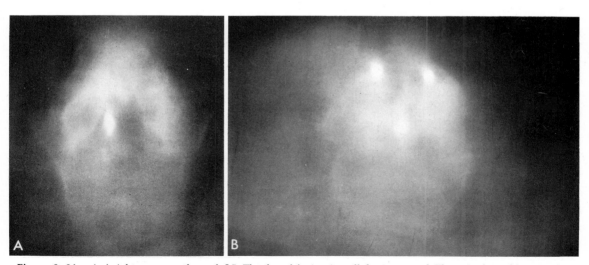

Figure 9–34. *A,* Axial tomogram through L5. The dorsal fusion is well demonstrated. The spinal canal is stenotic on a developmental basis. The diagnosis of spinal stenosis was apparently not appreciated and the patient had a bone fusion. Residual Pantopaque is seen in the spinal canal. *B,* Axial tomogram through L5. The dorsal symmetrical dense area represents Harrington rods. The ventral dense area represents residual Pantopaque. The vertebral canal is completely obliterated secondary to bony fusion overgrowth.

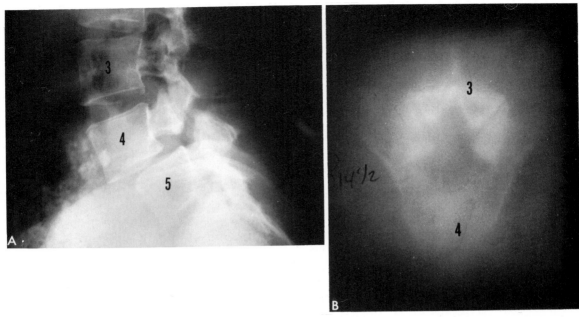

Figure 9–35. *A,* Lateral view of lumbar spine showing spondylolisthesis at the level of L4-L5. *B,* Axial tomogram through the level of L3-L4 showing "Christmas tree" shape of canal. The level of cut is just above defect in pars interarticular of L4. The superior articulating processes of L4 have become markedly hypertrophied due to redistribution of forces in weight-bearing.

Since transverse axial tomography shows only the bony configuration of the canal and not the associated soft tissue, the degree of lumbar stenosis may be even more marked than the tomograms indicate. Transverse axial tomography adds a new dimension to the evaluation of spinal pathology.

THE DIFFERENTIAL SPINAL BLOCK

Differential spinal anesthesia as described by Ahlgren involves the serial injections of increasing concentrations of an anesthetic into the subarachnoid space.[1] This has proved to be a great aid in differentiating be-

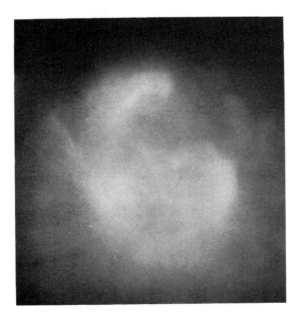

Figure 9–36. Axial tomogram through intraosseous level of L5. The defect in the dorsal arch on the left side is due to a previous laminectomy.

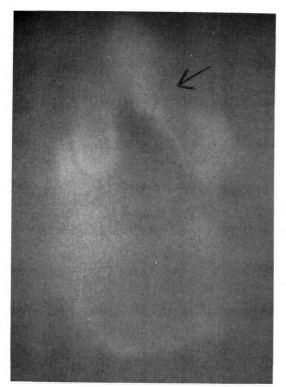

Figure 9–37. Axial tomogram through the level of articular segment of L4-L5. The deformity (arrow) of the lamina is a congenital abnormality.

tween organic and functional pain and is particularly useful in patients with strong emotional problems, in patients with a paucity of objective findings in the presence of severe pain and in patients with suspected malingering.

A subarachnoid tap is performed, using a 20 gauge needle, with the patient in the lateral recumbent position and the painful side down. Injections are made at 10 minute intervals of: 5 ml. isotonic saline (placebo); 10 ml. 0.2% procaine (sympathetic block); 10 ml. 0.5% procaine (sensory block); and 10 ml. 1% procaine (motor block). After each injection the patient is asked to evaluate his pain at rest, and then after a passive manipulation such as the straight leg raising test. Evaluation of vasomotor, sensory and motor function is also conducted to evaluate the efficacy of the anesthetic.

With the use of this test the etiology of pain can usually be ascribed to either an organic lesion or a functional basis. It is further possible to determine if the organic

pain is mediated principally by the sensory or sympathetic portion of the nervous system.

The results are most dramatic when the patient has either complete relief of pain with only saline or no relief with 1% procaine, when it produces motor paralysis or a sensory level several dermatomes above the pain site. In both of these circumstances, the etiology of the pain can be interpreted as being nonorganic or functional in nature.

CONGENITAL AND DEVELOPMENTAL ABNORMALITIES OF THE LUMBAR SPINE AND THEIR RELATIONSHIP TO DISC DISEASE

The relationship between congenital and developmental structural abnormalities of the spine to disc degeneration is poorly understood. Too often, fallacious reasoning has created misunderstandings in this field. A patient with back pain shows a structural abnormality on his x-ray and, therefore, it is assumed that this abnormality is the cause of his pain. Recent epidemiologic studies have dispensed with many of these misunderstandings.[58, 60] Only through large-scale radiographic investigation of both symptomatic and asymptomatic individuals can knowledge useful in terms of the etiology of back symptoms be generated. Relating one group of abnormalities, such as the congenital structural changes, to a second group of abnormalities, such as disc degeneration, either or both of which may be asymptomatic, becomes rather difficult.

Spondylolysis

The term spondylolysis refers to a defect in the pars interarticularis. This defect, seen often in childhood, is not congenital, since it is never seen at birth. There is significant evidence that an individual with a pars defect will have a 25 per cent greater likelihood of back difficulty than an individual without the defect.[65, 109, 124] It is also likely that a pars defect whether unilateral or bilateral will increase the incidence of disc degeneration.[124] Degeneration of the disc is accentuated by loss of the protection and stability of the posterior elements. Mechanical stresses, particularly torsional stresses which are most detrimental to the disc, are exerted upon the annulus, with resultant early breakdown.

Spondylolisthesis

In certain individuals with bilateral pars defects, a forward migration of the superior vertebra will occur. This is known as spondylolisthesis. This defect almost always leads to disc degeneration but, interestingly enough, extrusion of nuclear material at this level is very uncommon. In the authors' experience with the operative treatment of spondylolisthesis, extrusions have been noted above the level of the spondylolisthesis but not at the same level. One might speculate that, with the forward slip of the vertebrae, the posterior longitudinal ligament is drawn tight, thereby preventing nuclear herniation.

Increased Lumbar Lordosis

Theoretically, one might expect an increased lumbar lordosis to subject the lower lumbar discs to excessive shearing stresses and thereby lead to the earlier onset of lumbar disc degeneration. Several population studies have given no support to this hypothesis. Somewhat surprisingly, increased inclination of the lumbosacral joint seems to protect it against annular damage.[58, 60, 109] As previously stated, rotary stress seems to have greater significance than flexion extension stress, and thus the part played by lordosis may be minor.

Sacralization and Lumbarization

The transitional vertebra may be either a lumbarized sacral vertebra or a sacralized lumbar vertebra. There is a great variation in both symmetry and degree. The normal lumbar transverse process may be slightly increased in size or it may be solidly fused to the sacrum. This may occur either unilaterally or bilaterally. The more completely sacralized the lumbar vertebra, the more stable it will be. The disc between a transitional vertebra and the sacrum will usually be vestigial. Ruptures and degeneration of this disc are extremely uncommon. When disc degeneration or rupture occurs in relationship to a transitional vertebra it is almost always above the level of the transitional vertebra.

Spina Bifida

There is no evidence to indicate that spina bifida statistically predisposes an individual to back pain or disc degeneration. A few isolated cases have been reported in which a spina bifida occulta associated with a prominent spinous process of L5 produced compression of the cauda equina.[110]

Tropism of the Facets

Asymmetrical orientation of the lumbosacral facets is termed tropism. The studies of Farfan and Sullivan[33] indicate that the incidence of annular tears are related to the orientation of the facets. They found that asymmetrical articular processes led to asymmetrical degeneration. Disc protrusions tended to be on the side of the more oblique joint surface. Theoretically this occurs because of an abnormal rotary stress acting on the annulus producing degenerative changes. Approximately half of the torque resistance of the intervertebral joint is supplied by the posterior elements and of this, the greatest percentage is by the facet joints themselves. When both facets are oriented in a sagittal direction, rotational forces are inhibited and there is decreased torque. Theoretically, this is the best configuration. Conversely, when one facet is oriented in a sagittal direction and the other in a coronal direction, one not only loses rotational stability but a cam action is present as well. These suppositions are supported by studies relating facet orientation to disc herniation.[33]

LUMBOSACRAL TILT AND LEG LENGTH DISCREPANCY

Tilting of the pelvis may occur with abnormal development of the lumbosacral facets, with abnormal development of the sacrum and pelvis, and with inequality of leg length. There is no evidence to indicate that these entities contribute to back pain or disc degeneration.[58, 60]

CONSERVATIVE TREATMENT OF LUMBAR DISC DISEASE

The goals to be established in the non-operative treatment of lumbar disc disease should be threefold: 1. relief of pain; 2. increase of functional capacity of the patient; and 3. slowing of disease progression.

At our present stage of knowledge, the first two goals are frequently within reach of the treating physician; the last and most important is not. Reports on the efficacy of various types of conservative therapy vary tremendously. One of the most optimistic of these reports claims that in a group of 400 patients with acute disc lesions, only two required operative intervention after conservative therapy.[75] Our own experience has led us to become more cautious in responding to inquiries about the possible failure of conservative therapy and the necessity for operative intervention. Approximately 20 per cent of patients with a firm diagnosis of an acute disc lesion will ultimately require surgery, when followed over a period of years. This is in agreement with several reports in the literature.[46, 51, 66]

The quality of result of conservative treatment of patients with disc disease will depend in part on the criteria for including a patient in the study group. Colonna and Friedenberg, utilizing the strict criterion of myelographic demonstration of disc protrusion, found a relatively low recovery rate of about 30 per cent.[15] The question of efficacy of nonoperative treatment depends not only on the diagnostic and intellectual capabilities of the physician but also on his ability to educate the patient and render proper emotional support during his problem. Success will depend upon the willingness of patients to accept not only various levels of chronic and acute pain but also altered functional capacity. It must be kept in mind and emphasized to the patient that disc degeneration is not a lethal disease. If the patient is willing to live with his pain, it is his prerogative to persist with a course of conservative therapy despite the treating physician's feeling that it has failed and operative intervention is required. A decision for surgical intervention should not be made ex cathedra but by the patient and his physician, on the basis of mutual understanding, confidence and trust. The patient with a bona fide disc lesion, who does not respond to conservative therapy in a reasonable length of time, should be granted the benefit of surgical intervention, to allow him a more comfortable and active life.

The course of conservative therapy will be presented here as it evolved over a period of years and was found to be effective in a large patient population. The reasons for its efficacy are often hypothetical, but it has been shown on an empiric basis to be the most efficient approach to the problem of acute and chronic disc lesions.

Bed Rest

The most important element of therapy in acute disc lesions is an adequate period of bed rest. In most instances, this can be accomplished most effectively at home, where the patient is in comfortable and familiar surroundings, and is cared for by his family. Should he lack adequate facilities for good home care, he should be admitted to the hospital for this treatment. It is expected that the patient remain at complete bed rest, with the exception of bathroom privileges for bowel movements once or twice a day, either with the use of a bedside commode or a nearby toilet facility. A short period of ambulation necessary to reach the bathroom is frequently less stressful than the acrobatics required to utilize a bedpan. If a firm mattress is available, we feel that bed boards are not necessary, and in many instances will actually increase the level of discomfort noted by the patient.

While in bed, the patient should be placed in a position such that his hips and knees are flexed to a moderate but comfortable degree. This has been found to be particularly necessary in disc herniations of the L4–L5 level. The patient is cautioned against sleeping in a prone position, which will result in hyperextension of the lumbar spine. A natural or synthetic "sheepskin" will provide additional comfort for individuals placed at prolonged periods of bed rest.

The duration of this period of bed rest is of prime importance. Too frequently, patients are mobilized and allowed to return to work before the inflammatory reaction to a disc herniation has subsided. The patient is informed that after an acute disc herniation, a minimum of two weeks is required at complete bed rest whether at home or in the hospital. Subsequent to this a week to 10 days of gradual mobilization is instituted if he has had substantial relief of pain and is free of list and paravertebral muscle spasm. It should be mentioned, parenthetically, that any patient with a profound neurologic deficit or with a progressive neurologic deficit should undergo operative intervention; he is not a candidate for conservative therapy. It is unrealistic to expect a patient with a frank disc herniation to return to full activities in less than one month. Compromise on this point is frequently sought by the patient, but in the long run will not be to his benefit. It should be pointed out to the patient that operative intervention, in itself, requires a prolonged period of rehabilitation and that strict adherence to a conservative program may preclude the necessity of operative intervention.

Based on present day knowledge of the pathophysiology of disc degeneration, it is the authors' feeling that the modality of bed rest is important, so that the secondary inflammatory reaction to disc degeneration may subside; bed rest is not instituted with the expectation that an extruded fragment will return to its original place within the annulus. Once extruded into the annulus or beneath the posterior longitudinal ligament, a fragment of nuclear material does not return to its original location. In many instances, however, if the edema and hyperemia of the soft tissues and nerve roots surrounding the extruded fragment are allowed to subside, the patient will become free of his acute back pain and sciatica. This relief may or may not be permanent. The work of Nachemson has shown that only in the horizontal position is the disc free of significant stress.[82] The sitting position places a substantial burden upon the lumbar disc; therefore, patients must be clearly informed that sitting at a desk or in an armchair does not provide adequate relief from stress for the lumbar spine.

Drug Therapy

The intelligent use of drug therapy is an important modality in the treatment of lumbar disc disease. Three categories of pharmacologic agents are utilized: muscle relaxants, anti-inflammatory drugs and analgesics. Since resolution of inflammation about a degenerated disc is the prime goal of therapy, an anti-inflammatory drug might be expected to be of singular importance in the treatment of this problem. This is indeed the case. One of the most useful of these drugs is phenylbutazone (Butazolidin). In an acute disc herniation, patients are started on phenylbutazone at a level of 100 mg. four times daily with food or milk. The side effects of this drug are well known and include gastric irritation, fluid retention and blood dyscrasia.

Coating the stomach with milk or food is effective in preventing gastric irritation. Blood counts should be repeated at periodic intervals, and the patient cautioned about the appearance of ulcerations in the mouth or other manifestations of blood dyscrasia. In those individuals who have a gastrointestinal intolerance to phenylbutazone a less irritating analogue, oxyphenbutazone (Tandearil), may be utilized in an equivalent dosage scale. The appearance of any unpleasant side effect should alert the patient to immediately discontinue the drug and call his physician.

It has been the authors' experience that certain patients who fail to show a response to phenylbutazone may get dramatic relief from the use of a short course of systemic steroids.[84] They should be utilized only in patients who are hospitalized and can be observed for the many potential hazardous side effects of systemic steroids. Dexamethasone has been utilized in a dosage of 0.75 mg. four times daily, tapered over a one week period of time.

As patients resolve their acute disc herniations, they may have residual chronic symptomatology of low back pain which will require anti-inflammatory drugs, usually in lower dosages than those utilized for the acute lesion. A common dosage level for outpatient treatment is phenylbutazone three times daily. Periodic blood counts are obtained when this drug is utilized on an outpatient basis. If this drug has not shown itself to be effective in alleviating the symptomatology of a particular patient in a two week period, it should be discontinued, as it will probably not prove to be effective.

The use of muscle relaxants is effective in acute disc lesions in which muscle spasm is a prominent finding. Methocarbamol (Robaxin) and carisoprodal (Soma) are the drugs most commonly used for this purpose. Either of them may cause drowsiness. Soma is utilized in a dosage of 350 mg. three times daily, and Robaxin in a dosage of 1.5 gm. four times daily. Occasionally, in an extremely acute problem of marked paravertebral muscle spasm, therapy will be initiated with the use of 10 ml. of intravenous Robaxin, which is then continued with the oral form of the drug. This will frequently produce striking relief of both pain and limitation of motion. Muscle relaxants are rarely used in the chronic or subacute phase of disc degeneration.

The judicious use of analgesics is of extreme importance during the acute phase of disc disease. It is our feeling that if the pain is of such a severe nature that parenteral narcotics are required, then morphine sulphate is the drug of choice. The dosage should be adequate to insure substantial relief of the patient's symptoms. Patients must be reassured that pain medication is available for their use and that a stoic attitude is, therefore, not essential. Many times during the acute early phases of treatment, the narcotics will be ordered on a regular rather than a p.r.n. basis. This will relieve the patient of the burden of summoning and waiting for nurses to obtain pain medication. Constipation is an untoward side effect of many of the opiates, and a stool softener should be added to the regimen if prolonged use of narcotics is required. As pain subsides, oral codeine or non-narcotic analgesics may be substituted for more potent drugs.

It has been found of value to add a sedative or mild tranquilizer to the patient's regimen to alleviate any anxiety and make the prolonged period of bed rest more tolerable. Phenobarbital in 15 to 30 mg. doses, four times daily will accomplish this goal.

Flexion Exercises

Lumbar flexion exercise becomes important in the subacute or chronic phases of lumbar disc degeneration (Fig. 9–38). The use of lumbar flexion exercise is based on the theory expounded by Williams.[123] The overall aim is to reduce the lumbar lordosis. The reversal of the lumbar curve and full flexion of the lumbosacral joint will accomplish this goal. Subluxated or overriding facets of the apophyseal joints are placed in a position where they no longer overlap. Second, the spine is placed in a position of greater stability, where the shearing stresses are minimized at the lower lumbar levels. Third, the intervertebral foramina are widened, allowing maximum room for exit of the nerve roots. A fourth goal of lumbar flexion exercises is to strengthen the abdominal musculature and flexors of the spine. Both of these muscle groups have been shown to be important in supporting the spine and alleviating stress on the intervertebral disc. All of these goals and the reasons for the effectiveness of the lumbar flexion exercise program are theoretical and open to question. Their efficacy, however, on an empiric and clinical basis has been clearly shown.

Lumbar flexion exercises should not be instituted in acute disc herniations until the patient's symptoms have subsided to the point at which list and paravertebral muscle spasm are no longer noted and the major part of the acute symptomatology has subsided. This will usually be two to three weeks after the initiation of conservative therapy. Exercises are then started in a very gentle manner and are immediately discontinued if a flareup of the patient's symptomatology appears. They may be reinstituted at a later date, when the patient's tolerance for them has increased. It is not necessary, however, to wait until the patient is completely asymptomatic before instituting this program of exercises.

General Measures of Back Hygiene

Along with a program of lumbar flexion exercises, the patient with lumbar disc degeneration should be educated in certain measures of back hygiene which are in accord with the flexion management of these disorders. He should be instructed to sleep on his side or back, with his knees and hips in a position of flexion. He should be cautioned against the prone position, which hyperextends the lumbar spine. If the patient is in a hospital bed, Fowler's position should be utilized. When sitting in a chair, he should sit with the buttocks well forward and his spine in a flexed position. This position is sometimes referred to as "slumping," and is regarded with a sense of horror by many physical therapists. It is our feeling, however, that people will habitually assume this position because of the comfort it provides. Crossing the legs while seated will add further flexion to this position and is also desirable.

Lifting heavy loads above the waist should be prohibited, particularly those in which the patient is forced to rock back into a position of hyperextension. When picking up a load from the floor, the patient must be cautioned to utilize the musculature of his legs and bend from the knee and hips rather than the thoracic and lumbar spine.

Physical Therapy

The most frequently used modalities of physical therapy are the application of heat and the use of light massage of the lower lumbar spine during the acute phases of disc her-

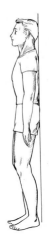

Lumbar spine exercises.

Two exercise sessions every day: (Morning and night *OR* afternoon and night).

Start with two (2) of each and gradually increase to ten (10) of each (twice a day), over a period of 10 days to two weeks.

1. Stand with back against wall and heels flat on the floor. Flatten "small" of back against wall by rotating pelvis up and forward.

    NOTE: No space between small of back and wall.

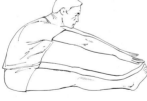

2. Lie on back with knees bent and feet flat on floor. Place hands on abdomen. Raise head and upper part of spinal column while contracting abdominal muscles.

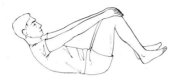

3. Lie on back. Separate legs. Bend knees and hips, and draw knees up toward axillae by clasping them with hands. *NOT TO BE DONE BY POSTOPERATIVE SPINE FUSION PATIENTS.*

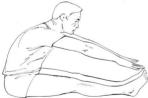

4. Sit on floor with legs outstretched. Touch toes without bending knees. When able to touch toes, stretch beyond toes. "Spring."

5. Lie flat on back. Without bending knees, lift one leg straight up, bending at hip; then the other; then both together.

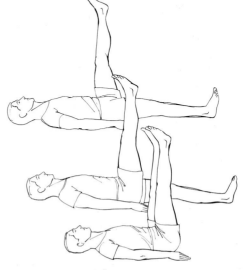

Figure 9–38. Lumbar spine exercises.

niation. Manipulation, with or without anesthesia, is not indicated in the treatment of lumbar disc disease. In many instances this will intensify rather than ameliorate the patient's symptomatology. The number of cases reported in the literature in which a profound neurologic deficit has occurred secondary to manipulation of the spine are too great in number to justify this technique. This is particularly true when relief can be obtained by more judicious means.

We have not found the use of pelvic traction desirable or necessary in the treatment of lumbar disc disease. It is a cumbersome apparatus which makes bed rest less comfortable. Its therapeutic value is highly dubious and probably nonexistent except for enforcing a program of bed rest.

BRACES AND CORSETS

Routine immobilization of the lumbar spine will rapidly lead to soft tissue contracture and muscle atrophy. For this reason the use of a rigid lumbar brace is seldom recommended. The young patient with degenerative disease is more advantageously treated with a program designed to increase his range of motion and strengthen his musculature rather than one based upon immobilization.

There are, however, certain instances in which the external support plays a useful role. The obese patient with poor abdominal musculature is frequently fitted with a firm corset with flexible metallic stays (Fig. 9–39). This corset serves the function of reinforcing his abdominal musculature and, thereby, increases his efficiency in utilizing the thoracic and abdominal cavities to support and extend the spine. The mechanism whereby the thoracic and abdominal cavities act as extensors of the spine is discussed in Chapter 2, Anatomy of the Spine. It would, of course, be preferable to train these patients to develop their abdominal musculature and shed their bodies of unneeded adipose tissue.

A secondary category of individuals for whom braces are utilized are elderly individuals with advanced multilevel degenerative changes. These patients will not tolerate an exercise program and indeed their symptomatology is frequently intensified by a program of mobilization. Depending upon the extent of their disease, a Knight–Taylor brace with shoulder straps or, possibly, a shorter lumbosacral brace with rigid metallic stays, is uti-

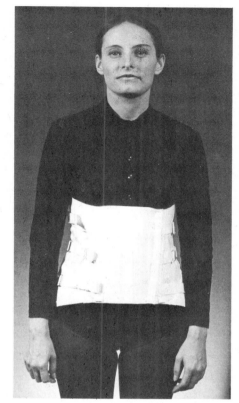

Figure 9–39. The lumbosacral corset with flexible metal stays utilized for abdominal and spinal support.

lized to partially immobilize the spine and place these arthritic joints at rest (Fig. 9–40). With bracing, marked relief of pain is rapidly achieved in these individuals. It is frequently possible to wean these people from their support, and this should be attempted, if possible, after their acute symptoms subside. This is to prevent further loss of muscle tone and stiffness in an already weakened spine.

Bracing is no longer utilized in the postoperative management of patients who have undergone spine fusion. If more than a two level spine fusion is undertaken (i.e., L3 to the sacrum or longer) the brace may be utilized.

Pregnancy and Lumbar Disc Problems

One of the most challenging problems confronting the orthopedic surgeon is the pregnant patient presenting with symptoms of disc degeneration. It is our feeling that the in-

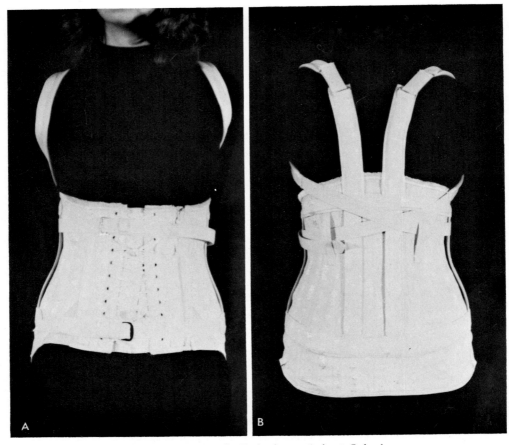

Figure 9–40.   Knight-Taylor brace; *A,* front, *B,* back.

tervertebral disc is placed under excessive stress during pregnancy for two reasons. The first of these is the obvious extra burden of carrying the fetus, and the second is the unusual ligamentous laxity found during pregnancy. This laxity is caused by the maternal production of relaxin or relaxin-like hormones. Relaxin is a hormone, found in many mammals, which produces the ligamentous laxity about the pelvis necessary for the birth of offspring that may be larger than the bony pelvic outlet. It is possible that a similar hormone, produced near term in humans, may be a cause of congenital hip dislocation and can certainly be of importance in producing relaxation of the ligamentous supporting structures of the spine.

The therapeutic modalities available during pregnancy are somewhat limited. For the most part one must depend upon bed rest and the use of a supporting corset. The physician hesitates to prescribe potent and potentially teratogenic drugs during pregnancy. Diagnosis is also somewhat hampered by the limited use of x-ray during the first trimester of pregnancy. Surgery, of course, is the court of last resort during pregnancy and is only indicated in the presence of serious neurologic findings. It is often necessary to prescribe long periods of bed rest for a pregnant patient in order for her to obtain a measure of relief. Use of a firm, flexible corset is of great help in alleviating the spine of excessive stress.

THE OPERATIVE TREATMENT OF LUMBAR DISC DISEASE

Of the many factors necessary for the successful operative treatment of lumbar disc disease, none is more essential than superb judgment as to when surgical intervention is desirable and to the selection of the proper surgical procedure. There is no single operative procedure that can be applied to all patients, and the type of surgery undertaken must be carefully designed to correct the particular pathologic entity causing the patient's symptoms. Simple laminotomy and disc excision will fail in a patient with spinal stenosis or lateral recess syndrome just as certainly as spinal fusion will fail to correct the symptoms of sciatica in acute disc herniations.

Indications for Surgery

PROFOUND OR PROGRESSIVE NEUROLOGIC DEFICIT

The most dramatic presentation of an acute disc herniation is the cauda equina syndrome, and this is the most certain indication for immediate surgical intervention. If bowel and bladder function are to be preserved, immediate decompression of the cauda equina is imperative. A delay of several hours may make the difference between total recovery and serious muscular impairment, with permanent dysfunction of the bladder and rectal sphincters.

Motor weakness requires more judgment in terms of urgency as a criterion for surgical intervention. Either complete paralysis of the quadriceps muscle or paralysis of the dorsiflexors of the foot (foot drop) is an indication for surgical decompression of the involved nerve root. The more prolonged the pressure on the nerve root, the less likely is the return of function. It should be stated, however, that this guideline is not absolute and, in the authors' experience, several cases have been seen in which the recommended decompression under these circumstances was not undertaken and the patient had a complete restoration of function with time. However, recommendations must be based on the plan that will yield the best likelihood of return of neurologic function. In the above circumstances surgery is indicated. When lesser degrees of motor weakness are present, extremely good judgment must be exercised as to when surgery should be recommended. If the weakness is mild to moderate, and compatible with adequate function of the extremity, a period of observation and conservative treatment is indicated. However, if the motor weakness is progressive in nature, and be-

comes significant in terms of function, then surgical intervention should be undertaken.

Sensory and reflex changes are helpful in terms of diagnosis, but are not in themselves indications for surgical intervention and are of no prognostic value in predicting the ultimate outcome of the disease. A persistent absence of an Achilles reflex in the face of lessening symptoms would certainly not be an indication for surgery.

UNRELENTING SCIATICA

Occasionally, an acute attack of sciatica will fail to respond to all forms of conservative treatment. The exact time course after which surgery should be recommended will vary from patient to patient, according to their pain tolerance and emotional stability, and the demand of their socioeconomic environment. In general, the authors do not recommend surgical consideration in acute sciatica before a period of four to six weeks. After this period of conservative therapy, with little or no improvement, surgical intervention would be justified.

RECURRENT EPISODES OF SCIATICA

In certain individuals, after an initial successful course of conservative treatment, the sciatica will recur and become incapacitating. There may be a complete absence of symptoms between the acute episodes, or low-grade sciatica may continue to a greater or lesser extent. If the recurrent episodes are not disabling, and if the intensity of the symptoms is within the patient's emotional tolerance and he is able to function at an acceptable level, then persistent conservative therapy is indicated. However, if the frequency and intensity of the attacks are severe enough to interfere with the individual's ability to follow gainful employment and enjoy the normal activities of daily living, then surgery should be undertaken. In general, the authors would consider surgery only after three recurrent episodes, but there is variation in this regard.

Great care must be taken to evaluate both the emotional stability of these patients and their reaction to pain. A patient who continues to have minor symptoms with conservative therapy but who has an overwhelming emotional reaction to this pain, particularly if an element of hostility is present, will usually do poorly even with surgery. If any uncertainty as to the emotional stability of the patient is present, psychiatric consultation is mandatory. This is not to say that patients with emotional problems, particularly patients with long-standing pain, should be denied surgical relief if significant pathology is present. It has been well demonstrated that long-standing pain will lead to depression even in basically stable individuals and that the depression will lift after the pain is alleviated.

In most instances, surgery will be undertaken for the relief of sciatic pain, and its effectiveness will depend on the discovery and relief of pressure upon the neural elements. Ideally, every operative procedure undertaken to relieve sciatica would reveal mechanical compression of the nerve roots. This is often not the case, and in these instances surgery will often fail. One might assume that the failure to discover mechanical compression is due to one of two factors, either an inadequate exploration or a non-mechanical cause for the sciatica. The former factor may be remedied by more thorough exploration and more complete understanding of the pathology. The latter, i.e., non-mechanical sciatica, can best be appreciated by an analysis of those factors present in the preoperative evaluation which best correlate with the presence or absence of demonstrable nerve root compression. The most thorough study in this regard is that of Hirsch.[54] In a review of some 3000 low back operations, he found that the most significant preoperative factors in the determination of mechanical nerve root compression were:

1. A well-defined neurologic deficit.
2. A positive myelogram.
3. A positive straight leg raising test.

When all of these factors are present, surgery will usually uncover mechanical compression and will be followed by a good result. If one or more of these factors are absent, great deliberation should be given before surgery is undertaken. This is not to say that one should not recommend surgery in the absence of a positive myelogram or in the absence of a neurologic deficit, but that careful evaluation of these cases should be undertaken. If, for instance, the patient has a well-defined neurologic deficit (such as an absent Achilles reflex), a positive straight leg raising test and a positive contralateral straight leg raising test, one might expect to find a herniated L5 disc compressing the S1 nerve root, despite the presence of a normal myelogram.

However, if two out of three critical factors are missing, such as a positive myelogram and a neurologic deficit, one might well expect a negative exploration and failure to relieve sciatica postoperatively.

Selection of the Operation

ACUTE DISC HERNIATION

In most individuals with acute disc herniations, the primary compelling symptom that leads to surgery is sciatica. Although the patient may have had many years of preceding troublesome but tolerable back pain, the leg symptoms ultimately will force him toward surgery. In individuals such as this, limited laminectomy with excision of the herniated material as well as excision of the nucleus of the abnormal disc is the procedure of choice. The approach may be limited, and in cases with a wide interlaminar space little or no bone need be removed. It is essential that the nerve root be completely explored well out through the foramen and be free of all external pressure at the termination of the procedure.

CHRONIC DISC DEGENERATION

BACK PAIN ONLY. Most individuals with chronic disc degeneration and back pain can be managed effectively with nonoperative treatment. The authors advocate a very conservative posture in regard to surgical treatment of patients with disc degeneration and back pain only. The rationale for this is that disc degeneration often becomes a diffuse process throughout the entire lumbar spine with the passage of time and, furthermore, it is extremely difficult to ascertain which of the several levels may be the source of the patient's pain production. An occasional individual will develop severe incapacitating back pain, intractable to medical therapy, which is clearly limited to one or two disc spaces. These individuals will obtain relief through arthrodesis of the spine. The procedure of choice is a bilateral spine fusion from the affected level to the sacrum. When surgery is undertaken for this type of diagnostic category a fusion of L4 to the sacrum is usually undertaken. Bone graft should not be placed in the midline over the lamina, as this will lead to thickening of the lamina with the possible late formation of spinal stenosis (Fig. 9–45). This diagnostic entity of spinal stenosis after midline spinal fusions is seen with greater frequency, as experience with spinal fusion increases.[96]

BACK AND LEG PAIN. Patients with chronic disc degeneration will present with a wide variety of ratios of back to leg pain. At one extreme is the individual with florid sciatica and negligible back pain. This individual requires decompression only if this can be accomplished without creation of instability during the operation. If a significant component of *back pain* is present, stabilization at the same time should be undertaken, with a bilateral lateral spine fusion incorporating the degenerated levels down through the sacrum. The type of pathology present will dictate the extent and type of decompression required. If midline ridging is the only abnormality present, and the nerve roots are free in the foramina, then complete laminectomy of the affected levels, with preservation of the facet joints will suffice. If an extrusion of disc material is present, this obviously should be removed but this is not usually the case in end stage disc degeneration. The disc space need not be entered in the majority of these individuals, since little nuclear material will be present. Although the symptoms may be unilateral, the authors would advise a complete laminectomy to prevent contralateral symptomatology in the future. If foraminal encroachment is present, a complete foraminotomy is indicated. If a narrow lateral recess is present, this must be unroofed completely out to the pedicle. In certain individuals, even after foraminotomy, and unroofing of the lateral recess, the nerve root will still be tightly tethered around a pedicle which has undergone a relative descent during disc degeneration. In these individuals, excision of the pedicle must be undertaken.

Occasionally, a lateral herniation or the presence of an aberrant ligament such as the corporotransverse ligament will cause a nerve root compression distal to the foramen. In the majority of these patients with chronic disc degeneration a minimum of two levels of decompression are undertaken, i.e., at L5 and at L4; but in developmental spinal stenosis a minimum of three levels are decompressed, extending up to L3. The decision as to how far craniad to proceed with decompression will depend also upon the operative findings, and we would not hesitate to advocate complete lumbar decompression from L1 to L5 if the pathology warrants.

A combined procedure in which a lateral spine fusion is undertaken at the same time as the decompression is indicated in the presence of significant low back pain or when stability is compromised by resection of the facet joints or pedicles. Laminectomy per se does not create sufficient instability to warrant fusion.

INDICATIONS FOR FUSION

The questions as to what is the ideal surgical procedure and what is the role of spinal fusion in a degenerated intervertebral disc are as yet unanswered. When reviewing the literature in this field, one is reminded of Josh Billings' cryptic statement, "It ain't what a man don't know that makes him a fool, but what he does know that ain't so." Eustace Semmes reviewed 1500 patients in whom only disc excision had been performed and found that 98 per cent considered themselves to have been benefited by their operation.[100] At the other end of the spectrum, Young and Love reviewed a series of 450 patients with a combined procedure and 558 patients with disc excision alone and found that the combined operation relieved both symptoms in 20 per cent more patients than did the operation for removal of the disc alone, and that there were three times as many failures to obtain relief of either back or leg pain when the fusion was not performed.[12] There are innumerable other follow-up studies in the literature that fail to resolve these questions. The answers will not be forthcoming until long term prospective studies are undertaken, in which patients in a definite diagnostic category are treated in a random and variable pattern. Until this is done, the proposed benefits of a considered spinal fusion will rest on less than solid grounds.

At our present stage of knowledge spinal fusion should be undertaken for the following indications:

1. Acute disc herniations with a protracted significant component of back pain.
2. Chronic disc degeneration with significant back pain and degeneration limited to one or two disc levels.
3. Surgical instability created during decompression with bilateral removal of the facet joints.
4. The presence of neural arch defects coincident with disc disease.

Surgical Technique

SIMPLE DISC EXCISION

It must be emphasized that the procedure described below is used in young people with evidence of acute single level soft disc herniation in whom radicular symptoms predominate. This method is designed to minimize the postoperative recovery time, yet effectively treat the source of nerve root compression, which is anticipated to be frankly herniated or extruded disc material.

ANESTHESIA. This operation may be performed under spinal, epidural, local or general endotracheal anesthesia. In view of the safety of modern anesthetic techniques, general anesthesia is preferred. Optimum muscle relaxation with myoneural blocking agents is possible, and the patient is freed from the anxiety of awareness during the operative procedure. In a relatively calm patient, spinal anesthesia is particularly safe and satisfactory. There is some question, however, on the advisability of following a lumbar myelogram with the intrathecal injection of still more foreign chemicals. Some have suggested that this combination, in addition to possibly causing intraoperative bleeding, may contribute to the later development of arachnoiditis. This supposition, however, remains unproved.

POSITION AT OPERATION. The patient is placed in a kneeling position as described on page 492. The abdomen lies free and the intra-abdominal pressure is reduced, thereby minimizing epidural venous bleeding. This position has proved to be of benefit, and since its adoption epidural bleeding has virtually been eliminated as a cause of concern during surgery. When operative procedures were done in a prone position with pressure on the abdomen, it was not infrequent for the surgeon to visualize distended epidural veins in the operative field. With the use of the abdomen-free kneeling position, however, the epidural veins are collapsed and offer little problem when encountered. Elastic stockings are used routinely.

PREPARATION AND ANTIBIOTICS. Prophylactic antibiotics are not used for simple disc excision. The back may be shaved at any interval prior to surgery. After the patient is positioned, the back is scrubbed with an antiseptic soap solution for 10 minutes. Subsequently, an antiseptic solution is applied several times by the surgeon prior to draping.

INCISION. Because this technique emphasizes a minimum of soft tissue dissection, to enhance early ambulation and recovery, accurate placement of the incision is required. Three criteria are utilized to place the incision, which is ordinarily 4 cm long, directly over the affected disc:

1. Notation of the level of the iliac crest on the plain lumbar spine films.

2. Observation of the skin mark by the myelographic spinal puncture needle and correlation of this scar with the level of needle insertion on the myelographic studies.

3. Palpation of the last spinous process, which is usually S1. By a combination of these landmarks, the operator can ordinarily satisfactorily locate the precise spinous process of concern. The incision runs from the centers of the spinous processes of the vertebrae between which the affected disc lies. Through this small incision the paraspinous muscles are dissected free from the lamina on the appropriate side and held in place with a Taylor retractor. This retractor fits nicely through the incision and its point comes to rest on the lateralmost extension of the lamina, just beneath the facet joints. The Taylor retractor may either be fixed to the drape or held by a roller gauze looped under the surgeon's foot. Palpation of the lamina at this point will ascertain the appropriate level, since L5 is the lowest vertebra to have a definitive lamina or ligamentum flavum, or both. In addition, the operator may grasp the spinous process with a large towel clip. The sacral spinous process does not move, whereas the other lumbar lamina will be somewhat mobile on normal articulations. This maneuver, incidentally, can demonstrate a particularly "loose" lamina suggestive of spinal instability or spondylolisthesis.

The ligamentum flavum beneath the superior lamina is separated and a thumbnail-sized opening is rongeured on the inferior margin of the superior lamina (Fig. 9–41). At this point, magnifying loupes of two and one-half power are applied, which greatly enhance the surgeon's ability to delineate fine structures. The ligamentum flavum is opened with a #15 scalpel blade and a long cottonoid pattie is inserted between the ligamentum flavum and the epidural tissue. A long, thin cottonoid pattie is easily accepted in this space, thereby separating the dura from the subsequent dissection of the ligamentum flavum. The remaining ligament can be excised by sharp dissection or

Ligamentum flavum

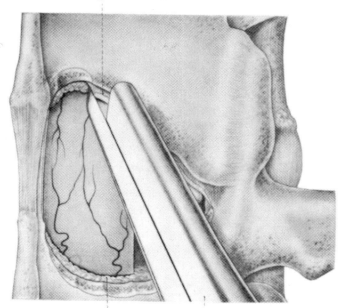

Figure 9–41. The lamina and underlying ligamentum flavum removed together with the punch rongeur. (From Kempe, L. G.: Operative Neurosurgery. Vol 2. New York, Springer Verlag, 1970.)

Epidural fat   Removing lamina and lig. flavum

removed piecemeal with the Kerrison punch rongeur (Fig. 9–41). Epidural fat, if present, is removed gently with forceps. At this point, the dura is clearly evident through the laminectomy incision. A separate thin band of liga-mentum flavum which runs along the lateral-most portion of the spinal canal may have to be removed separately.

The operator is now prepared to inspect the nerve root (Fig. 9–42). This is the most

Cut edge of sup. lamina   Extruded nucleus pulposus

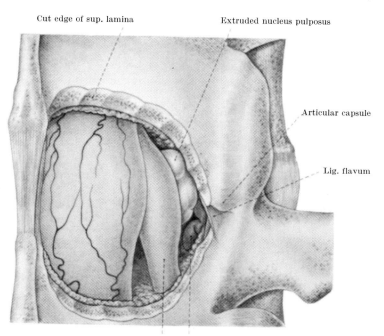

Figure 9–42. The nerve root and ex-truded disc prior to further dissection. This, of course, is the ideal situation, but frequently retraction of the nerve root and further exploration are re-quired to visualize the offending disc material. (From Kempe, L. G.: Operative Neurosurgery. Vol. 2, New York, Springer Verlag, 1970.)

Articular capsule

Lig. flavum

Nerve root   Epidural vein

significant portion of the procedure because only by palpation can one assume that the appropriate nerve root is under pressure and thereby responsible for the radicular symptoms. Under loupe magnification, the nerve root is retracted medially with a Freer nasal septum elevator. A thinner instrument with similar contour, the Penfield dissector, can separate the inferior surface of the nerve root dura from the floor of the spinal canal. When there is a significant disc herniation, these two structures are frequently adherent. If difficulty is encountered in retraction of the nerve root, the operator can assume that there is pressure caused by bulging or extruding disc material. If frank extrusion is encountered at this point, an effort should be made to remove it fairly early in the dissection in order to avoid retraction injury to the nerve root. The extruded fragment should be removed intact, if possible, since portions of a fragmented extrusion may be difficult to find subsequently. If a bulging disc is encountered, as is most frequently the case, 1 × 1 cm cottonoid patties with radiopaque strings can be put in the epidural space after the nerve root is gently retracted over the dome of the disc. Such pat-

ties, above and below the disc herniation, can gently retract the nerve root and thereby avoid the hazards of a metal root retractor in the hands of an assistant. Ultimately, with nerve root retractor in place, an area of herniated disc at least 1 cm² should be visible. It may be necessary to extend the laminectomy lateralward to get sufficient room. Removal of significant portions of the intervertebral facet joint is not necessary in order to expose the usual disc herniation.

The largest possible incision into the annulus fibrosus and disc material is made with a number 15 knife blade on a long thin handle. This is often accompanied by a spontaneous extrusion of the nucleus pulposus. Straight and angled intervertebral disc rongeurs are inserted into the disc material (Fig. 9–43). The surgeon should at all times be aware of the depth to which the rongeur is being inserted. Although the jaws of the rongeur are operated by the right hand (for a right-handed surgeon) the left hand holds the shaft of the disc rongeur and prevents it from plunging when vigorous "bites" of disc material are extracted. A sense of bottoming is felt when the jaws of the rongeur are closed. The jaws are

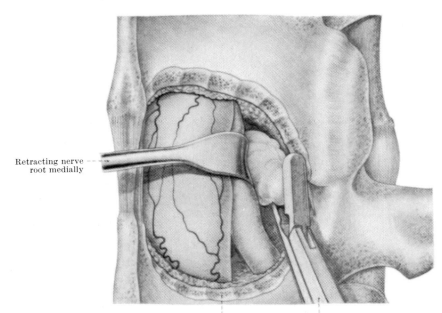

Retracting nerve root medially

Cut edge of inf. lamina   Removing ruptured nucleus pulposus

Figure 9–43. Removal of the disc extrusion while the nerve is retracted. We recommend retraction of the nerve root with cotton pledgets whenever possible to avoid trauma to the nerve root. (From Kempe, L. G.: Operative Neurosurgery. Vol 2. New York, Springer Verlag, 1970.)

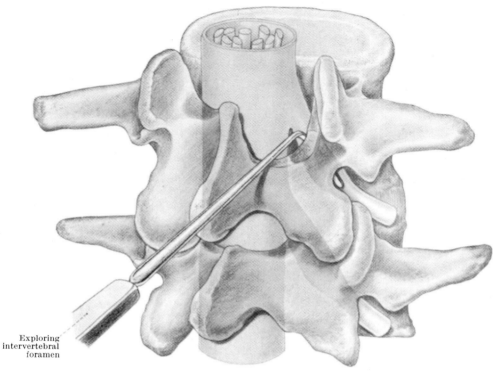

Exploring
intervertebral
foramen

Figure 9–44. Exploration of the intervertebral foramen with a probelike instrument to detect further causes of nerve root impingement, a necessary step in all cases, particularly when disc excision fails to "loosen" the root. (From Kempe, L. G.: Operative Neurosurgery. Vol 2, New York, Springer Verlag, 1970.)

then opened and advanced a few millimeters into the disc material prior to its excision. The jaws of the disc material should be in contact with the cartilaginous plates of the superior or inferior vertebra during the piecemeal removal of disc material. This technique, along with the surgeon's undivided concentration, will prevent plunging of the disc rongeur into the retroperitoneal space. When the central and lattermost portions of the nucleus pulposus have been removed, the interspace is entered with a right angled dural separator and the residual, more fibrotic disc material is separated from the annulus. It is forced into the center of the interspace and retrieved separately with disc rongeurs. Angled curets are then inserted into the interspace, and the disc material is scraped from the cartilaginous plates and again retrieved. Care is taken to effect as complete an excision of the disc material as is possible. The right angled dural elevator is then placed between the nerve root and the site of the former disc herniation in the epidural space. Any residual bulging is flattened by forceful

collapse of the elevated area into the interspace.

At this point a careful inspection of the epidural space around the nerve root is made with an appropriate instrument. The nerve root should now be movable with a minimum of force. If there is resistance to movement or tension the procedure is not complete: a search must be made for extruded disc fragments, perhaps more remote from the laminectomy (Fig. 9–44). If the nerve root continues to be tense, a "foraminotomy" may be performed. With a Kerrison punch rongeur, bone is excised along the course of the exiting nerve root. This could require removal of the medial portion of the interarticular facet joint. This sacrifice must be made, however, if the nerve root cannot be freed in any other way. Our experience indicates that significant portions of this joint can be excised at one level, unilaterally, without subsequent problems. If persistent tension on this nerve root is due to an underlying spondylotic spur, foraminotomy may be the only technique by which the nerve root can be decompressed. Ultimately, the foraminotomy may extend well out beyond the confines of the spinal canal to the point at which the nerve root curves around the pedicle. If there is evidence of nerve root tension at this point, pedicle removal may be required. At this point, the nerve root is usually quite free. It is not unusual, however, to expose 2 to 3 cm of nerve root prior to effecting the desired "loose" feeling.

WOUND CLOSURE. After the disc material has been radically removed and the nerve root is free, the entire exposed dura is covered with a piece of flattened Gelfoam. The paraspinous muscles are approximated with 00 chromic suture and subcutaneous closure is obtained with 00 chromic suture and wire or nylon on the skin. The postoperative management is the same as described for the other laminectomy techniques which follow.

LUMBAR DECOMPRESSIVE LAMINECTOMY AND FORAMINOTOMY

This procedure is applied for most cases of symptomatic chronic disc degeneration, for large acute disc herniations with high degree myelographic block, for multiple myelographic disc defects, particularly when the symptomatic disc is uncertain, and for situations of multiple nerve root involvement. The operation is designed to decompress the lumbar theca and appropriate nerve roots, especially when it may be impossible to actually remove the anteriorly placed source of compression.

ANESTHESIA. Since this operation is more commonly performed in older individuals, we prefer general endotracheal anesthesia, with appropriate cardiovascular monitor.

POSITION AT OPERATION. Again the kneeling position, with abdomen free, is preferred (as described previously).

INCISION. The incision is midline, and ordinarily covers several of the lower lumbar vertebrae. When the edges of the incision are open and retracted with hemostats, the fascia of the paraspinous muscles is incised at its point of contact to the spinous processes. With a broad, sharp periosteal elevator, the paraspinous muscles are stripped subperiosteally from the spine. Frequent packing with dry sponges maintains hemostasis as the dissection continues. Large self-retaining retractors are then applied, and the appropriate spinous processes and laminae are identified.

Utilizing the sharp angled bone cutter, the paraspinous processes of the appropriate laminae are removed. Using large curets, soft tissue between the laminae is scraped free and the laminae themselves are gently rongeured. When there is evidence of great pressure, this procedure must be done very carefully with pointed rongeurs. When the myelogram indicates foraminal involvement, particularly with a relatively compression free central lumbar theca, the laminae and ligamentum flavum can be removed with a large, right angled Kerrison punch rongeur. Ultimately, the appropriate laminae are removed to the level of the medial surface of the pedicles. If a central decompression is desired, and there has been no significant evidence of radiculopathy, the nerve roots may be inspected for looseness and the procedure can then be terminated. If there have been radicular symptoms, as is usually the case with the ordinary indications for surgery, the appropriate nerve roots should be inspected. If difficulty in retracting the nerve root is encountered, one ordinarily palpates an anteriorly placed bulging, chronically degenerated disc. Although it may be possible to remove portions of this disc material, or even an extruded fragment, it is frequently feasible to decompress the root only by the performance of an extended foraminotomy (as described above). The history, neurological examination and myelogram will indicate which nerve roots must be explored and foraminotomized. If multiple extensive foraminotomies must be done, the procedure is ordinarily followed by a lateral spine fusion. When the nerve roots are free, the entire exposed dura is covered with Gelfoam.

WOUND CLOSURES. After a sponge count, the paraspinous muscles are approximated with 0 chromic gut, and the skin closed in two layers. If meticulous hemostasis is obtained, closed drainage is not necessary. Postoperative management is similar to that indicated below for the fusion procedure.

GELFOAM MEMBRANE

Scar formation about the dural sac and nerve roots after surgical intervention constitutes one of the most frequent causes of postoperative pain. In our experience this scar formation is almost always present to a greater or lesser extent. It acts as a constrictive force about the neural elements and also tethers the nerve roots to the spine. For reasons that are not well explained, this scar formation causes

Figure 9–45. This drawing illustrates iatrogenic spinal stenosis due to a midline spinal fusion. The decortication of lamina and application of bone graft in the midline creates spinal stenosis through two mechanisms. The first of these is thickening of the lamina and the second is overgrowth of the fusion mass at the cranial end of the fusion dipping into the interspace and compressing the neural elements.

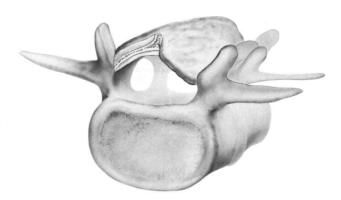

symptomatology in certain patients and not in others. It may be present for several months or a year before the symptoms become apparent. Surgical removal of this scar tissue in the past has usually led to its recurrence in a short time. Thus, it was with great interest that surgeons concerned with the spine greeted the recent research of MacNab[74] on the etiology and prevention of postoperative scar formation in the neural canal. In the experimental animal, he clearly showed the relationship of postoperative dural scar to surgically exposed muscle. This tendency toward scar formation could be markedly inhibited by the interposition of a resorbable Gelfoam membrane. Attention to atraumatic technique and complete hemostasis were also of obvious importance.

No clinical reports are as yet available on this procedure. However, the authors have utilized this type of Gelfoam membrane interposed about all areas of exposed dura and nerve root during the past three years in over 300 cases of nerve root decompression. No ill effects have become evident, although the period of follow-up evaluation is as yet too short to make a general recommendation as to the use of this technique.

LATERAL SPINE FUSION

When arthrodesis of the spine is necessary, the authors currently recommend the use of bilateral lateral fusion. Many variations of this technique have been reported in the past.[27, 118, 121] There are several advantages in the use of a lateral fusion. Foremost among these are the certainty of obtaining a solid fusion, the ability to perform the fusion in the face of absence of the posterior elements and the prevention of iatrogenic spinal stenosis (Figs. 9–45 and 9–46).

ANESTHESIA. This operation may be performed under spinal anesthesia, but with the exception of unusual circumstances we would routinely advise endotracheal intubation and general anesthesia. Cardiac monitors are frequently used on elderly individuals and in the presence of a history of cardiovascular disease. After placement of the endotracheal

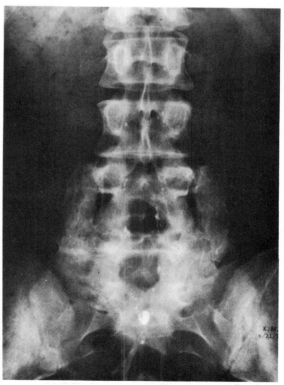

Figure 9–46. Well formed bilateral lateral spinal fusion from L4 to the sacrum. Note the massive appearance of the bone graft from the transverse process of L4 to the ala of the sacrum. No graft material is placed in the midline.

tube, both lungs are auscultated to be certain that aeration is taking place.

POSITION AT OPERATION. This procedure is performed in the prone position. If decompressive laminectomy or disc excision is to be performed at the same time, the kneeling position is utilized to ensure collapse of the epidural veins and to minimize abdominal compression (Fig. 9–47). If only a spinal fusion is to be performed, the patient is placed on a flat operating table, with lateral rolls beneath the chest and abdomen to allow breathing space. The anterior iliac crest is centered over the kidney rest, permitting flexion of the table, if desired to reduce the lumbar lordosis. Elastic stockings are placed on the patient to prevent thrombophlebitis.

ANTIBIOTICS. The use of antibiotics to prevent surgical infection is controversial. Although the authors do not recommend antibiotics in most surgical procedures, the magnitude of a lateral spine fusion is such that we feel antibiotics to be a desirable precaution. Cephaloridine (Loridine) is utilized preoperatively, intraoperatively, and postoperatively for 72 hours. A typical regimen would be to administer Loridine, 0.5 gm IM at 10:00 P.M. the night prior to surgery, 0.5 gm IM on the morning before surgery and 1 gm intraven-

ously during the course of the operation. Postoperatively 0.5 gm would be ordered intramuscularly every 6 hours for 72 hours. It is also recommended that the wound be irrigated frequently during the operative procedure with an antibiotic solution of bacitracin and polymixin. With the use of the above program and with careful, rapid surgical technique, an infection rate below 1 per cent has been constantly maintained.

INCISION. A hockey stick incision is utilized, with the lower pole deviating to the side where the iliac crest graft will be obtained. If an L4 to the sacrum fusion is to be performed, the incision starts above the third lumbar spinous process, continues in a caudal direction to the sacral spinous process and then deviates gradually 2 inches in a lateral direction (Fig. 9–48). The horizontal component of the lower end of the incision allows easy access to the ilium to obtain graft material. The vertical limb of the incision is carried directly down to the fascia in the midline, without the creation of layers. Absolute hemostasis is obtained at this step. Then, utilizing the electric cutting knife, the fascia is incised from above the third spinous process to the lower portion of the sacrum. Subsequently, utilizing a broad sharp periosteal elevator, the

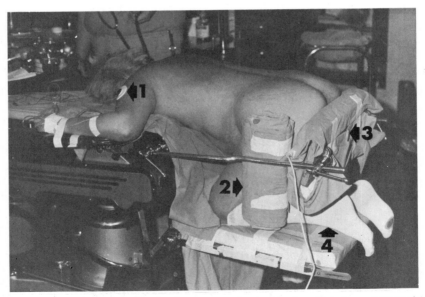

Figure 9–47. Kneeling position utilized for laminectomy and spinal fusion. Note how, even in this obese patient, the abdomen is completely free preventing any pressure on the vena cava.
  1. EKG monitoring is used because of the difficulty of listening to the heart sounds in this position.
  2. Lateral padding is used to stabilize the patient and prevent pressure on the side bars.
  3. The patient is stabilized caudally by the use of a seat to prevent extreme flexion at the knees and hips.
  4. Elastic stockings or elastic bandages are used to prevent pooling of blood in the calf area.

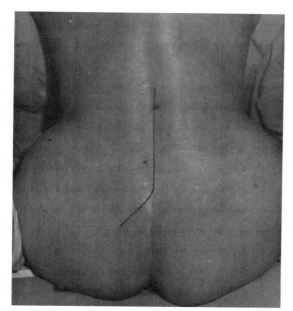

Figure 9–48. Hockey stick incision used for a two level spinal fusion from L4 to the sacrum. Incision extends from the third lumbar spinous process to the sacrum and then deviates laterally to allow exposure of the iliac crest.

directed cranially or caudally, allowing it to cut the soft tissues cleanly from bone. It should be stressed that a large curet is infinitely safer than a small one in this area.

If nerve root exploration and decompression is to be undertaken, it may start at this juncture. If not, attention is then turned to exposure of the transverse processes. Using either the electric knife or a sharp periosteal elevator, the fascia is incised directly laterally to the facet joints of L3–L4. As this fascia is incised, the periosteal elevator can sweep laterally along the superior articular facet of L4, and down onto the fourth transverse process. Paraspinal muscles can then be swept laterally, exposing the entire length of the transverse process. When the process is cleaned of soft tissue and completely exposed on its dorsal aspect, this area should be packed with a sponge to control bleeding. The incision in the fascia should then be continued in a caudal direction and, utilizing the L4–L5 facet joint as a landmark, the fifth transverse process should be exposed in a similar manner. All ligaments and muscles should be dissected well laterally, forming an uninterrupted gutter between the transverse processes and the ala of the sacrum. After the fifth transverse process is exposed, cleaned and packed, the fascia incision is continued down to a point distal and lateral to the superior articular facet of the sacrum. Dissection lateral to this element will expose the ala of the sacrum. Many dense ligaments are adherent in this area, and must be dissected from the sacrum in order to clearly expose the ala. It is essential to clearly visualize both the transverse processes and the ala in order to obtain an optimal preparation of the fusion bed. The sponges previously used to obtain hemostasis about the transverse processes and the ala of the sacrum are then removed, and a careful decortication of the transverse processes, the lateral portion of the pedicles and the lateral portion of the articular facets is performed. This is best accomplished with large, sharp curets. Some care is required in order not to fracture the transverse process. The ala of the sacrum is best decorticated with a narrow, round gouge. The lateral portion of the superior articular facet of the sacrum should also be decorticated. It is not necessary to excise the facet joints. This process of exposure and decortication is repeated on both sides of the spine. The wound is again carefully packed, and the midline fascia closed with a towel clip.

paraspinal muscles are stripped subperiosteally from the spine. This dissection is carried to the facet joints. As this dissection progresses, the wound is packed tightly with sponges to control bleeding. When this is completed, the sponges are removed and large self-retaining retractors are placed to expose the posterior elements of the spine. At this point, the surgeon should orient himself carefully through the sacrum and the lower lumbar vertebrae to be certain he is working at the correct levels.

Utilizing a large, sharp angled bone biter, the spinous processes of the sacrum, the fourth and fifth lumbar vertebrae, and a portion of the third spinous process are removed. The soft tissues are then meticulously dissected and removed from the posterior elements of the spine down to the ligamentum flavum. This is accomplished with large sharp curets. This dissection is most easily accomplished when started laterally at the facet joints and the tissues swept toward the midline, where they are removed with the scalpel. The correct use of the curet is mandatory. Pressure should never be exerted in a downward direction. Rather the curet should be

BONE GRAFT. The posterior iliac crest is exposed by dissecting away the layer of adipose tissue with a large sponge. The fascia is incised in line with the posterior iliac crest, and the crest then dissected subperiosteally. The gluteal muscles are carefully dissected from the lateral wing of the ilium. Care must be taken to remain beneath the periosteum or dramatic bleeding which is difficult to control can occur. A broad reverse retractor is then inserted to clearly expose the lateral portion of the ilium. Utilizing sharp, curved gouges, long strips of cortical and cancellous bone are removed from the ilium until the inner wall of the ilium is exposed. Large amounts of bone are readily obtained from this area. This graft material should be cut into strips approximately 1 to 2 ml in width and saved in blood-soaked sponges (Fig. 9–49).

PLACEMENT OF THE GRAFT MATERIAL AND CLOSURE OF THE WOUND. The midline wound is then reexposed and the self-retaining retractors are reinserted. All the sponges are removed from the wound and the wound

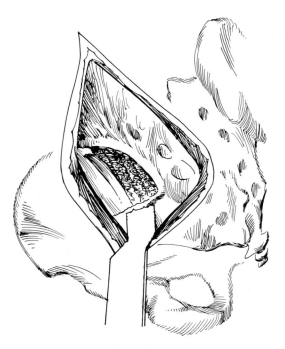

Figure 9–49. Technique of obtaining autogenous graft material from the posterior iliac crest. A large spiked retractor is utilized to expose the posterior surface of the ilium. Long strips of cortical and cancellous bone are then obtained, utilizing curved gouges. The graft material is saved in blood-soaked sponges and transferred to the previously prepared bed within five minutes.

checked with careful finger palpation to be certain that none of the recesses harbor a hidden sponge. At this point, the preliminary sponge count should be obtained. The graft material is then placed in the trough which has been created from the fourth transverse process to the ala of the sacrum bilaterally (Fig. 9–50).

The wounds should be frequently irrigated with antibiotic solution and, at this point, all devitalized tissue debrided. The double limb suction drain is inserted with one limb deep in the midline wound and the other at the iliac crest donor site. The fascia is then closed, utilizing #1 chromic suture. Subcutaneous closure is obtained with 00 chromic suture and the skin approximated with interrupted 000 wire.

POSTOPERATIVE MANAGEMENT. The patient is allowed out of bed and walking the day after surgery. If there is difficulty in voiding, the patient may be allowed to stand at his bedside on the night of surgery. This may circumvent the need for catheterization with its attendant risk of infection. An exercise program is started on the second or third postoperative day, with deep knee bends and tuck exercises with the knees being drawn to the chest. No external support is utilized in the way of braces or corsets. This program of early mobilization has not been shown to lower the rate of successful fusion and has many dramatic advantages. Psychologically, the patient becomes attuned to an optimistic course and early return to productive life. The paraspinal muscles rapidly resume their normal tone, and the resolution of edema and hematoma occurs quickly.

The suction drains are withdrawn and the dressings removed at 48 hours. The wound remains exposed to the air after this point. It is sprayed with Betadine (povidone-iodine) twice daily. Narcotics or mild analgesics are utilized for the first few postoperative days as needed. Antibiotics, as previously noted, are administered for 72 hours postoperatively. The sutures are removed and the patient discharged at 10 days.

Subsequent to discharge, the patient is encouraged to gradually increase his level of activity. He is advised that the pain in his spine should be his guideline to his level of activity and that this should not be exceeded. Automobile riding is prohibited for the first several weeks. Heavy lifting is also discouraged. After four to six weeks, the patient may return to light work, at least on a part-time

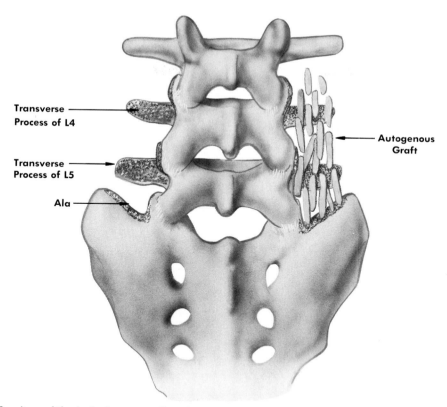

Transverse Process of L4

Transverse Process of L5

Ala

Autogenous Graft

Figure 9–50. Area of the bed of raw cancellous bone for a lateral spine fusion from L4 to the sacrum. The bed is shown on the left and the graft material is in place on the right. In actuality a much larger volume of graft material is utilized. The bed includes the transverse processes, the ala of the sacrum, the lateral portion of the pedicle and the lateral portion of the superior articular facets.

basis. After three months, most patients are able to return full time to sedentary and moderately active employment. Heavy physical labor is prohibited for six months. The same is true of vigorous athletics.

The patient is re-evaluated at six-week intervals for the first three months and then at three-month intervals for the first year. As recovery progresses, the patient is placed on a more vigorous program of flexion exercises and is again instructed as to the essential aspects of back hygiene. He is encouraged to return to a normal way of life as rapidly as possible.

ANTERIOR INTERBODY FUSION

This type of fusion should be reserved for certain patients who have had multiple surgical procedures through the posterior approach to the spine, which have failed. Dense posterior scarring, wide resection of the posterior elements of the spine, and a failed lateral spinal fusion are indications for consideration of this technique. The major disadvantage inherent in this surgical approach is the inability to carefully explore and decompress nerve roots, when this is required.

This operation should be performed by a spinal surgeon and an abdominal surgeon together, unless the spinal surgeon has had extensive experience with the anterior approach.

ANESTHESIA. A naso-gastric tube is utilized to prevent abdominal distention. Endotracheal anesthesia is preferred with the patient in the Trendelenburg position.

APPROACH. The retroperitoneal approach described by Harmon is utilized. A left paramedian incision is made, the anterior rectus sheath opened and the muscle retracted laterally. The retroperitoneal space is entered and the peritoneum dissected bluntly from the undersurface of the posterior rectus sheath.[48] The peritoneum is mobilized and, as the lower lumbar spine is exposed, the ureter is left in its peritoneal bed and reflected to the right. The sacral promontory is identified by palpation. It is essential not to damage the sympathetic nerves coursing over the sacrum. The major sympathetic chains on either side of the lumbar vertebrae are carefully dissected and retracted in a lateral direction. The L5 interspace is exposed by retracting the left iliac artery and vein to the left, and the right iliac artery and vein to the right. To expose the fourth lumbar vertebra, the left artery and vein are displaced to the right side of the spine. Spiked retractors are driven into the body of the vertebra to maintain exposure.

ANTERIOR DISC EXCISION AND FUSION. The anterior longitudinal ligament is elevated as a flap, with the base attached on the left. Exposure can be improved at this time by hyperextension of the operating table and spine. Then, utilizing the sharp osteotome, curets, and rongeurs, the entire disc is excised and a trough created in the opposing surfaces of the vertebral body above and below. The dimensions of this space are then measured, and three cortical-cancellous grafts are obtained from the left iliac crest. The grafts should be slightly larger than the notch so that firm impaction can be obtained. After insertion of the three grafts the spine can be brought to a neutral position, locking the grafts in place (Fig. 9–51). The previously created flap of anterior longitudinal ligament can be reattached or, if this is not possible, excised. The wound is closed in a routine manner after hemostasis is obtained. An excellent comprehensive discussion of the role, techniques and results of anterior disc excision and fusion was recently presented by Goldner.[41]

POSTOPERATIVE MANAGEMENT. The nasogastric tube is removed after peristalsis returns. Elastic stockings are utilized during and after surgery, to prevent thrombophlebitis. The management in other respects is similar to that after lateral spinal fusion.

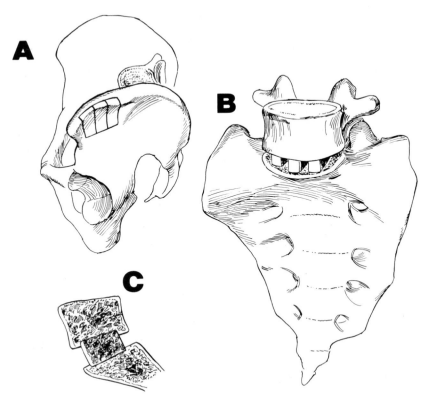

Figure 9–51. Technique of anterior lumbar fusion. After excision of the intervertebral disc, cortical cancellous grafts from the iliac crest are inserted into countersunk panels created in the adjacent vertebral end plates.

Complications of Lumbar Disc Surgery

The basic precept of all surgeons is "above all, do no harm." The prevention of complications in spine surgery demands an awareness of all the potential hazards, a thorough knowledge of standard and variational anatomy, and meticulous surgical technique. Despite elaborate precautions and great care, however, these complications may occur, but should be recognized early and treated appropriately.

COMPLICATIONS DURING OPERATION

VASCULAR AND VISCERAL INJURIES. Injuries to the great vessels, including the aorta, inferior vena cava, and iliac vessels, as well as other visceral structures, occur from penetration of the anterior portion of the annulus with surgical instruments. These injuries carry serious implications, with a mortality rate of almost 55 per cent.[28] The majority of these injuries occur while trying to clean the anterior portion of the disc space with a curet or a pituitary rongeur. An erroneous estimation of the depth of the interspace will lead to the instrument penetrating the annulus and traumatizing one of the large vessels. Immediate laceration through the wall of the muscle may occur with massive hemorrhage; partial injuries to the wall of a vessel, with delayed hemorrhage may occur; or laceration of both artery and vein may occur, with a resultant arteriovenous fistula. The aorta and vena cava lie in approximation to the L4 disc space, while the iliac vessels lie in approximation to the L5 disc space.

Prevention of these injuries will be enhanced if adequate exposure is undertaken during the surgery. If adequate exposure and hemostasis are not obtained prior to entering the disc space, continuous epidural bleeding will obscure the field of vision and make it difficult to estimate the depth of the disc space. The depth with which an instrument penetrates the disc space should never exceed one and one-eighth inches. The surgeon who performs occasional spinal surgery should have his instruments marked in this regard. Even skilled surgeons, however, must constantly keep this dimension in mind while working in the depths of the disc space. A third, and most important, precaution is that every instrument tip should be against bone while cleaning a disc space. Pituitary rongeurs should not be closed unless the rasp of metal upon bone is felt, nor should the stroke of a curet be continued unless this reassuring sensation is felt.

Awareness of the possibility of this complication is important, and prompt surgical intervention is the only effective treatment. Profuse bleeding from the disc space, or hypovolemic shock disproportionate to the observable blood loss, should alert the surgeon to this possibility. The general circulatory signs of an arteriovenous fistula following back surgery, of course, should alert the physician to the possibility of a fistula.

The management of this complication is immediate laparotomy and repair of the vascular injury. The spinal wound should be closed immediately with towel clips and a sterile plastic drape. Blood and fluid replacement should begin immediately, and the patient turned to the supine position while a vascular surgeon is summoned.

INJURIES TO THE NEURAL ELEMENTS. Tears of the dura may occur during laminectomy and decompression, while gaining access to the spinal canal. Packing cottonoids between the dura and the bony elements of the canal will prevent this mishap. Much more difficulty will be found in cases in which previous surgery has been performed, with the formation of extensive scar tissue around the dura. Even with utmost care occasional tears of the dura will occur. Should this injury occur it is important to promptly repair the defect with fine silk sutures. Failure to perform an adequate repair may result in the formation of a fistula or spinal extradural cyst.

Nerve root injuries may occur from excessive retraction, laceration, or thermal burns.

Excessive retraction with metallic instruments can be avoided by gently packing the nerve roots with cotton pledgets. If this is properly performed, the nerve root can be adequately displaced medially without the necessity of repeated instrumentation, as described in the section on the technique of disc excision.

Lacerations of the nerve root usually occur through inadequate visualization and failure to recognize a flattened nerve root over an extruded disc. These injuries can be prevented by adequate visualization and careful control of bleeding. There is no particular advantage in attempting to identify a nerve root and disc herniations through a minute opening in the spinal canal. When any difficulty whatsoever is encountered in recognizing the pertinent anatomy such as the nerve root and disc herniations, the laminectomy should be widened so that the nerve root can be identified with confidence proximal to the disc herniation. An incision into the annulus should never be made until the nerve root at that level is positively identified and retracted. A wide exposure will facilitate this procedure.

Thermal burns can be prevented by employing electrocautery only when a nerve root has been retracted and with a fine tip bovie forceps. Extreme care should be used when setting the current level, and this should be checked on muscular tissue before coagulation within the spinal canal.

COMPLICATIONS DURING THE IMMEDIATE POSTOPERATIVE PERIOD

These complications are not unique to spine surgery, and follow the basic precepts of good surgical physiology. Pulmonary atelectasis, with failure to adequately expand the lungs postoperatively, is frequently seen in patients after endotracheal anesthesia. This is seen in the first three postoperative days and is a common cause for temperature elevations. The physical findings may be minimal, and even chest x-ray may not be revealing, with minor episodes of atelectasis. The best prevention and treatment is early mobilization of the patient, frequent encouragement toward coughing, and deep breathing. The anxious patient or the patient who cannot be rapidly mobilized should be routinely placed on intermittent positive pressure breathing. Blow bottles are of some help.

INTESTINAL ILEUS. Intestinal ileus is an occasional complication of low back surgery. It will produce abdominal distention, nausea with vomiting and respiratory distress, and auscultation will reveal the absence of bowel sounds.

Treatment should include nasogastric suction, with intravenous fluids and electrolytes until restoration of bowel function is indicated by peristalsis and the passage of flatus.

URINARY RETENTION. This common complication is seen in the immediate postoperative course, and is due to a combination of anxiety, pain, the supine position, and nerve root irritation prior to and during surgery. The great danger is the excessive use of urethral catheters, with the subsequent danger of infection. Great efforts are made to manage this

problem without the use of catheterization. Male patients are allowed to stand at bedside as early as the night of surgery, and female patients are allowed to use a bedside commode. If this is unsuccessful, parenteral urecholine should be utilized. Only when these two measures fail is catheterization undertaken.

WOUND INFECTION. Wound infection is a complication dreaded by all surgeons. It should be suspected when pain or temperature elevation occurs during the latter part of the first postoperative week. If there is any significant suspicion of infection, the wound should be cultured either through needle aspiration or swab, and immediate gram stain and culture performed. If an organism is identified, treatment should be instituted immediately. In the presence of a significant infection, the patient should be returned to the operating room and the wound reopened, thoroughly debrided and irrigated. A closed irrigation system should be introduced and the wound closed. This should be utilized for 10 to 14 days, together with parenteral antibiotics appropriate for the specific organism cultured. Minor infections should be drained promptly and treated with a specific antibiotic. It should be emphasized that the primary treatment of a surgical infection is surgery. Antibiotics are not adequate in themselves for collections of purulent material.

THROMBOPHLEBITIS. Thrombophlebitis is seen with decreasing frequency since the routine use of early mobilization. Its onset is heralded by a feeling of pain, tightness, and swelling in the affected extremity. Physical examination will reveal tenderness along the course of the vein, swelling, a positive Homans' sign and a possible temperature elevation. Treatment is immediately instituted, with intravenous heparin, warm compresses to the leg and elevation of the extremity. The incidence of this complication is so low after spinal surgery that routine postoperative anticoagulation is not indicated, unless the patient has had a prior episode of thrombophlebitis.

TECHNICAL COMPLICATIONS RESULTING IN PERSISTENT SYMPTOMATOLOGY

INADEQUATE NERVE ROOT DECOMPRESSION. Not infrequently, a patient continues with unrelenting sciatica postoperatively, and upon reexploration it becomes evident that the true pathology was not uncovered at the time of primary surgery. This complication can be prevented only if the variety of pathologic entities causing nerve root compression are understood and appreciated by the surgeon. To simply look for an acute disc herniation through a small fenestration and consider this adequate treatment in all cases is to invite persistent pain. The most common conditions in which nerve root compression is not relieved are unrecognized disc lesions at another level, unrecognized lateral recess syndrome, unrecognized migrated free fragment of disc material, unrecognized foraminal encroachment, and unrecognized tethering of a nerve root about the pedicle. These errors can be avoided with a generous laminectomy and wide exposure whenever doubt exists as to the true nature of the pathology. Careful exploration of the nerve root should be undertaken, from its origin at the dural sac well out into the foramen. A large, malleable cervical dilator is found useful in exploring foramina. Right angle nerve root elevators can be used with advantage to explore beneath a nerve root and dural sac, and will rule out central protrusions and migrated fragments. When doubt arises as to the level of the protrusion, exploration of two or three disc spaces should be undertaken. An additional half hour spent in careful exploration may save the patient years of misery and disability. The importance of an adequate and meticulous exploration cannot be overemphasized. It should be added parenthetically that no additional morbidity has been experienced with wide laminectomy.[61]

FIBROSIS AROUND THE NERVE ROOTS AND DURA. Scar formation will occur with great regularity about the dura and nerve roots after surgical exploration. The reasons why this will cause symptoms in one patient and not in others are not understood at the present time. The scar tissue can act as a tethering force as well as a constricting force about the nerve roots. Some hope for prevention of this complication is given by the recent work of MacNab, with the use of a gelfoam membrane, as described in the earlier section on Surgical Technique.

Careful hemostasis and gentle handling of the neural tissue will also decrease the amount of scar tissue formation.

PSEUDARTHROSIS. Pseudarthrosis is a dreaded complication of spinal fusion. The incidence of this complication has decreased markedly with the advent of the lateral spine fusion. In a recent study by DePalma and Rothman, a group of 39 patients with radiographically demonstrable pseudarthrosis were studies. Of this group, only 17 were symptomatic. Thus, it is the authors' recommendation that a significant trial of conservative therapy be instituted before surgical correction is undertaken. The prevention of pseudarthrosis is based on adequate surgical technique and attention to the general physiology of the patient, and particularly to the treatment of anemia.[92]

DISC SPACE INFECTION. Disc space infection should be considered when there is a rapid dramatic recurrence of severe back pain one to six weeks after excision of an intervertebral disc. The patient may or may not have a temperature elevation, and frequently the only laboratory abnormality will be an elevated sedimentation rate. Serial radiographic examination will reveal loss of height of the disc space, irregular destruction of the end plate and, ultimately, sclerotic reaction.[116]

Diagnosis can usually be made by radiographic and clinical findings without biopsy or needle aspiration of the disc space. Treatment demands complete immobilization in a plaster spica from the lower rib cage to above the knees. Large doses of parenteral antibiotics effective against staphylococcal organisms are utilized for a period of two to three months. Those patients who do not respond to conservative therapy should undergo debridement of the disc space through a retroperitoneal abdominal approach.

ARACHNOID CYST. If dural tears are unrecognized or are not repaired an arachnoid cyst may be formed, and can on occasion assume dramatic size. Treatment of these lesions necessitates operation and excision of the cyst.

INSTABILITY OF A MOTOR UNIT. Instability of a motor unit may be present preoperatively or after the excision of an intervertebral disc. There is some evidence to suggest that this instability is associated with failure of relief of symptoms after disc excision.[38]

In the face of persistent back pain and sciatica after disc excision and radiographically proven instability, lateral spine fusion should be undertaken to stabilize the spine. This potential for instability is not in itself an adequate justification for fusion of all spines after disc excision. The criteria for a combined procedure and spinal fusion are outlined in the discussion on indications for spinal surgery and the selection of the appropriate operative procedure.

IMPINGEMENT SYNDROME. After midline spinal fusion certain patients develop symptoms at the site of contact of the fusion mass against the spinous process of the vertebra, directly cranial to the fusion. The clinical picture is one of pain on extension of the spine, with point tenderness at the area of the impingement. This usually also can be demonstrated radiographically.

Treatment of this entity requires resection of the lower portion of the spinous process involved.

RETAINED FOREIGN BODIES. With the use of accurate sponge counts and radiographic tagging of sponges and cotton pledgets, this complication should be rather rare. Occasionally, a cotton pledget will be detached from its identifying string and, if unrecognized, may be retained in the wound. These foreign bodies may cause a local inflammatory reaction, and for this reason reexploration should be undertaken, with removal of the foreign body. Bone wax sometimes causes a granulomatous reaction and persistent drainage from a wound. This material should be used sparingly and may require removal.

IATROGENIC SPINAL STENOSIS. As our temporal perspective increases, many instances are being noted of cauda equina compression secondary to overgrowth of lamina and fusion masses, when midline fusion techniques have been utilized. Not only will the bone graft material hypertrophy, but also the lamina will appear to increase in thickness, under the stimulus of decortication and grafting (Fig. 9–45). The neural canal and foramina may be encroached. Treatment requires midline decompression.

PELVIC INSTABILITY. The creation of pelvic instability after removing iliac bone for grafting, and fatigue fractures at the site of the graft removal are rare complications of spinal fusion but should be considered in patients with persistent back pain after spinal fusion.[17] Fatigue fractures will heal spontaneously. Pelvic instability may require sacroiliac fusion.

Results of Operative Treatment of Lumbar Disc Disease

Over three decades have passed since the advent of surgical treatment of lumbar disc disease. Improvement in the efficiency of surgical treatment must be predicated on accurate knowledge of the quality of result which can be expected with each technique and diagnosis. Long-term follow-up is essential in this area, and studies of this type are now available in the literature.[26, 126] The pressing need at the present time is for an accurately constructed prospective study using various surgical techniques for each of the specific diagnostic entities under consideration. Retrospective studies grouping all disc diseases into one diagnostic category are of limited value.

DePalma and Rothman have reported their experience over a period of 20 years, with over 1500 patients who had undergone surgery for lumbar disc degeneration.[26] These patients were called back for personal interview, physical examination and repeat radiographic examination, including stress films. In order to minimize bias, the evaluations were performed by physicians other than the operating surgeon.

Examination of the population distribution curve revealed that the average age at surgery was 40, with a normal frequency distribution above and below this level. This age distribution is in keeping with the more recent pathologic concepts of disc degeneration. The average age of follow-up evaluation was 48, the average follow-up period was 8 years. One hundred and ninety-five patients were followed for a period of 10 years or longer (Table 9–2).

Relief of symptoms was the most important criterion for success in terms of low back surgery. Patients were questioned about the degree and temporal nature of their relief of back and leg pain. Their evaluation as to the subjective worth of their surgery was also elicited.

In individuals with L5 disc degeneration, 15 per cent had persistent back pain, 7 per cent had persistent sciatica, and 14 per cent had both back pain and sciatica. The results are approximately the same with L4 disc degeneration and two-level disc degeneration (Table 9–3). When questioned as to overall

TABLE 9–2. POPULATION

Mean age surgery	40 years
Mean age follow up	48 years
Mean follow up	8 years
Range follow up	1–20 years
Ten year or greater follow up	195 patients

TABLE 9–3. PERCENTAGES OF DISC DEGENERATION PATIENTS SHOWING SYMPTOMS AT FOLLOW UP

	L5–S1	L4–L5	Both
Preoperative			
Back pain	10	7	7
Leg pain	5	0	4
Both	85	93	89
Postoperative			
Back pain	15	17	11
Leg pain	7	7	4
Both	14	17	20

TABLE 9–5. PERCENTAGE CHANGES IN PHYSICAL FINDINGS AFTER SURGERY

Loss of all reflex change	25
Loss of all motor deficit	50
Loss of all sensory deficit	50
Loss of abnormal curve	
Muscle spasm	
Tenderness	90 or more
Limited motion	
Straight leg raising	

relief of their pain, approximately 60 per cent of individuals in each category stated that they had obtained complete relief of back and leg pain, approximately 30 per cent considered themselves partially relieved, and 2 to 3 per cent were a total failure with no relief whatsoever. Of the patients with disc degeneration at L4 or L5, 88 per cent felt their surgery worthwhile; the percentage was less when both disc spaces were affected (Table 9–4).

Physical findings were evaluated at follow-up and compared to preoperative findings. The nonspecific findings such as muscle spasm, tenderness and limitation of motion, and straight leg raising disappeared in 90 per cent of those individuals who showed these findings preoperatively. Neurologic deficits returned to normal less often postoperatively. Motor and sensory deficits which had been present preoperatively disappeared in 50 per cent of the patients. Only 25 per cent of the patients lost their preoperative reflex changes. This is somewhat better than the results reported by Knutsson, in which only 33 per cent of patients lost their sensory deficit, 24 per cent lost their motor deficit and 2½ per cent lost their reflex abnormalities[67] (Table 9–5).

Certain general observations were noted which are also of interest. An attempt was made to select those factors which would be of poor prognostic significance for the patient undergoing back surgery.

In regard to diagnosis, high discs (i.e., above the L4–L5 level) did more poorly in regard to relief of symptomatology. One operative category appeared to fare more poorly; lumbosacral fusion combined with disc excision alone at the L4–L5 level. At one time this operation was felt to be appropriate when a degenerated L4–L5 disc was found together with evidence of an unstable lumbosacral mechanism. The correlation of physical findings with quality of result revealed that a negative straight leg raising test in the preoperative examination tended to correlate with a poor result. This observation was also noted by Hirsch.[54] He noted that laminectomy and exploration were negative more often when the straight leg raising test, neurologic examination and myelogram were negative. He further observed that with negative exploration the quality of result was poor regardless of the operative procedure performed.

PSEUDARTHROSIS

The overall rate of solid fusion in the above series was 92 per cent, with an incidence of pseudarthrosis of 8 per cent. Following the advent of the lateral fusion technique, the incidence of pseudarthrosis in two level fusions is 6 per cent.[25] The incidence of pseudarthrosis in one-level fusions utilizing the lateral technique is less than 1 per cent. In our study group, 39 patients were discovered whom we could classify radiographically as having definite pseudarthrosis. In the hope of learning in detail what the diagnosis of pseudarthrosis portends for a patient, we studied these individuals in detail. They were compared with a matched group of 39 patients, each having an identical diagnosis and opera-

TABLE 9–4. PATIENTS WITH DISC DEGENERATION SHOWING SUBJECTIVE RELIEF AT FOLLOW UP

	L5–S1	L4–L5	Both
Total	62	67	59
Partial	30	24	28
Temporary	4	7	11
None	3	3	2
Surgery worthwhile	88	88	75

TABLE 9–6.   PERCENTAGE OF PATIENTS
WHO CONSIDERED SURGERY
WORTHWHILE

Pseudarthrosis	Solid Fusion
82	92

TABLE 9–8.   PERCENTAGES OF PATIENTS
WITH BACK PAIN AT FOLLOW UP

	Pseudarthrosis	Solid Fusion
Preoperative	92	97
Postoperative	44	38

tion in whom the fusion was solid. By comparing these two matched groups, we can state with some degree of precision the implication of pseudarthrosis for the patient who has undergone a spinal fusion.

In an overall subjective evaluation of the worth of their surgery, 82 per cent of the patients who had developed pseudarthrosis felt that their surgery was worthwhile, whereas 92 per cent of the group who had solid fusions felt that their surgery was worthwhile (Table 9–6). Little difference was found between the pseudarthrosis group and the solid fusion group when they were asked specifically about their overall relief from symptomatology. Fifty-six per cent of patients in the former group and 61 per cent in the latter group obtained total relief. It is interesting to note that, although there was a slight decrease in the number who obtained total relief in the pseudarthrosis group, three patients who achieved solid fusions obtained no relief, and all patients who developed pseudarthrosis obtained at least partial or temporary relief (Table 9–7).

When back pain alone was considered, of the 92 per cent of patients in the pseudarthrosis group who originally had back pain, 44 per cent still had the symptoms at follow-up evaluation. In the solid fusion group, of the 97 per cent of patients who originally had back pain, 38 per cent had significant back pain at follow-up evaluation (Table 9–8).

Sciatica was eliminated more consistently than back pain at follow-up evaluation. Of the 79 per cent of patients in the pseudarthrosis group who had sciatica, only 25 per cent had their symptoms at follow-up evaluation. In the

solid-fusion group, of the 85 per cent of patients who originally had sciatica, only 20 per cent had their symptoms at follow-up evaluation (Table 9–9). The subjective factors noted above were submitted to Chi-square analysis and in no case was a significant difference noted between the pseudarthrosis and the solid fusion group. It seems justifiable to draw certain conclusions from the above information. One of two situations must exist: either the pseudarthrosis represents a fibrous stabilization which is essentially as effective as bony fusion, or the fusion component of these procedures was not essential. The former is not unreasonable, as the amount of motion demonstrated on flexion-extension films of pseudarthrosis is usually minimal, and is often less than 2 ml. The latter conclusion, however, remains in question.

It would furthermore seem prudent to carefully observe patients with pseudarthrosis for a rather prolonged period of time before reoperating in an attempt to achieve union. There seems little rationale for submitting patients to multiple attempts at repair of pseudarthrosis if, as a group, there is little difference in their subjective result when solid fusion is obtained.

The overall picture obtained is that a certain number of patients who have undergone spinal fusion continue to have back pain and less frequently sciatica, whether or not their fusion has become solid. The success rate, as judged by objective evaluation, is slightly greater in that group which has achieved solid fusion. Pseudarthrosis, of itself, does not appear to be the dreaded complication that is

TABLE 9–7.   PERCENTAGE OF PATIENTS
RECEIVING RELIEF FROM SYMPTOMS

	Pseudarthrosis	Solid Fusion
Total	56	61
Partial	34	26
Temporary	10	5
None	0	8

TABLE 9–9.   PERCENTAGE OF PATIENTS
WITH SCIATICA AT FOLLOW UP

	Pseudarthrosis	Solid Fusion
Preoperative	79	85
Postoperative	25	20

often portrayed. A more precise definition of the role of spinal fusion, and evaluation of the essentiality of achieving this fusion, will depend on the availability of long term prospective studies of spinal surgery.

As one reviews the overwhelming amount of written material pertaining to spinal surgery, certain precepts become clear, and certain requirements evident, if good results are to be obtained.

REQUIREMENTS FOR SUCCESSFUL SPINAL SURGERY

1. Accurate knowledge of the variable pathology of disc degeneration.
2. Accurate diagnosis of nerve root compression.
3. Adherence to the proper criterion for surgical intervention.
4. Selection of the proper operative procedure.
5. Skillful execution of the surgical procedure by an experienced spinal surgeon.
6. The prompt recognition and treatment of complications.
7. Careful postoperative care and rehabilitation.

If every patient undergoing spine surgery had the benefit of these principles, the quality of surgical result would improve dramatically, and the grey veil of apprehension, fear and anxiety that has surrounded spinal surgery for years would be lifted.

INDUSTRIAL, COMPENSATION, AND LEGAL BACK INJURIES

Even the novice physician quickly becomes aware that the patient who has sustained his low back injury at work in a compensation setting or in a circumstance with legal involvement may be much less responsive to operative or nonoperative treatment than the patient who sustains his injury in a less complex and encumbered situation. There have been a multitude of studies dealing with this problem which have reinforced this observation. One of the more recent, comprehensive, and incisive reviews of this topic is that of Beals & Hickman.[11] The more jaded observer will feel that these patients are often frank malingerers, while the more psychiatrically oriented physician will feel that these patients are attempting to answer their emotional problems through their somatic complaints. There is little doubt that, in addition to the patient's physical injury, a number of other aspects of this problem, including the psychiatric, sociologic, economic and vocational forces will determine the patient's recovery and return to work. It has been shown that a large proportion of the effort and expense emanating from industrial injuries is focused on a minority of cases. The average cost of an industrial back injury when surgery was involved has been estimated by Leavitt to be approximately $10,000.[69]

Several key factors must be understood and appreciated in the approach to the patient with a significant industrial back injury.[11]

1. As time progresses (from the time of injury), patients often increasingly elaborate and exaggerate their symptoms, with less evidence of depression. The neurotic triad of hypochondriasis, depression and hysteria displays an evolutionary pattern, in which early are shown severe depressive reactions with mild hypochondriasis and hysteria and later are shown less depression and greater hypochondriasis and hysteria.

2. The chronic neurotic individual is often aggravated by surgical intervention.

3. Emotional and sociologic inadequacies of patients with back symptoms may predispose them to conversion symptoms. Through this mechanism they may resolve their psychological conflicts and convert them to a somatic presentation.

4. Patients who are psychologically disabled will not return to work despite recovery from physical disability.

5. Operative intervention may be helpful in these patients when medically indicated by the strict objective criteria outlined earlier in this chapter and when not contraindicated by gross psychopathology.

The role of surgery must be highly selective, and requires great judgment. When less than the most rigorous criteria for surgical intervention are utilized, failure is preordained. A review of lumbar laminectomies performed on compensation patients at the Philadelphia General Hospital during the years 1969 and 1970 reveals that of 13 individuals who underwent lumbar laminectomies, eight remain totally disabled, two remain partially disabled, one died and two returned to active working status: of the two who returned to active work only one considered himself improved by the surgery.[77]

Thus, it would seem quite clear that industrial back injuries are complex problems, involving not only anatomic but also psychiatric considerations, sociologic fragility and the economic and legal milieu of the patient. Effective recovery of these individuals will be predicated upon appreciation of this situation by the treating physician and a multidisciplinary approach to these problem cases.

CHEMONUCLEOLYSIS

Chemonucleolysis is the term used to describe injection of the enzyme chymopapain into the intervertebral disc as a method of treatment of back pain and sciatica. The use of this technique in humans was first described by Lyman Smith.[105, 106, 107] Over a period of 10 years, the clinical reports of other investigators in this area have tended to substantiate the efficacy of this technique as first reported.[14, 36, 85] It is not possible at this juncture to be precise about the quality of the long-term result after chemonucleolysis, since true randomized treatment studies using chemonucleolysis and laminectomy in identical patient diagnostic categories have not evolved. Additionally, we are limited to a 10 year period of follow-up on individuals subjected to this procedure.

Indications for Chemonucleolysis

Chemonucleolysis may serve as an intermediate treatment level between conservative therapy and operative intervention. It may be thought of as the last step of conservative treatment. The same criteria utilized for surgical intervention in acute soft disc herniations are utilized for chemonucleolysis. In general, those patients who are expected to fare best with laminectomy have also shown the best results with chemonucleolysis. Patients with multiple previous operative interventions, those with advanced bony structural degenerative changes, and those with predominant back pain have responded less well than have patients with acute disc herniations. Patients should be prepared to undergo surgical laminectomy if their sciatica is not relieved by chemonucleolysis.

Mode of Action

Chymopapain, the major proteolytic component of papaya latex, rapidly dissolves portions of the water-insoluble components of nucleus pulposus from normal or prolapsed discs in vitro.[112] Injection of this enzyme into the disc is thought to hasten the degradation of chondromucoprotein, to relieve excessive and uneven intradiscal pressures. This simple concept, although a useful explanation, may not be accurate. MacNab, after myelographic and surgical study of patients who had undergone chemonucleolysis, states that the structural alterations in the disc may not be significant in relief of sciatica.[72] It is his feeling that alteration of the surface charge may be the more critical factor in pain relief.

Safety

As with any new therapeutic procedure the desire of the treating physician to do no harm is paramount. It appears that this technique is proving itself extremely safe. The problems encountered relate to allergy to the dye used for discogram, allergy to chymopapain, anesthetic risks, disc space infection, and neurologic deficit. With the use of proper precautions, all these risks are slight, and within acceptable boundaries.

Technique

The basic technique of chemonucleolysis has been outlined by Lyman Smith[105] and has changed little to the present time. General anesthesia is employed. The patient is placed, right side up, on an x-ray table. A bolster or plastic kidney rest is placed beneath the left flank. Although this procedure can be performed with routine x-ray equipment, an image intensifier is desirable. The skin is prepared and draped as for a surgical procedure. Eighteen gauge, 6 inch needles are introduced into the lower three lumbar discs. The lateral approach is utilized. The needles are directed from a point 8 cm lateral to the posterior spine of L4, 45 degrees caudal for the L5 disc. At the higher disc levels, the 45 degree, anterior inclination of the needle is utilized at the appropriate level. The needles are placed and, using the image intensifier, check roentgenograms are taken confirming their exact position in both planes. One-half to 1 ml of Reno-grafin is then injected into the discs to be investigated. A period of observation is useful to allow detection of any allergic reaction to the contrast material. Depending on the result of this discogram and the previous myelogram, the appropriate discs are then injected with chymopapain in a dosage of 2 to 4 mg. Smaller doses are utilized for a degenerated disc and larger doses for a protruded disc. A further period of observation after the injection of chymopapain is also important, to rule out allergic reactions to the chymopapain. The patient is then taken to the recovery room for observation, and subsequently returned to his bed. Postoperative management is similar to that after laminectomy.

Recommended Precautions

Certain precautions are advised to prevent problems which have been described with chemonucleolysis. A careful history of allergy is important, particularly to radiographic dyes, iodine and meat tenderizer. The lateral approach is recommended rather than the transdural approach, to decrease the chance of neurologic injury, although a midline approach may on occasion be necessary because of the structural configuration of the lower disc spaces. Sterile procedure is also mandatory during this undertaking, to decrease the risk of discitis.

Results

The results to be expected after chemonucleolysis have been described by several clinical investigators.[14, 22, 36, 85, 106, 107] A classification of end results has been proposed by MacNab, with four end result categories: excellent—no pain, no restriction of activities; good—occasional back or leg pain of insufficient severity to interfere with the patient's ability to do his normal work or his capacity to enjoy himself in his leisure hours; fair—improved functional capacity, but handicapped by intermittent pain of sufficient severity to curtail or modify work or leisure activities; poor—no improvement or insufficient improvement to enable increase in activities, further operative intervention required. The most recent series of 100 patients reported by Nordby indicated that chemonucleolysis re-

TABLE 9–10. EFFECTIVENESS OF CHEMONUCLEOLYSIS

	Author			
	Nordby	Smith	Ford	Day
Result (per cent)				
Excellent	13	>88	>59	33
Good	61			44
Fair	16	4	22	8
Poor	10	8	19	1
No. of patients	100	112	126	86

sulted in 13 per cent excellent results and 61 per cent good results, with a total of 74 per cent falling into these two satisfactory groups. If the 16 per cent considered a fair result are to be included in a satisfactory group, then the level of satisfactory results reaches 90 per cent. No patients were made worse by this treatment. Table 9–10 allows for comparison of the various series reported by investigators in this area.

Summary

Chemonucleolysis appears to be emerging as a useful tool in the treatment of lumbar disc degeneration on an intermediate level between traditional conservative care and surgical excision of the offending disc. The short-term effectiveness of this therapy appears good, although its effect beyond a 10-year period remains unknown.

The advantages which may evolve from chemonucleolysis are:

1. Decreased perineural scar formation.
2. Avoidance of surgical complications such as wound infection, nerve root injury, and blood transfusion.
3. Decreased morbidity and faster recovery.
4. Few patients are made worse by this procedure.

The disadvantages are:

1. Possibility of not discovering an intraspinal neoplasm which would be apparent on laminectomy.
2. Inability to deal effectively with osseous pathology and extruded, migrated disc material.
3. The possibility of allergic reaction.

MANAGEMENT OF FAILURES OF LUMBAR DISC SURGERY

One of the most difficult tasks in medicine is the management of the patient who has failed to gain lasting relief from spinal surgery. These patients often present with a perplexing history and physical examination, show evidence of both depression and anxiety and, understandably, are reluctant to put faith in their treating physician. Having once gone through a major surgical procedure with unsatisfactory results, they are torn between continuing with a life of pain and disability or seeking salvation through operative treatment which has on one occasion fallen short of its goals. They not infrequently fall into the hands of unscrupulous practitioners and charlatans, only to meet further disappointment. If a physician is to accept responsibility for these individuals, he must be willing to invest many hours in their evaluation, develop a methodical approach to their diagnosis and treatment and, finally, be willing to accept less than perfect results. These problems are indeed a trial for both the patient and his treating physician.

Diagnosis

As in all other areas of medicine, the first step in effective treatment is rendering an accurate diagnosis. A thorough differential diagnosis of the causes of persistent back pain after surgery must be pursued, with each cause being considered or eliminated on a rational basis.

ERROR IN ORIGINAL DIAGNOSIS

Lumbar laminectomy and disc excision will obviously fail to alleviate a patient's symptomatology if a herniated disc was not the true cause for his symptoms. This statement, although obvious, needs great emphasis. Disc degeneration, with or without herniation, is such a ubiquitous process that its very presence does not imply that it is the cause for a patient's disability. We have seen many instances in which a myelogram revealed a herniated disc in the lower lumbar spine, when in actuality, the cause of the patients' symptoms was either tumor or infection in the upper lumbar or lower thoracic area (Fig. 9–52). One cannot end his diagnostic search with the appearance of an abnormal myelogram. If there is any inconsistency between the myelographic appearance and the patient's symptomatology further diagnostic investigation must be considered. After a failed back operation, this problem becomes compounded. The authors have made it a policy to personally telephone the surgeon who performed the original operation in order to obtain an accurate description of the pathology found. All too often operative reports fail to yield a true description of the operative findings. Usually greater candor will be obtained in personal discussions. If this type of information is not obtained, one can fall into the trap of "operating on operations." By this we mean the patient who is reexplored after failed disc surgery and in whom at the time of reexploration only perineural scarring is found and removed. A spine fusion is performed at this operation only to have the patient continue with symptoms. At some future date, a nonunion of the fusion occurs, and further surgical intervention is undertaken to repair the nonunion. As might be expected, this also fails to alleviate the patient's symptoms, with the further specters of cordotomy, thalamic surgery and insertion of dorsal column stimulators appearing on the horizon. This entire cycle, of course, might have been prevented if it had been ascertained that no nerve root compression was demonstrated at the original laminectomy. The point of this is that great effort must be made to ascertain whether at any time definite evidence of disc herniation with nerve root compression was demonstrated. If not, further search must be made for nonmechanical causes of the patient's back pain and sciatica. Tumor, infection, and arthritic disorders of the spine must be considered as well as the other nondiscogenic problems.

Technical Causes for Failure of Lumbar Disc Surgery

The technical complications which may lead to persistent symptomatology after surgery have been described in detail earlier (see page 497), but will be outlined here.

1. Inadequate nerve root decompression.
2. Fibrosis about the nerve roots and dura.
3. Pseudarthrosis.
4. Disc space infection.
5. Arachnoid cyst.
6. Instability of a motor unit.
7. Impingement syndrome.
8. Retained foreign bodies.
9. Iatrogenic spinal stenosis.
10. Pelvic instability.

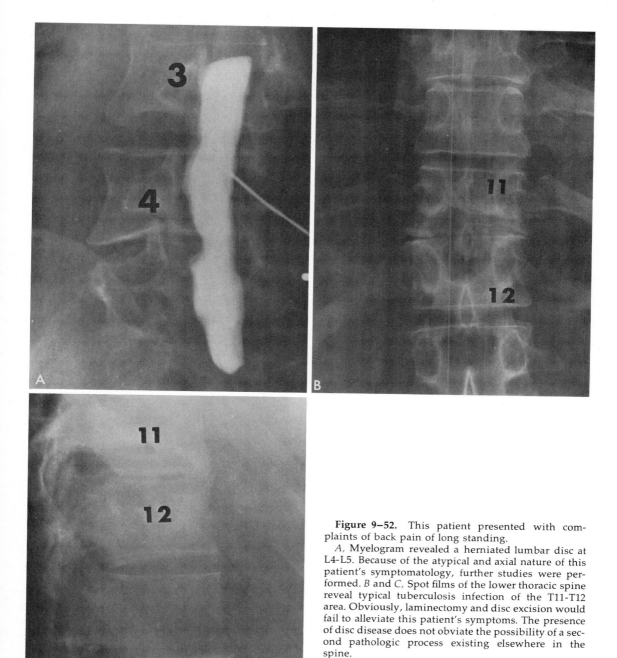

Figure 9–52. This patient presented with complaints of back pain of long standing.

A, Myelogram revealed a herniated lumbar disc at L4-L5. Because of the atypical and axial nature of this patient's symptomatology, further studies were performed. *B* and *C,* Spot films of the lower thoracic spine reveal typical tuberculosis infection of the T11-T12 area. Obviously, laminectomy and disc excision would fail to alleviate this patient's symptoms. The presence of disc disease does not obviate the possibility of a second pathologic process existing elsewhere in the spine.

Other Causes for Recurrent Symptoms

NEW HERNIATION AT ANOTHER LEVEL. One will on occasion see patients who have had a disc herniation treated successfully, with complete relief of symptoms, and who after a pain-free interval, develop signs and symptoms of a further disc herniation at a different level. These patients should not be considered in the category of failed spinal surgery. Their diagnosis is usually clear cut and should respond well to the appropriate treatment, whether nonoperative or surgical.

RECURRENT HERNIATION AT THE SAME LEVEL. If the nuclear material is incompletely evacuated at the first operation patients may develop recurrent herniations at the original site. These patients, after a period of pain relief, develop recurrent sciatica in the original nerve root distribution. It is difficult, if not impossible, to differentiate these symptoms from those of perineural scar formation. On occasion, myelography may be helpful but often it is not, owing to scar formation which has formed and tethers the nerve root.

CONTRALATERAL NERVE ROOT IRRITATION DUE TO BUCKLING OF THE ANNULUS AT THE LEVEL OF DISC EXCISION. Certain patients during their first two to three months of convalescence after discectomy will note symptoms of nerve root irritation in the contralateral leg. This is often due to settling of the disc space after excision of nuclear material, with buckling of the annulus and irritation of the contralateral nerve root. In our experience, these symptoms usually subside with rest and anti-inflammatory drugs, and do not require further surgical intervention.

PSYCHONEUROSES. Anxiety and depression frequently cause failures of spinal surgery. On the other hand, failed spine surgery, not too surprisingly, often leads to profound depression. Understanding and analysis of the problem is essential in the successful management of these patients, and cannot be ignored. A complete discussion of this problem will be found in Chapter 18.

Diagnostic Evaluation

A logical and systematic approach to failed spine surgery is usually undertaken on an in-patient basis, with a multidisciplinary approach. Despite the wide spectrum of physicians involved and the multitude of special tests undertaken, one individual must assume overall responsibility for the patient's care, and develop a meaningful relationship with the patient.

As a routine, we advise in-patient evaluation by our medical, neurosurgical, orthopedic and psychiatric services. Each adds a valuable facet to our understanding of the patient, and all have been helpful in our experience.

Radiographic examination of the lumbar spine is routinely performed with anterior, posterior, oblique and lateral views. Flexion-extension films are helpful in demonstrating instability or nonunions of fusions. Despite the known shortcomings of postoperative myelograms, we almost routinely repeat this procedure to rule out spinal neoplasms or persistent compression of the neural elements.

Electromyography is not performed routinely but may be useful in certain instances to document neurologic deficit.

Subsequent to psychiatric consultation, psychological testing may be performed at the psychiatrist's discretion. The differential spinal block (see page 474) is particularly helpful in differentiating organic versus nonorganic causes for the patient's symptoms.

Therapy

The recurrence of symptoms, in and of itself, is not justification for repeated surgical intervention. Conservative therapy should be instituted as outlined earlier (see page 476). If conservative treatment is successful in achieving an acceptable level of pain relief to the patient, no further consideration of surgical intervention need be undertaken.

If pain persists, despite conservative treatment, the patient must then decide if the level of pain is enough to warrant further surgical intervention. This presumes that the diagnostic entity under consideration is amenable to surgical treatment. At this point, the limitations of surgical intervention must be clearly spelled out to the patient. We caution that one of three patients undergoing salvage surgery of this type will receive little or no benefit from their procedure. Although this may be somewhat pessimistic, we are anxious that patients realize that surgical intervention at this point cannot guarantee success. It should be pointed out to patients that with permanent limitation of their activities, they may be able to bring their symptoms within tolerable bounds.

There will be a group of patients whose pain is intolerable and has not responded to conservative treatment, who would in all likelihood not respond to further surgical intervention in the lumbar spine. They should be considered for surgical procedures designed primarily for pain relief as discussed in Chapter 17.

OPERATIVE PROCEDURE FOR FAILED DISC SURGERY

When called upon to re-explore a nerve root and disc space that has had previous surgery, it is not uncommon for us to find a mixed type of pathology. Usually, extensive fibrosis is present about the dura and nerve root, extending well into the foramen. Protrusions at the disc space itself may consist of both a bulging annulus and nuclear material. Varying amounts of bone will have been resected at the time of the primary or secondary laminectomy. We feel compelled to excise the scar tissue and perform a radical exploration of the nerve root well beyond the foramen. This will often call for a foraminotomy and wide laminectomy. All nerve roots that are involved clinically and myelographically are explored. At this juncture, the amount of instability created is difficult to evaluate. In an attempt to render a definitive operation to the patient, we will usually perform a lateral spinal fusion at the completion of the decompressive portion of the operation.

In those patients whose primary symptom is back pain, nerve root exploration may not be mandatory. There are certain clear indications for spinal fusion in the absence of sciatica. The first of these is severe incapacitating back pain after disc excision. Assuming no other pathologic process is producing the pain, one might reasonably expect good success in those individuals with localized disc degeneration.

Iatrogenic instability produced through the intervention of the surgeon at the time of the primary procedure is a second indication for spinal fusion. With the more complete knowledge of the pathology of the spine, and more radical exploration of nerve roots, the spinal surgeon will often find it necessary to resect facet joints, complete laminae, and pedicles. While resection of these elements is not often necessary to achieve nerve root decompression, the resultant spine may be quite unstable. This situation demands fusion. Certain individuals will also develop instability after a simple disc excision. Careful statistical analysis of this problem would indicate that extensive motion after discectomy will tend toward persistent back pain, while restriction of interspace motion will tend toward a satisfactory result.

The third indication for spinal fusion is the presence of a neural arch defect that was not stabilized at the primary operation.

The Surgical Treatment of Spondylolisthesis in Adults

The clinical picture of spondylolisthesis evolves gradually as one studies the transition from late adolescence to early adulthood. For a complete discussion of the etiology, classification, and treatment of this disorder in childhood and adolescence the reader is referred to Chapter 5, Congenital Anomalies of the Spine. Upon reaching maturity, the fear of further anterior migration is no longer present and is only a minor consideration in terms of surgical treatment. After employing the usual forms of non-operative therapy, such as limitation of activities, a lumbosacral corset, and spinal exercises, certain individuals will remain incapacitated by low back pain and leg pain secondary to spondylolisthesis. It is these individuals who should be considered as candidates for surgery. Progressive deformity and neurologic deficits are subsidiary considerations for the most part.

It is unrealistic to recommend one surgical procedure for the entire spectrum of clinical disorders associated with spondylolisthesis. Great confusion exists in the literature, and advocates are found for simple nerve root compression by resection of the loose neural arch on the one hand and spinal fusion on the other. In deciding on the optimal mode of surgical treatment, one must consider the age of the patient, the anatomic configuration of the spine in regard to the degree of slip and size of the transverse processes, and the clinical pain pattern, i.e., back pain only, leg pain only, or both. Despite the frequency of this disorder and the large amount of surgery performed on an annual basis for this problem, there exists in the literature no randomized prospective study of the surgical treatment of spondylolisthesis by the diverse methods of treatment available. In the absence of this essential information, one must be guided by his personal experience and skill, as well as by the limited amount of information available from the retrospective studies conducted in the literature.

A plan of approach to this problem in adults is outlined below; the authors have found it to be generally satisfactory, and it has been supported by the work of others interested in this problem.

BACK PAIN ONLY

Most patients with spondylolisthesis have back pain and lumbar insufficiency as primary symptoms. Approximately one third will, in addition, have sciatica. This ratio is constant in both children and adults.[68a] A successful spinal fusion will usually alleviate symptoms in those individuals who have only back pain.[50a, 89a, 110a] This is most effectively achieved by the technique of posterolateral fusion (for technique see page 491). The extent of the fusion will depend both on the degree of slip and the size of the fifth transverse process. When the degree of slip is minor and the fifth transverse process is large, the fusion need extend only from L5 to the sacrum.[124b] When the degree of slip is large and the transverse process small, the fusion mass should be carried from the sacrum to the fourth transverse process. When any doubt exists as to the adequacy of the fifth transverse process, the surgeon should not hesitate to extend the fusion to L4 in order to obtain a more adequate bed.

BACK PAIN AND LEG PAIN

Those individuals with both back and leg pain require both decompression, by excision of the loose neural arch and excision of the fibrocartilage mass at the defect site, and stabilization of the spine by fusion, for optimal relief of symptoms. This appears to combine the excellent relief of sciatica produced by the decompression as advocated by Gill with the stability and relief of back pain afforded by the spinal fusion.[40a] This combined procedure is the most common operation utilized by the authors for spondylolisthesis today. It has yielded excellent results in our hands as well as others'. Rombold reports 93 per cent satisfactory long term results with this approach.[89a] As previously stated, the extent of the fusion should be determined by the size and accessibility of the fifth transverse process.

PATIENTS OVER AGE 60 WITH PREDOMINANT LEG PAIN

In older patients in whom leg pain is a predominant symptom, simple resection of the loose posterior elements and nerve root de-

compression as advocated by Gill appears to be a satisfactory approach.[40a] The enthusiastic reports by Gill for the treatment of spondylolisthesis have not been uniformly supported. Amuso and co-authors noted only 64 per cent satisfactory results utilizing the same criteria for grading as Gill.[4a] However, the older individual with limited demands on his spine, and greater intrinsic stability at the level of the spondylolisthesis, will usually obtain satisfactory relief of pain. Further progression of the slip, after resection of the posterior elements, a valid fear in children, does not appear to be a problem in adults.[4a, 40a] Certain adults will show a minimal amount of further anterior migration but the small amount of further migration does not appear to correlate with the quality of clinical result.

NON-UNION OF SPINAL FUSION

Those individuals who have a pseudarthrosis after a midline spinal fusion, and whose symptoms justify the need for further surgery, are recommended to have a lateral spine fusion. In those who have had a lateral spine fusion which has failed, the anterior approach to the spine is then utilized, as described on page 496. If the primary approach to the spondylolisthesis has been the anterior approach and non-union has resulted, a posterolateral spine fusion is then utilized.

DEGENERATIVE SPONDYLOLISTHESIS

Degenerative spondylolisthesis (and retrospondylolisthesis) does not represent a true defect in the posterior neural arch but rather malalignment of the vertebra associated with disc degeneration and instability of both the disc itself and the posterior facet joints. For a discussion of this relationship the reader is referred to page 460. The surgical treatment of this disorder is considered together with disc degeneration, as outlined on page 484.

References

1. Ahlgren, E. W., et al.: Diagnosis of pain with a graduated spinal block technique. J.A.M.A. *195*:125–128, 1966.
2. Ahlgren, P.: Lumbale Myelographic mit Conray Meglumin 282. Fortschr. Rontgenstr. *111*:270–276, 1969.
3. Ahlgren, P.: Lumbar myelography with Dimer-X. IX Symposium Neuroradiologicum, Goteberg, Aug. 1970. Book of abstracts, p. 135.
4. Ahlgren, P.: Postmyelografiske eller postoperative arachnoiditiske forandringer efter Conturex-, Conray- og Dimer-X-myelografier (Danish).

Dansk Selskab for Diagnostisk Radiologi. October 27, 1972.

4a. Amuso, S. et al: The Surgical Treatment of Spondylolisthesis by Posterior Element Resection. J.B.J.S. 52A:529–536, 1970.

5. Archer, V. W.: The Osseous System. Chicago, Year Book Medical Publishers, 1963.

6. Armstrong, J. R.: Lumbar Disc Lesions. Baltimore, The Williams & Wilkins Co., 1965.

7. Autio, E., Suolanen, J., Norrback, S., and Slatis, P.: Adhesive arachnoiditis after lumbar myelography with meglumine iothalamate (Conray). Acta Radiol. 12:17–24, 1972.

8. Barr, J. S. et al.: Evaluation of end results in treatment of ruptured lumbar intervertebral discs. Surg. Gynec. Obstet. 125:250–256, 1967.

9. Battista, A.: Subarachnoid cold saline wash for pain relief. Arch. Surg. 103:672–675, 1971.

10. Baumgartner, J., Bonte, G., Braun, J. P., Caron, J., Cecile, J., Fischgold, H., Gonsette, R., Hirsch, J. F., Legre, J., Metzger, J., Serre, H., and Simon, J.: La radiculographic lombo-sacree a l'iothalamate de methyl glucamine (Contrix 28). Bilan de 847 examens. Rev. Rhumat. 36:549–554, 1969.

11. Beals, R., and Hickman, N.: Industrial injuries of the back and extremities. J. Bone Joint Surg. 54A:1593–1611, 1972.

12. Begg, A. C. et al.: Myelography in lumbar disc lesions. Brit. J. Surg. 34:10–157, 1946.

13. Branemark, P. et al.: Tissue response to chymopapain. Clin. Orthop. 67:52–67, 1969.

14. Brown, J. E.: Clinical studies on chemonucleolysis. Clin. Orthop. 67:94–99, 1969.

15. Colonna, P. C., and Friedenberg, Z.: The disc syndrome. J. Bone Joint Surg. 31A:614–618, 1949.

16. Coventry, M. B. et al.: The intervertebral disc, its microscopic anatomy and pathology. J. Bone Joint Surg. 27:460, 1945.

17. Coventry, M. B., and Tapper, E.: Pelvic instability. J. Bone Joint Surg. 54A:83–101, 1972.

18. Crelin, E. S.: A scientific test of the chiropractic theory. Amer. Sci. 61:574–580, 1973.

19. Cronqvist, S., and Fuchs, W.: Lumbar myelography in complete obstruction of the spinal canal. Acta Rad. Diag. 2:145–152, 1964.

20. Dandy, W. E.: Concealed ruptured intervertebral discs. J.A.M.A. 117:821–823, 1941.

21. Daum, H. F. et al.: Protrusions of the lumbar disc. South. Med. J. 52:1479–1484, 1959.

22. Day, P. L.: Lateral approach for lumbar discogram and chemonucleolysis. Clin. Orthop. 67:90–93, 1969.

23. DePalma, A., and Gillespy, T.: Long term results of herniated nucleus pulposus treated by excision of the disc only. Clin. Orthop. 22:139–144, 1962.

24. DePalma, A., and Prabhakar, M.: Posterior-posterobilateral fusion of the lumbo-sacral spine. Clin. Orthop. 47:165–171, 1966.

25. DePalma. A., and Rothman, R.: The nature of pseudarthrosis. Clin. Orthop. 59:113–118, 1968.

26. DePalma, A., and Rothman, R.: Surgery of the lumbar spine. Clin. Orthop. 63:162–170, 1969.

27. DePalma, A., and Rothman, R.: The Intervertebral Disc. Philadelphia, W. B. Saunders Co., 1970.

28. Desausseure, R. L.: Vascular injuries coincident to disc surgery. J. Neurosurg. 16:222–229, 1959.

29. Edeiken, J., and Hodes, P.: Roentgen Diagnosis of Disease of Bone. Baltimore, The Williams & Wilkins Co., 1967.

30. Edeiken, J., and Pitt, M.: The radiologic diagnosis of disc disease. Ortho. Clin. N. Amer. 2:405, 1971.

31. Emmett, J., and Love, J.: Vesical dysfunction caused by protruded lumbar disc. J. Urol. 105:86–91, 1971.

31a. Epstein, J., Epstein, B., Rosenthal, A., Carras, R., and Lavine, L.: Sciatica caused by nerve root entrapment in the lateral recess: The superior facet syndrome. J. Neurosurg. 36:584–589, 1972.

32. Falconer, M. A. et al.: Observations on the causes and mechanisms of symptom production in low back pain and sciatica. J. Neurol. Neurosurg. Psychiat. 11:13–26, 1948.

33. Farfan, H. F., and Sullivan, J. D.: The relationship of facet orientation to intervertebral disc failure. Canad. J. Surg. 10:179–185, 1967.

34. Fernstrom, U., and Goldie, I.: Does granulation tissue in the intervertebral disc provoke low back pain. Acta Orthop. Scand. 30:202–206, 1960.

35. Fincham, R. W. et al.: Neurologic deficits following myelography. Arch. Neurol. 16:410–414, 1967.

36. Ford, L.: Clinical use of chymopapain in lumbar and dorsal disc lesions. Clin. Orthop. 67:81–87, 1969.

37. Ford, L. T., and Key, J.: An evaluation of myelography in diagnosis of intervertebral-disc lesions in low back. J. Bone Joint Surg. 32A:257–266, 1950.

38. Froning, E. C., and Frohman, B.: Motion of the lumbosacral spine after laminectomy and spine fusion. J. Bone Joint Surg. 50A:897–918, 1968.

39. Gardner, W. J.: Specialization in intraspinal surgery. Surg. Gynec. Obstet. 121:838–839, 1965.

39a. Gargano, F. P., Jacobson, L., and Rosomoff, H.: Transverse axial tomography of the spine. Neuroradiology 6:254–258, 1974.

40. Gesler, R. M.: Pharmacologic properties of chymopapain. Clin. Orthop. 67:47–51, 1969.

40a. Gill, G., Manning, J. G., and White, H. L.: Surgical treatment of spondylolisthesis without spine fusion. J. Bone Joint Surg. 37A:493–520, 1955.

41. Goldner, J. L. et al.: Anterior disc excision and interbody spine fusion for chronic low back pain. Ortho. Clin. N. Amer. 2:543–568, 1971.

42. Gonsette, R.: An experimental and clinical assessment of water-soluble contrast medium in neuroradiology: a new medium—Dimer-X. Clin. Radiol. 22:44–56, 1971.

43. Greenfield, G. B.: Radiology of Bone Diseases. Philadelphia, J. B. Lippincott Co., 1969.

44. Hadley, L. A.: Anatomico-Roentgenographic Studies of the Spine. Springfield, C. C Thomas Co., 1964.

45. Haft, H. et al.: Larger volume pantopaque myelography. Radiology 74:605–610, 1960.

46. Hakelius, A.: Prognosis in sciatica. Acta. Orthop. Scand. 129:6–76, 1970.

47. Halaburt, H., and Lester, J.: Leptomeningeale forandringer efter lumbale myelografier med vandoploselige kontraststoffer (Danish). Dansk Selskab for Diagnostisk Radiologi. October 27, 1972.

48. Harmon, P. H., and Abel, M.: Correlation of multiple objective diagnostic methods in lower lumbar disc disease. Clin. Orthop. 28:132–151, 1963.

49. Harmon, P. H.: Congenital and acquired variations including degenerative changes of the lower lumbar spine; role in production of painful back and lower extremity syndrome. Clin. Orthop. 44:171–188, 1966.

50. Hartmann, J. T. et al.: Discography as an aid in eval-

uation for lumbar and lumbo-sacral fusion. Clin. Orthop. *81*:77–81, 1971.

50a. Henderson, E. D.: Results of the Surgical Treatment of Spondylolisthesis. J.B.J.S. *48A*:619, 1966.

51. Henderson, R. S.: The treatment of lumbar intervertebral disc protrusion. Brit. Med. J. *2*:597–598, 1952.

52. Highman, J.: Complete myelographic block in lumbar degenerative disease. Clin. Radiol. *16*:106–111, 1965.

53. Hirsch, C. et al.: Studies on structural changes in the lumbar annulus fibrosus. Acta Orthop. Scand. *22*:184–231, 1952.

54. Hirsch, C.: Efficiency of surgery in low back disorders. J. Bone Joint Surg. *47A*:991, 1965.

55. Hirsch, C.: Reflections on the use of surgery in lumbar disc disease. Ortho. Clin. N. Amer. *2*:493–497, 1971.

56. Hitselberger, W., and Witten, R.: Abnormal myelograms in asymptomatic patients. J. Neurosurg. *28*:204–206, 1968.

57. Holt, E.: The question of lumbar discography. J. Bone Joint Surg. *50*:720–726, 1968.

58. Horal, J.: The clinical appearance of low back disorders. Acta Orthop. Scand. Suppl. *118*:7–109, 1969.

58a. Howorth, B.: Low backache and sciatica. J. Bone Joint Surg. *46A*:1515, 1964.

59. Hudgins, W. R.: The predictive value of myelography in the diagnosis of ruptured lumbar discs. J. Neurosurg. *32*:152–162, 1970.

60. Hult, L.: The Munkfors Investigation. Acta Orthop. Scand. (Suppl.) *16*: 1954.

61. Jackson, R. K.: The long term effects of wide laminectomy for lumbar disc excision. J. Bone Joint Surg. *53B*:609–616, 1971.

62. Jockheim, K. A.: Lumbaler Bandscheibenvorfall. Berlin, Springer-Verlag, 1961.

63. Jones, M., and Newton, T.: Inadvertent extra-arachnoid injections in myelography. Radiology *80*:818–822, 1963.

64. Jones, R. A., and Thomson, J.: The narrow lumbar canal. J. Bone Joint Surg. *50B*:595–605, 1968.

65. Kettelkamp, D., and Wright, D.: Spondylolisthesis in the Alaskan Eskimo. Paper presented at the Meeting of the Western Orthopedic Assn., Portland, Oregon, Oct. 6, 1970.

66. Key, J. A.: The conservative and operative treatment of lesions of the intervertebral discs in the low back. Surgery *17*:291–303, 1945.

67. Knutsson, B.: Aspects of the neurogenic electromyographic records of voluntary contraction in cases of nerve root compression. Electromyography *2*:238–242, 1962.

68. Lansche, W. E., and Ford, L. T.: Correlation of the myelogram with clinical and operative findings in lumbar disc lesions. J. Bone Joint Surg. *42A*:193–206, 1960.

68a. Laurent, L., and Einola, S.: Spondylolisthesis in children and adolescents. Acta Orthop. Scand. *31*:45–64, 1961.

69. Leavitt, S. et al.: The process of recovery patterns in industrial back injuries. Indust. Med. *40*:7–15, 1971.

70. Levine, M. E.: Depression, back pain, and disc protrusion. Dis. Nerv. Sys. *32*:41–45, 1971.

71. Lombardi, G., and Passerini, A.: Spinal Cord Diseases. Baltimore, The Williams & Wilkins Co., 1964.

72. MacNab, I. et al.: Chemonucleolysis. Can. J. Surg. *14*:280–289, 1971.

73. MacNab, I.: Negative disc exploration. J. Bone Joint Surg. *53A*:891–903, 1971.

74. MacNab, I.: Personal Communication, 1972.

74a. MacNab, I., and Doll, D.: The blood supply of the lumbar spine and its application to the technique of intertransverse lumbar fusion: J. Bone Joint Surg. *53B*:628–638, 1971.

75. Marshall, L. L.: Conservative management of low back pain: A review of 700 cases. Med. J. Australia *1*:266–267, 1967.

76. Mason, M., and Raab, J.: Complications of Pantopaque myelography. J. Neurosurg. *19*:302–311, 1962.

77. Menkowitz, E., and Whittaker, R.: Personal communication, 1973.

78. Mixter, W. J., and Barr, J. S.: Rupture of the intervertebral disc with involvement of the spinal canal. N. Eng. J. Med. *211*:210–215, Aug. 1934.

79. Meschan, I.: Roentgen Signs in Clinical Practice. Philadelphia, W. B. Saunders Co., 1966.

80. Mossanyi, L. et al.: Pathologic mechanisms and clinical changes of the spine in old age. Geront. Clin. *3*:24–31, 1961.

81. Mulvey, R.: An unusual myelographic pattern of arachnoiditis. Radiol. *75*:778–780, 1960.

82. Nachemson, A.: The load on lumbar disks in different positions of the body. Clin. Orthop. *45*:107–122, 1966.

83. Nash, C. L. et al.: Post-surgical meningeal pseudocysts of the lumbar spine. Clin. Orthop. *75*:167–177. 1971.

84. Naylor. A., and Turner, R.: ACTH in treatment of lumbar disc prolapse. Proc. Royal Soc. Med. *54*:14–16, 1961.

85. Nordby, E. J., and Lucas, G. L.: A comparative analysis of lumbar disc disease treated by laminectomy or chemonucleolysis. Clin. Orthop. *90*:119–129, 1973.

86. Parrish, T. F.: Lumbar disc surgery in patients over 50 years of age. South. Med. J. *55*:667–669, 1962.

87. Pearce, J., and Moll, J.: Conservative treatment and natural history of acute lumbar disc lesions. J. Neurol. Neurosurg. Psychiat. *30*:13–17, 1967.

88. Ratheke, L.: Uber Kalkablagerungen in den Zwischenwirbelscheiben. Fortschr. Roint. genstr. *45*, 1932.

89. Riccitelli, M. L.: Low back pain and sciatica in elderly patients. J. Am. Geriat. Soc. *13*:80, 1965.

89a. Rombold, C.: Treatment of spondylolisthesis by posterolateral fusion. J. Bone Joint Surg. *48A*:1282, 1966.

90. Ross, J. C., and Jackson, R. M.: Vesical dysfunction due to prolapsed disc. Brit. Med. J. *3*:752–754, 1971.

91. Rothman, R.: The clinical syndrome of lumbar disc disease. Ortho. Clin. N. Amer. *2*:436–475, 1971.

92. Rothman, R. et al.: The effect of iron deficiency anemia on fracture healing. Clin. Orthop. *77*:276–283, 1971.

93. Rothman, R. et al.: Spinal extradural cysts. Clin. Orthop. *71*:186–192, 1970.

94. Sacks, S.: Anterior interbody fusion of the lumbar spine. Clin. Orthop. *44*:163–170., 1966.

95. Scham, S., and Taylor, T.: Tension signs in lumbar disc prolapse. Clin. Orthop. *75*:195–203, 1971.

96. Schatzker, J. and Pennal, G.: Spinal stenosis. J. Bone Joint Surg. *50B*:606–618, 1968.

97. Schobinger, R.A., Krueger, E. G., and Sobel, G. L.:

Comparison of intraosseous vertebral venography and Pantopaque myelography in diagnosis of surgical conditions of the lumbar spine and nerve roots. Radiology 77:376, 1961.

98. Schultz, E., and Brogden, B.: The problem of subdural placement in myelography. Radiology 79:91–95, 1962.

99. Schultz, E., and Miller, J.: Intravasation of opaque media during myelography. J. Neurosurg. 18:610–613, 1961.

100. Semmes, E.: Ruptures of the Lumbar Intervertebral Disc. Springfield, C. C Thomas Co., 1964.

101. Shapiro, J. et al.: Differential diagnosis of intradural and extradural spinal canal tumors. Radiology 76:718–731, 1961.

102. Shealy, N. C.: Dangers of spinal injections without proper diagnosis. J.A.M.A. 197:1104–1106, 1966.

103. Simon, S. D. et al.: Lumbar disc surgery in the elderly. Clin. Orthop. 41:157–162, 1965.

104. Skalpe, I. O.: Lumbar myelography with Conray Melgumin 282. Report of 100 examinations with special reference to the adverse effects. Acta neurol. (Scand.) 47:569–578, 1971.

105. Smith, L.: Chemonucleolysis. Clin. Orthop. 67:72–80, 1969.

106. Smith, L.: Enzyme dissolution of the nucleus pulposus in humans. J.A.M.A. 187:137, 1964.

107. Smith, L.: Enzyme dissolution of the nucleus pulposus. Nature, 198:1311, 1963.

108. Spangfort, E.: Lasegue's sign in patients with lumbar disc herniation. Acta Orthop. 42:459, 1971.

109. Splitoff, C.: Roentgenographic comparison of patients with and without backache. J.A.M.A. 152:1610, 1953.

110. Stark, W. A.: Spina bifida occulta and engagement of the fifth lumbar spinous process. Clin. Orthop. 81:71–72, 1971.

110a. Stauffer, R., and Coventry, M.: Posterolateral lumbar spine fusion. J. Bone Joint Surg. 54A:1195–1204, 1972.

111. Stinchfield, F., and Cruess, R.: Indications for spine fusion. Instructional Course Lectures 18:41–45, 1961.

112. Stern, I. J.: Biochemistry of chymopapain. Clin. Orthop. 67:42–46, 1969.

113. Stewart, W. J.: Lateral discograms and chemonucleolysis in the treatment of ruptured or deteriorated lumbar discs. Clin. Orthop. 67:88–89, 1969.

114. Taren, J.: Unusual complication following Pantopaque myelography. J. Neurosurg. 17:323, 1960.

115. Taylor, T., and Akeson, W.: Intervertebral disc prolapse. Clin. Orthop. 76:54–79, 1971.

116. Thibodeau, A. A.: Closed space infection following removal of lumbar intervertebral disc. J. Bone Joint Surg. 50A:400–410, 1968.

117. Tillinghast, A. J.: Roentgenologic evaluation of osseous change in the spine of the elderly. Clin. Orthop. 26:74–77, 1963.

118. Truchly, G. et al.: Posterolateral fusion of the lumbosacral spine. J. Bone Joint Surg. (A) 44A:505–512, 1962.

119. Verbiest, H.: A radicular syndrome from developmental narrowing of the lumbar vertebral canal. J. Bone Joint Surg. 36B:230–237, 1954.

120. Verbiest, H.: Further experiences on the pathologic influence of a developmental narrowness of the bony lumbar vertebral canal. J. Bone Joint Surg. 37B:576–583, 1955.

120a. Verbiest, H.: Further experience on the pathological influence of a developmental narrowness of the bony lumbar canal. J. Bone Joint Surg. 37B:576–583, 1955.

121. Watkins, M. B.: Lumbosacral fusion results with early ambulation. Surg. Gynec. Obstet. 102:604–606, 1956.

122. Watkins, M. B.: Postero-lateral bone grafting for fusion of the lumbar and lumbo-sacral spine. J. Bone Joint Surg. 41A:388–395, 1959.

123. Williams, D. C.: Examination and conservative treatment for disc lesions of the lower spine. Clin. Orthop. 5:28–35, 1955.

124. Wiltse, L.: The effect of common anomalies of the lumbar spine upon disc degeneration and low back pain. Ortho. Clin. N. Amer. 2:569, 1971.

124a. Wiltse, L. L.: Spondylolisthesis: Classification and etiology. A.A.O.S. Symposium on the Spine. St. Louis, C. V. Mosby Co., 1969, pp. 143–167.

124b. Wiltse, L. L., and Hutchison, R.: Surgical treatment of spondylolisthesis. Clin. Orthop. 35:116–135, 1964.

125. Young, D.: Complications of myelography. N. Eng. J. Med. 285:156–157, 1971.

126. Young, H., and Love, J.: End results of removal of protruded lumbar intervertebral discs with and without fusion. Instructional Course Lecture 16, 213–216, 1959.

CHAPTER 10

Acceleration Extension Injuries of the Cervical Spine

IAN MACNAB, F.R.C.S.(Eng.), F.R.C.S.(Can.)
The Wellesley Hospital

INTRODUCTION

Acceleration extension injuries of the neck were first recognized as a clinical entity with the introduction of catapult-assisted take-offs of aircraft. Many pilots developed persisting neck pain of sufficient severity to warrant medical discharge from the service. Some even lost consciousness on takeoff and crashed. It became apparent that the lesion was due to hyperextension of the neck, produced by sudden acceleration. It was found that by increasing the height of the back of the seat in order to support the head, extension strains were prevented and the problem was overcome. Acceleration injuries of the neck were not commonly seen again until the massive invasion by motor vehicles of the urban areas in the late 1940's. By the 1950's rear-end collisions constituted about 20 per cent of all motor vehicle accidents in the North American continent.

At law, the striking vehicle was almost invariably considered to be at fault, and this fact took away the burden of proof of liability. The injury sustained rarely presented objective stigmata of an organic lesion. The blameless client incapacitated by subjective symptoms, the evidence of which could not be proved or disproved, was manna for the plaintiff's attorney, pestilence for the defense attorneys, and a paid vacation for the unscrupulous patient. The introduction of the term "whiplash" by Crowe in 1928 lent an evil connotation to the injury, and many patients became more disabled by the diagnosis than by the injury.[7]

The emotional overtones associated with the lesion converted it into a cause rather than a clinical syndrome. Lawyers and doctors alike took sides on philosophical rather than scientific grounds, and little attempt was made to elucidate the pathomechanics of injury, the pathological changes that might ensue, and the symptoms and signs that might reasonably result from such changes. One of the first attempts to assess the forces applied to the neck was by Severy.[16] Using anthropomorphic dummies, he showed that in a 15 mph collision the head would accelerate with the force of 10 G. The demonstration that victims of rear-end collisions were indeed subjected to severe strains of the neck prompted several clinicians to review the problem more objectively.[1, 3, 8, 11, 13]

MECHANISM OF INJURY

When a car is struck from the rear it is suddenly accelerated in a forward direction. As this occurs, the upright of the front seat is pushed against the trunk of the occupant, and the upright bends backward to a degree varying with the weight of the occupant and the rate of acceleration. If there is no head rest, there is nothing pushing the head forward as the car accelerates, so that in the first few milliseconds following impact, the trunk of the occupant is moved forward in relation to the head. At the limit of stretch of the soft tissues of the neck, the head falls backward, and an extension strain is applied to the neck. The force of this hyperextension strain is intensified by the forward recoil of the front seat.

As the neck is hyperextended and the head rotates, the maxilla rotates away from the mandible, and the mouth is flung open, to a degree that may strain the temporomandibular joint.

Backward rotation of the head stretches the anterior cervical muscles, and when their tone is overcome there is nothing to resist the extension movement except the anterior longitudinal ligament and the anterior fibers of the annulus. If the rate of stretch of the muscles is very rapid, there may be insufficient time for relaxation of the muscle fibers, and muscle ruptures may occur. When the car stops accelerating, the head will rebound forward and this forward movement may be accelerated by contraction of the neck flexor muscles because of induction of the stretch reflex on the extension phase of movement. If the car now hits the car in front, sudden deceleration will occur. Sudden deceleration of this type will increase the rate at which the head is thrown forward and will produce forward movement ·of the body of the occupant, with the result that the head may strike the windshield, the steering wheel or the dashboard.

The force of the impact tends to "compress" the car—in effect making it into a shorter but taller vehicle. A vertical component of force is, therefore, also present, pushing the occupant up in the air. This may result in the occupant striking his head against the top of the car, or being thrown over the back of the front seat.

It is important to recognize this vertical component of force in the construction of head rests. If the head rest is not level with the top of the occiput, then, because the occupant is pushed upward by the impact, his head will fall back over the top of the head rest.

In rear-end collisions then, injury results from the relative acceleration of the head and the trunk of the occupant, and the degree of injury is dependent on the *rate* of acceleration. Many factors influence the rate of acceleration

and must be specifically sought for when assessing the severity of injury.

Acceleration depends on the force applied and the inertia of the vehicle that has been struck. The force is dependent upon the weight and speed of the striking vehicle, so that a streetcar traveling at 3 mph can apply as much force and initiate the same degree of acceleration as a compact car traveling at 40 mph. The inertia of the car that has been struck will depend not only on its weight but also on factors that will allow it to roll easily; for example, slippery road conditions, whether the brakes were on, automatic or standard transmission. A car that is moving slowly will accelerate more rapidly than one that is stationary.

The amount of damage sustained by the car bears little relationship to the force applied. To take an extreme example: If the car was stuck in concrete, the damage sustained might be very great but the occupants would not be injured because the car could not move forward, whereas, on ice, the damage to the car could be slight but the injuries sustained might be severe because of the rapid acceleration permitted.

In impacts up to 15 mph the right-front-seat passenger stands in greater danger of injury than does the driver, because the driver can brace himself to some extent by holding on to the steering wheel. Over 20 mph the force of acceleration is such that the pelvis of

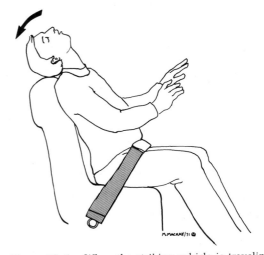

Figure 10–1. When the striking vehicle is traveling faster than 20 m.p.h. the steering wheel may prevent the trunk of the driver from sliding forward, and the extension strain to the neck is correspondingly greater.

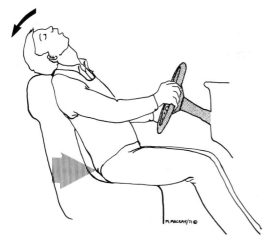

Figure 10–2. A lap belt, by preventing the trunk from sliding forward, may aggravate the extension strain suffered by the cervical spine.

the front-seat passenger slides forward on the seat, the trunk is now reclining at an angle, and the extension strain on the neck is correspondingly less. However, the steering wheel prevents the trunk of the driver from sliding forward any distance and, therefore, at this speed of impact, the driver may be more seriously injured than the front-seat passenger (Fig. 10–1). Similarly, safety belts, by preventing forward movement of the trunk, tend to aggravate the injury (Fig. 10–2).

In high-speed impact the force with which the occupant's body strikes the seat tends to break the upright of the front seat (Fig. 10–3). As the car accelerates, the occupant is lying almost horizontally and a traction rather than

an extension strain is applied to the neck. Paradoxically, then, the occupant is less likely to be severely injured in a high speed collision. Experimentally, the author has shown, using model cars with monkeys as passengers, that the injuries received are significantly less when the car is constructed in such a manner that on impact with the rear bumper, the upright of the front seat tilts back 30°.

PATHOLOGY

In an attempt to understand the pathological changes that take place, animals were subjected to an extension strain on the neck produced by sudden acceleration.[14] Because of the difficulties of obtaining a standard force, it was decided to use the force of gravity. Anesthetized animals were strapped to a steel platform attached to two vertical guide rails and the platform was dropped over distances varying from two to 40 feet. On striking the bottom of the runway, the animal's head and neck were suddenly extended over the edge of the platform producing an acceleration strain as in a rear-end collision. The degree of force applied to the neck could be varied by altering the height of the drop. It is realized, of course, that this apparatus does not accurately reproduce the forces involved in rear-end collisions, but the method was used to determine whether recognizable acceleration extension injuries did indeed occur.

By altering the height of the drop, various lesions resulted. Muscle injuries were noted, varying in severity from minor tears of the sternomastoid to more severe tears of the longissimus colli. Any tear of the longissimus

Figure 10–3. With high speed impact the upright of the front seat may break. Because the trunk of the occupant falls backwards, an extension rather than an acceleration strain is applied to the neck.

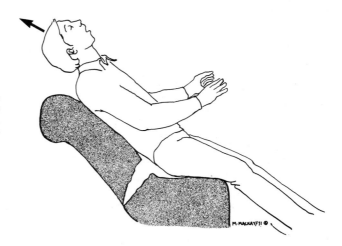

colli, no matter how small, was associated experimentally with a retropharyngeal hematoma. Hemorrhages were also seen in the muscle coats of the esophagus. Damage to the longissimus colli was occasionally associated with damage to the cervical sympathetic plexus.

One of the most interesting lesions seen in the experiments conducted was tearing of the anterior longitudinal ligament and separation of a disc from the associated vertebra (Fig. 10–4). This lesion never occurred without damage to the anterior cervical muscles. The disc injury in the monkeys could not be detected on x-rays, even after a passage of several months.

Wickstrom also studied the pathological lesions resulting from experimental acceleration extension injuries of the neck in primates.[20] He noted damage to the brain and its covering, consisting of hemorrhage and edema. He reported sprains of apophyseal joints, subchondral fractures of facets, hemorrhages in muscles, ruptures of muscle, hemorrhage about the cord and cervical nerve roots, and hemorrhage under the anterior and posterior longitudinal ligaments. Some animals subsequently showed evidence of concussion, with impaired neuromuscular control. Wickstrom stated that the severity of the pathological changes found were directly related to the rate of acceleration of the head.

It is always difficult and at times dangerous to translate the findings of experimental investigation into the sphere of clinical experience. However, I would like to suggest that these experiments show that recognizable lesions can be produced. They suggest that the lesions can vary from very minor injuries, such as a tear of the muscular fibers, to serious lesions, such as separation of the disc or damage to the posterior joints. It is reasonable to presume that the same variation is seen clinically, with the majority of patients sustaining minor injuries only, but some suffering lesions of more serious significance.

THE SYMPTOM COMPLEX

A knowledge of the pathomechanics of the injury and of the lesions produced experimentally makes it easier to understand the symptoms commonly complained of. Patients with serious injuries usually experience some pain immediately after the accident, although significant discomfort may be postponed for as long as 24 hours. Later, the pain radiates from the neck to one or both shoulders and down the arms. The patient may not have any pain in the neck and, indeed, the pain may be experienced solely in the shoulders or in the arms, or in the back of the head. The pain may radiate to the interscapular region and to the chest and into the suboccipital region. Occipital headaches are common, and these may radiate over the vertex, or bitemporally, or may be associated with retro-ocular pain. This pattern of pain radiation is of no value in localizing the site of the lesion. The same pattern of pain radiation can be reproduced by the experimental injection of hypertonic saline into the supraspinous ligament at any point from C1 to C7. Similar pain patterns can be produced on clinical discography at any cervical segment. It is important to emphasize that the presence of persisting suboccipital pain does not necessarily indicate a local lesion at the atlantoaxial region—it may be referred pain, arising from any damaged cervical segment.

Similarly, pain radiating down the arm does not necessarily indicate nerve root pressure. It is commonly another manifestation of referred pain. Disc herniation with root irritation and impairment of root conduction rarely results from a whiplash injury of the neck. Pa-

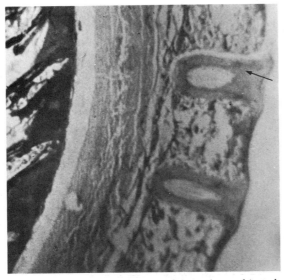

Figure 10–4. Cervical spine of a monkey subjected to an acceleration extension strain of the neck. Note the separation of the disc from the vertebral body of C5.

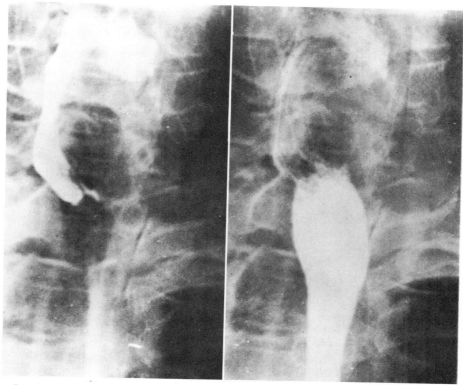

Figure 10–5. Barium swallow showing obstruction of the esophagus produced by a large retropharyngeal hematoma.

tients frequently complain of subjective numbness in relation to the ulnar border of the hand and, indeed, in some instances there may be diminution of appreciation of pin prick involving the ring and little fingers. This is rarely the result of root pressure or even, as suggested by Simmons, a traumatic ulnar neuritis.[17] Much more commonly, it is due to scalenus spasm secondary to the painful lesions in the neck.

Other symptoms commonly complained of are the following.

DYSPHAGIA. Dysphagia complained of shortly after the accident is probably attributable either to pharyngeal edema or to a retropharyngeal hematoma (Fig. 10–5). The latter can be seen on a routine lateral x-ray of the spine by observing the forward displacement of the air shadow of the pharynx. The early onset of dysphagia is of serious prognostic significance. Dysphagia occurring after the passage of several weeks, however, is usually emotional in origin.

BLURRING OF VISION. Intermittent blurring of vision of short duration is a common symptom, which may be caused by damage to the vertebral arteries, or which may reflect damage to the cervical sympathetic chain. Blurring of vision by itself is of no prognostic significance, but if it is associated with Horner's syndrome it indicates a serious soft tissue injury.

TINNITUS. Many patients complain of a buzzing in the ears or a "plopping" sensation. The pathogenesis of this symptom is not clear. It may result from a temporomandibular injury; it may be caused by a temporary shutoff of the vertebral arteries at the time of injury; or it may reflect direct damage to the inner ear. Persistent tinnitus, usually associated with some loss of hearing in the upper range, is difficult to prove to have been caused by the accident, as these patients rarely have had any audiometric testing prior to their accident. Usually, tinnitus by itself is of no prognostic significance.

DIZZINESS. Early severe vertigo, caused by vertebral artery spasm or an inner ear disturbance, generally indicates a severe extension strain. The "veering" that many patients

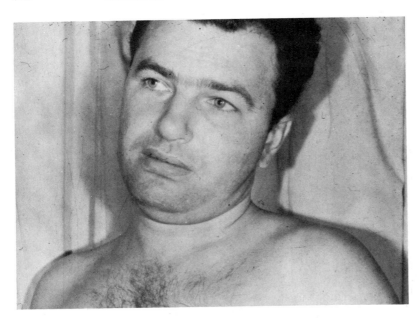

Figure 10–6. This patient with marked spasm of the left sternomastoid complained of a "veering" type of dizziness.

complain of is probably attributable to interference with the neck righting reflex, induced by spasm of the supporting cervical muscles (Fig. 10–6). Vertigo can be aggravated experimentally by the injection of hypertonic saline into the sternomastoids. This symptom subsides when the neck movements are regained. Some patients experience severe vertigo on rotation of the head, and may indeed lose consciousness. In such instances, the possibility of vertebral artery compression must be investigated. In most patients, the brunt of the extension force is experienced in the mid cervical region. In older patients with preexisting degenerative changes of the C5-C6 and C6-C7 levels, the movement in the mid-cervical spine is decreased. In such instances, the major injury occurs in the upper cervical spine, particularly at the atlantoaxial level.

These older patients frequently also have concomitant atherosclerotic changes involving the vertebral arteries, and it is in this group that the various types of vertebral artery syndromes may develop. Some may go on to present the Wallenburg syndrome (lateral medullary syndrome), caused by thrombosis of a posterior inferior cerebellar artery. Some may die from basilar artery thrombosis.

MUSCLE RUPTURES. As the head starts to rotate backward, the sternomastoid muscles contract. If the moment rotating the head backward is too great, the muscles are passively stretched rapidly and do not have a chance to elongate and at the same time maintain tension. In such instances the muscle will rupture, with the formation of a hematoma. Frankel reported a 36-year-old man in whom the right sternomastoid was nearly twice as large as the left.[9] Hemorrhage and edema of the strap muscles may give rise to hoarseness and dysphagia, and a similar lesion in the longus colli may make it difficult for the patient to lift his head from the pillow.

Lesions of the Upper Cervical Nerve Roots

The superficial branches of the cervical plexus (the great auricular nerve, the superficial cervical nerve, and the supraclavicular nerves) pierce the cervical fascia and wind around the posterior border of the sternomastoid to reach the skin. They may be stretched as the neck is extended, particularly if extension is combined with rotation. Traction injuries to these nerves may result in patches of hypoesthesia or dysesthesia associated with a dry skin. There may be tenderness at the point where the nerves emerge through the fascia, and percussion at this point may result in paresthesia radiating over the area of skin distribution. This phenomenon may persist for several months after injury.

TEMPOROMANDIBULAR JOINT SYMPTOMS

As mentioned previously, when the head rotates backward the mouth is flung open, and this may result in temporomandibular joint strain; indeed, the joint may be dislocated.[10] As the jaw is flung open the masticatory muscles are stretched, resulting in a reflex rapid closing of the mouth. The closing of the mouth may be sufficiently forceful to break teeth.

Patients with strain of the temporomandibular joint complain subsequently of pain on chewing and of painful limitation in the ability to open their mouths. It is important to note that these symptoms are aggravated by halter traction and, indeed, cervical traction may by itself produce a temporomandibular arthropathy in the presence of malocclusion.

Significance of Symptoms

Although there is general agreement on the type of symptoms to be expected, widely divergent views are held on the significance of these symptoms, and these diverging viewpoints, rigidly held and hotly contested, are usually based on impressions only. In an endeavor to make these impressions more factually significant, the progress of 575 patients was carefully followed by the author. Many physicians believe that "whiplash syndrome" patients are a group of hysterical, neurotic, if not frankly dishonest people. However, there are certain disturbing features, apparent from an analysis of the case histories available, that make it difficult to accept the fact that litigation neurosis is the *sole* explanation of the long drawn out disability in every instance.

Some patients in the author's study had associated injuries. In addition to injuring their necks, they sprained their ankles or broke their wrists. Normal painless function returned to their ankles and wrists in the expected period of time. These patients did not complain for month after month about painful ankles or wrists, but they did still complain of neck pain. It is difficult to understand why litigation neurosis in these instances should be confined to the neck.

When forward flexion of the neck is produced by acceleration or deceleration, the head stops moving when the chin touches the chest. Similarly, in lateral flexion, movement stops in the normal cervical spine when the ear hits the shoulder. In both these modalities of cervical movement, the range of movement occurring is within physiological limits and, in normal necks, even at the extreme of movement, no strain is applied to the intervertebral joints. In extension injuries to the neck, however, there is no block to movement until the occiput hits the chest wall, and this is far beyond the physiologically permitted limit. In the series of rear end collisions analyzed, there were five patients who, at the moment of impact, were facing the back of the car. As a result of the impact, they experienced an uncontrolled flexion of the neck but none complained of neck pain. Of 69 patients who were passengers in vehicles involved in side collisions, as a result of which one presumes that they had a lateral flexion movement applied to the neck, only seven suffered neck pain, and only in two did significant disability persist for more than two months.

If neck pain following acceleration injuries is purely neurotic in origin, it is difficult to understand why patients commonly get neurotic if their head is thrown backward and rarely get neurotic if it is jolted forward or sideways. These findings suggest that the persistence of pain following forced extension of the neck is related in some way to the fact that the neck can, and may, move beyond the physiologically permitted limit.

An interesting observation on the significance of litigation neurosis comes from a followup of these patients after settlement of court action (Table 10–1). There were 266 patients in whom all the legal problems had been settled two or more years before followup. As in any review of this type, it was impossible to get all these patients back for study. Only 145 patients were examined personally and, of these, 121 were continuing to have symptoms. It is obvious that in a followup such as this, in which attendance for review seems pointless, time consuming, and difficult, the patients most likely to attend are those with continuing

TABLE 10–1. ANALYSIS OF RESULTS TWO YEARS AFTER SETTLEMENT OF COURT ACTION

Total number of patients available for review	266
Number of patients reviewed	145
Number of patients with symptoms	121
Persistence of symptoms two years after settlement	121 of 266 (45%)

symptoms. To avoid bias of this type, it is necessary that we regard all patients who did not come back as having been completely cured. On this basis, it can be said that out of 266 patients, 121 continued to have some measure of symptoms. That is to say, satisfactory conclusion of settlement or court action failed to relieve symptoms in 45 per cent of the group studied. The group studied is not representative of every whiplash injury. It is a special group, which consists of patients referred for specialist opinion because of the severity of symptoms or because of undue persistence of symptoms, and represents, therefore, the more severe disabilities, whether they be physiogenic or psychogenically induced.

The results at first sight may appear to be grossly at variance with Gotten's often quoted review. In 1956 Gotten published a survey of 100 cases of whiplash injuries reviewed after settlement of legal action.[12] It was stated in this review that 88 per cent had "largely recovered," and only 12 per cent were still significantly disabled. Reading this review the other way around, one can say that out of 100 patients reviewed, many had some sort of symptoms and, even after the passage of several years, 12 per cent, a significant number, were seriously disabled and 3 per cent were still losing time from work.

In other followup studies reported, the results are remarkably constant. The majority of patients improve with the passage of time, and they can learn to live with their intermittent residual discomforts.[4, 18] However, about 12 per cent are left with discomfort of sufficient severity to interfere with their ability to do their work and with their capacity to enjoy themselves in their leisure hours.

It can be fairly stated, therefore, that careful followup reviews strongly support the contention that significant soft tissue damage may indeed result from acceleration extension injuries and, because of this, it is not surprising that symptoms may be prolonged.

CLINICAL MANAGEMENT

Sudden death has been reported as the result of acceleration extension injuries of the neck. Serious vascular injuries resulting from extension strains have been reported several times.[5, 6, 15] As mentioned previously, occlusion of the posterior inferior cerebellar artery has also been reported following acceleration extension injuries of the neck. No one doubts the clinical picture in these patients because of the positive and undeniable physical findings. However, many clinicians are still reluctant to accept the fact that relatively minor lesions associated with disabling and persisting symptoms, may result from this type of injury.

When a patient breaks his neck, even though the injury may involve litigation, an emotional or functional overlay is not common. Similarly, when patients break their wrists or sprain their ankles, even if the lesion is associated with an acceleration extension injury of the neck, normal painless function usually returns to the ankles and wrists in the expected period of time without functional overlay. Surely, these observations suggest that broken necks are treated adequately, sprained ankles are treated adequately, broken wrists are treated adequately; and surely these findings suggest that, by failure to treat a whiplash injury adequately, the physician himself may be responsible for producing some of the so-called litigation neurosis.

If the physician in his treatment is to avoid an iatrogenic neurosis he must accept the possibility of significant injury and be prepared to investigate its probability. The first stage must be a careful painstaking history.

Many factors modify the injury received and, when assessing the significance of the symptoms, the physician must learn as much as he can about the details of the accident. The rate of acceleration is of vital importance. It is necessary to know therefore the answers to the following questions. What was the type of vehicle in which the patient was sitting and the relative weight of the vehicle that struck the car? What were the road conditions — slippery or dry? Was the car moving at the moment of collision? How far was the vehicle pushed forward? Did it hit the car in front? What happened to objects in the car — did the glove compartment door fly open? Were objects on the front seat thrown into the back seat?

It is necessary to know whether the patient was driver or passenger. As mentioned previously, at low impact speeds the right front passenger is more vulnerable to injury. If the driver can anticipate the accident he may have time to brace himself and hold firmly to the steering wheel, thereby decreasing the subsequent neck movements.

It is important also to know the position of the patient's head at the moment of impact.

The physiologically permitted range of extension is much less when the neck is rotated (Fig. 10–7A and B). Normally, at the limit of extension, the occipitomental line is approximately 20 to 30 degrees above the horizontal when the chin is pointing straight forward. If the neck is rotated to 45 degrees, the degree of extension permitted is only about half this range. Because the permitted physiological range of extension is very short when the neck is slightly rotated, the posterior joints can soon be pushed beyond the physiological range, and injury results from an extension strain.

Experimentally in cadavers, rupture of the anterior longitudinal ligament is much more readily produced when the head is rotated before an extension strain is applied to the neck.

If driver and passenger both have their heads turned, talking to one another, then the presence of right-sided pain in the driver and left-sided pain in the passenger can lend "an air of artistic verisimilitude to an otherwise bald and unconvincing narrative."

The movement of the patient is also important. Did his head hit the roof? Did he feel his head snap back? In severe injuries, the neck may be extended to such a degree that the occupant faces the rear of the car. Some information as to the severity of the forces involved may be gathered by asking the patient what happened to his hat, glasses, or even false teeth, as a result of the impact. In one patient in the series studied, a plastic Spanish comb she was wearing was thrown against the rear window and broken. Conversely, if the patient was wearing a hat and glasses and neither was dislodged, it is reasonable to presume that the head was not jolted around vigorously.

Significant injuries almost invariably give rise to some pain immediately after the accident. The pain may temporarily subside, and then gradually intensify over the next few hours. It is important to enquire specifically about this time period. Patients who have been seriously emotionally upset by the experience will frequently state that they were unable to sleep on the night of the accident—not because of the pain but because they constantly relived their frightening experience.

If seen shortly after the accident, patients with significant injury will have evidence of damage to the soft tissues at the front of the neck, with tenderness on palpation. The physician must be wary of the patient who bitterly complains of pain in the neck presenting marked tenderness over the spinous processes posteriorly, without any discomfort on palpating the anterior structures.

At the conclusion of the history, the physician should have a clear impression of the patient who has been injured, as well as of the injury that has been sustained. A clear record of the physical findings must be made—permitted range of movement of the neck, sites of tenderness, and evidence of nerve root irrita-

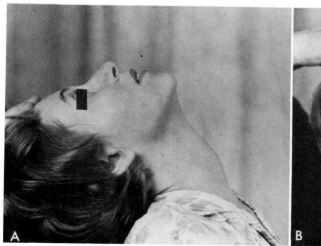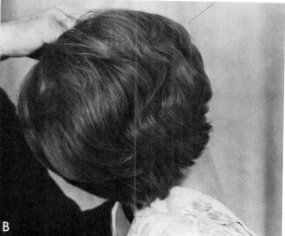

Figure 10–7. *A,* Normally at the limit of extension a line drawn from the occiput to the tip of the chin would be 45° above the horizontal. *B,* When the neck is rotated 45° the permitted range of extension of the neck is decreased by about 50 per cent.

tion or impairment of root conduction. It must be remembered that apparently bizarre areas of diminution of appreciation of pin prick, such as the side of the face or behind the ear, may result from stretching of the superficial cervical nerves (Fig. 10–8).

Radiological findings must be interpreted with care. Loss of cervical lordosis can be demonstrated in normal subjects by just lowering the chin (Fig. 10–9, *A* and *B*). The apparent flattening of the cervical curve so commonly seen is usually caused by the position in which the patient holds his head when the lateral view is taken. Changes in the pattern of movement on flexion and extension do not necessarily indicate damage to the discs or posterior joints but may merely reflect restricted movement because of pain or fear of pain. Rarely, crush fractures of the posterior joints can be seen, and these are best demonstrated with a pillar view.

If the patient appears to have sustained a significant injury as evidenced by the nature of the impact, by marked spasm of the sterno-

mastoid, or by complaints suggestive of damage to the anterior soft tissues of the neck, the neck should be splinted. If the neck needs splinting at all, it needs splinting well. The best way to do this is to apply at least three soft cervical ruffs. The only way to rest the neck completely is to remove the weight of the head, and the only way this can be achieved is to confine the patient to bed and insist that he remain recumbent. If, in 12 to 24 hours, the patient is relatively symptom free, he may get up, otherwise he should stay in bed for a week. Traction may be given at this stage, but only if it relieves pain. If patients are asked to stay in bed for a week, it is essential that they be given some form of sedation, otherwise, because they feel relatively well, they are unlikely to carry out this form of seemingly unreasonable therapy. Their only symptom is pain; therefore, the need for rest in bed must be explained to them, or they will not cooperate.

The majority of these patients at the end of this rest period, should be able to go to work. They should be given instructions on how to avoid extension strains to the neck during the activities of daily living (see Neck Sparing Routine, below). Most important, they must be told the difference between hurting themselves and harming themselves. They must be told that many things they may do during the day may hurt them, but that a "flare up" of pain does not necessarily signify increasing damage to the neck. They should be told that, if they restrict their activities because of fear of harm, they are mistaken. Many patients, fearful of harming themselves, restrict their activities unnecessarily, in the honest but mistaken belief that this was their physician's advice. Their problems are compounded of apprehension and misapprehension, and it is important to deal firmly with both.

NECK SPARING ROUTINE

Sleeping

If you have discomfort at night the following changes may be helpful. Sleep on your back with the back and neck supported by five pillows, so that you are in the reclining or semisitting position. It is important when doing this to try to keep the neck and the rest of the spine in a straight line. If you still have discomfort, or if you are unable to

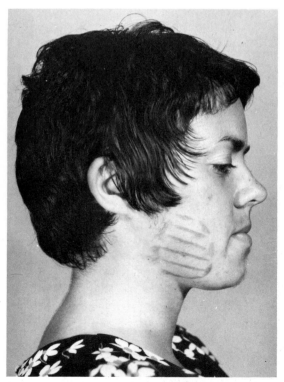

Figure 10–8. Area of loss of appreciation of pin prick, demonstrated by a patient following an acceleration extension injury of the neck.

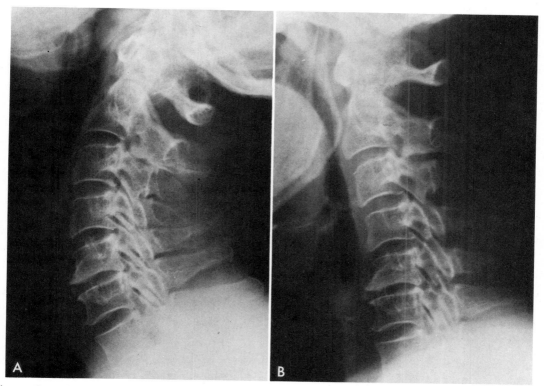

Figure 10–9. The normal cervical lordosis seen on the lateral view (A) can be obliterated just by lowering the chin (B).

sleep on your back, it will be necessary for you to wear a soft, supporting collar. This can be provided for you. *Go to bed early*. Even if you do not sleep the whole time, it is advisable to try to get 10 hours rest at night during the acute phase of your trouble.

Sitting

Avoid adopting any position in which your head is tilted backwards, for example, resting your chin on your hand. Try to sit with your neck and spine in a straight line—your shoulders braced back and your chin tucked in—the sort of posture you expect your children to adopt when you tell them to "sit up straight."

Tension

Any form of emotional tension will aggravate the pain. It does so because in states of tension we adopt the "fight position," with the chin thrust forward. When such situations arise, make a deliberate effort to relax the muscles. Be more conscious than ever of the need to keep your chin tucked in and the neck and spine in a straight line.

Driving

Prolonged driving commonly aggravates pain in the neck. This is caused by a combination of tension and bad sitting posture. Avoid the tendency to thrust your chin over the top of the steering wheel. If you are short, sit on a firm cushion so that you do not have to crane your neck to see out of the window. Bring the seat as close as possible to the steering wheel so that you can sit with your back supported by the back of the car seat, with your spine held straight.

Reaching

Avoid reaching or looking up at high objects—both activities demand that you tilt your neck backwards. If this is repeated or prolonged it will hurt your neck.

Lifting

Avoid carrying any object weighing over 10 lbs. When your neck is painful do not wear heavy overcoats. Do not pull, or attempt to move, heavy objects of furniture.

Sports

When your symptoms are severe, all sports should be avoided. Golf, bowling and gardening put severe strains on the neck. Swimming—except for swimming on the back—will aggravate the pain. Diving should be avoided until you are completely free from all symptoms.

Patients should not be given unnecessary and expensive medication. As the cost of medication rises, so does the cost of injury. Mild analgesia to take the edge off their discomforts, and mild sedation to take the edge off their anxieties, are all that are required. The nature and the purpose of the drugs must be explained to the patient. It is both dishonest and bad medicine to give the patient a tranquilizer, pretending it is something to take his "neck spasms" away. If he is disabled by a psychogenic magnification of his symptoms, he must be told so, and must be told that he is being given sedation to treat this aspect of his problem.

Physiotherapy, if ordered, must be along rational lines. Heat in all modalities, massage, and traction may make the patient feel easier temporarily but do nothing to speed the resolution of the underlying lesions. If attendance at the physiotherapy department makes the patient take time from work, it is probably harmful in that it firmly engraves on the patient's mind the severity of the lesion. Traction can be used at home but should only be prescribed if the patient gets relief from pain while traction is actually being applied and for some time afterward. Traction is not curative, its function is solely to make the patient more comfortable and to lessen the use of analgesics. The patient must be told this. If the patient does not feel comfortable in a soft homemade ruff-type collar, then there is no point in ordering any other kind. If he does indeed feel better in a collar and can work more efficiently while wearing it, there is no psychologically sound reason for withholding it.

If the patient's problems are severe enough to warrant putting him to bed for a week, then he will probably have daily discomfort for six weeks. If at the end of six weeks the patient is still conscious of some measure of discomfort all day long, then he may well have intermittent discomfort for a further six months to a year. The patient must be told the expected duration of symptoms. There is nothing more demoralizing than to expect a cure day by day from some new pill or from some new apparatus at the physiotherapy department. Unless the physician honestly believes that his patient will get better in a week or 10 days as a result of the treatment employed, he must tell the patient what to expect. However, the patient must be told at the same time that the lesion in the neck alone, and the discomforts derived from it, do not provide sufficiently adequate reason to withdraw completely from the activities of daily living.

The patient may not be seen for several months after the injury, at which time assessment of the severity of the injury and the cause of the continuing disability becomes much more difficult to determine. The physician must ask himself, "Why is *this* patient so disabled by the pain of which he complains?" Many patients are genuinely fearful of perpetuating the damage sustained and, therefore, being permanently crippled. For this reason alone they assiduously avoid any activity that may provoke discomfort. Their disability is exaggerated by ignorance. Patients may have become disconsolate because of failure of medical therapy. Week after week they have confidently expected that their discomfort will subside as a result of treatment prescribed; and week after week their hopes have been dashed as their symptoms continue. The failure of therapy, with the continuance of pain, engraves on their minds the severity of the injury they received. One such patient, on being told that she had not been subjected to a serious injury of the neck, asked "If there is nothing much wrong with me, why is it costing so much to get me better?"

False faith in ineffectual treatment brings on the symptoms of secondary depression. These patients are tired all the time and sleep does not refresh them. They are more easily provoked to anger and tears, and become intolerant of faults they recognize in others. They lose their sense of fun.

If it becomes apparent that the patient's disability results from a psychogenic magnification of the symptoms derived from his basic underlying physical disorder, and that in better emotional health he would not be significantly troubled, let alone disabled, then the physician must tell the patient his honest opinion of the nature and cause of the continuing disability. This should be recognized early and a psychiatric opinion sought early.

In such instances, a Pentothal pain study is of vital importance.[19] In this test, the patient is given Pentothal to the stage of corneal areflexia and then is allowed to rouse slowly to the stage at which he will respond by wincing and grimacing to noxious stimulae such as pinprick. At this stage, a physical examination is carried out. Previously tender areas are palpated and the range of movement of the neck is assessed. If, at this stage, it is not possible to elicit areas of muscle tenderness, and a full range of painless passive movements can be demonstrated, in a neck which previously showed movements markedly restricted by pain, one may reasonably conclude that there is little physiogenic basis for the patient's complaints. If, on the other hand, physical examination evokes a withdrawal response, there is a significant anatomical basis for the patient's pain, despite the obvious manifestation of an emotional breakdown.

In teaching patients to live within the limits of minor discomforts the attitude of the physician is of paramount importance. He must accept the possibility of injury, and investigate its probability in each patient. He must not be perfunctory in treatment, yet, he must never overtreat the patient. His treatment should not interfere with the patient's daily routine. Very few come to surgery. If the patient's pain persists for more than two years and interferes significantly with his ability to do his job or his capacity to enjoy himself in his leisure hours, and if it can be shown by a Pentothal pain study that there is a significant physiogenic basis for symptoms, then the patient requires more detailed investigation, in an attempt to localize the site of the pathological lesion. Flexion and extension x-rays may reveal restricted mobility at one segment. This is of significance only if the movements can be made without invoking marked muscle spasm. Abnormal mobility may be demonstrated, associated with a backward and forward glide of the vertebral bodies on flexion and extension.

Frequently, the radiological signs are inconclusive and the involved segment can only be demonstrated by discography. It must be emphasized that the radiological pattern of the discogram is of little diagnostic significance. The important finding is the reproduction of the pain pattern experienced by the patient. To obtain a significant finding, discography must be performed meticulously. Repeated puncturing of the anterior longitudinal ligament, by probing with the needle, may produce too much pain and obscure the results of the investigation. If severe pain is produced

by forceful injection of one disc, then pain usually will be produced at every other disc injected, and the findings of the examination will be meaningless.

The anterior longitudinal ligament should be infiltrated with local anesthetic before any disc is injected. Needles are inserted into all the discs and accurately centered in the nucleus pulposus before any injection. A relatively non-irritating type of water-soluble or radiopaque dye is used (e.g., Conray), and 0.5 ml is injected into each disc. The injection is stopped immediately if the patient experiences any discomfort. No further discs should be examined until the pain subsides. If the pain persists, local anesthetic is injected. When the patient is comfortable, the next disc is injected with radiopaque dye. When all have been injected, the disc or discs that produced some pain on minimal injection, are reinjected with saline, to define clearly the pain pattern produced. If the trial injections fail to produce pain at any one level, then each disc is reinjected with a further 0.5 ml of dye, taking the same precautions. Significant findings can only be obtained by a careful, painstaking examination of this type.

Patients whose symptoms stem from one or at the most two adjacent disc units will respond well to an anterior cervical discectomy and fusion.

In teaching the remainder of the patients to accept and live within the limits of minor discomfort, the physician must be honest about the treatment he is giving, about the patient's physical and mental well being and about the prognosis; and, above all, he must take care not to fan the flames of hostility that these patients so commonly exhibit, and thereby initiate, aggravate or perpetuate a financially motivated exaggeration of symptoms.

References

1. Abbot, K. H.: Whiplash injuries. (Letter to editor.) J.A.M.A. *162*:917, 1956.
2. Billig, H. J.: The mechanism of whiplash injuries. Int. Rec. Med. *169*:3, 1956.
3. Braaf, M. M., and Rosner, S.: Symptomatology and treatment of injuries of the neck. New York J. Med. *55*:237, 1955.
4. Braaf, M. M., and Rosner, S.: Whiplash injuries of the neck: Symptoms, diagnosis, treatment and prognosis. N.Y. State J. Med., *58*:1501, 1958.
5. Carpenter, S.: Injury of neck as cause of vertebral artery thrombosis. J. Neurosurg. *18*:849, 1961.

6. Coburn, D. F.: Vertebral artery involvement in cervical trauma. Clin. Orthop. *24*:61–63, 1962.

7. Crowe, H. E.: Injuries to the cervical spine. Paper presented at the meeting of the Western Orthopaedic Association, San Francisco, 1928.

8. DePalma, A. F., and Subin, D. K.: A study of the cervical syndrome. Clin. Orthop. *38*:135, 1965.

9. Frankel, V. H.: Cervical Pain. New York, Pergamon Press, 1972.

10. Frankel, V. H.: Temporo-mandibular joint syndrome following deceleration injury to the cervical spine. Bull. Hosp. Joint Dis. *26*:1, 1969.

11. Gay, J. R., and Abbot, K. H.: Common whiplash injuries of the neck. J.A.M.A. *152*:1698, 1953.

12. Gotten, N.: Survey of one hundred cases of whiplash injury after settlement of litigation. J.A.M.A. *162*:856, 1956.

13. Jackson, R.: Mechanism of cervical root irritation. Dallas Med., *38*:71, 1952.

14. Macnab, I.: Acceleration injuries of the cervical spine. J. Bone Joint Surg. *46A*:1797–1799, 1964.

15. Schneider, R. C., and Schemm, G. W.: Vertebral artery insufficiency in acute and chronic spinal trauma. J. Neurosurg. *18*:348, 1961.

16. Severy, D. M., Mathewson, J. H., and Bechtol, C. P.: Controlled automobile rear-end collisions, an investigation of related engineering and medical phenomena. Canad. Serv. Med. J. *11*:727, 1955.

17. Simmons, E. H.: Ulnar nerve neuritis associated with whiplash injuries. Paper given at the meeting of the Canadian Orthopaedic Association, Hamilton, Canada, 1969.

18. Thiemeyer, J. S., Duncan, G. A., and Hollins, G. G.: Whiplash injuries of the cervical spine. Virginia Med. Monthly, *85*:171–174, 1958.

19. Walters, J. A., The Psychogenic Regional Pain Syndrome and its diagnosis. "PAIN" (Ford Hospital Symposium) Knightson and Dunke Eds. Little, Brown & Company Inc. Boston, 1966.

20. Wickstrom, J., Martinez, J., and Rodiguez, R.: Quoted by Frankel, V. H., *In* Cervical Pain. New York, Pergamon Press, 1972.

CHAPTER 11

Fractures and Dislocations of the Spine

HORACE A. NORRELL, M.D.
University of Kentucky

INTRODUCTION

There are 10,000 new cases of spinal cord injury annually in the United States. Faced with this serious problem we are still groping for most of the answers specifically related to the injured spinal cord. Nevertheless, important advances have been made in the general care of patients with spinal cord injury. Many of these advances in care have originated from specialties not primarily interested in spinal cord injury. Optimal patient care today depends upon the availability, interest and cooperation of many specialists. Of greatest importance to the acute injury victim are the constant and vigorous effort and attention to minute details which can only be provided by the responsible surgeon. The surgeon accepting such a responsibility must critically analyze his own ability as well as those of his colleagues and his institution to provide exemplary care based on modern treatment techniques. If dissatisfied with the results of this analysis, he should either make the necessary corrections or decide not to accept the responsibility of care of spinal cord injury victims. Recognizing the need for such highly critical and specialized care in the United States, centralized spinal cord injury centers are now being developed.

INITIAL EVALUATION OF THE SPINAL INJURY VICTIM

From the time of a suspected spinal injury, every precaution must be taken to avoid further injury to the spinal cord. Rogers noted that 10 per cent of his patients developed symptoms of spinal cord compression or an increasing neurological deficit after the original injury—during emergency care, during the time when the diagnosis was being established, during definitive treatment or following spinal reduction.[71] Geisler reported a 3 per cent incidence of delayed spinal cord injury resulting from failure to recognize the injury to the spinal column.[26] Quite frequently, the delayed injury occurred following hospital admission. Every attempt should be made to avoid such catastrophes, and their legal consequences, by careful management during each stage, from evacuation from the injury site until the patient's final release from medical care.

An accident capable of generating forces sufficient to injure the spine or spinal cord frequently produces a concomitant extraspinal injury. Many of the associated wounds are immediately life-threatening, and their treatment takes precedence over the spinal injury. The surgeon responsible for managing the spinal injury must be immediately available to coordinate the resuscitative effort by establishing diagnostic and treatment priorities, while taking the necessary steps to prevent further spinal cord injury. The responsible surgeon must not only be an expert in the management of spinal injuries but also be well-versed in modern resuscitative techniques. All too frequently, the responsible surgeon must point out that the "neurogenic shock" occurring with cervical spinal cord transection may cause mild hypotension but is not responsible for a continuing fall in blood pressure, or that the usual tachycardia accompanying hemorrhagic shock might be abolished by the spinal cord injury. Once the life-threatening emergencies have apparently been conquered, the responsible surgeon must not be lulled into a false sense of security and overlook the delayed appearance of other serious extraspinal injuries.

History and Physical Examination Related to the Spinal Injury

Beyond the general history and physical examination, the surgeon is particularly interested in the cause and extent of the injury to the spinal cord. Frequently, a history obtained from the patient or a witness will both help to reveal the mechanism of spinal injury and establish the earlier neurological state.

A careful examination of the spinous processes may reveal abnormal separation, mobile processes, or evidence of direct trauma to the region. Examination of the head, including the vertex, of the face, or even of the buttocks, might reveal abrasions or contusions, demonstrating the point of impact which produced the spinal injury.

Many of the reports of recovery from apparently complete spinal cord transection are probably the result of a hasty and incomplete initial neurological assessment. A more careful examination might have shown minimal motor or sensory preservation, indicating an incomplete lesion. The initial, complete neurological assessment must be deftly performed and carefully recorded so as not to delay further treatment. Each sensory modality, including pinprick, position, touch, deep pain, vibration, as well as motor function, including deep and superficial reflexes, must be tested. A careful sensory examination of the perineum is necessary to detect occasional sacral sensory preservation. For cervical injuries, a careful motor and sensory examination of each cervical spinal cord segment must be performed and repeated at frequent intervals to assess function at and around the level of the spinal cord injury. When examining the cervical spinal cord segment function, it may be difficult to differentiate between spinal cord and nerve root signs at the level of the injury, since there is little disparity between the vertebral level and the corresponding spinal cord segments. Occasionally, nerve root dysfunction may result from nerve root avulsion produced by a traction injury to the brachial plexus. This must be differentiated from a primary spinal injury. For fractures of the lumbar spine or thoracolumbar junction, particular attention is devoted to evaluation of the conus medullaris and cauda equina.

Such careful examinations are essential not only to determine the immediate status of the neurological lesion but also to perform any retrospective analysis of the patient's course. (See specific injuries for a more detailed discussion.)

INITIAL RADIOGRAPHIC EXAMINATION

Once the patient's general condition has stabilized, adequate radiographs must be obtained to delineate the extent of the spinal injury. During this phase, the patient must be accompanied by a surgeon who is not only competent in managing any emergency which may arise but who is also capable of ordering and interpreting appropriate radiographs. In patients with cervical spinal injury, we frequently apply tong traction in the emergency room before the original radiographs are obtained. This assures a greater degree of cervical spinal immobility during the initial evaluation and treatment phase. Whitley also advocates this practice, while Schneider and others are opposed.[78, 96]

Even in patients with obvious traumatic myelopathy, the offending spinal deformity can be overlooked on the initial radiographs. Braakman analyzed 36 cases of cervical spine subluxation, with unilateral or bilateral facet locking, in which diagnosis had been delayed for longer than two weeks.[11] The most common causes for failure in diagnosis were: 1) radiographs of inadequate quality; 2) failure to show all cervical vertebrae; and 3) failure to recognize locked facets, despite the fact it was clearly shown by radiographs of good quality.

Failure to demonstrate all of the cervical vertebrae accounted for 16 per cent of the diagnostic failures in Braakman's series. This difficulty is commonly encountered with a transverse lesion of the lower cervical spinal cord because these patients often lie with hunched shoulders. Downward pull on the patient's arms is often necessary to demonstrate the lower cervical vertebrae. Occasionally, this technique will fail to demonstrate the cervicothoracic junction, and additional techniques must be employed. If radiographs beyond the routine anteroposterior, lateral and the open-mouth view of the cervical spine are required the surgeon must coordinate the effort. The patient's condition must not be jeopardized, either by the lack of adequate radiographs or by the delay or manipulation required to obtain additional, and possibly unnecessary, radiographs. Even when apparently indicated, flexion and extension views are rarely obtained during the initial radiographic assessment; muscle spasm and voluntary guarding, creating spinal immobility, may produce a spurious result. When necessary, flexion and extension views are taken after the acute pain and spasm have subsided. (Essential radiographic views will be discussed with specific injuries.)

ADDITIONAL DIAGNOSTIC STUDIES

There is no unanimity of opinion regarding the value of the Queckenstedt test, myelography, or discography in the evaluation and management of spinal cord injuries.

QUECKENSTEDT TEST. Spinal puncture with a Queckenstedt test (bilateral jugular vein compression, with observation of spinal fluid manometrics) is performed to determine the patency of the subarachnoid space, particularly at the level of the spinal cord injury. Many surgeons routinely employ the Queckenstedt test in acute spinal injury victims, basing the need for immediate surgical exploration on the presence of a spinal manometric block.

In a series of 20 consecutive patients with acute cervical spinal cord injury, Braakman performed serial manometric studies, beginning on admission and repeated one, two, four, and nine days after admission.[12] He found that if a spinal fluid block was present, it would usually resolve spontaneously within several days, irrespective of the nature of the vertebral injury. He was unable to establish any

clear difference between the recovery of those patients in whom a spinal fluid block existed and those in whom it did not. Twenty-four hours following injury, a spinal fluid block was present in 12 of the 20 patients.

Significant extramedullary spinal cord compression may exist in the presence of completely normal manometrics.[30, 65] On the other hand, the block may be due entirely to intramedullary swelling of the spinal cord. There may be complete myelographic obstruction at the level of the injury, despite normal manometrics. This condition can be explained by the limitations on the Queckenstedt test imposed by the caliber of the spinal puncture needle. As long as there is a patent passage through the subarachnoid space as large as the needle caliber, no manometric block can exist. The cerebrospinal fluid may flow around an almost complete obstruction, yet the viscous Pantopaque will be obstructed. A change in position of the cervical spine required for myelography may also convert an incomplete block to a total obstruction of the subarachnoid space.

In view of the unreliability of the Queckenstedt test in either predicting the immediate status of the spinal cord or influencing the final outcome of the injury, I find very little justification for using the procedure in acute spinal injury victims.

MYELOGRAPHY. Myelography is not without hazard to patients with acute spinal cord injury, particularly those with cervical fracture-dislocation. Raynor found some degree of spinal redislocation during myelography in four of five patients studied.[68] Although abnormalities are seen frequently during myelography, the anatomical interpretation is commonly difficult and not helpful in the final analysis. After carefully considering the patient's neurological status and correlating it with the highest quality radiographs, myelography should be performed if questions or inconsistencies exist. Myelography is rarely indicated in patients with complete lesions. Specific indications for myelography are discussed with treatment.

When myelography must be performed, a lateral spinal puncture performed at the atlantoaxial interval allows the patient to remain supine throughout the procedure.[41] The disadvantage of this procedure is the poor visualization of the ventral aspect of the subarachnoid space, a most important area when dealing with acute spinal injuries.

Tomopneumomyelography appears to have overcome many of the objections raised to positive contrast myelography. Larson has shown the utility of this procedure, demonstrating specific anatomical changes with great clarity.[51]

DISCOGRAPHY. Raynor and Verbiest have stressed the diagnostic value of discography when dealing with acute spinal cord injuries.[68, 91] Discography may also be performed during an anterior cervical operation by directly inserting a needle into a questionably abnormal intervertebral disc.[65] Although I do not use discography, the intraoperative technique is appealing, for it might eliminate the false-positive abnormalities frequently encountered with the percutaneous technique.[36]

GENERAL CARE OF THE SPINAL INJURY VICTIM

Although this chapter is primarily devoted to the injured spine and spinal cord, dysfunction of other organ systems produced by spinal cord injury cannot be ignored, since this is so intimately related to the patient's welfare. One or more chapters could be devoted to general care, but would be superfluous for this book's readers. This review is limited to those problems occurring during the acute injury phase, in which either recent important advances have been made or glaring deficiencies exist.

Respiratory Problems Associated with Spinal Cord Injuries

The reduction in early mortality from spinal cord injury is, for the most part, related to improvements in respiratory care. The problems of pulmonary insufficiency secondary to the neurological lesion are often compounded by direct injuries to the chest and lung parenchyma, as well as by the aspiration of blood or vomitus. Gastrointestinal atony accompanying the spinal cord injury may have serious pulmonary consequences. Abdominal distention further reduces the already impaired ventilation by impeding diaphragmatic excursion, and vomiting caused by gastric distention is likely to result in aspiration in the patient immobilized by a spinal injury. Inability to cough further complicates this problem. A nasogastric tube must be inserted in the emergency room and the gastric contents aspirated.

During emergency resuscitation, oral tracheal intubation, when performed by an expert, can be accomplished with little change in the position of the cervical spine. In situations of less emergency, endotracheal intubation by the nasal route offers even less hazard of further injury to the cervical spinal cord. An endotracheal tube may be left safely in position for several days until the pulmonary problem has been corrected, or until continuing problems necessitate a tracheostomy. The use of volume-pressure-controlled ventilators in conjunction with endotracheal intubation is another important aspect of treatment. Respirators are essential for the treatment of pulmonary insufficiency directly related to the neurological dysfunction as well as the frequent complication of atelectasis. Almost every patient with a significant cervical spinal cord injury will require ventilatory assistance at some stage. Patients are frequently successfully maintained on ventilators for long periods of time. The success of this treatment depends upon meticulous pulmonary care and the adjustment of ventilation based upon the results of frequent arterial blood gas and pH determinations.

We have reduced the incidence of serious antibiotic-resistant pulmonary infections by withholding antibiotics until a specific indication arises. Prophylactic antibiotics are not administered to any patient, even those with prolonged tracheal intubation, by an endotracheal tube or tracheostomy. Although pathogenic organisms are common in the frequently taken tracheal cultures, we do not treat bacterial colonization (the appearance of any potential pathogen, in the absence of purulent tracheobronchial secretions or clinical evidence of infection).[16] Once an infection is encountered, it is treated vigorously with appropriate antibiotics, based upon sensitivity studies.

In 1970, we reported four patients with acute cervical spinal cord injury who developed marked cardiorespiratory instability, manifested by cardiac asystole and respiratory arrest in response to tracheal stimulation by a suction catheter. Although asystole persisted for as long as seven seconds, cardiac activity invariably resumed spontaneously. This reflex was not related to hypoxia and was not abolished by large doses of atropine. Subsequently, Krieger reported a similar reflex but abolished it by the administration of one milligram of atropine given every four hours.[48]

Much of our understanding of the respiratory dysfunction occurring with acute lesions of the cervical spinal cord has come from the study of patients who have had a high cervical cordotomy performed, particularly those with bilateral lesions. In the past, there was no adequate explanation for the cause of death, during sleep, of the acute cervical spinal cord injury victim who was apparently having no unusual problems. We now know that these deaths are related to the syndrome of sleep apnea.[48, 49] This condition must be recognized and treated before the fullblown syndrome occurs. It begins with vague subjective sensations of lethargy associated with sighing respirations; the patient may complain of an inability to get enough air. He may be confused. At this time, objective clinical evidence of respiratory impairment may be lacking on physical examination. The novice examiner might ascribe the symptoms to an anxiety reaction, and even precipitate apnea by the administration of a sedative. The patient usually goes on to hypoventilate, and then becomes apneic when asleep. If the apnea is recognized before the patient dies and he is awakened, breathing resumes but hypoventilation persists and sleep apnea recurs. The administration of oxygen is particularly hazardous to patients with this syndrome.[50]

Arterial blood gas studies and vital capacity measurements are not reliable guides to the presence or severity of this syndrome. It is caused by a faulty respiratory control mechanism, manifested by a decrease in response to carbon dioxide.[47, 49]

In patients with even the slightest cervical spinal cord injury, we carefully observe the ventilatory pattern. If hypoventilation, irregular breathing, sighing or unexplained air hunger occurs, even in the presence of normal arterial blood gases, we insert an endotracheal tube and employ controlled mechanical ventilation; controlled respiration is usually necessary for three to 10 days. Before the endotracheal tube is removed, intermittent mandatory ventilation is employed for 24 hours; the respirator is discontinued and the patient's response is carefully observed for another 24 hours.

Early Care of the Urinary System

The initial insertion of an indwelling urethral catheter into the bladder of the spinal cord injury victim is frequently the genesis of an almost never-ending series of urinary tract complications. These include acute and chronic infections, not always limited to the genitourinary system, hydronephrosis, renal and vesical stones, and a variety of penoscrotal lesions. Many patients, even after a complete return of neurological function, continue to be plagued by chronic urinary problems which were introduced during the initial treatment phase.[37]

Urinary drainage is best managed by Guttmann's intermittent non-touch technique, which requires a scrubbed and gowned surgeon.[28] In an analysis of 476 spinal cord injury patients managed by this technique, 62 per cent were discharged from the hospital with sterile urine. Most patients either regained urinary control or adequate reflex bladder emptying within six to seven weeks after injury.

Guttmann's treatment regimen is probably the best available today, yet it is rarely practiced in the United States. The technique requires medical or specialized paramedical personnel on duty at all times. The administrator of a hospital not constantly providing care for a large number of spinal cord injury victims is usually unwilling to provide the funds for the hiring of appropriate personnel, despite the importance of an intermittent catheterization program. Centralization of acute spinal injury care might provide administrative justification for the personnel necessary to provide appropriate care of the urinary system.

Comarr analyzed the urinary status of 408 patients with spinal cord lesions (almost all traumatic).[20] Intermittent catheterization was begun at the time of injury in very few patients; but even after a delayed start using this technique 78 per cent of the patients became catheter free. When the percentage of catheter-free patients was analyzed according to the neurological lesion, there was no numerical difference between catheter-free patients with upper motor neuron lesions and those with lower motor neuron lesions. Intermittent catheterization was begun at four-hour intervals, and the time extended depending upon the progress of the bladder. Comarr emphasized that the technique was not applicable to females. Even in patients with established urinary infections who were started on intermittent catheterization many developed sterile urine. Comarr concluded: 1) that intermittent catheterization is preferable to bladder training with an indwelling catheter; 2) that intermittent catheterization must be started from the onset of spinal cord injury to achieve the best results; and 3) that from the onset, the non-touch technique is mandatory.

Faced with a seemingly insoluble problem of establishing a non-touch technique program, at Kentucky we have been investigating another approach to the management of the urinary system. Indwelling urethral catheters are not used. Instead, a small-gauge Silastic indwelling suprapubic catheter, attached to a closed drainage system, is inserted by the percutaneous technique. This method is not comparable to the open insertion of a suprapubic tube, which was condemned after World War II. In patients with complete or near complete spinal cord transection, the external urinary sphincter is resected by the transurethral route. Continence is provided, since the internal sphincter is spared. Early in the course of treatment, the suprapubic catheter is clamped and allowed to drain at intervals. As bladder tone returns, urination begins; when the residual volume becomes minimal, the suprapubic tube is removed. We are presently performing an analysis of patients managed by this technique and consider it experimental.

Protein and Electrolyte Disturbances

Transection of the spinal cord produces a profound systemic catabolic response; the pathophysiology and treatment of this problem have received widespread attention, but as yet no method has been found to prevent it.[7] The reduction of serum proteins and hematocrit in the acute spinal cord injury victim should not be ignored, since this may be responsible for some potentially dangerous problems, particularly those related to peripheral edema, electrolyte disturbances and possibly pulmonary congestion. The hematocrit is maintained at at least 35 per cent by the administration of packed erythrocytes. Serum protein determinations are frequently obtained, and the level maintained at 6 gm per 100 ml by the administration of salt-poor human albumin. The protein balance is soon restored to normal, and it is seldom necessary to administer more than 50 grams of albumin.

A patient with a cervical spinal cord injury may develop a profound hyponatremia (110–120 mEq/l), which may respond to sodium replacement or diuretics.[48, 52] Occasionally, when the hyponatremia is the result of inappropriate antidiuretic hormone (ADH) secretion, the administration of sodium will not correct the deficit. The syndrome of inappropriate ADH secretion includes: 1) hyponatremia, 2) continued renal excretion of sodium, 3) hyperosmolar urine in relationship to a hypo-osmolar serum, and 4) normal renal and adrenal function. Occasionally, the problem will be compounded by the use of mechanical ventilation.[96] The syndrome is corrected by withholding fluids until the hyponatremia is reversed. Since we have taken a more aggressive attitude toward the maintenance of a near-normal serum protein level, the syndrome of inappropriate ADH secretion seems to be a less frequent problem.

In patients with spinal cord injury, hyperkalemia, resulting in ventricular fibrillation, may appear immediately following the administration of succinylcholine.[84] The likely explanation for the sudden increase in serum potassium levels is that the denervated muscle cell membrane is altered, resulting in an atypical response to depolarization (a nonselective increase in cell membrane permeability to sodium and potassium) produced by succinylcholine. It is unwise to use succinylcholine in any patient with spinal cord injury, particularly during the vulnerable period which commences at about seven days after injury and extends for about 90 days.

Decubitus Ulcers

Decubitus ulcers or pressure ulcers are an unacceptable complication in any patient with a spinal cord injury. During rehabilitation, the spinal injury victim is made so acutely aware of the problems attending the development of a decubitus ulcer that he will demand everything possible to prevent it. During the acute injury stage, the patient is frequently immobile, unaware of the problem, and unable to prevent the formation of an ulcer. Even a mention of decubitus ulcers may seem out of place in a modern discussion of spinal cord injuries. Yet, recently, more than one third of the acute and subacute spinal cord injury patients transferred from other hospitals to Rancho Los Amigos Hospital arrived with decubitus ulcers.[98]

Turning the patient every two hours, without jeopardizing the spinal cord, can be accomplished by using turning frames, circle beds, the Stoke Mandeville bed, or a regular hospital bed. The majority of our patients are managed on sheep skins in a regular hospital bed; the patient is rotated and propped with pillows, and meticulous skin care is provided.

Injury to the Carotid and Vertebral Arteries Occurring Secondary to Cervical Spinal Injuries

Injury to the carotid and vertebral arteries associated with spinal injuries is infrequent. Nevertheless, the importance of recognizing such injuries warrants a discussion.

Vertebral artery thrombosis occurs most commonly as a result of injury to the vessel as it enters the foramen transversarium of the sixth cervical vertebra. Stretching of the artery against the bone during extension causes intimal damage, which may result in a propagating thrombus. Neurological signs are related to vascular insufficiency in the brainstem. Simeone recently reviewed vertebral artery injuries in the neck.[81]

During an anterior exploration for a cervical fracture-dislocation we encountered a totally divided vertebral artery with a bone fragment interposed between the proximal and distal ends of the vessel. Following removal of the fragment, brisk bleeding appeared from both ends of the vessel. The artery was ligated and the patient demonstrated no signs of ischemia. Tears of the vertebral artery are apparently rare even in fatal injuries to the craniospinal junction. Davis found only two ruptured vertebral arteries in 50 autopsies, cases in which the craniospinal junction was carefully examined.[23] Although tears of smaller cervical branches of the vertebral arteries occurred quite commonly.

Carotid artery injury occurs most commonly following blunt cervical trauma, but may also result from hyperextension of the cervical spine. With hyperextension, intimal damage most frequently appears at the level of the anterior arch of the atlas or the transverse process of the third cervical vertebra, presumably from the vessel being stretched over the bony prominences. Patients with carotid artery injury frequently display a latent period between the time of injury and the onset of symptoms, in all likelihood related to a progressive thrombosis, beginning at the site of intimal injury. Present consensus favors the nonoperative treatment of acute carotid artery thrombosis.[90]

Not all vascular injuries causing neurological problems result from thrombotic occlusion of the injured vessel. Heilbrun demonstrated multiple intracranial emboli arising from a traumatized area within the cervical carotid and vertebral arteries.[32]

Schneider, particularly interested in concomitant spinal cord and brain stem injuries, pointed out the difficulty in differentiating between vascular and compressive injuries involving the cervicomedullary junction.[78]

INJURY TO LOWER CERVICAL SPINE AND SPINAL CORD

Mechanism

The surgeon responsible for treating the patient with a spinal injury must be able to deduce the mechanism producing the injury by correlating the history, physical findings and the appropriate radiographs. Proper management of the patient is dependent upon an intelligent understanding of the mechanism producing the injury for the following reasons: 1) Certain fractures and/or dislocations which are notoriously unstable pose an immediate threat of further injury to the spinal cord, requiring particular caution on the surgeon's part. 2) Specific neurological syndromes may occur in the presence of few or no radiographic abnormalities. 3) Additional necessary radiographic information beyond routine anteroposterior and lateral projections can be systematically and safely obtained if a particular mechanism of injury is suspected. 4) Appropriate and safe reduction of dislocations depends upon an understanding of how the dislocation occurred. 5) Lengthy immobilization in tong traction may be unnecessary with certain injuries while, on the other hand, early operation or prolonged immobilization may be required for other injuries.

CLASSIFICATION OF MECHANISMS OF INJURY AND NEUROLOGICAL SYNDROMES

Rarely is the spinal injury the result of a single moment of force. Commonly, rotation and axial compression are added to either flexion or extension forces. Selecki emphasized that a classification based entirely on either radiographic or clinical evidence is improper.[79] He performed a series of important experiments using the entire intact cervical spine of cadavers. Roaf's earlier experiments employed the "basic spinal unit," which was composed of two vertebrae and the intervertebral disc with the surrounding ligaments.[69] Rightfully, Selecki was critical of most conclusions drawn from Roaf's experiments utilizing such short spinal segments. Realizing the limitations of cadaver experiments, Selecki has, nevertheless, added much to our understanding of the pathology occurring as a result of cervical spinal trauma. He emphasized that the term "compression fracture," referring to the vertebral body injury, is used mainly as a descriptive radiologic term and may create confusion as to the injury mechanism. In reality, fractures of a lamina or pedicle may result from compression also, but they are not termed compression fractures in radiological terminology. Compression is probably a component of most spinal injuries and may occur with flexion, extension or rotation. It is unlikely that the term "compression fracture" can be purged from the radiologist's vocabulary, but the surgeon must be aware of the term's implications. Similarly, "burst fracture," used by Holdsworth,[34] implies an injury resulting entirely from a force delivered directly along the axis of the spine, fixed in an anatomically neutral position. Selecki takes exception to this explanation, since flexion or extension components of the injury can frequently be demonstrated. In his experiments, all injuries were created primarily by compression forces, and all the main varieties of spinal fractures and dislocations were obtained, demonstrating the multiplicity of injuries produced by compression.

The publications of Holdsworth and Whitley are modern classics dealing with the mechanisms of injury.[34, 97] However, the more recent work of Selecki has simplified the classification of cervical spinal injuries according to the following broad categories of injury mechansims: 1) extension, 2) flexion, 3) extension with rotation, 4) flexion with rotation, and 5) lateral flexion. My discussion will be based upon his classification.

EXTENSION INJURIES. From his clinical series Selecki concluded that extension injuries to the cervical spine occur three times more commonly than flexion injuries. Whitley, primarily interested in radiographic abnormalities, found flexion and extension injuries to occur with almost equal frequency. This discrepancy probably arises from the fact that extension injuries frequently occur in the absence of radiographic abnormalities. Extension injuries occur primarily when a force is applied to the forehead, face or chin, most commonly during falls, diving into shallow water (although this more commonly results in a flexion injury), or in rear-end collision. Blows to the vertex, with the spine in a neutral position, usually result in extension injuries to the lower cervical spine, caused by the force vectors compressing the lordotic spine into further extension. Many patients suffering extension injuries will have forehead abrasions or facial fractures demonstrating the point of impact responsible for the spinal injury.

The radiographic findings associated with extension injuries may be minimal (widening of an intervertebral disc space) or entirely absent. However, Selecki emphasized that the degree of ligamentous and intervertebral disc injury is always greater than might be expected from the radiographic examination. A small triangular chip of bone from the anterior inferior angle, or the superior end plate of a vertebral body appearing on the lateral radiograph is a characteristic feature of extension injuries. This fracture occurs secondarily to a tear in the anterior longitudinal ligament resulting in avulsion of the anterior bone fragment (Fig. 11–1). Eventually, calcification of the ligament may be seen at the point of rupture. Herniations of disc material into the spi-

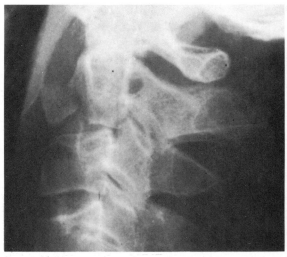

Figure 11–1. Hyperextension resulted in a tear in the anterior longitudinal ligament and avulsion of the anteroinferior body of the axis.

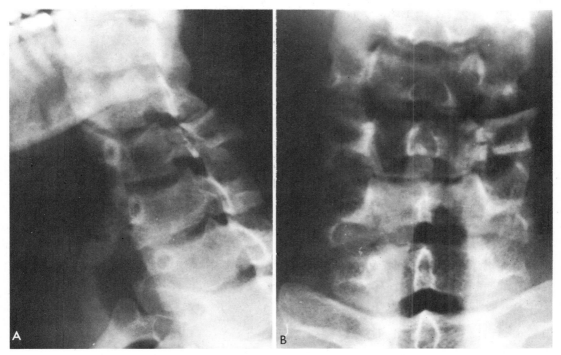

Figure 11–2. An extension injury resulted in the unilateral fracture of the C5 pedicle. *A*, In the oblique projection the displacement of the articular facets is demonstrated. *B*, In the anteroposterior projection the vertebral body is tilted toward the side of injury due to loss of articular facet support to the left. Rotational forces probably account for the unilateral injury.

nal canal are quite rare with extension injuries; Braakman was unaware of any report of posterior intervertebral disc herniation occurring with extension injury.[12]

Whitley described fractures of the posterior elements, resulting from extension injuries. If such fractures occur, the inferior articular facets of the vertebra may be impacted. On the lateral radiograph, the inferior facets tend to be horizontal and the lateral mass appears almost triangular. Occasionally, the facets may appear horizontal, without actually being fractured. This results from a fracture through the pedicles, which produces dorsal displacement of the separated posterior elements (Fig. 11–2). The force, if severe, may tear the intervertebral disc and anterior longitudinal ligament, dislocating the cervical spine.[34] Forsythe also pointed out that, on rare occasions with extension injuries, the upper vertebral body may eventually be displaced forward and the dislocation might be mistaken for a flexion injury.[25]

In patients with neurological deficit and a history of extension injury, it is particularly important to note any radiographic changes of cervical spondylosis or a narrowed sagittal diameter of the spinal canal. In these patients devastating neurological signs appear with minimal radiographic abnormalities. Taylor first performed experiments demonstrating the infolding and forward bulging of the ligamentum flavum produced by hyperextension.[87] He believed this to be the most commonly responsible mechanism for hyperextension injury to the cervical spinal cord, although earlier he described temporary subluxation as the usual cause of spinal cord injury with hyperextension. Similar experiments performed using spines with cervical spondylosis demonstrated simultaneous impingement on the central portion of the spinal canal by the ventral transverse ridges and the dorsal ligamentum flavi.

Brieg extended Taylor's experiments in 1960, demonstrating that the posterior indentations occurring during hyperextension were not only caused by the bulging ligamentum flavum but that dorsal folds within the dura also played a significant role in producing the deformity with the spinal canal.

Neurological Problems Associated with Extension Injuries. In a most severe injury I found total anatomical spinal cord transection at the upper cervical levels in a young patient who had a hyperextension injury without spinal disruption. Hyperextension of the cervical spine commonly results in the syndrome of acute central cervical spinal cord injury. The central cord injury syndrome, however, is not invariably the result of hyperextension;[9] flexion injuries resulted in approximately one half of the cases of central spinal cord injury reported by Braakman.[12] The syndrome is characterized by motor impairment greater in the upper than in the lower extremities, bladder dysfunction and varying degrees of sensory loss, usually minimal, below the level of the lesion. The lower extremities tend to recover motor power first, bladder function returns next, followed by strength in the upper extremities, and finally finger movement. Schneider postulated a structural distortion of the spinal cord which was greatest in the central portion of the cord, accounting for the neurological syndrome.[74] He believed that the central "hematomyelia" and surrounding edema common at all lesions was secondary to the mechanical distortion. A more likely explanation for the typical spinal cord lesion is a minor mechanical insult followed by progressive central hemorrhagic destruction. In all likelihood, the mechanical trauma results in minimal anatomical disruption, but sets off a series of metabolic changes which ultimately result in varying degrees of central cord necrosis.[63] Lesions identical to those of central cord injury have been produced experimentally both by occluding the arterial blood supply to the cervical spinal cord in dogs and by direct non-disruptive trauma.[63, 100]

FLEXION INJURIES. Flexion injuries most commonly result from head-on automobile collisions, shallow water diving accidents, blows to the occiput with the head held in neutral position, or blows to the vertex with the victim's chin on the chest. Stress is placed upon the intraspinous ligaments and ligamentum nuchae which may result in rupture of these structures, or fractures of their posterior bony attachments (spinous processes) or both. Probably the most common cause of a spinous process fracture (or, rarely, multiple process fractures) particularly at the cervicothoracic junction is avulsion by an unusually forceful contraction of the attached muscles. These fractures occur commonly in diggers, hence the name "shovelers' disease," "shovelers' fracture" or "clay shovelers' fracture."[73] Flexion injury may produce only widening of the posterior aspect of the interspace or an increase in the distance between the spinous processes.[97] An early stage of flexion injury with a relatively low range of compression is responsible for the anterior vertebral body wedge fracture. Dislocation rarely occurs at this stage of injury.[79]

If the injuring force has a forward and upward (cephalad) component, the damage will be primarily ligamentous; when a shearing force predominates, vertebral subluxation with a facet overriding occurs. With significant subluxation, the anterior longitudinal ligament may be stripped from the surface of the lower vertebral body, avulsing a portion of the anterosuperior portion of the lower vertebral body.[97] If overriding of the articular facets is complete, locking occurs (Fig. 11–3). With incomplete subluxation the vertebral bodies may spontaneously become realigned, yet remain unstable. Intermittent subluxation may then occur, particularly with normal flexion. Braakman uses the term "sprain" to designate an injury in which there is evidence that the periarticular ligaments have been lacerated, yet it is impossible to determine whether or not complete temporary subluxation occurred at the moment of injury.[12]

If the force of trauma is delivered along the vertebral axis, with the cervical spine in early flexion (loss of the lordotic curve), a "burst fracture" may occur (Fig. 11–4). Holdsworth classified these as vertical compression injuries, stating that "the vertebral body is shattered from within outward, in which case the ligaments are frequently not damaged."[34] Portions of the intervertebral disc are commonly forced into the vertebral bodies. Cheshire, disagreeing with Holdsworth, believes that ligamentous injury frequently accompanies burst fractures.[18] In 1956, Schneider described a similar fracture, the "tear-drop fracture."[76] Characteristically, there is a separation, downward and forward displacement of the anteroinferior margin of the involved vertebral body. Of greater importance is the second component of the tear drop—the posteroinferior margin (fragment) is displaced into the spinal canal (Fig. 11–4). Burst fractures, vertical compression fractures and tear-drop fractures are, for practical purposes, synonymous.

Neurological Problems Associated with

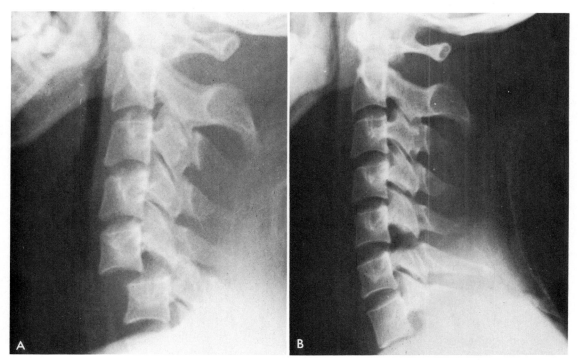

Figure 11–3. *A,* Complete dislocation of C5 with bilateral facet locking could not be reduced by traction. *B,* Operative reduction was achieved by removing the leading surface of the superior articular facets of the lower vertebra; note removed portion of the facets.

Flexion Injuries. When complete dislocation and locking of the articular facets occur, the laminal arch of the upper vertebra comes forward, compressing the dorsal aspect of the spinal cord against the posterosuperior surface of the next lower vertebral body (Fig. 11–5). Signs of spinal cord injury are usually profound, although 20 per cent of Whitley's patients escaped without spinal cord injury.[97] Those victims escaping cord injury frequently experience nerve root injury owing to the deformation of the intervertebral foramina at the site of articular facet locking. Serious spinal cord lesions can mask associated root lesions and, thereby, prevent their recognition.

Schneider described the syndrome of acute anterior spinal cord injury.[75] This injury is characterized by immediate complete motor paralysis, hypoesthesia, and hypoanalgesia below the level of the spinal cord lesion; there is preservation of the sense of motion and sense of position, but partial loss of the sense of touch and vibration. The neurological pattern was found in acute injury to the anterior portion of the cervical spinal cord to be associated with destruction or compression by extruded intervertebral discs, or fracture-dislocations. Later, Schneider described the injury in association with "tear-drop" fractures.[76]

At the University of Kentucky, in an analysis of 20 patients having flexion injuries resulting in "burst" fractures of the vertebral body, eight had a complete transverse spinal cord lesion.[61] Seven patients demonstrated complete or almost complete motor paralysis with preservation of one or more sensory modalities. A pure acute anterior spinal cord syndrome was found in only one patient in our series, although a minor variation of the syndrome occurred in two additional cases. The Brown-Sequard syndrome occurred in one patient. I agree with Braakman, who concluded that there is no strict relationship between a particular neurological picture and a certain type of vertebral injury, if central cord injury from hyperextension is excluded.[12]

EXTENSION INJURIES WITH ROTATION. These injuries usually result from blows to the lateral aspect of the face or head, causing rota-

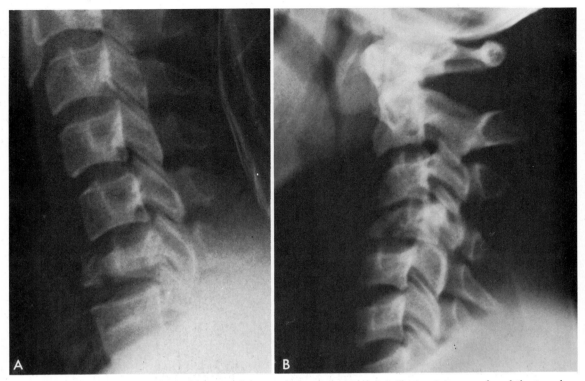

Figure 11–4. Two different burst fractures of the cervical vertebral body. *A,* Flexion injury produced the tear drop fragments on both the anterior and posterior inferior surface of C5. *B,* With a greater axial component of the force the articular facets are fractured in addition to the vertebral body.

tion of the spine. The blow may be delivered to the vertex of the skull with the spine rotated and extended. There is usually an axial component of the force which is mainly absorbed by the articular facets on the side opposite the facial trauma. This produces a unilateral fracture of the articular facet pedicle or lamina, which may best be demonstrated on oblique radiographs or by an anteroposterior projection with caudal angulation of the x-ray tube (Fig. 11–6).[1] Whitley states that the spinal cord damage is frequently unilateral with such lesions;[97] however, this was not confirmed by Selecki's experiments.[79]

FLEXION INJURIES WITH ROTATION. The direction of the external force is similar to that producing extension rotation injuries, except that the cervical spine is forced into flexion. The characteristic abnormality is either unilateral facet locking or unilateral facet fracture.[46] Unilateral locking usually occurs in the lower cervical spine. Damage to the ligaments and intervertebral disc is less severe than in bilateral locking, with bony injury being more common. Frequently, the superior articular facet opposite the injury is fractured, as may be the vertebral body immediately below the locking (Fig. 11–7).[10] The sagittal diameter of the spinal canal is reduced, but not to the degree seen with bilateral locking, thus the frequency of serious spinal cord injury is less (Fig. 11–5). The radiographic features of unilateral locking of the articular facets are quite characteristic, but the diagnosis is frequently overlooked owing to the fact that too much attention is given to the vertebral body shift and too little to the facet abnormalities. In the lateral projection, subluxation of the upper vertebral body is less than one half of the sagittal diameter of the vertebral body, and the facets are displaced on one side. Hence, the superimposition of the facet joints at each level, normally seen in the lateral projection, is interrupted at the level of the unilateral facet interlocking; cephalad to the level of the dislocation the entire axis of the cervical spine is rotated, producing an appearance somewhat similar to that obtained in a standard oblique

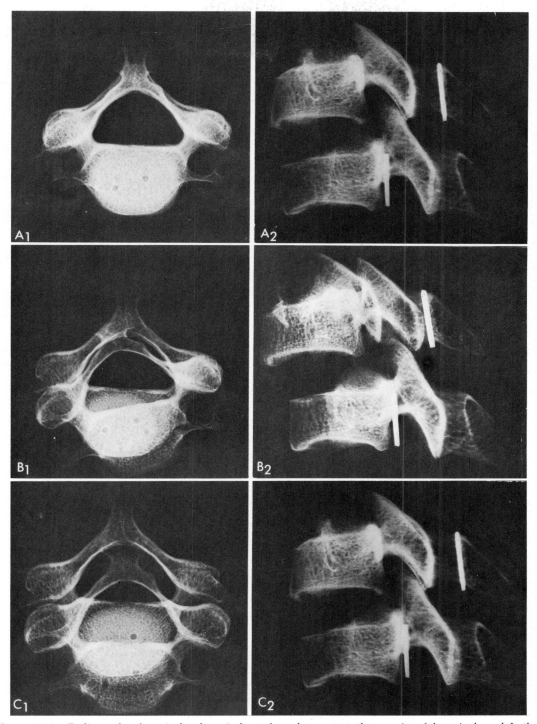

Figure 11–5. Radiographs of two isolated cervical vertebrae demonstrate the capacity of the spinal canal. In the lateral projection radiopaque markers have been placed at the apex of the laminal arch on the superior vertebra and on the posterior midsagittal surface of the inferior vertebral body. *A,* Normal configuration. *B,* Rotary subluxation with unilateral facet locking slightly reduces the sagittal diameter. *C,* With complete dislocation and with bilateral facet locking, the sagittal diameter of the spinal cord is greatly reduced.

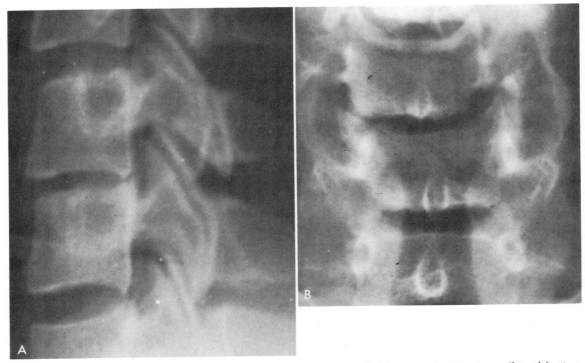

Figure 11–6.   An extension-rotation injury, probably also having an axial force, resulted in: *A*, a unilateral fracture (impaction) of the inferior articular facet of C6 (no fracture line is seen, only the asymmetry of articular facets); and *B*, a fracture of the right uncinate process of the C6 vertebral body (same patient). The fracture line from the uncinate process extends across the vertebral body.

projection (Fig. 11–8). On the anteroposterior projection, the spinous processes are displaced to the side of the interlocking, and the intervertebral disc space may also be inclined to the side of the interlocking, because of the cephalad displacement of the superior vertebral body. If necessary, oblique radiographs can be taken to further clarify the abnormality.

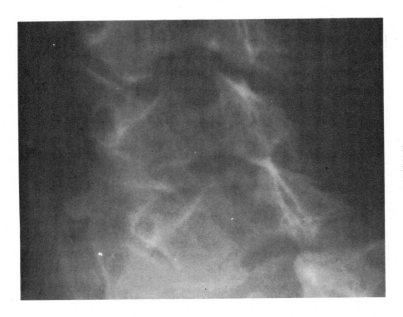

Figure 11–7.   A fracture of the superior articular facet of C6 produced an isolated C7 radiculopathy. The separated bone fragment can be seen in the intervertebral foramen.

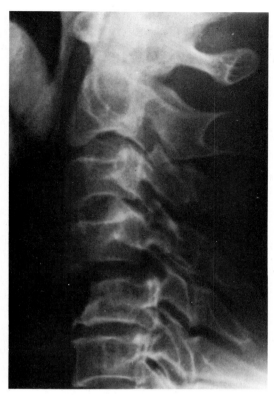

Figure 11–8. A flexion-rotation injury resulted in unilateral locking of the articular facets at the C5-C6 level. Note the obliquity of the spinal segments above the level of the subluxation.

LATERAL FLEXION INJURIES. A rare injury, seen almost exclusively in children, is the result of a force delivered directly to the lateral apsect of the cervical spine and skull. The injury results in wedging of the lateral aspect of a vertebral body and its associated lateral mass. The injury can best be visualized in the anteroposterior projection radiographs; tomography in this plane may be helpful.

TREATMENT OF FRACTURES AND DISLOCATIONS OF THE LOWER CERVICAL SPINE

Treatment of all injuries to the cervical spine and spinal cord must be aimed at: 1) preservation of the functionally and/or anatomically intact spinal pathways; 2) restoration of alignment of the spinal canal, relieving spinal cord compression; 3) establishment of spinal stability; and 4) freedom from postinjury pain.

Although everyone agrees that restoration of spinal canal alignment is essential, the speed with which this should be accomplished remains somewhat controversial. In many patients with cervical spinal fractures, spinal canal alignment is rapidly reestablished when tong traction is applied and a small amount of weight is added. When dealing with dislocations, particularly when one or both of the facets are locked, the treatment is not so simple, yet progression of the neurological lesion is common when the dislocation is not reduced.[12] Guttmann is opposed to the "forceful conservative procedure" of manipulation.[27] I certainly agree with Guttmann's philosophy, but, on the other hand, I believe that almost every dislocation can be corrected within a few hours following injury by the aggressive and judicious combination of tong traction and proper positioning of the victim's spine. Others concur with these ideas, stressing the importance of achieving spinal realignment as quickly and safely as possible. Although manipulation under general anesthesia has been advocated, this has generally not found acceptance in the United States. If the patient's general condition permits, reduction of dislocation is begun in conjunction with the initial radiographic assessment and continued in an Intensive-Care-Unit, with the patient under constant surgical observation. Frequent, high quality radiographs or the use of a television-fluoroscopic image intensifier during this stage is essential to avoid further spinal cord injury. Braakman has emphasized that excessive skull traction resulting in abnormal widening between the vertebral bodies on both sides of an injured motor segment can lead to progression of the cord injury.[12]

The following maneuver has been quite successful in reducing bilateral facet locking. Beginning with 20 pounds of weight on the tongs, under close radiographic control, traction is increased, in increments of 10 or five pounds, until the trailing edge of the inferior articular facets (upper vertebral body) are almost perched upon the leading edge of the superior articular facets (lower vertebral body). To reach this state in 90 minutes or less, a final weight of 80 pounds or more may be required. Countertraction is applied by bandaging the legs to the lower end of the bed. When appropriate vertebral distraction has been accomplished, the neck is brought into slight flexion, which will further disengage the facets. This maneuver is followed by slight extension, simultaneously reducing the amount of traction, reestablishing the continuity of the spinal canal. Unilateral facet locking may be more difficult to reduce but, again, adequate separation of the interlocking must be achieved before any attempt is made to slightly flex and rotate the head away from the side of locking to accomplish reduction. Frequent radiographs are taken during the reduction, and the patient must be cautioned to immediately report any new neurological symptoms which might result from the technique. I favor abandoning the procedure immediately if progression of neurological signs appears during closed reduction. Increased pain in the neck or in the scapular region is quite common during closed reduction, but this immediately subsides after reduction has been accomplished. The importance of reducing facet locking for relief of nerve root signs and symptoms has been stressed by Braakman.[10] In his series, small amounts of traction weight (less than 10 kg) invariably resulted in failure to reduce the dislocation. When adequate traction failed to relieve the dislocation operative reduction was recommended. Cloward and Verbiest recommend open reduction through the anterior approach, using skull traction and local pressure on the anteroinferior surface of the dislocated vertebral body.[19, 91] Occasionally, reduction will be impossible from the anterior approach, particularly when unilateral locking has occurred. When open reduction is necessary, I prefer a posterior reduction, which is accomplished by removing the upper surface of the superior articular facet which holds the overriding inferior articular facet. One patient in my series, with bilateral facet locking, required an anterior exploration two days following open posterior reduction owing to the progressive development of a Brown-Sequard syndrome produced by a large fragment of herniated intervertebral disc compressing the spinal cord. Chronic untreated (old) facet locking is discussed in the section on Delayed Progressive Neurological Loss.

The third aim in the treatment of spinal injuries is to establish spinal stability. Stability is defined as the absence of any abnormal mobility between any pair of vertebrae, when lateral radiographs are taken in flexion and extension at the conclusion of the treatment of a fracture or fracture-dislocation.[18] Stability, when applied to an acute fracture or dislocation, refers to the predicted ultimate stability of the spine following appropriate treatment, not the immediate state. Stability, when used in the acute sense, is speculative, based upon experience. Predicted stability, as a basis for treatment of spinal injuries, has always provided argument between advocates of early surgical spine fusion and those who favor treatment by long-term skeletal traction. Most authors agree that the primary factor contributing to instability is ligamentous injury, most commonly sustained by anterior dislocation. Another factor contributing to the instability is the poor healing properties of the torn intervertebral discs.[6, 73] Bilateral facet dislocations are very unstable, according to Holdsworth, since tearing of the system of dorsal ligaments, intervertebral disc, capsules of the facet joints and posterior longitudinal ligaments renders the spine completely unstable.[35] Cheshire found instability of the cervical spine in approximately 6 per cent of such injuries, which is a surprisingly low figure.[18]

Holdsworth classified "burst fractures" as stable, stating that the body is shattered by the axial force but the ligaments are rarely injured. However, the frequent flexion component of injury produces ligamentous injury, rendering the spine unstable. Schneider reported a group of patients with delayed progressive neurological deficit caused by unstable flexion teardrop fractures.[76] In a retrospective analysis of 63 similar cases, Cheshire found an instability incidence of only 4.8 per cent.[18] Flexion subluxation accompanied by a fracture of the lower vertebral body was the most unstable injury in Cheshire's series; instability occurred in 21 per cent of these cases.

Although I strongly recommend early anterior cervical fusion for fracture-dislocations of the cervical spine, my advocacy of this technique is not primarily based upon the frequency of instability following adequate tong traction.[60] It is difficult to refute the good results obtained by the proponents of long-term tong traction. Tong traction is a safe and effective technique of patient management, requiring the same skill, careful planning and painstaking attention to details as that provided by the surgeon practicing early operation. Certain patients have contraindications to early anterior fusion (25 per cent in the Kentucky series), and must be treated by tong traction immobilization. The plan for traction immobilization must be individualized for each patient's injury. Certain patients, e.g., some extension injuries, or minor anterior wedge fractures, require only a short period of, or no traction immobilization, while others require eight weeks of continuous traction. Generally speaking, the more unstable fractures require the longest periods of tong traction immobilization. Brav has clearly shown that most treatment failures from tong traction result from an inadequate period of traction immobilization. The Minerva jacket cannot be accepted as a substitute for tong traction, but should be used, as bracing, following an appropriate period of tong traction.

In contrast to the Minerva jacket, the halo traction apparatus, fixed with either plaster or pelvic pins, provides excellent immobilization of the injured cervical spine, allowing early ambulation. Although the halo apparatus seems to be growing in popularity in early treatment of cervical spine trauma, little has been written about the results of this technique for either primary treatment of fractures or dislocations or early postoperative immobilization.[89] Most reports deal chiefly with the results of halo immobilization following spinal fusion for nontraumatic disorders, only mentioning its use in the management of traumatic lesions.[58]

In patients with analgesia resulting from spinal cord injury, the application of the halo apparatus fixed with a body cast is not advised, since skin necrosis is liable to occur at pressure points beneath the cast. The halopelvic apparatus may help to avoid this problem. Until there has been a careful analysis of traumatic injuries treated by the early application of halo traction, and of the indications and contraindications established, I believe that only surgeons with extensive experience both in the treatment of spinal injuries and in the use of halo traction should choose this form of treatment. For technique see page 91.

The management of hyperextension injuries with minimal or no radiographic changes, resulting in a central spinal cord injury syndrome, requires special mention. It has been my policy to perform a myelogram, several days after admission, if the lesion is incomplete. Rarely is any abnormality other than spondylosis discovered. If an extramedullary mass is discovered, anterior operation is recommended. For the complete spinal cord lesion, myelography is less important and may be omitted. Surgery is not performed upon patients with central spinal cord injury syndrome and generalized cervical spondylosis.

Experimental Techniques and Their Application in Humans

Reestablishment of axonal anatomical continuity following spinal cord injury remains a distant hope. Recent research has provided important information regarding the treatment of spinal cord injuries in which the anatomical continuity of the spinal cord has not been interrupted. As early as 1911, Allen, employing a standardized low-force injury to the spinal cord of animals, recognized the progressive damage caused by edema and hemorrhage, and even performed a myelotomy to relieve "high intramedullary pressure," finding that some animals made uneventful recoveries following surgery.[4] It was not until 1969 that the work of White renewed interest in the morphological and functional significance of the progressive changes occurring within the spinal cord following experimental trauma (Table 11-1).[94] The minimal force delivered to the spinal cord capable of causing paraplegia in an experimental animal produced no immediate histological changes at the injury site, but within 15 minutes small zones of pericapillary hemorrhages could be seen in the central gray zone immediately beneath the impact area. Within eight hours the lesion progressed to an elongated central hematoma surrounded by an area of hemorrhagic necrosis within the white matter. Kelly, in 1970, demonstrated the rapid decline of the tissue oxygen saturation, following experimental nondisruptive spinal cord trauma.[42] It remained for Osterholm, in 1972, to explain the pathophysiology of progressive autodestruction of the traumatized spinal cord.[63] An analysis of the injured tissue revealed profound increases in the norepinephrine levels, which were universally associated with massive central hemorrhages. This concentration of norepinephrine began immediately following spinal cord injury and reached a maximal level when central hemorrhages appeared. Osterholm hypothesized that the norepinephrine liberated earliest at the injury site depressed or halted electrical transmission, but higher levels of norepinephrine produced vasospasm, which arrested spinal cord perfusion, and thus resulted in autodestruction.

The experimental treatment of nondisruptive spinal cord lesions actually preceded the renewed interest in the morphology and pathophysiology of the lesions. Albin demonstrated that local cord cooling was helpful, if

**TABLE 11–1. SEQUENTIAL CHANGES,
EXPERIMENTAL NONDISRUPTIVE SPINAL CORD TRAUMA**

Time	Anatomical	Physiological	Biochemical
Immediate 1 Minute	None	Evoked response blocked at injury site	
5 Minutes	Central gray matter venules distended with blood	Decreasing gray matter blood flow	Significant rise in tissue norepinephrine
15 Minutes	Axonal changes appear in white matter—electron microscopy (E.M.) Gray matter pericapillary hemorrhages	Marked reduction in gray and white matter blood flow	Tissue oxygen reduced by 50%
30 Minutes	Progressive	Some return of white matter blood flow	Maximum reduction in tissue oxygen
1 Hour	Coalescence of gray matter Hemorrhages	Decrease in white matter blood flow	Maximum accumulation of norepinephrine
4 Hours	Gray matter infarction Blood vessel necrosis White matter edema E.M.—Breaks in myelin sheaths	Progressive decreased flow	Norepinephrine levels decreasing
8 Hours	Elongated central hematoma Non-hemorrhagic necrosis of white matter	Blood flow limited to periphery of white matter Progressive increased flow	Persistent hypoxia
24 Hours		Blood flow normal in non-necrotic white matter	

utilized within specific time limits, in reversing experimental traumatic paraplegia.[2] These effects were attributed to the prevention of edema by hypothermia. More recently, Tator performed similar experiments comparing normothermic and hypothermic spinal cord perfusion.[86] Normothermic perfusion provided the same protection as that previously attributed to hypothermia; the benefits were at least partly due to the perfusion itself. The perfusion may be responsible for diluting the excess norepinephrine at the injury site.

Osterholm controlled accumulation of norepinephrine at the injury site through a biochemical blockade, using alpha methyl tyrosine, which significantly reduces norepinephrine synthesis.[64] This exerted a potent protective effect against the development of progressive hemorrhagic necrosis. Alpha methyl tyrosine is extremely toxic and cannot be used in humans. Studies published in 1974 have not confirmed the elevated norepinephrine levels following experimental spinal cord trauma. The Journal of Neurosurgery has devoted its January 1974 (Volume 40) issue to experimental spinal cord injury. The work of Hedeman and Naftchi deals specifically with the

catecholamine levels following experimental trauma.[31a, b, 57a]

Kelly administered hyperbaric oxygen (two atmospheres) to animals with experimental spinal cord injury, finding the technique as effective as hypothermic perfusion in reversing experimental paraplegia.[44] Ducker also demonstrated similar protective effects, produced by the systemic administration of dexamethasone; intrathecal depomethylprednisolone was less effective.[24]

Experience with Newer Techniques in Humans

Although many neurosurgeons are using localized spinal cord cooling in spinal cord injury patients, the procedure must still be classified as experimental. Despite the fact that some of White's patients with functionally complete lesions showed improvement following hypothermic perfusion, he cannot categorically advise the procedure. If localized spinal cord hypothermia is to be performed, it must be performed early after the injury, and the spinal cord must appear anatomically intact. White emphasized the importance of careful patient assessment before and after spinal cord hypothermia, if any meaningful data are to be obtained.[95]

In view of the experimental data demonstrating the protective effects of glucocorticoid steroids, patients with any degree of spinal cord injury should receive steroids as soon as possible following injury. I have used dexamethasone, 10 mg initially, followed by 4 mg every four hours, in adults. I have used neither dehydrating agents (mannitol or urea) to reduce swelling nor low molecular weight dextran to improve the microcirculation. Myelotomy has been used in the past during the acute phase of injury but, to my knowledge, is not presently being employed.

It will be practically impossible to statistically prove the effectiveness of any form of therapy for human spinal cord injury. Unlike the controlled trauma in animal experiments, the lesions in humans are more diverse. During the early stages after injury, when appropriate therapy must be instituted, the anatomical or physiological completeness of the spinal cord is rarely known. Although motor and sensory function may be entirely lacking by neurological examination below the level of an apparently complete transverse spinal cord lesion, it is occasionally possible to demonstrate sensory conduction in the spinal cord by using averaged cortical evoked potential (CEP). In the past, the neurologic examination has been the only effective technique to determine the functional integrity of the spinal cord; averaged CEP, although still largely experimental, will possibly become an important tool in the evaluation and management of patients during the acute phase of spinal cord injury.

Treatment of Patients with Progressive Neurological Signs During the Stage of Acute Injury

Almost everyone considers progression of neurological signs as an indication for operation in patients with spinal cord injury. Three patients in the Kentucky series of 141 with cervical spinal cord injuries (1964–1971) required an emergency operation for progressive neurological signs. Two of these patients had flexion injuries with "tear-drop" fractures, and the third developed a Brown-Sequard syndrome 48 hours following the open reduction of locked facets. All three patients had anterior operations (two vertebral body replacements and one Cloward procedure) and were found to have disc and/or bony fragments compressing the spinal cord. All rapidly improved following operation. Laminectomy was originally advocated for progressive neurological signs, and without doubt has been successful in arresting the progression of neurological signs in many patients. A more rational approach to the problem of progressive neurological deficit is an anterior operation rather than laminectomy, for the anterior approach most frequently provides direct access to the lesion producing the progressive neurological deficit. Rarely, progression of neurological signs will result from intramedullary hemorrhage and edema. The management of this condition is discussed under "Experimental Techniques."

The Disadvantages of Laminectomy in the Treatment of Acute Cervical Spinal Cord Injuries

The routine performance of laminectomy on patients with cervical spinal cord injury is to be condemned. No longer can the attitude of "everything possible has been done" or "it cannot hurt" be accepted. Guttmann, Harris, and Verbiest have emphasized not only the futility but also the dangers of routine laminectomy following cervical spinal cord trauma.[27, 30, 91] Furthermore, laminectomy and dentate ligament section may not relieve compression if there is a significant kyphos, particularly if there is an extruded disc fragment anterior to the spinal cord. The importance of the role of dentate ligament section in "decompression" of the spinal cord has been questioned by the work of Brieg.[14] He has demonstrated that the dentate ligaments do little to fix spinal cord movement in the dorsal-ventral plane; however, the spinal cord is fixed in the axial plane by the dentate ligaments. There is no proof that decompression plays any role in arresting the progression of intramedullary spinal cord hemorrhage and edema.

Recently, in a retrospective survey of a group of patients admitted to a rehabilitation unit, Morgan found that 65 per cent of patients were made worse by laminectomy performed later than 48 hours following injury, and 23 per cent were worse following laminectomy done within 48 hours of injury.[56] No report was given on the number of patients having laminectomy for progression of neurological signs. Improvement in relationship to operation was difficult to assess, since improvement of incomplete lesions is common, regardless of the treatment. In the group having laminectomy, acceptable alignment of the spine was not achieved in 40 per cent of the patients with incomplete lesions, despite the fact that many patients had primary fusions. Morgan has further investigated the group of patients having laminectomy following flexion injuries and found that laminectomy removes the last vestige providing stability to the injured spine, producing a markedly unstable deformity as a final result.[57]

Anterior Fusion for Fractures and Dislocations of the Cervical Spine

The advantage of anterior cervical fusion for injuries to the cervical spine have been clearly stated.[19, 30, 34, 92] The ultimate objective in the treatment of any patient with a spinal cord injury is the restoration of the patient's condition to the highest level of function dictated by his neurological damage. In terms of morbidity, the patient should be restored to a functional state in the shortest possible time and with the least discomfort. Early anterior operation (mean time following injury — five days) in most patients affords almost immediate mobility of the patient, avoiding many of the physical and psychological complications attending prolonged bed confinement associated with spinal cord injury.[30] Along with Perret, I recommend early operation; in contrast, Braakman recommends delayed surgery (two weeks or more) for fear of contributing to the patient's respiratory insufficiency. Such problems should be anticipated in patients with and without operation, and most can be prevented with meticulous respiratory care.[12]

In contrast to Verbiest,[92] many surgeons have not excluded patients with complete transverse spinal cord lesions from their early operative group.[30, 34, 79] The strongest arguments favoring early operation upon patients with complete lesions — a group destined to remain permanently quadriplegic — is early mobilization and institution of physical therapy, plus decompression of the nerve roots at the level of injury.

Through an anterior approach, bone and disc fragments compressing the spinal cord and nerve roots are easily removed; however, the importance of removing these fragments for nonprogressive spinal cord lesions continues to elicit controversy. Guttmann believes that the intraspinal fragments have little bearing on the ultimate neurological recovery and "if nature is given a chance, by proper positioning of the broken spine, the displaced vertebra and fragment in the great majority of cases will find their correct place." I disagree with his philosophy, based upon the following observations. In 10 autopsy cases, Harris found acute posterior protrusions of the intervertebral disc, and in four additional cases there was severe compression of the cervical spinal cord by bone fragments.[30] Four patients had had almost complete lesions which became complete and three others had complete lesions which ascended to produce respiratory failure. Raynor discovered bone and/or disc fragments in the spinal canal in one third of the cervical spine injury patients he studied.[68] In cases of "tear-drop" fractures, reduction following adequate traction is usually inadequate, and the degree of spinal cord compression found at anterior operation is almost always greater than suspected from the radiographs. In my series of patients with crushed vertebral bodies treated by vertebral body replacement, 12 of 20 patients had significant bony or disc material compressing the spinal cord. There was little correlation between the neurological status and the presence of bone or disc fragments within the spinal canal; six patients had complete spinal cord lesions, and six had incomplete lesions. It is impossible to obtain statistical proof that relief of spinal cord compression ultimately produced a neurological recovery superior to nonoperative treatment. The report of Verbiest suggests that persistent spinal cord compression may play an important role in delaying neurological recovery.[92] Some patients, who had not improved with up to three and one half months of nonoperative treatment, promptly recovered following an anterior reduction of a dislocation or correction of the kyphosis, combined with the removal of intraspinal disc material. The exact mechanism by which improvement is afforded is unknown, but is thought most likely to be relief of vascular compression. Every possible effort that does not jeopardize the patient's safety should be made to reduce spinal cord compression in the hope that it will have a favorable influence upon the neurological recovery. Removal of spinal cord compression in a patient with an acute complete transverse lesion has no beneficial effect upon the recovery of spinal cord function below the transverse lesion, but preservation of nerve root function immediately above the lesion, and the possible prevention of an ascending spinal cord lesion by removal of spinal cord compression is another matter.

Pierce has stressed the importance of sparing even one root level and significantly improving the patient's rehabilitation potential when dealing with a complete transverse spinal cord lesion.[66] In the past, probably too little attention has been paid to nerve root function at the level of injury in patients with complete spinal cord transection. In an analysis of patients requiring vertebral body replacement, all patients with a complete spinal cord transection had some degree of impaired motor root function at the level of the fractured body.[61] Motor root function invariably improved with the passage of time. Frequently, the degree of nerve root compression found during an anterior operation is most impressive, and this can easily be relieved by operation. Braakman has shown the importance of reducing locked facets for the optimal recovery of nerve root function, even in patients with complete spinal cord transection.

In contrast to laminectomy, the anterior surgical approach to the spinal cord, if properly performed, offers little hazard of further injury to the spinal cord. In none of Verbiest's 41 surviving patients was there evidence that the operation had aggravated the neural deficit. In our analysis of 58 anterior cervical operations for trauma, we could detect no loss of neurological function following operation. For technique see pages 116 to 120.

Complications Following Anterior Cervical Operations

"There is indeed great danger that one becomes so inspired by the novelty of the technique of approach, by the handsome radiopgraphic pictures that can be obtained postoperatively, that one loses sight of the indication and pays little attention to the neurological results."[12] The surgeon performing anterior operations for traumatic conditions of the cervical spine must not disregard Braakman's important statement; only by heeding this can complications be avoided. In the Kentucky series of acute closed fracture-disloca-tions of the lower cervical spine (excluding atlas and odontoid process), 58 of 115 patients (50 per cent) had an anterior cervical fusion performed.

The most common problem encountered following surgery is respiratory insufficiency. This condition may not be a direct complication of surgery, since it frequently appears in the nonoperative group of patients (see General Care). Verbiest reported postoperative respiratory obstruction secondary to retropharyngeal hematoma or edema. Although some of our patients have experienced some difficulty in swallowing for a short time from retropharyngeal swelling, the airway has not been threatened.

Graft displacement following operation can be avoided by proper graft placement and by recognizing the degree of fixation afforded by inserting an appropriate bone graft. With certain injuries, particularly anterior dislocations associated with torn posterior ligaments and vertebral body fractures which are accompanied by facet fractures, it may be difficult to achieve immediate firm fixation during an anterior operation; these patients require up to three weeks' recumbency. I agree neither with Perret, who believes all patients need to be kept in skeletal tongs for two to three weeks following an anterior fusion nor with Verbiest, who recommends four weeks' traction following surgery.[65, 92] Rarely are my patients kept recumbent following operation; graft displacement or loss of vertebral alignment has not been a real problem.

Postoperative wound infections must be avoided. Only one superficial infection occurred in our series of 58 anterior operations.

Contraindications for Early Anterior Operation

Respiratory insufficiency is the most common contraindication to early anterior operation. In many patients, the respiratory problems can be corrected with an endotracheal tube and ventilatory assistance for 48 to 72 hours. Operation is performed only after the respiratory problem has been corrected. If a tracheostomy is required, the patient is no longer considered a candidate for anterior fusion. In our experience, individuals requiring early tracheostomy usually have a protracted need for respiratory assistance which, in most instances, precludes early anterior fusion; these patients' fractures are managed with tong traction. Tracheostomy, rarely required following operation, may be accomplished four days after the fusion without any great fear of infecting the fusion wound, as long as the two wounds do not communicate through the subcutaneous spaces.

Posterior Cervical Fusion for Acute Injuries to the Cervical Spine

Rogers and Forsythe, as proponents of early posterior fusion for cervical spine injuries, were the forerunners of today's advocates of anterior fusion.[25, 71] The philosophy of early rehabilitation and prevention of further injury to the nervous system by posterior fusion has today largely been replaced by a philosophy of anterior fusion. The posterior approach, however, is still indicated for locked facets which cannot be reduced by traction; in which case, operative reduction may be combined with posterior cervical fusion. For technique see pages 127 to 131. Others prefer the anterior approach, even when the facets are locked, for spinal reduction and fusion.[19, 92] Posterior fusion for lesions at C1–C2 will be discussed in a later section.

PROGNOSIS FOLLOWING CERVICAL SPINAL CORD INJURY

Mortality

Modern patient-care techniques no longer permit us to complacently accept the death of a patient with a cervical spinal cord injury. No patient's death should be allowed to pass without a careful analysis of what could have been done to prevent it. Early mortality following operation varies from 15 per cent in Verbiest's series to 10 per cent in Perret's series. Guttmann's nonoperative series mortality was 7.6 per cent, which is not comparable to most operative series. Verbiest and Perret did not report their nonoperative deaths, while Guttmann's figures represent a more selected series of patients referred to a spinal injury center.

In the Kentucky series, considering deaths within 60 days as directly attributable to the acute effects of injury, there were 13 deaths (nine per cent) among the 141 patients admitted with significant cervical spine injuries (sprains and minor fractures excluded). Nine patients died from the complications associated with progressive pulmonary insufficiency related to complete transverse lesions. Three patients died of the effects of severe head injury and spinal cord injury, and one patient died from pulmonary embolism. Only one patient did not have a complete transverse lesion. In the operative group there were three deaths following 76 cervical spine operations, an operative mortality of 3.9 per cent; all those who died had complete spinal cord lesions. There were 24 patients in the operative group who had a complete lesion of the cervical spinal cord, representing a 12.5 per cent operative mortality in this group.

Considering all patients, operative and nonoperative cases, with "severe neurological damage," Harris reported 13 deaths in 70 patients, a mortality rate of 18 per cent.[30] In the Kentucky series, there were 92 patients with severe neurological damage, and 13 deaths, an overall mortality rate of 14 per cent.

Prognosis for Neurological Recovery

COMPLETE LESIONS

The prognosis for ultimate recovery can largely be predicted by the neurological state during the acute phase of injury. Braakman observed 71 patients who were admitted within several hours after injury; all had complete transverse cervical spinal cord lesions — a complete, flaccid paralysis, complete sensory loss, and reflex loss below the level of injury.[12] Within six hours after surgery, five patients had some return of function, and two additional patients regained function from six to 24 hours following injury. At 24 hours following injury, 64 of the 71 patients still had a complete neurological lesion which remained unchanged. Thus, if a complete traumatic lesion is still present at 24 hours following injury, it is almost certainly irreversible. A tonic flexor plantar response, with a short interval between stimulus and the response, or priapism, were particularly poor prognostic signs.

INCOMPLETE LESIONS

Spinal cord concussion is extremely rare, and is mentioned only for the sake of completeness. Following injury, there may be a complete loss of motor and sensory function below the level of injury. The signs completely resolve within a matter of minutes to a few hours. Concussion may occur following minor trauma in patients with congenital anomalies of the craniospinal junction, particularly when spinal instability exists.

Almost all cases of incomplete injury to the spinal cord can be divided into: 1) the anterior cord syndrome, 2) the central cord syndrome, 3) the Brown-Sequard syndrome (cord hemisection), or 4) the posterior cord syndrome.

In a careful, long-term analysis of incomplete lesion of the cervical spinal cord, Bosch found that 60 per cent of the patients with an acute central cervical spinal cord syndrome ultimately became ambulatory and achieved functional use of their hands; somewhat less (53 per cent) regained bladder control.[9] Late during the course of treatment about one fourth of the patients developed progressive neurological deterioration, characterized by increasing spasticity. In my experience, this condition is not usually due to spinal cord compression. However, a careful investigation is warranted to exclude a correctable lesion.

The prognosis for recovery from the anterior cord syndrome is extremely poor. In Bosch's series, of 12 patients with this condition, none recovered voluntary motor, bladder or bowel function.[9] In patients with complete motor paralysis with minor degrees of sensory preservation, whose signs do not fulfill the diagnostic criteria of the anterior cord syndrome, the expected functional recovery is also quite poor.[12]

About 90 per cent of patients with Brown-Sequard syndrome recover all function; the posterior spinal cord syndrome is also associated with a good prognosis for complete recovery.

Recovery of nerve root function is good following appropriate treatment. If the neurological deficit is due to destruction of anterior horn of the spinal cord or root avulsion, rather than a compressive lesion of the nerve root, then return of motor function will be poor.

Delayed Progressive Neurological Loss

Harris clearly outlined the most common causes of late progression of neurological signs.[31] These include lack of treatment resulting from failure to recognize and diagnose the condition—either the fault of the surgeon or the patient who did not seek medical attention—and inadequate treatment—although the lesion was recognized initially, management was improper—which includes failure to obtain late radiographs to determine spinal stability.

Either pain at the site of an old injury or the appearance or progression of neurological signs usually brings the patient with the chronic lesion to the attention of the surgeon. Treatment must be carefully planned to avoid further damage to the nervous system. Holdsworth has emphasized that manipulative reduction of an old dislocation is impossible and operative reduction is fraught with hazard to the spinal cord. In the presence of a normal neurological examination, he stated that it is often better to leave the spine unreduced, or, if the neck is painful, it should be fused in the deformed position. In discussing dislocation with locked facets, Braakman advised operative reduction if the dislocation was from two to four weeks old.[11] Reduction was contraindicated if the dislocation was more than six weeks old, because the chance of success was poor and the attempted reduction might aggravate the neurological symptoms. In one case, neurological signs appearing three and one-half years following bilateral dislocation were successfully treated by laminectomy without reduction.

Spinal instability is the most common cause of the delayed onset of pain and progressive neurological difficulty. Instability may result in increasing subluxation, angulation, deformity, or the development of traumatic arthritis with excess callus, all of which produce a dynamic compression of the spinal cord and nerve roots. It is rare for pain or progressive neurological deficit to occur as a result of a fixed deformity unless it be due to arachnoiditis.[11, 19, 76] This does not condone the acceptance of deformity as a final result in the treatment of fracture-dislocations. Occasionally, new symptoms may result from the development of spondylosis at the interspace above or below a fused interspace presumably secondary to hypermobility of the joint adjacent to the treated injury.

The demonstration of a pseudoarthrosis may be accomplished by obtaining flexion and extension views of the spine; occasionally, cineradiography or laminography will also be helpful. Myelography at this stage is almost always indicated to further clarify the etiology of the trouble. Anterior interbody fusion offers a successful approach to late progressive deformity or instability. In unstable "teardrop" fractures, vertebral body replacement may be required, and is preferable to laminectomy and dentate ligament section.

FRACTURES AND DISLOCATIONS OF THE ATLAS AND AXIS

The Atlas

Atlantal fractures most commonly result from a blow to the vertex of the skull by a semicompressible or soft object, with the vertebrae below the atlas fixed in a rigid vertical alignment. Most commonly, slight extension of the head at the craniospinal junction produces a fracture of the posterior arch of the atlas at its weakest points, the vertebral artery grooves just behind the lateral masses (Fig. 11–9),[80] Fractures at this site make up approximately two thirds of all atlantal fractures, while the remaining one third are burst fractures. The anatomical configuration of the atlas makes it especially liable to burst fractures. The wedge-shaped lateral masses, having centrally directed apices, articulate with the skull above and the axis below. Both lateral masses are joined by the relatively thin anterior and posterior arches, which are easily fractured when the lateral masses are driven apart by a force applied to the vertex (Fig. 11–9B). In addition to separation, the force is frequently severe enough to produce compression of the lateral masses. Goeffrey Jefferson's name is rightfully attached to the burst fractures of the atlas. His comprehensive in-

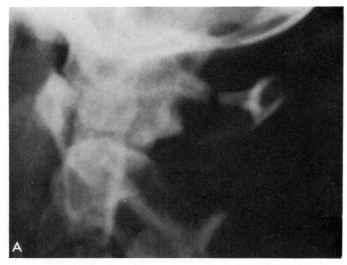

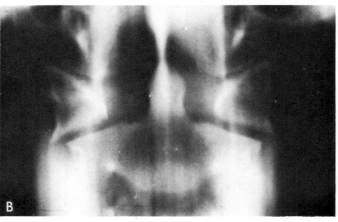

Figure 11–9. Two fractures of the posterior arch of the atlas (A) are accompanied by separation of the lateral masses (B). A fracture through the anterior arch must be present for the separation to occur.

vestigation, reported in 1920, left little to be added to the mechanism of injury and pathology of fractures of the atlas.[38]

Symptoms associated with fractures of the atlas include occipital and suboccipital pain along with neck stiffness. These symptoms are not unique to fractures of the atlas but also occur with fractures of the axis and injuries to the ligaments connecting these structures. Signs of spinal cord injury are rarely observed with fractures in this area, since the spinal canal is wide in proportion to its neural contents, and when burst fractures occur the fragments are centrifugally separated. Fractures of C1 rarely produce immediate death of the victim.[23]

Lateral radiographs usually reveal posterior arch fractures, and the open-mouth anteroposterior projection is sufficient to diagnose burst fractures; further clarification may be obtained by anteroposterior tomograms. The hazard of radiographic overinterpretation in this area, caused by rotation and lateral bending, has been pointed out by Sherk.[80] Frequently, fractures of the atlas are accompanied by fractures of the lower cervical spine. These must not be overlooked. Occasionally, only a single fracture line will be seen across the posterior arch. In all likelihood, a second fracture will be present, but not seen on the radiographs. It is most difficult to produce a single fracture in a rigid circle (atlas). If displacement of the posterior arch has occurred, more than one fracture is necessarily present. Uncomplicated fractures of the posterior arch pose no particular problem in therapy. Support of the neck in a brace results in healing. Even if fibrous union takes place, results of treatment are excellent.

Burst fractures require careful treatment, if proper healing is to occur. The same anatomical configuration of the atlas that results in the burst fracture accounts for the problems encountered in properly aligning the fragments. The axial pull of the cervical muscles attached to the skull tends to maintain and exaggerate the separation of the lateral masses. Only by judicious use of tong traction can appropriate alignment be established and healing take place. This usually involves a minimum of eight weeks in tong traction, the amount of traction weight being dictated by the position of the fragments. Treatment by traction is usually followed by three to four months of external support. Again the Minerva jacket cannot be substituted for tong traction.

TRAUMATIC DISLOCATIONS OF THE ATLAS WITHOUT FRACTURE

Immediately fatal cervicomedullary junction injuries often result from atlantal displacement secondary to ligamentous rupture without fracture.[23]

A less severe injury is traumatic rotary fixation of the atlantoaxial joint. Although Wortzman reported 23 cases without associated fractures, Abel described fractures in 31 of his 47 cases.[1, 101] The etiology of this condition is poorly understood; it is thought to be due not to ligamentous rupture but to damage to the atlantoaxial joints, or possibly the joint capsules. Persistent asymmetry of the odontoid process in its relationship to the lateral masses of the atlas, not correctable by rotation, is the radiologic criterion of diagnosis (Fig. 11–10). This appearance persists after signs and symptoms have disappeared and the late deformity enables the differentiation from torticollis and muscle spasm. Symptoms usually disappear spontaneously, but three of 23 patients in Wortzman's series required cervical spine fusion for persistent pain.

Systemic disease states, including rheumatoid arthritis, Down's disease and pharyngeal infections in children, result in spontaneous atlantoaxial dislocation secondary to relaxation of the transverse ligament of the atlas.[53, 85, 88] Such changes should not be attributed incorrectly to traumatic dislocation.

The Axis

ODONTOID PROCESS

Fractures of the odontoid process frequently are not shown or are overlooked on the initial radiographic examination. Occipital and suboccipital pain, identical to that described with fractures of the atlas, is a common symptom. Occasionally, a patient with an undiagnosed odontoid fracture will enter the emergency ward supporting his chin with one hand and the occiput with the other. Such patients usually give a history of a neck injury resulting in suboccipital pain associated with a feeling of impending doom.

The mechanism of injury producing a fracture of the odontoid process is not clearly understood. Selecki produced a fractured odontoid process in a cadaver spine by compression forces comparable to a blow to the vertex with the spine held in extension; in ad-

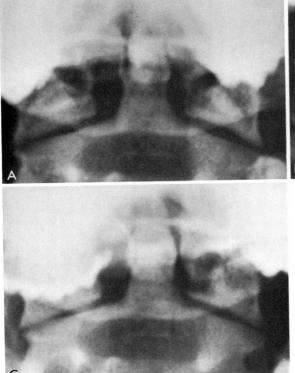

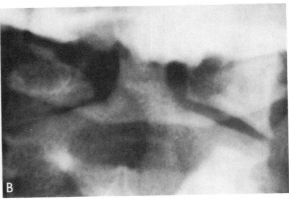

Figure 11–10. Rotation fixation of the atlantoaxial joint. *A,* In the neutral position there is an approximation of the left atlantal articular mass to the odontoid process. With 15° rotation of the head to the right *(B)* and to the left *(C)* the abnormality persists. In the normal spine, turning the head to the left would increase the distance between the left atlantal articular mass and the odontoid process.

dition, there were other fractures of the upper cervical spine.[79] Blockley was unable to produce an odontoid process fracture in cadavers.[8] Schatzker pointed out that the fracture is usually the result of a high velocity force and not the result of simple shearing force transmitted by the powerful transverse ligament or an avulsion produced by the alar ligaments.[72] He believes fractures of the odontoid occur as a result of a combination of these forces; displacement results from the shearing force.

The open-mouth anteroposterior and lateral radiographs are used as screening views of the odontoid process. The radiographic diagnosis of fractured odontoid process may be difficult to establish even in the presence of excellent radiographs. If doubt exists, tomography must be obtained, and then, occasionally, a question may remain. Delayed diagnosis caused by overlooking the fracture on the original radiographs is not rare.

Fractures of the odontoid process most commonly occur at the base. The fracture line traverses the base of the odontoid process at the level of the groove on each side which separates the odontoid process from the lateral mass (Fig. 11–11). Twenty-five per cent of the fractures occur higher on the odontoid process, approximately midway between the base and tip of the process.[72] In young children, the fracture line usually runs through the epiphyseal plate, a level somewhat lower than the usual base fracture in adults.[8] In a child, the fracture may be overlooked on the anteroposterior radiograph, since the epiphyseal line is normally radiolucent. Displacement of the odontoid process on the lateral radiograph establishes the diagnosis. This should not be confused with developmental anomalies of the odontoid process.

Two publications dealing with odontoid process fractures are mentioned chiefly for historical interest, since these often-quoted articles are misleading. In 1928, Osgood and Lund reported a mortality rate of over 50 per cent associated with fractures of the odontoid process, creating a continuing impression that such fractures have an extremely high mortality.[62] Fractures of the odontoid process resulted in death of the acute injury victim in four of 50 autopsied cases from the Baltimore Medical Examiner's Office, but the mortality rate in treated patients is low.[23] The second publication, by Amyes and Anderson in 1956, has given rise to an erroneous conclusion that following treatment non-union was rare.[5] In a review of 63 cases, treated by a variety of techniques, the authors reported that all but three fractures healed or "became immobilized" after four to nine months; no distinction was made between bony union and fibrous union. Neither article reflects modern treatment or diagnostic statistics.

Fractures of the body of the atlas with or without displacement of the odontoid process are not considered true odontoid process fractures. Bony union usually occurs in these body fractures; whereas, the incidence of non-union following true odontoid process fractures remains high. Schatzker, in a careful study of 37 cases of odontoid process fractures, found a 63 per cent overall incidence of non-union.[72] When posterior displacement of the odontoid process accompanied the fracture, 89 per cent of the cases were found to result in non-union; 42 per cent of the undisplaced fractures went on to non-union. These findings have been confirmed in a small number of patients reported by Solovay.[83] Tomograms should be obtained as a routine posttreatment evaluation of patients with odontoid process fractures.

The incidence of hypermobility of the atlantoaxial joint following non-union is unknown, but pseudoarthrosis (fibrous union) of the odontoid process does not imply gross instability.[8, 72] Schatzker concluded that an incidence of 64 per cent non-bony union after apparently adequate closed treatment (six weeks in skull traction followed by six weeks in a Minerva jacket) was unacceptable.[72] He advised posterior atlantoaxial fusion in all patients who expect to lead a normal life, subjected to the ordinary hazards of living. In contrast, Braakman is opposed to operative intervention in any cases of odontoid fracture.[12] He prefers tong traction followed by at least three to four months of plaster immobilization.

I favor posterior bony fusion of the atlas through C3 for fractures of the odontoid process. The surgical technique has been demonstrated by Alexander.[3] Inclusion of the occiput in the fusion is completely unnecessary. Successful posterior cervical fusion certainly does not insure that an odontoid process fracture will heal by bony union; in Schatzker's series 60 per cent of the fractures treated by surgical fusion failed to unite, despite the immobilization produced by a successful posterior fusion. Rogers also reported non-union of the odontoid following surgical fusion of the atlas to the axis.[71]

More recently, Kelly has advocated posterior fixation, using the combination of acrylic and wire, and McLaurin reported on simply wiring the atlas and axis; neither group

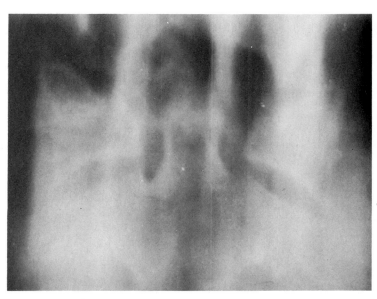

Figure 11–11. This undisplaced fracture, low across the base of the odontoid process, could only be demonstrated by laminagraphy.

used bone grafts.[43, 54] In three of McLaurin's 12 patients, the wire was found to be broken on followup radiographs. Internal wire fixation can hardly be considered permanent, since the wire frequently breaks from fatigue or becomes loose at the site of its bony attachment owing to pressure absorption. I question the advisability of not using bone grafts since non-union of the odontoid process is so common, even after a successful posterior bony fusion. For technique see pages 124 to 127.

OTHER FRACTURES OF THE AXIS

HANGMAN'S FRACTURE. In 1965, Schneider reported a series of patients with bilateral arch fractures of the axis, without an odontoid fracture, with or without dislocation of the atlas on the third cervical vertebra (Fig. 11–12).[77] Such fractures are almost identical to those produced by judicial hanging when a submental knot was employed, hence, the descriptive name "hangman's fracture." Automobile accidents account for the majority of modern-day hangman's fractures.

The mechanism by which the fracture-dislocation occurred in judicial hangings was extensively discussed in Schneider's publica-

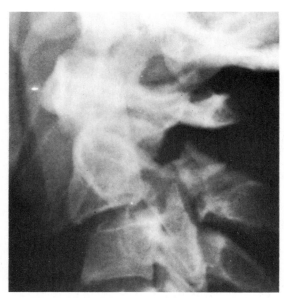

Figure 11–12. A bilateral pedicle fracture of the axis (Hangman's fracture) is the result of a hyperextension injury, but frequently results in a forward subluxation of the axis on C3.

tion. The weakest point of the "cervicocranium" (a functional unit composed of the cranium, atlas and axis) is the junction of the neural arch of the axis with the body. In judicial hanging, the hyperextension and distraction caused by the force of the "drop," and the position of the submental knot produced the neural arch fractures, allowing marked separation of the cervicocranium from the more caudal cervical spine. The extension component of the injury was also responsible for the frequent disruption of the intervertebral disc between the axis and the third cervical vertebra, as well as the occasional avulsion fracture of the anteroinferior surface of the axis, or the anterosuperior surface of the third cervical body.

Death from judicial hanging probably resulted from a combination of marked stretching and tearing of the spinal cord and compression produced by the marked dorsal displacement of the cervicocranium. Cornish agreed that this fracture, which he termed "traumatic spondylolisthesis," is mainly the result of extension; but vertical compression may be an additional force in the modern-day fracture.[22]

The neurological deficit resulting from the modern version of the fracture is, fortunately, less dramatic than that previously obtained by the hangman. Only two fatalities resulted from hangman's fractures in the autopsy series of fatal craniospinal injuries.[23] The apparent low incidence of serious spinal cord injury resulting from hangman's fracture is presumably due to the generous anteroposterior diameter of the spinal canal in the upper cervical region and the absence of the strong distractive force occurring with hanging. Schneider reported medullary and pontine neurological signs in three of his patients, and attributed these to ischemia, produced either by vertebral artery insufficiency or to small-vessel impairment. All of these signs eventually disappeared.

The hangman's fracture is rarely overlooked on the initial lateral radiograph. When present, a more careful search for other cervical vertebral fractures should be made, since the incidence of multiple fractures is frequent. Once the diagnosis of hangman's fracture has been established, skull tongs are applied, chiefly to provide immobilization. Any forward dislocation which has occurred between the axis and the third cervical is easily corrected by positioning the head with minimal weight on the tongs (five pounds or less). Cornish warned that skull traction is illogical "in that it runs parallel in effect to the most deadly form of judicial hanging."

If dislocation is present on the original radiograph, indicating disruption of the intervertebral disc, the patient is a candidate for early anterior interbody spinal fusion. In the absence of dislocation, the patient, in traction, is allowed several days to recover from the acute pain and muscle spasm; then, flexion and extension views are obtained under the supervision of the surgeon. If dislocation occurs, anterior interbody fusion is performed, and the patient, wearing a neck brace, is immediately allowed out of bed. If no dislocation occurs, the tongs are removed, and he is fitted with a cervical brace and allowed to be out of bed. Radiographs are repeated at increasing intervals until bony union has occurred. In three of 14 cases reported by Cornish, early ambulation without operation was allowed, based upon absence of dislocation on flexion and extension radiographs.[22] Schneider prefers treatment by skeletal traction for six weeks, followed by bracing for another two months. Satisfactory bony union occurs at the fracture site following all appropriate forms of treatment. Inadequate treatment may result in a chronic subluxation of the axis on the third cervical body.

THORACOLUMBAR FRACTURE DISLOCATIONS

Fractures and Dislocations Involving the Thoracic Spine T1–T9

This portion of the thoracic spinal canal contains the spinal cord and its associated thoracic nerve roots. The physiological response to trauma of this spinal cord segment is identical to that described in the cervical spinal cord. The spinal canal below T9 or T10 contains roots of the cauda equina, a unique arrangement in the spinal canal; fractures below T9 are considered in a separate category.

Closed fractures involving the T1–T9 segment of the spine are rare, accounting for only 25 per cent of all fractures of the thoracic and lumbar spine (excluding anterior wedge fractures in older patients, particularly females, which may or may not be traumatic).[93] Fractures commonly result from a strong

force being directly applied to the dorsal surface of the thoracic spine. The upper portion of the spine may be sheared from the lower part by fractures of the articular processes and rupture of the ligaments. Such fractures are frequently immobilized by the attached rib cage.[34] Simple wedge fractures, from extreme flexion, also occur in this portion of the spine, are stable, and rarely result in injury to the spinal cord. Burst fractures of the T1–T9 area of the spine are rare, since the relatively fixed dorsal kyphosis usually results in anterior flexion wedge fractures even from a force transmitted directly along the vertical axis of the spine. In my experience, if the force of the injury is sufficient to produce a spinal cord injury at this level, the lesion is usually complete. This has been confirmed by others.[26]

Immediate laminectomy is contraindicated for traumatic myelopathy in the thoracic region for the same reasons discussed in the section on cervical spinal cord injury. Stability usually poses no problem, and there is rarely an indication for any operative procedure, including fusion, during the acute injury phase. Late instability has been recorded following laminectomy for flexion compression fractures of the thoracic spine.[70] Progressive neurological deficit rarely occurs following injury to the thoracic spinal cord. Although I have had no experience with the transthoracic anterior approach to the thoracic spinal cord for traumatic lesions producing progressive spinal cord compression, this approach has great appeal. Cook, using Hodgson's technique, described transthoracic anterior approach for traumatic lesions, but his two operations involved the lower thoracic and lumbar spine.[21, 33] The need for such an operation in the T1–T9 region following trauma will indeed be rare. For technique see pages 135 to 140.

For the patient with either a complete transverse spinal cord lesion or no neurological deficit and an apparently stable fracture, we have tended to allow early mobilization after the pain of the acute injury has subsided. In the rare patient with an unstable injury caused by marked separation of the bony segments, six weeks' recumbency or an anterior fusion is indicated. In patients with a partial spinal cord lesion, even if the bony injury is judged stable, I avoid early mobilization, treating them with four to six weeks' bed rest for fear of producing further spinal cord injury.

Fractures and Dislocations Involving the Thoracolumbar Junction and Lumbar Spine

Holdsworth was particularly interested in fractures of the thoracolumbar junction and spent many years studying patients with these fractures, which were common from coal mining accidents around Sheffield, England. The worker in a low tunnel would be hit in the thoracic spine by falling coal, forcing the thoracolumbar spine into extreme flexion.

MECHANISMS OF INJURY

Fractures of the thoracolumbar junction are generally considered to be the result of: 1) flexion compression; 2) axial compression; 3) lateral rotation, which is rather unique to this portion of the spine; or 4) tension stress (discussed with Lap Seat Belt Injuries). Holdsworth considered flexion compression fractures to be stable, but Roberts added that instability may result when there is posterior ligamentous disruption.[70] Weitzman reported that if severe wedging occurred (a loss of anterior height of greater than 50 per cent), the fracture should be considered unstable.[93] Dis-

location with facet locking, which commonly occurs in the cervical region, is rare at the thoracolumbar junction or in the lumbar area. In contrast to the more horizontal facet joints of the cervical region, the lumbar facets are vertically situated, making overriding almost impossible.

The lateral rotation fracture is produced by the superior vertebral body being forcefully rotated on the next lower vertebra. The superior vertebral body and intervertebral disc remain attached to a typical slice fragment of the upper surface of the lower vertebra; one or both articular facets are usually fractured and dislocation may occur (Fig. 11–13). Tension stress injuries usually occurring with lap seat belt injuries will be discussed in a separate section.

NEUROLOGICAL MANIFESTATIONS

Holdsworth extensively studied the neurological manifestations of the thoracolumbar junction injuries; frequently, both the terminal spinal cord (conus medullaris) and the roots of the cauda equina are affected.[34] Complete paraplegia, with a level at the first lumbar cord segment, is due to a combination

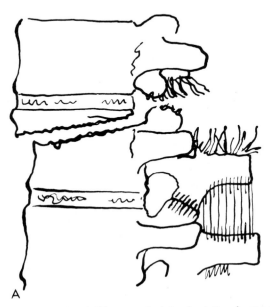
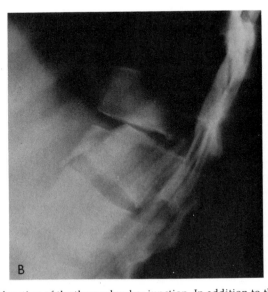

Figure 11–13. *A,* Diagram of a lateral rotation fracture-dislocation of the thoracolumbar junction. In addition to the slice fracture through the vertebral body, the posterior ligaments are avulsed. *B,* Rarely is the radiographic picture identical to the diagram. The fracture line is commonly spiral and not parallel to the x-ray beam. Usually, the fracture results in an anterior displacement of only a portion of the vertebral body. Forward dislocation of the vertebra above the level of the fracture with disruption of only the upper one third of the fractured vertebral body is characteristic.

of damage to both the conus, containing the sacral spinal cord segments, and to all of the cauda equina roots. A thoracolumbar junction fracture which produces only sacral motor and sensory deficit is entirely due to conus damage, with sparing of the lumbar cauda equina roots. Combinations of a complete conus lesion and incomplete cauda equina injury can be explained by varying degrees of root escape. It is particularly important to recognize the difference between the conus lesion (spinal cord) and the cauda equina lesion (nerve root), since the prognosis for recovery in each is quite different. Holdsworth emphasized the importance of repeated examinations for the detection of any residual motor or sensory function of the sacral segments of the cord, which, if present, has good prognostic significance.[34] As in other areas of the spinal cord, if no function of the conus is present within 24 hours following injury, the lesion is probably complete. Also, presence of the anal or bulbocavernosus reflex in the absence of motor power or sensation is indicative of an upper motor neuron lesion and is a poor prognostic sign.

Since the position of the conus medullaris is variable in its relationship to the lower thoracic and upper lumbar vertebrae, I have arbitrarily chosen T10 as the upper vertebral level to be considered in the treatment of thoracolumbar injuries.

TREATMENT

Probably no other area of spinal fracture treatment offers a greater dilemma than the thoracolumbar junction. Holdsworth, recognizing the potential for neurological recovery and the frequent instability of the fractures at this site, believed stability at the fracture site to be of paramount importance. His chief concern was the unstable rotational fracture-dislocations at the thoracolumbar junction. His patients without neurological deficit were treated on a plaster bed for 12 weeks. When paraplegia existed from fractures at the thoracolumbar junction, Holdsworth recommended open reduction with double plating of the spinous processes, followed by eight to 12 weeks' recumbency. He considered vertical compression fractures of the thoracolumbar junction to be stable, and patients with this fracture were treated by eight to 12 weeks of recumbency. In contrast to Kaufer, Holdsworth did not recommend internal fixation for all fracture-dislocations below the thoracolumbar junction.[40] Kaufer recommended early internal fixation for all lumbar fracture-dislocations, with or without neurological deficit. Holdsworth's entire treatment regimen was based upon the premise that proper alignment and ultimate stability were all important. He chose to ignore the importance of residual intraspinal bone fragments, so common with burst fractures. Guttmann, reviewing the English experience with open spinous process plating, condemned it on the basis that it did not prevent redislocation and late angulation.[29] He preferred "postural reduction" for all thoracolumbar fractures and dislocations, but admitted that delayed major redislocation did occasionally occur, producing increasing neurological symptoms. In this event, late operation was required to achieve fixation. Guttmann also chose to ignore the role of intraspinal fragments or other lesions causing compression of the cauda equina nerve roots. In addition to direct compression injury, the roots of the cauda equina may prolapse through dural and arachnoidal tears at the level of vertebral disruption; root scaring would prevent full recovery.[31]

In the United States, patients having thoracolumbar junction and lumbar spine fractures with neurological deficit have generally been treated by early laminectomy aimed at providing an optimal chance for recovery for the injured cauda equina roots, yet laminectomy may result in spinal instability.[67] Roberts studied a group of patients with profound neurological deficit from thoracolumbar fractures, almost all having had an early laminectomy.[70] Burst fractures remained stable, but all rotational fractures at the thoracolumbar were unstable and were accompanied by a progressive spinal deformity. Occasionally, minor wedge flexion fractures showed progressive spinal deformity, seemingly as a result of laminectomy. Progressive deformity of the lower thoracic and lumbar spine may be due to a continuing anterior collapse of the vertebral body secondary to avascular necrosis of the damaged vertebral body (Kummell's disease).[29, 74] Despite the progressive deformity, instability is rarely demonstrated by flexion and extension radiographs. This further emphasizes the necessity for a long-term clinical followup, including radiographs, in all patients with spinal injuries. Progressive angulation should be treated by an anterior vertebral body replacement.

Kelly and Whitesides, recognizing the frequent instability following laminectomy and the importance of retained intraspinal fragments, have utilized Hodgson's technique of anterior spinal decompression and fusion when anterior instability threatens the conus or the cauda equina roots.[45] For the delayed progressive anterior deformity, the anterior spinal fusion is the procedure of choice. We have chosen this approach as the primary mode of treatment in a small number of patients with neurological deficit. All had potentially unstable injuries, or intraspinal bone fragments at the thoracolumbar junction. The removal of the involved vertebral body and adjacent intervertebral discs provides access to the anterior dura, allowing decompression of the cauda equina and the simultaneous insertion of a tibial bone graft. The results thus far have been gratifying, both in neurological recovery as well as in absence of late deformity.[15] We have not performed this operation below L2 and doubt that the necessity would often arise, since most fractures at the lower levels are stable. For technique see pages 140 to 146.

From 1966 through 1970, we, in conjunction with the orthopedic surgeons, utilized twin Harrington rods in the treatment of 21 patients with thoracolumbar fracture-dislocations. Katznelson has reported a smaller series of nine patients in which Harrington rods were used following thoracolumbar trauma.[39] In our patients with unstable fracture-dislocations and complete spinal cord transection, above the origin of the cauda equina, no laminectomy was performed; Harrington rods were inserted and a posterior bony fusion performed. In patients with cauda equina injury, a laminectomy was performed; an intradural exploration provided access to bony fragments and permitted the repair of dural lacerations. Harrington rods were then inserted, and a posterolateral bony fusion was performed. All patients were allowed to move about out of bed, as dictated by their neurological status, soon after operation. Three patients required late removal of loose Harrington rods, and two patients with fracture-dislocations at the thoracolumbar junction developed progressive anterior vertebral collapse due to failure of the rods and the bony fusion. In the majority of patients with incomplete lesions of the conus medullaris and cauda equina, the neurological status was worse immediately following operation. I do not know whether this was due to the laminectomy or the manipulation required to reestablish spinal alignment with the Harrington rods. The neurological loss produced by surgery was ultimately regained in all patients. The correction of the spinal deformity following operation was frequently impressive. Nevertheless, based upon our total experience, we have abandoned the procedure.

For stable wedge compression fractures of the thoracic and lumbar spine, in a patient without neurological deficit, we have allowed early ambulation. Symptomatic results and anatomical reduction are similar to, or perhaps better than, those achieved by hyperextension casting, although Guttmann still opposes early mobilization.[27, 93] Initially, the patient is kept comfortably at bed rest until the acute symptoms of pain and ileus subside. Then he is allowed to roll about in bed and begin hyperextension exercises. One week following injury, the patient is usually walking. Hyperextension exercises are continued, with the patient avoiding flexion, for the first three weeks. No bracing is used.

Fractures of the lumbar transverse processes may occur as a result of direct trauma, or indirectly as a result of muscular pull. Frequently, the muscular pull will greatly displace the fragments so that bony fusion will not occur.[74] Fractures of the transverse process are particularly painful, but only a short term of immobilization is necessary in the treatment of this injury.

Lap Seat Belt Injuries

Lap seat belt injuries are discussed separately from other injuries to the thoracolumbar spine, since both the mechanism producing the injury and the resulting fracture-dislocations are unique. In addition, characteristic soft tissue wounds frequently accompany the injury. Lap seat belts have largely been replaced by a shoulder and lap restraint system, which should reduce the number of characteristic lap belt injuries. In an extensive review of injuries associated with wearing seat belts, Williams concentrated primarily upon the extraspinal injuries.[99] He was able to collect 87 cases of lap belt injuries, with 42 victims having intra-abdominal injuries. Characteristically, the intra-abdominal injuries include intestinal contusions and seromuscular tears and perforations; mesenteric tears are also common. Only one third of the victims had abdominal-wall ecchymoses at the site where the lap seat belt crossed the lower abdomen, although this pattern was seen in 20 of Smith's 24 cases.[88] The lap belt, which should be worn below the iliac crests, usually produces injury to the abdominal wall or peritoneal contents by being worn above the iliac crests or by migrating above the crests during the accident.

Smith has extensively studied the spinal injuries associated with lap seat belt accidents. Normally, the flexion axis of the intact lumbar spine is through the center of the intervertebral discs. In the presence of a lap seat belt, the axis of spinal flexion is shifted forward to the point at which the restraining belt is in contact with the abdominal wall and iliac crests. The forward shifting of the flexion axis is thought to be responsible for the rather unique fractures and dislocations occurring with lap belt injuries. With the entire spine posterior to the flexion axis, all components are subjected to tension stress, resulting in bony or ligamentous failure during distraction (Fig. 11–14).

In reviewing 24 cases, it was found that the spinal disruption occurred between the first and second lumbar vertebra in all but six cases.[82] In 20 typical cases, there was a consistent pattern of separation of the posterior spinal elements, while anterior vertebral body compression was either absent or minimal. In

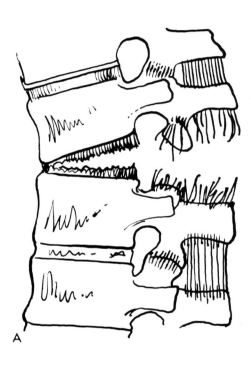

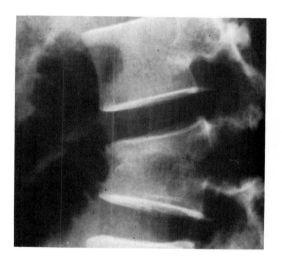

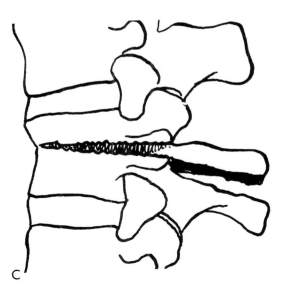

Figure 11–14. Trauma sustained while wearing a lap seat belt is responsible for tension stress injuries resulting in either *A,* ligamentous disruption without fracture or *B* and *C,* the Chance fracture extending through the vertebral body, transverse processes and posterior elements.

some patients, separation of the posterior elements had occurred entirely as a result of rupture of the posterior ligaments and intervertebral disc, without any evidence of neural arch fracture. Occasionally, one or both superior articular facets were avulsed.

In five patients, the line of disruption passed entirely through bone, producing a horizontal fracture line extending across the vertebral body, continuing posteriorly through the pedicles, transverse processes, laminae, and spinous processes. The intraspinous ligaments remained intact, and there was little or no bony displacement. This fracture was first described by Chance and now his name has become an eponym associated with this fracture (Fig. 11–14).[17]

Severe neurological deficit appeared only four times in Smith's 24 cases, and none occurred with a Chance fracture. Most commonly, the neurological injury is the result of extreme dislocations resulting from ligamentous rupture. These injuries are quite unstable in contrast to the Chance fracture. Surgical treatment should follow the guidelines expressed for other lumbar fractures.

Delayed Neurological Signs Associated with Stable Thoracolumbar Injuries

Progressive neurological deficit due to spinal instability or deformity has already been discussed. Delayed surgical exploration or reexploration of the cauda equina and conus may be indicated in patients with static, partial lesions. Ransohoff's basic indication for reexploration is the persistence of disabling neurological signs which have remained fixed for at least six months.[67] A myelogram is performed, and if it is abnormal, surgical exploration is performed. The surgical goal is to relieve all extradural compression and to release dural-arachnoidal adhesions. Ransohoff believes that the intradural aspect of the operation is the most important. The dural-arachnoidal adhesions are dissected, with the aid of the operating microscope; no attempt is made to separate individual roots. The dural covering is reconstituted by primary closure or a dural substitute. In Ransohoff's series, all 15 patients demonstrated neurological improvement over the preoperative state, and in over 80 per cent of the patients, this improvement was functionally significant.[67]

Harris emphasized the neurological significance of a fixed deformity in partial conus or cauda equina lesions. He pointed out that fixed gross displacement should be corrected, since this is not the condition for the neural tissues to achieve recovery of function.

COMPOUND WOUNDS OF THE SPINE AND SPINAL CORD

The minority of spinal injuries encountered in civilian practice are compound wounds; only 15 per cent (41 of 273) of the spinal injuries treated at the University of Kentucky were compound wounds. Bullet wounds, usually from low velocity hand guns, account for most civilian compound spinal injuries.

War wounds, created by shell fragments or high velocity bullets, cause extensive soft tissue destruction and bony fragmentation. Such injuries must be treated by established technique of extensive wide debridement.[55] This technique is not necessarily applicable to civilian injuries. My discussion will be limited to compound injuries encountered in civilian practice, particularly low velocity bullet wounds.

Yashon reviewed 65 cases of civilian gunshot wounds resulting in spinal cord injury.[102] If there was immediate and complete loss of neurological function below the level of injury, recovery did not occur, with or without laminectomy. With incomplete spinal cord injury, progressive recovery, anticipated following closed injury, did not occur with compound wounds, although only five patients with incomplete lesions were observed over a long term. Recovery was only slightly better in 23 patients with injury to the conus medullaris and cauda equina. Surgery probably has less to offer in terms of improving neurological recovery in compound wounds than it does in closed injury of the spinal cord.

Certain similarities exist between acute closed and compound spinal injuries: 1) The presence or absence of a block on Queckenstedt test has little or no bearing on the ultimate prognosis; 2) laminectomy does little to improve ultimate recovery of neurological function; and 3) a normal-appearing spinal cord seen at operation, in the face of a functionally complete lesion, does not improve the prognosis for ultimate neurological recovery.

Gunshot wounds producing spinal cord injury often are associated with serious intra-abdominal or intrathoracic injuries. The appropriate treatment of these immediately life-threatening extraspinal injuries should take precedence over any surgical procedure on the spine. Tetanus prophylaxis must be accomplished according to the principles governing any gunshot wound.

Myelography has a very limited role in the management of patients with compound spinal wounds. The likelihood of producing arachnoiditis is great when Pantopaque is introduced into bloody cerebrospinal fluid, a common finding with compound wounds.

In the past, gunshot wounds have been operated upon chiefly as a prophylaxis against central nervous system infection. The necessity for debridement has possibly been overemphasized, since none of Yashon's nonoperative group (30 per cent of his entire series) developed infection—all received antibiotics.[102] At Kentucky, we have not operated upon 36 per cent of our patients with bullet wounds causing spinal injury, and there have been no infections in this group.

Indications for surgery include: 1) an entrance wound in the paraspinous region, close to the point of spinal injury, providing a short, direct pathway for micro-organisms, or a potential subarachnoid-cutaneous fistula; 2) a situation in which fecal contamination from the peritoneal cavity might have access to the subarachnoid space; 3) marked bony comminution within the spinal canal, or a missile located within the canal, both of which may act as a foreign body nidus within the subarachnoid space; 4) high velocity missile wounds (from high-powered rifles); 5) the occurrence of progressive neurological deficit; 6) cauda equina injury; and 7) the rare, persistent subarachnoid-pleural fistula. In general, I have not operated upon critically ill patients, or on those in whom the bullet apparently did not enter the spinal canal, although major neurological deficit may be present. Surgery for debridement and dural closure is performed when the patient's general condition permits; haste is unwise. If surgery cannot safely be performed within 48 hours following injury, the need for it should be even more seriously questioned. All patients not having surgery receive prophylactic antibiotics; I have not administered post-operative antibiotics to patients having early surgery, when there has been appropriate tetanus immunization and no gross wound contamination.

Spinal instability, even following laminec-tomy, is not a problem with civilian gunshot wounds, since the injury rarely produces total bony or ligamentous disruption.

References

1. Abel, M. S.: Occult Traumatic Lesions of the Cervical Vertebrae. St. Louis, Warren H. Green, Inc., 1965, 148 pp.
2. Albin, M. S., White, R. J., Acosta-Rua, G., and Yashon, D.: Study of functional recovery produced by delayed localized cooling after spinal cord injury in primates. J. Neurosurg. 29:113–120, 1968.
3. Alexander, E., Jr. and Davis, C. H., Jr.: Reduction and fusion of fracture of the odontoid process. J. Neurosurg. 31:580–582, 1969.
4. Allen, A. R.: Surgery of experimental lesion of the spinal cord equivalent to crush injury of fracture dislocation of spinal column. J.A.M.A. 57:878–880, 1911.
5. Amyes, E. W., and Anderson, F. M.: Fracture of the odontoid process, a report of sixty-three cases. Arch. Surg. 72:377–393, 1956.
6. Bailey, R. W., and Badgley, C. E.: Stabilization of the cervical spine by anterior fusion. J. Bone Joint Surg. 42A:565–624, 1960.
7. Benes, V.: Spinal Cord Injury. London, Bailliere, Tindall, and Cassell, 1968, pp. 132–136.
8. Blockey, N. J., and Purser, D. W.: Fractures of the odontoid process of the axis. J. Bone Joint Surg. 38B:794–817, 1956.
9. Bosch, A., Stauffer, S., and Nickel, V. L.: Incomplete traumatic quadriplegia, a ten-year review. J.A.M.A. 216:473–478, 1971.
10. Braakman, R., and Vinken, P. J.: Unilateral facet interlocking in the lower cervical spine. J. Bone Joint Surg. 49B:249–257, 1967.
11. Braakman, R., and Vinken, P. J.: Old luxations of the lower cervical spine. J. Bone Joint Surg. 50B:52–60, 1968.
12. Braakman, R., and Penning, L.: Injuries of the Cervical Spine. Amsterdam, Excerpta Medica, 1971, 262 pp.
13. Brav, E. A., Miller, J. A., and Bouzard, W. C.: Traumatic dislocation of the cervical spine, Army experience and results. J. Trauma 3:569–582, 1963.
14. Brieg, A.: Biomechanics of the Central Nervous System. Stockholm, Almqvist and Wiksell, 1960, 183 pp.
15. Brocklehurst, G., and Norrell, H.: Unpublished work, 1972.
16. Bryant, L. R., Trinkle, J. K., Mobin-Uddin, K., Baker, J., and Griffen, W. O.: Bacterial colonization profile with tracheal intubation and mechanical ventilation. Arch. Surg. 104:647–651, 1972.
17. Chance, G. O.: Note on a type of flexion fracture of the spine. Brit. J. Radiol. 21:452–453, 1948.
18. Cheshire, D. J.: The stability of the cervical spine following the conservative treatment of fractures and fracture-dislocations. Paraplegia 7:193–203, 1969.
19. Cloward, R. B.: Treatment of acute fractures and fracture-dislocation of the cervical spine by vertebral-body fusion, a report of eleven cases. J. Neurosurg. 18:201–209, 1961.

20. Comarr, A. E.: Intermittent catheterization for the traumatic cord bladder patient. J. Urol. *108*:79–81, 1972.
21. Cook, W. A.: Transthoracic vertebral surgery. Ann. Thoracic Surg. *12*:54–68, 1971.
22. Cornish, B. L.: Traumatic spondylolisthesis of the axis. J. Bone Joint Surg. *50B*:31–43, 1968.
23. Davis, D., Bohlman, H., Walker, A. E., Fisher, R., and Robinson, R.: The pathological findings in fatal craniospinal injuries. J. Neurosurg. *34*:603–613, 1971.
24. Ducker, T. B., and Hamit, H. F.: Experimental treatment of acute spinal cord injury. J. Neurosurg. *30*:693–697, 1969.
25. Forsyth, F., Alexander, E., Davis, C., and Underdal, R.: Advantages of early spine fusion in the treatment of fracture-dislocations of the cervical spine. J. Bone Joint Surg. *41A*:17–36, 1959.
26. Geisler, W. O., Wynne-Jones, M., and Jousse, A. T.: Early management of patients with trauma to the spinal cord. Med. Serv. J. Can. *22*:512–523, 1966.
27. Guttmann, L.: Initial treatment of traumatic paraplegia and tetraplegia. *In* Harris, P. (ed): Spinal Injuries. Edinburgh, Morrison and Gibb Ltd, 1965, pp. 80–92.
28. Guttmann, L., and Frankel, H.: The value of intermittent catheterization in the early management of traumatic paraplegia and tetraplegia. Paraplegia *4*:63–84, 1966.
29. Guttmann, L.: Spinal deformities in traumatic paraplegics and tetraplegics following surgical procedures. Paraplegia *7*:38–58, 1969.
30. Harris, P.: Some neurosurgical aspects of traumatic paraplegia. *In* Harris, P. (ed): Spinal Injuries. Edinburgh, Morrison and Gibb Ltd, 1965; pp. 101–112.
31. Harris, P., and Whatmore, W. J.: Spinal deformity after spinal cord injury. Paraplegia *6*:232–238, 1969.
31a. Hedeman, L. S., Shellenberger, M. K., and Gordon, J. H.: Studies in experimental spinal cord trauma. Part I: Alterations in catecholamine levels. J. Neurosurg. *40*:37–51, 1974.
31b. Hedeman, L. S., and Ranajit, S.: Studies in experimental spinal cord trauma. Part 2: Comparison of treatment with steroids, low molecular weight dextran, and catecholamine blockade. J. Neurosurg. *40*:44–51, 1974.
32. Heilbrun, M. P., and Ratcheson, R. A.: Multiple extracranial vessel injuries following closed head and neck trauma, case report. J. Neurosurg. *37*:219–223, 1972.
33. Hodgson, A. R., Stock, F. E., Fang, H. S. Y., and Ong, G. B.: Anterior spinal fusion, the operative approach and pathological findings in 412 patients with Pott's disease of the spine. Brit. J. Surg. *48*:172–178, 1960.
34. Holdsworth, F.: Fractures, dislocations and fracture-dislocations of the spine. J. Bone Joint Surg. *52A*:1534–1551, 1970.
35. Holdsworth, F. W.: Early operative treatment of patients with spinal injury. *In* Harris, P. (ed): Spinal Injuries. Edinburgh, Morrison and Gibb Ltd, 1965, pp. 93–100.
36. Holt, E. P.: Fallacy of cervical discography; Report of 50 cases in normal subjects. J.A.M.A. *188*:799–801, 1964.
37. Jacobson, S. A., and Bors, E.: Spinal cord injury in Vietnamese combat. Paraplegia *7*:263–281, 1970.
38. Jefferson, G.: Fracture of the atlas vertebra. Report of four cases and a review of those previously recorded. Brit. J. Surg. *7*:407–422, 1920.
39. Katznelson, A. M.: Stabilization of the spine in traumatic paraplegia. Paraplegia *7*:33–37, 1969.
40. Kaufer, H., and Hayes, J. T.: Lumbar fracture-dislocation. A study of twenty-one cases. J. Bone Joint Surg. *48A*:712–730, 1966.
41. Kelly, D. L., and Alexander, E.: Lateral cervical puncture for myelography. J. Neurosurg *29*:106–110, 1968.
42. Kelly, D. L., Lassiter, K. R. L., Calogero, J. A., and Alexander, E.: Effects of local hypothermia and tissue oxygen studies in experimental paraplegia. J. Neurosurg. *33*:554–563, 1970.
43. Kelly, D. L., Alexander, E., Davis, C. H., and Smith, J. M.: Acrylic fixation of atlantoaxial dislocations. A technical note. J. Neurosurg. *36*:366–371, 1972.
44. Kelly, D. L., Lassiter, K. R. L., Vongsvivut, A., and Smith, J. M.: Effects of hyperbaric oxygenation and tissue oxygen studies in experimental paraplegia. J. Neurosurg. *36*:425–429, 1972.
45. Kelly, R. P., and Whitesides, T. E., Jr.: Treatment of lumbodorsal fracture-dislocations. Ann. Surg. *167*:705–717, 1968.
46. King, D. M.: Fractures and dislocations of the cervical part of the spine. Aust. N.Z. J. Surg. *37*:57–64, 1967.
47. Krieger, A. J., Christensen, H. D., Sapru, H. N., and Wang, S. C.: Changes in ventilatory patterns after ablation of various respiratory feedback mechanisms. J. Appl. Physiol. *33*:431–435, 1972.
48. Krieger, A. J., and Rosomoff, H. L.: Respiratory and autonomic dysfunction in patients with diseases of the cervical spinal cord. Presented Am. Assn. Neurological Surgeons, Boston, April 20, 1972.
49. Kuperman, A. S., Krieger, A. J., and Rosomoff, H. L.: Respiratory function after cervical cordotomy. Chest *59*:128–132, 1971.
50. Kuperman, A. S., Fernandez, R. B., and Rosomoff, H. L.: The potential hazard of oxygen after bilateral cordotomy. Chest *59*:232–235, 1971.
51. Larson, S. J., Kim, Y. K., and Reigel, D. H.: Gas myelography in the management of spinal cord injury. Scientific exhibit. Clinical Congress, American College of Surgeons, San Francisco, October 2, 1972.
52. Long, D. M., and Story, J. L.: Hyponatremia following bilateral cervical cordotomy. J. Neurosurg. *25*:623–627, 1966.
53. Lourie, H., and Stewart, W. A.: Spontaneous atlantoaxial dislocation. A complication of rheumatoid disease. New Eng. J. Med. *265*:677–681, 1961.
54. McLaurin, R. L., Vernal, R., and Salmon, J. H.: Treatment of fractures of the atlas and axis by wiring without fusion. J. Neurosurg. *36*:773–780, 1972.
55. Meirowsky, A. M.: Neurosurgical management. *In* Meirowsky, A. M. (ed): Neurological Surgery of Trauma. Washington, Office of the Surgeon General, Department of the Army, 1965, pp. 307–325.
56. Morgan, T. H., Wharton, G. W., and Austin, G.: The results of laminectomy in patients with in-

complete spinal cord injury. Paraplegia 9:14–23, 1971.

57. Morgan, T. H.: Personal communication, June 23, 1972.

57a. Naftchi, N. E., Demeny, M., Decreschito, V., Tomasula, J. J., Flamm, E. S., and Campbell, J. B.: Biogenic amine concentrations in traumatized spinal cords of cats. J. Neurosurg. 40:52–57, 1974.

58. Nickel, V. L., Perry, J., Garrett, A., and Heppenstall, M.: The halo. J. Bone Joint Surg. 50A:1400–1409, 1968.

59. Norrell, H. A., Wilson, C. B.: Early anterior fusion for injuries of the cervical portion of the spine. J.A.M.A. 214:525–530, 1970.

60. Norrell, H., and Wilson, C. B.: Letter to the editor. J.A.M.A. 215:2114, 1971.

61. Norrell, H.: The role of early vertebral body replacement in the treatment of certain cervical spine fractures. Proc. 18th Spinal Cord Injury Conf. U. S. Veterans Administration, 35–39, 1971.

62. Osgood, R. B., and Lund, C. C.: Fractures of the odontoid process. N. Eng. J. Med. 198:61–72, 1928.

63. Osterholm, J. L., and Mathews, G. J.: Altered norepinephrine metabolism following experimental spinal cord injury. (Part I) Relationship to hemorrhagic necrosis and post-wounding neurological deficits. J. Neurosurg. 36:386–394, 1972.

64. Osterholm, J. L., and Mathews, G. J.: Altered norepinephrine metabolism following experimental spinal cord injury. (Part II) Protection against traumatic spinal cord hemorrhagic necrosis by norepinephrine synthesis blockade with alpha methyltyrosine. J. Neurosurg. 36:395–401, 1972.

65. Perret, G., and Green, J.: Anterior interbody fusion in the treatment of cervical fracture dislocations. Arch. Surg. 96:530–539, 1968.

66. Pierce, D. S.: Spinal cord injury with anterior decompression, fusion, and stabilization and early rehabilitation. J. Bone Joint Surg. 51A:1675, 1969.

67. Ransohoff, J.: Lesions of the cauda equina. Clin. Neurosurg. 17:331–344, 1970.

68. Raynor, R. B.: Discography and myelography in acute injuries of the cervical spine. J. Neurosurg. 35:529–535, 1971.

69. Roaf, R.: A study of the mechanisms of spinal injuries. J. Bone Joint Surg. 42B:810–823, 1960.

70. Roberts, J. B.: Stability of the thoracic and lumbar spine in traumatic paraplegia following fracture or fracture-dislocation. J. Bone Joint Surg. 52A:1115–1130, 1970.

71. Rogers, W. A.: Fractures and dislocations of the cervical spine. An end-result study. J. Bone Joint Surg. 39A:341–376, 1957.

72. Schatzker, J., Rorabeck, C. H., and Waddell, J. P.: Fractures of the dens (odontoid process), an analysis of 37 cases. J. Bone Joint Surg. 53B:392–405, 1971.

73. Schmonl, G., and Junghans, H.: The Human Spine in Health and Disease. 2nd ed. (Am) New York, Grune & Stratton, 1971, pp. 242–306.

74. Schneider, R. C., Cherry, G., and Pantek, H.: The syndrome of acute central cervical spinal cord injury with special reference to the mechanism involved in hyperextension injuries of the cervical spine. J. Neurosurg. 11:546–577, 1954.

75. Schneider, R. C.: The syndrome of acute anterior spinal cord injury. J. Neurosurg. 12:95–122, 1955.

76. Schneider, R. C., and Kahn, E. A.: Chronic neurological sequelae of acute trauma to the spine and spinal cord. (Part I) The significance of the acute-flexion or "tear-drop" fracture-dislocation of the cervical spine. J. Bone Joint Surg. 38A:985–997, 1956.

77. Schneider, R. C., Livingston, K. E., Cave, A. J. E., and Hamilton, G.: "Hangman's fracture" of the cervical spine. J. Neurosurg. 22:141–154, 1965.

78. Schneider, R. C.: Concomitant craniocerebral and spinal trauma, with special reference to the cervicomedullary region. Clin. Neurosurg. 17:266–309, 1970.

79. Selecki, B. R., and Williams, H. B. L.: Injuries to the Cervical Spine and Cord in Man. Glebe, New South Wales, Australasian Medical Publishing Co. Ltd, 1970, 191 pp.

80. Sherk, H. H., and Nicholson, J. T.: Fractures of the atlas. J. Bone Joint Surg. 52A:1017–1024, 1968.

81. Simeone, F. A., and Goldberg, H. I.: Thrombosis of the vertebral artery from hyperextension injury to the neck. Case report. J. Neurosurg. 29:540–544, 1968.

82. Smith, W. S., and Kaufer, H.: Patterns and mechanisms of lumbar injuries associated with lap seat belts. J. Bone Joint Surg. 51A:239–254, 1969.

83. Solovay, J., and Brice, G. B.: Laminagraphy in the follow-up of fractures of the odontoid process. Am. J. Roentgen. 83:645–652, 1960.

84. Stone, W. A., Beach, T. P., and Hamelberg, W.: Succinylcholine-induced hyperkalemia in dogs with transected sciatic nerves and spinal cords. Anesthesiology 32:515–520, 1970.

85. Sullivan, A. W.: Subluxation of the atlanto-axial joint: Sequel to inflammatory processes in the neck. J. Pediatrics 35:451–464, 1949.

86. Tator, C. H., and Deecke, L.: Normothermic vs. hypothermic perfusion in the treatment of acute experimental spinal cord injury. Surg. Forum 23:435–438, 1972.

87. Taylor, A. R.: The mechanisms of injury of the spinal cord in the neck without damage to the vertebral column. J. Bone Joint Surg. 33B:543–547, 1951.

88. Tishler, J., and Martel, W.: Dislocation of the atlas in monogolism. Radiology 84:904–906, 1965.

89. Thompson, H.: The halo traction apparatus: A method of external splinting of the cervical spine after injury. J. Bone Joint Surg. 44B:655–661, 1962.

90. Towne, J. B., Neiss, D. D., and Smith, J. W.: Thrombosis of the internal carotoid artery following blunt cervical trauma. Arch. Surg. 104:565–568, 1972.

91. Verbiest, H.: Surgery of the cervical vertebral body in cases of traumatic deformity or dislocation. In Harris, P. (ed): Spinal Injuries. Edinburgh, Morrison and Gibb Ltd, 1965, pp. 112–120.

92. Verbiest, H.: Anterolateral operations for fractures and dislocations in the middle and lower parts of the cervical spine. Report of a series of 47 cases. J. Bone Joint Surg. 51A:1489–1530, 1969.

93. Weitzman, G.: Treatment of stable thoracolumbar spine compression fractures by early ambulation. Clin. Orthop. 76:116–122, 1971.

94. White, R. J., Albin, M. S., Harris, L. S., and Yashon, D.: Spinal cord injury: Sequential morphology and hypothermic stabilization. Surg. Forum 20:432–434, 1969.

95. White, R. J., Yashon, D., Albin, M. S., and Demian, Y. K.: The acute management of cervical cord trauma with quadriplegia. To be published in J. Trauma.

96. White, W. A., and Bergland, R.: Experimental inappropriate ADH secretion caused by positive pressure-respirators. J. Neurosurg. 36:608–613, 1972.

97. Whitley, J. F., and Forsyth, H. F.: Classification of cervical spine injuries. Am. J. Roentgen. 83:633–644, 1960.

98. Wilcox, N. E., Stauffer, E. S., and Nickel, V. L.: A statistical analysis of 423 consecutive patients admitted to the Spinal Cord Injury Center, Rancho Los Amigos Hospital, 1 January 1964 through 31 December 1967. Paraplegia 8:27–35, 1970.

99. Williams, J. S.: The nature of seat belt injuries. J. Trauma 11:207–218, 1971.

100. Wilson, C. B., Bertan, V., Norrell, H. A., and Hukuda, S.: Experimental cervical myelopathy. (Part 2) Acute ischemic myelopathy. Arch. Neurol. 21:571–589, 1969.

101. Wortzman, G., and Dewar, F. P.: Rotary fixation of the atlantoaxial joint: Rotational atlantoaxial subluxation. Radiology 90:479–487, 1968.

102. Yashon, D., Jane, J. A., White, R. J.: Prognosis and management of spinal cord and cauda equina bullet injuries in sixty-five civilians. J. Neurosurg. 32:163–170, 1970.

CHAPTER 12

Infectious Disease of the Spine

A. R. HODGSON, O.B.E., F.R.C.S.E., F.A.C.S., F.R.A.C.S.
University of Hong Kong

NON-TUBERCULOUS INFECTIONS OF THE SPINE

History

The early history and bibliography of this condition were well documented by Wilensky in 1929.[107] The early authors recognized two important points: 1) The difficulty of making the diagnosis; and 2) the dangerous complication of spinal cord involvement. The later articles are summarized by Griffiths and Jones.[36]

Frequency

Formerly, invasion of the spine by pyogenic organisms was rarely diagnosed clinically. Postmortem reports suggest that it is more frequently involved than the clinical frequency suggests. In other words, small, subclinical lesions may occur and heal without giving rise to symptoms and signs. Modern methods of diagnosis, including needle biopsy and open biopsy, have led to an increase in the frequency of accurate diagnosis of this condition. This may be illustrated by quoting the ratio of cases of spinal osteomyelitis to general osteomyelitis reported over the years.

1899 *Hahn*   1 case of pyogenic spinal infection in 661 cases of osteomyelitis = .15 per cent.[38]

1929 *Wilensky*   9 cases of pyogenic spinal infection in 578 cases of osteomyelitis = 1.5 per cent.[107]

1936 *Kulowski*   60 cases of pyogenic spinal infection in 1500 cases of osteomyelitis = 3.94 per cent.[60]

1961 *Robinson and Lessof*   10 cases of pyogenic spinal infection in 292 cases of osteomyelitis = 3.42 per cent.[85]

Kulowski emphasized that all patients suffering from sepsis, and I would add to this *particularly* if the sepsis be in the pelvis or abdomen, should be watched carefully for the appearance of spinal complications and, if such patients die, the entire spine should be examined at autopsy.[60]

Sex

These infections are more common in the male, as demonstrated by the following figures:

1906 Donati   68% male[25]
1915 Volkmann   72% male[102]
1929 Wilensky   55% male[107]
1936 Kulowski   74 male, 28 female[60]
1971 Griffiths and Jones   15 male, 13 female[36]

Osteomyelitis in general is more common in the male, but an added factor may be the frequency of pelvic infections in the male ac-

567

cording to Carson and Henriques, among many others.[13, 43]

Age

The age incidence has been increasing over the years. See Table 12-1.

Bremner and Neligan described five cases occurring in children between the ages of nine months and two and a half years.[9] They draw attention to the benign form of this condition, the uniformity of the clinical picture, and the rapid recalcification in the x-ray.

Finch describes the case of a child aged three weeks suffering from a staphylococcal osteomyelitis of the spine.[31]

Site of Vertebral Involvement

The usual seat of the infection in the vertebra is the vertebral body. Griffiths and Jones found it to be involved in every one of their 28 cases.[36] Other sites have been described, probably because of their rarity: the odontoid process, in cases described by Makins and Abbott, Frank, and Leach et al.;[32, 64, 70] the articular process, in one case described by Shehadi;[89] and the transverse processes, in two cases described by Makins and Abbott.[70] The posterior arches of vertebrae have been described by Makins and Abbott in two cases.[66]

Causative Organism

Many different kinds of organisms have been found to cause spinal osteomyelitis. The most common is *Staphylococcus aureus*. A list of some of the organisms is given.

> *Staphylococcus aureus* and *albus*[31]
> *Streptococcus viridans* and *pyogenes*
> *Actinomyces*[29]
> *Aerobacter aerogenes*
> *Escherichia coli*
> *Clostridium perfringens*
> *Proteus*
> *Pyocyaneus*
> *Brucella*[80]
> *Gonococcus*
> *Micrococcus tetragenus*
> *Pneumococcus*
> *Pseudomonas*[105]
> *Serratia marcescens*[21A]
> Enteric group[35, 100, 101]
> > *Salmonella typhosa*
> > *S. paratyphi A* and *B*
> > *S. suipestifer*
> > *S. typhimurium*
> > *S. enteritidis*
> > *S. panama*
> > *S. oranienburg*

Level of Vertebral Involvement

The level of vertebral involvement has usually been recorded by various spinal segments such as cervical, thoracic and lumbar, not by individual vertebra, which is the method of preference. The most frequent segment involved is the lumbar, followed by the thoracic, with cervical and sacral about equal in frequency. Garcia and Grantham have produced a barograph indicating each vertebra involved; although the number is not large, there

TABLE 12-1. INCIDENCE OF NON-TUBERCULOUS INFECTIONS OF THE SPINE ACCORDING TO AGE

	Makins and Abbot[70] 1896	Daverne[20] 1903	Donati[25] 1906	Wilensky[107] 1929	Kulowski[60] 1936	Stone and Bonfiglio[95] 1963	Griffiths and Jones[36] 1971
Under 10 years	5	12	15	2	1	—	} 5
10–20 years	11	6	24	—	32	—	
20–30 years	3	9	11	3	15	—	} 8
30–40 years	—	—	—	4	21	1	
40–50 years	—	—	—	—	14	1	
50–60 years	—	—	—	—	11	3	} 15
60–70 years	—	—	—	—	4	9*	
Total	19	27	50	9	98	14	28

*One over seventy.

is a suggestion of a curve similar to that found in the level of involvement in spinal tuberculosis.[33]

Pyogenic Spondylitis Complicating Posterior Disc Excision

In 1958, Sullivan, Bickel and Svien reported on infections of the spine following removal of the intervertebral disc at operation.[96] Further reports were made by Stern and Crandall in 1959. This condition does not differ sufficiently in management to justify separate description.

Associated Bony Lesions

Kulowski states that lesions in the lower lumbar spine are frequently associated with sacroiliac joint infection, and that other bones may be affected.[60]

Associated Disease

Infection in people suffering from diabetes mellitus is common. This condition was found in five of 15 of Stone and Bonfiglio's cases and ten of Garcia and Grantham's cases.[33, 95] It seems mandatory to perform fasting blood sugar measurements in all cases.

Primary Focus

In general, osteomyelitis, skin infections, boils and impetigo may be the primary focus. However, spinal osteomyelitis often occurs after urinary infections and infections occurring after catheterization and prostatectomy and other pelvic and abdominal infections. Many authors believe the infections to be carried by venous pathways to the vertebral plexus, of which the vertebral body is such an integrated part.

Involvement of the Contents of the Spinal Canal

This occurs in approximately 15 per cent of cases and carries a high mortality. The infection may occur as an epidural infection, either localized or diffuse, or it may penetrate the dura, producing a meningomyelitis.[1, 6, 48] The onset is acute, and spinal root pain is present in about one third of the cases. When the first signs of interference of the function of the spinal cord appear, urgent decompression of the spine is called for.

Symptoms and Signs

GENERAL

The usual symptoms and signs of a general infection should be looked for. Fever varies with the acuteness of the attack, and temperature may be deceptively low. Malaise and loss of weight are usual but in the mild form the patient is surprisingly well. The patient likes to rest a good deal, as he finds the pain to be less when he rests and more when he is active. In the acute form, septicemia may arise. Erythrocyte sedimentation is always markedly raised: an average of 87 mm per hour in Garcia and Grantham's cases.[33] The white blood count may be surprisingly normal, although in the acute form it is raised. In cases in which antibiotics have been prescribed early, the signs and symptoms may be masked and diagnosis made difficult. Anorexia, fretfulness in children, or limping and hip pain in lumbar disease may be noted.

LOCAL

Pain in the spine at the site of the infection is the most constant symptom, and Kulowski found it to be present in all his cases.[60] It is aggravated by movement and may persist as a throbbing ache during rest. Tenderness on deep palpation or percussion of the spinous process is usually elicited, and the process may be slightly prominent. Spinal rigidity on movement, and muscle spasm are common. Abscesses are frequent and may be divided into two types: deep paravertebral, which are difficult to detect on clinical examination, and superficial, which are readily detected clinically. Hip contracture owing to irritation or fibrosis of the psoas muscle is frequent in lumbar disease. Severe kyphotic spinal deformity is not common. In the lumbosacral region, thrombosis of the iliac veins may occur. There may be a limitation of the straight leg lifting test.

Associated Urinary Tract Infection

Carson drew attention to the frequency of infection of the urinary tract; all of his cases had infection.[13] Five of the first six of Turner's cases had urinary tract infection.[99] Henriques, reviewing the literature of infective bone involvement complicating postoperative sepsis in the pelvis, showed that the bone involvement was almost invariably of the spine, irrespective of the causative organism.[43] He postulated spread by way of the vertebral veins and their connections, as suggested by Batson in 1940.[4] Robinson and Lessof found infection following operation upon the urinary tract in five of the 10 cases that they reported.[85] This association has been noted by many: Henson and Coventry, Leigh, Kelly and Weems, Liming and Youngs, Alderman and Duff and DeFeo, among others.[2, 21, 44, 65, 68] Lame described osteomyelitis of the spine following operations on the rectum and sigmoid.[61, 62] Sherman and Schneider reported three cases following septic abortion or postpartum infection.[90]

X-ray Appearances

It is important to x-ray the whole spine, taking anteroposterior, lateral, and right and left oblique views. Tomograms are essential. Myelography is essential if neurological symptoms and signs are present. Angiography and lymphangiography may be required in some cases. It is of great importance that serial x-rays be taken at regular intervals so that the progress of the disease may be followed.[28]

The vertebrae in the thoracolumbar area are most often involved; frequency of vertebral involvement decreases the farther up the spine one goes. Involvements of the odontoid, the transverse process of the cervical vertebra, and the posterior elements of the spine have been described but are rare.

EARLY SIGNS

Early signs include paravertebral abscess shadow, caused by pus or edema, and narrowing of the intervertebral disc. A small area of erosion producing a lytic defect, usually in the superior and/or inferior aspects of the vertebral bodies, is the earliest bony change to be seen (Fig. 12–1, A and B); however, it cannot be discerned within a month of onset of symptoms, and it may take longer. Tomograms will show these bony changes before straight x-rays.

LATER SIGNS

Erosion may produce destruction of the vertebral bodies, which may result in spinal deformity of lateral deviation or kyphosis (Fig. 12–2, A-D). Abscess formation occurs in sites similar to those of paravertebral tuberculous abscess, but are usually smaller. The vertebral body may sustain a pathological fracture and collapse in the same manner as concertina collapse of tuberculous spondylitis.

Reactive sclerosis or increased density, bony bridging, lack of significant osteoporosis, rapid evolution of radiological changes, and complete disc destruction suggest that the lesion may be pyogenic; the diagnosis should be confirmed by recovery of the causative organism from the lesion.

Osteomyelitis in the thoracic spine may involve the lung, presenting characteristic changes on x-ray of the chest.

Occasionally, the appearance of a densely sclerotic or ivory vertebra will be seen in the healing stage. The infection involves two adjacent vertebrae and this may be of help in distinguishing it from malignancy. Spontaneous vertebral fusion is a common finding after the passage of time.

Diagnosis

This may be a perplexing problem on clinical grounds alone. Accurate diagnosis depends on careful bacteriological and microscopic examination of the pus and tissue, which can be obtained by needle biopsy or open biopsy, using anterior spinal approaches. It is very important to identify the causative organism and determine its sensitivity to antibiotics as soon as possible, so that the correct antibiotic therapy may be used. We agree with Stone and Bonfiglio that none of the serological tests help to identify staphylococcal infections with constancy.[95] Blood culture is usually positive in the pyrexia stage. The erythrocyte sedimentation rate is always raised, often to very high levels. Serological tests are helpful in diagnosing Salmonella infections. Polymorphonuclear leukocytosis occurs in acute cases; it is absent in chronic cases, in which there may be leukopenia. A

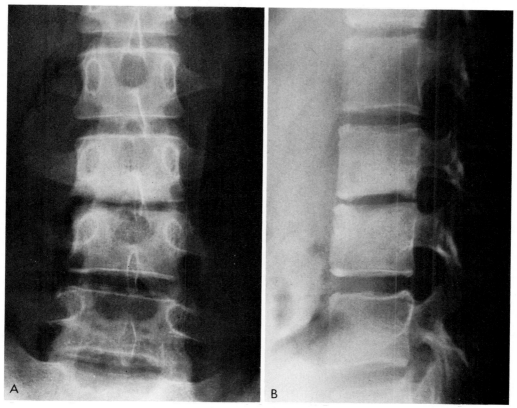

Figure 12–1.   Early pyogenic infection of the spine. *A,* The 13-year-old patient presented with slightly kyphotic apex (L2) and slight pain. She had been treated with antibiotics for urinary tract infection. Note narrowing of the intervertebral disc, and sclerosis with erosion of cartilaginous plate. *B,* Lateral view of same patient, showing same x-ray findings.

negative tuberculin test usually excludes tuberculosis infection.

DIFFERENTIAL DIAGNOSIS

Conditions which must be considered in differential diagnosis include acute pachymeningitis, perinephric abscess, meningitis, suppurative arthritis of the hip, tuberculosis of the spine, and malignancies, either primary or secondary.

Treatment

Two methods of treatment are advocated, conservative and operative. The early writers tended to advocate conservative treatment, but they were quite prepared to approach the posterior elements of the spine and to evacuate abscesses as they appeared.[70] Some more recent authors favor rest and antibiotic treatment in some cases and operative treatment in others. Mayer was an early advocate of operation upon the bodies of the vertebrae.[71] Waisbren recommends the giving of gamma globulin with antibiotics in cases which are not responding to therapy.[103] Kulowski advises operative intervention in all cases where suppuration is evident, and if there is any doubt he suggests exploration.[60] Wiltberger was forced to operate upon a case of osteomyelitis of the bodies of L4–L5 of three years' duration which was resistant to conservative therapy.

Present thoughts on treatment vary a good deal, which is not surprising in a condition sufficiently uncommon and infrequent that adequate experience has not been gained in its management. In Hong Kong, we have had considerable experience in the management of osteomyelitis of the spine caused by tuberculosis, and we use the same principles in other forms of spinal osteomyelitis.

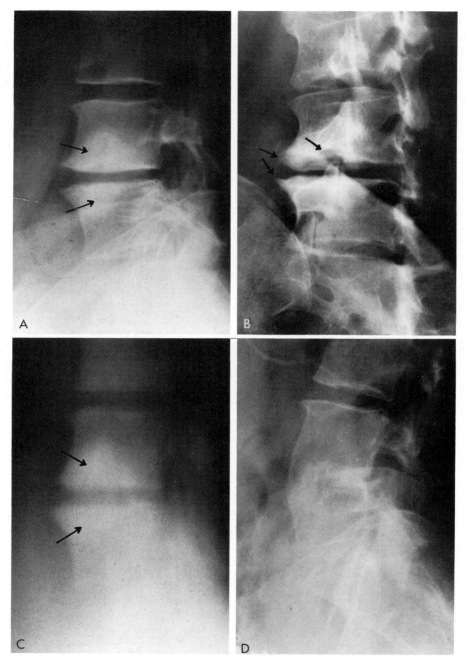

Figure 12–2. *A,* Lateral view of patient with mild infection of contiguous sides of L4-L5. Note increased density. *B,* Oblique view of same case. Note increased density and erosion of undersurface of L4. *C,* Lateral tomogram of same patient. *D,* Lateral view showing result 10 years after debridement and anterior fusion.

The most important step is to recover pus for culture and sensitivity tests. This may be done by vertebral biopsy or at open operation. If open operation is performed, it may be pos-

sible to diagnose the organism with the naked eye from the appearance of the pus. Some authors reserve operative intervention for those cases which do not respond to conservative treatment; a drawback is that it is not always easy to know whether the case is responding or not, and one may find that as time has passed the disease has progressed so that a more severe pathology and a more difficult operative problem result. We prefer to operate early, and to decompress the abscess and evacuate the pus and send it for identification of organism and sensitivity tests. If the stability of the spine is impaired, we stabilize it by an anterior graft. In the cervical spine, skull traction or halopelvic distraction apparatus are useful methods of stabilizing the cervical spine.

Complications are dealt with as they arise. Paraplegia should be treated by careful evaluation of cause using myelogram and tomogram. The cause of the paraplegia is removed at operation by costotransversectomy, anterolateral approach or transthoracic approach. Spinal fusion is not usually needed as the spine usually fuses spontaneously.

Griffiths and Jones state that most of their cases recovered after rest and antibiotic treatment.[36] Skull traction is employed in cases with cervical spine involvement; and plaster of paris beds and halo-pelvic distraction apparatus are utilized at other spinal levels in Hong Kong. Operative intervention has been employed in five cases, with one anterior graft fused.

Mortality Rate

Mortality varies with the type of disease; acute disease carries a higher mortality than does chronic. Following is a list as recorded by various authors: note that mortality was markedly higher prior to the introduction of antibiotics.

TUBERCULOSIS OF THE SPINE

History

An Egyptian mummy of Nesperehân, a Priest of Amûn of the 21st Dynasty, is stated to show tuberculous caries of the thoracic spine, with pronounced kyphosis and a psoas abscess.[27] An illustration of the mummy shows a reversal of the height-width ratio in the vertebral bodies of the lumbar spine; this suggests that the disease occurred during childhood. The date is circa 3000 B.C. Other examples of mummies with skeletal changes suggesting spinal tuberculosis have been described.[22]

The first written description of the disease, given by Hippocrates (c. 450 B.C.), contains a recognizable description of spinal tuberculosis and mentions that the prognosis in disease below the diaphragm is better than that above, an observation which is still true.[47]

It is to Percivall Pott that we owe the first full description of the condition, and this included autopsy findings.[82]

Incidence

The disease has become rare in countries in which there are adequate housing, nutrition and preventive medical measures. It is still prevalent in the densely populated parts of Asia and Africa, and parts of South America.

Site Frequency

Perusal of the site frequency in this disease shows that the spine is involved in over half of the cases of bone and joint tuberculosis. Our figure in 1000 consecutive cases of bone and joint tuberculosis is 58.7 per cent;

Makins and Abbot, 1896 — Mortality 70%[70]
Carson, 1930 — 4 out of 4 survived[13]
Kulowski, 1936 — 15 + 10 out of 102 died[60]
Butler et al., 1941 — 15 out of 16 died[11]
Wiltberger, 1952 — 1 out of 1 survived[106]
Pritchard and Robinson, 1961 — 15 out of 15 survived[84]
Stone and Bonfiglio, 1963 — 15 out of 15 survived[95]
Griffiths and Jones, 1971 — 3 out of 28 died[36]

this is in great contrast with the frequency of vertebral involvement in non-tuberculous infections of the skeleton, which varies between two and five per cent, according to the author.[60] This difference is very significant and will be discussed further under Etiology.

Site of the Lesion

The different parts of the spine are not equally liable to be involved in tuberculosis. Authors have been in the habit of dividing the regions of the spine into cervical, cervicothoracic, thoracic, thoracolumbar, lumbar, lumbosacral and sacral, and this I do not consider a very good way. We prefer to make use of a barograph on which each involved vertebra is indicated by one unit. It will be seen in Figure 12–3 that the peak of the barograph in our 587 consecutive cases of spinal tuberculosis is at L1 vertebra, and that the curves drop evenly away from each side of the peak. This indicates that the infection probably enters the spine at the level of L1. This will be considered further when we deal with Etiology.

Age and Sex Distribution

Males usually outnumber females in most series, but the ratio is similar to that in most populations in which males usually predominate.

The age of involvement varies according to many factors, but usually in an overcrowded, undernourished population the child is exposed to a massive infection early in life and develops the disease in childhood. Twenty years ago in Hong Kong, 70 per cent of spinal tuberculosis patients were under 10 years of age. In well-housed and well-nourished people, the child is usually not exposed to any infection till school age, and it may be that the patient will have reached adulthood before becoming exposed to infection, and subsequently being infected. In some cases, people from a country where tuberculosis has been wiped out, lacking resistance to the disease, have gone to live in a country where the disease is prevalent and contracted the disease. With improvement of antituberculosis measures throughout the world, there is a gradual shift in the age incidence upward.

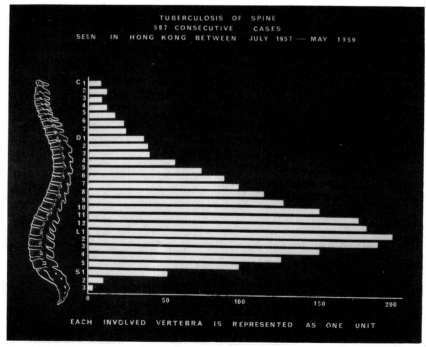

Figure 12–3. Barograph of 587 consecutive cases of spinal tuberculosis occurring in a series of 1000 consecutive cases of bone and joint tuberculosis.

Etiology

There are certain interesting statistical facts which emerge when a large series of consecutive cases of spinal tuberculosis is considered which demand an explanation and in this explanation is the clue to the etiology.

The First Fact. The barograph in the series of 587 cases of spinal tuberculosis occurring in a series of 1000 consecutive cases of bone and joint tuberculosis showed a statistically significant curve with a peak at L1 (Figure 12–3).

The Second Fact. In pyogenic osteomyelitis, the spine is involved in under five per cent of cases, while in spinal tuberculosis the spine is involved in 58.7 per cent.[60] If pyogenic osteomyelitis is an arterial blood-borne disease, can the tubercle bacillus spread by the same route and give such a marked difference in percentage involvement? This could be explained if the tubercle bacilli and the vertebra had some special affinity for each other. All attempts to produce spinal tuberculosis in experimental animals by injecting tubercle bacilli locally into the vertebrae and into the left ventricle of the heart, and producing local spinal injury at periods of time afterwards, as described by Blacklock, failed to produce any spinal disease.[7] We considered the matter carefully and for some time, and the most probable explanation that we could suggest was that a different pathway of spread, either venous or lymphatic, might occur in spinal tuberculosis.

The Third Fact. Other interesting observations which had to be explained were the occurrence of double and triple spinal foci, and spinal lesions associated with tuberculous hip disease and bilateral hip disease (Figure 12–4). The different pathway would have to explain these findings.

A clue appeared in an article by Henriques, in which he reviewed the literature and showed that osteomyelitis complicating infections following upon urological operations usually occurred in the spine, sometimes in the hip joint and occasionally elsewhere in the skeleton.[43] He contended that the pathway of these infections from the primary focus to the spine was by way of the venous pathway, as suggested by Batson.[4] Although the nature of the organisms varied greatly, they settled mainly in the spine. This led us to start a series of animal experiments in which we injected organs in the abdomen and pelvis with tubercle bacilli and sacrificed the animals at periods of time afterwards. We used monkeys, rabbits and rats, and injected mainly the kidney, but also the ovary, the prostate in male monkeys, as well as other parts of the pelvis and abdomen. We were surprised and delighted to find that we could produce a primary infection in the injected organ, usually the kidney, and a secondary lesion in the spine.

We were able to make sections of these animals and to trace the infection from the kidney to the spine by way of the fourth venous plexus. The infection penetrated the lumbar vertebra at the same level as the primary lesion, in monkeys, using the kidney as the primary site, this was usually the second lumbar vertebra, for the monkey has six vertebral bodies in the lumbar spine, and the kidney lies opposite the second. We were able to trace the infection which penetrated the vertebra to the spinal canal and passed upward along the vertebral veins and could produce lesions in vertebral bodies at a higher level. Spread downward was usually along the anterior surface of the vertebral bodies; usually there was no penetration to the lumbar vertebral canal.

We became interested in the fourth venous plexus described anatomically by Breschet, but whose importance as a pathway between the abdomen and pelvis and the cephalic parts of the body for spread of malignant metastases and infections was emphasized by Batson.[4, 10] We made latex injection studies of the plexus in rats, rabbits, monkeys and humans. In the quadruped animal, this plexus is poorly formed and consists mainly of two lateral veins with scanty communications between them. In the biped, the plexus is much larger, with many communications between the two lateral veins. The plexus is an important bypass for venous blood from the lower limbs, pelvis and abdomen when the normal pathway of the inferior vena cava is obstructed, as in the valsalva maneuver, coughing and sneezing, and physical stress which requires holding the breath. A good anatomical description of this plexus in humans is given by Clemens, and the physiological significance has been described by Batson, Herlihy, Eckenhoff, and others.[5, 16, 26, 45, 46]

Living Pathology

In the direct operative approach, using anterior approaches which have been de-

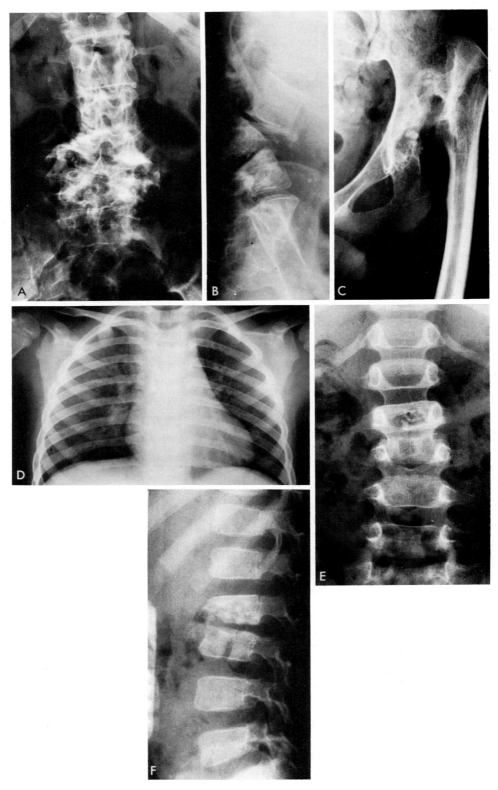

Figure 12–4. *See opposite page for legend.*

scribed previously, we have been able to observe all stages of the disease at the different
levels of the spine and at all ages.[30, 48-50, 54, 55]
Postmortem reports have been small and
sporadic. The only large series reported is
that of Auerbach and, excellent as this report
is, it, by necessity, deals with the final stage of
the disease.[3] In the living patient, we are able
to recognize all stages of the disease, in
particular the early granulation tissue and
necrotic phase, and to assess tissue bleeding
and avascularity.

Pre-pus Phase

The earliest phase is the stage of granulation tissue (Fig. 12–5), which consists of
Langhan's giant cells, epithelioid cells and
round cells. The granulation tissue seems to
have a very close relationship with, and possibly arises from, the veins and is proliferative
in character. We are not sure whether this
spread of granulation tissue takes place in the
lymphatics, in association with the vein, or in
the vein itself. Two findings in our experimental animals suggest that in these animals
the spread was venous. The first finding was in
serial sections of a rabbit, in which a large vein
was found to be thrombosed; however, a few
sections more distally the same vein was
found to be patent. In other animals, we were
able to trace the infection into the spinal cord,
which is stated not to have a lymphatic supply.

When granulation tissue proliferates
greatly, the cells start to swell and the walls of
the cells rupture, presumably from deficient
nutrition; pus forms from the debris of these
cells, and this is the start of a paraspinal
abscess formation.

Very rarely, we have seen a coagulation
necrosis of the tissues surrounding the spine,
instead of a paravertebral abscess. This necrosis appears to be due to a host hypersensitivity to the products of the tubercle bacillus.

We believe that these necrotic tissues in time
become pus and the lesion becomes a paravertebral abscess.

THE PARAVERTEBRAL ABSCESS AND ITS CONTENTS

Once pus forms, we are dealing with a
paravertebral abscess, which is a most important finding in spinal tuberculosis. It was not
till 1940 that Swett, Bennett and Street drew
attention to the "dominant role of the abscess
in the disease."[97] They pointed out that a patient demonstrating an abscess clinically had
active disease and without an abscess no disease. We have failed to diagnose an abscess
clinically and found one at operation in 10 per
cent of our cases, and these have mostly been
cases of lumbar disease, in which the abscess
is more difficult to detect on x-ray.

Pus. As we have seen, pus is the first
content of the abscess and perhaps the most
important. In the early months, particularly in
children, the pus is fluid. The color is a characteristic green-yellow and may contain small
fragments of bone, cartilaginous plate, sloughs
and granulation tissue. As the duration of the
disease lengthens, the pus obtains the consistency of toothpaste and is whiter in color; as
time goes on it becomes caseous, and may
become gritty, solid and off-white in color
after many years.

The paravertebral abscess can become
very large, and often contains a liter or more
of pus. The pressure of the pus has been
measured and is usually in the area of 20 mm
of water, but we have not been happy that this
is an accurate method of measurement. There
is no doubt that the pressure of pus causes the
stripping of the paravertebral tissues seen particularly in the thoracic region; it may play a
part in the production of aneurysmal syndrome and cause some reduction in blood supply to the peripheral portion of the vertebral
body.

Sequestra. As we have seen, the

Figure 12–4.   Spinal tuberculosis. *A,* L3-L4 anteroposterior view. *B,* L3-L4 lateral view. Note that the L3 and L4 vertebral bodies have merged into one, a characteristic finding in this disease. Note also the suggestion of calcification of
the nucleus pulposus of the intervertebral disc in L5 which occasionally occurs. *C,* Patient had associated involvement
of the left hip, which had dislocated. *D,* Hilar shadows suggestive of tuberculosis infection of hilar glomus. *E,* Anteroposterior x-ray of same case. *F,* Lateral view showing tuberculosis including the contiguous surfaces of L2-L3.

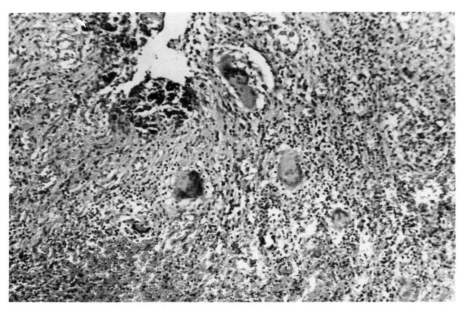

Figure 12–5. Tuberculosis of the spine. Histological section of granulation showing Langhans' giant cells, round cells, epithelial cells, and some calcification.

abscess strips the coverings of the thoracic vertebral bodies or renders them partially or completely avascular. Portions or complete vertebrae die, and any moderate or even minor jar to the spine may cause a pathological fracture of the dead bone and so form a sequestrum. The sequestra may be quite large, measuring from an inch to an inch and a half, but, usually, they are small and difficult to find in the pus; if it were not for the fact that they block the instrument used to suck the contents of the abscess out at the time of operation they might be missed. The larger sequestra tend to detach from the posterior portion of the vertebral body and may be retropulsed onto the spinal cord and become a cause of pressure paraplegia in Pott's paraplegia. Sequestra formation is very frequent in spinal tuberculosis but does not occur in the pre-pus stage of the disease (Fig. 12–6).

The Intervertebral Disc

The intervertebral disc does not become involved as a primary focus, as it is an avascular structure; when this does occur, it is a peripheral involvement and the disc may, and often does, become detached from the destroyed vertebral bodies on either side and may be found loose in the abscess in a fairly complete state.

The x-ray observation that narrowing of the intervertebral disc may be an early sign of spinal tuberculosis is true, but the deduction that "therefore the intervertebral disc is involved primarily in the disease" is not so. What takes place is that the vertebral bodies on either side of the disc are infiltrated with granulation tissue and lose their blood supply, and the disc loses its nutrition and becomes narrow. Indeed, in tuberculosis, the cancellous bone in the vertebral body can be completely destroyed and still present a normal x-ray picture, but tomograms will show the lytic lesion.[42] Occasionally, an intervertebral disc may calcify.

Granulation Tissue

We have described and discussed the formation of granulation tissue. Within the abscess it may be found as pachymeningitis externae, as described by Charcot, lying in close relationship with the dura.[14] If healing takes place, this may turn into fibrous tissue and bone and it may strangulate the cord, causing paraplegia. This paraplegia is recognized clinically by the presence of sensory changes and is rare. This tissue may be found in the cancellous spaces of the vertebral bodies, and usually clothes the internal surface of the abscess wall; with healing it turns into fibrous tissue.

Revascular Phenomenon

This condition was first noted on x-ray and named ivory vertebrae by Souques, Lafaurcade and Terris in 1924. The condition is described on x-ray as a vertebral body which has a normal shape and size but which has a definite increased resistance to x-rays, so the shadow is very white and little of the normal trabecular pattern may be seen.[92] Cleveland and Bosworth described this condition in tuberculosis of the spine and named it avascular necrosis.[17] The phenomenon occurs mostly in the lumbar vertebrae and has long been associated with healing of the disease.

At operation, we found these vertebrae to be very hard, and there was some difficulty in cutting through the bone. Histological studies showed that this was a reossification and revascular phenomenon. The sections showed that the bony lamellae were very much thicker than normal, some three times the normal thickness, and the cancellous spaces were decreased in size. On microscopic examination, these laminae were found to be sandwich-like, the filling being of dead bone which stains very poorly and which has empty lacunae. On either side is new bone, staining well, with lacunae filled with osteocytes, which is new bone growing along the surface of the dead bone and completing the sandwich. In time, the laminae remodel and the vertebra returns to normal density.

Harris and Bobechko described a similar finding in rabbits following division of the femoral neck.[40]

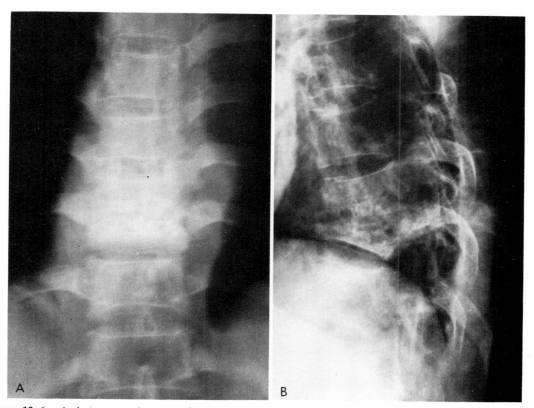

Figure 12–6. *A,* Anteroposterior x-ray showing sequestra between intervertebral bodies. Note bilateral paravertebral abscesses. *B,* Lateral x-ray of same patient, showing sequestration between intervertebral bodies.

"Aneurysmal Syndrome"

This term was coined by Ghormley and Bradley in 1928 and is a characteristic finding in the thoracic spine, particularly in children; it is usually associated with a long paravertebral abscess.[34] We have been able to study this condition at operation and in postmortem specimens; this erosion is usual in the sides and sometimes the posterior portion of the vertebrae, and it occurs in the cervical region. We feel that it is caused by the stripping of the paravertebral ligaments and periosteum, and the resultant loss of blood supply allows that portion of the vertebral body whose nutrition comes from the periosteal vessels to be attached by the tuberculous disease. (Fig. 12–7); this results in a circumferential destruction of the superficial portion of the vertebral body. Schulthess in 1904 described this as superficial anterior spondylitis, regarding it as a significant, if rare, form of spinal tuberculosis. It would appear that this is aneurysmal syndrome under another name.

Concertina Collapse

This name has been given to a state which occurs when a single vertebral body, weakened by permeation with granulation tissue, collapses. As it does so, it tends to protrude radially and may cause paraplegia. This can be confused with the similar x-ray appearance in secondary carcinoma of the vertebral body (Fig. 12–8).

Penetration of the Organs

The paravertebral abscess lies deep within the body and finds difficulty in discharging itself through the body. In an attempt

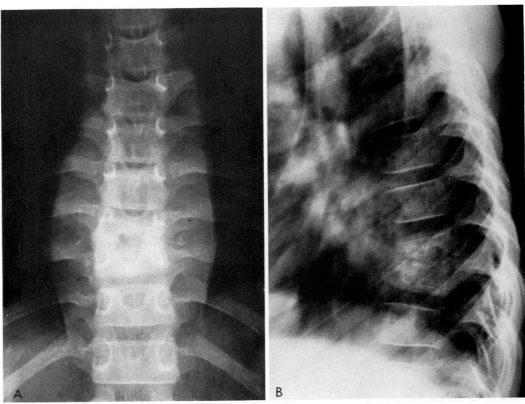

Figure 12–7. *A,* Anteroposterior x-ray showing involvement of D8-D9 by tuberculous disease and a large fusiform abscess. *B,* Lateral x-ray shows tuberculous infection of D8-D9. Note the erosion of the cortex of the vertebral bodies shown in D7, the so-called aneurysmal syndrome. The extent of the abscess denotes the extent of spinal involvement.

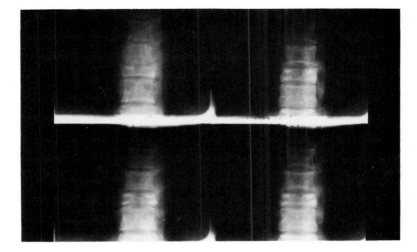

Figure 12–8. Concertina collapse.

to do this, many of the organs of the body have been penetrated, among them the trachea, esophagus, vena cava, bronchus, lung, pleura, pericardium mediastrium, aorta, liver, kidney, ureter, abdominal cavity, intestine, urinary bladder, vagina and rectum.

The most frequently involved organ is the lung, and this is described by Fang, Ong and Hodgson.[30] They reported 327 consecutive cases of thoracic spinal tuberculosis in which there were 32 lung penetrations. The sequence of events appears to be fibrin adhesion formation between the visceral pleura covering the lung and the parietal pleura covering the abscess. This leads to lung collapse in the region of the adhesion formation. The pus penetrates the adhesion area into the collapsed lung, and it is usually sufficient to clear out the abscess in the collapsed lung, spray it with antitubercular drugs and close it. In one case, a wedge resection had to be carried out. In another of our cases, the abscess ruptured into a bronchus during induction of anesthesia and, fortunately, the anesthetist was able to evacuate the pus by suction.[55] Cases have been reported wherein the patient has coughed up pus and sequestra.[105]

Other Spinal Changes

VERTEBRA WITHIN A VERTEBRA. O'Brien, while reviewing the first 500 cases of tuberculosis of the spine in which anterior fusion had been performed, found a case in which this appearance was seen.[75] He explains it, and I think correctly, by saying that the central outline of the vertebral body is that of the vertebral body at the time of operation, showing signs of osteoporosis, and can be compared in appearance with an x-ray taken just before operation. The normal bone which has grown since then has grown forward and upward, but not backward. This suggests that once a bone is osteoporotic in a child it has no hope of recovering, and that osteoporosis is a permanent state of affairs. It also suggests that there is no backward growth of the vertebral body and the obvious result, if there were, would be to narrow the spinal canal.

LATERAL DEVIATION OF THE SPINE. Lovett gives Bartow the credit for describing this in 1889.[69] They drew attention to the main features of the condition, which occurs commonly early in the disease and is confined to the lower thoracic and lumbar vertebrae. Lovett devised an instrument to measure the angle of deviation and found a maximum of 8 degrees in four of the 30 cases he described. In discussing the paper, A. J. Steele states: "If the destruction were greater on one side than on the other, we would have a lateral deviation which was permanent." This is exactly what happens, there is unilateral destruction of the vertebral body. In the experimental animal one can trace the infection from the kidney involved to the side of the vertebrae on which the kidney lies, where a unilateral lesion occurs; and this explains why it is common, occurs early in the disease, and is confined to lower thoracic and lumbar vertebrae.

RIB CHANGES. Kyphosis follows the destruction of the vertebral bodies, and if this occurs in the thoracic region the ribs approximate posteriorly and their inclination forward and downward is changed to a more horizontal direction. If the anterior destruction is extensive, the ribs approximate posteriorly, and the spine may hang on the ribs posteriorly. This changes the shape of the ribs, compressing them from above and below.

BONY BRIDGING. Leri was one of the early authors to describe this condition, in 1912.[67] He observed that the paravertebral ligaments may calcify or ossify when they sustain increased tension, when they are torn, and when they are involved in lesions of vertebral bone or joints. We have had the opportunity to remove these bony bridges at the time of operation and the condition appears, on histological examination, to be due to ossification of the paravertebral ligaments (Fig. 12–9). The condition is more common in the lumbar spine. Its frequency is stated to be 10 per cent. Cofield states that it is confined to patients over the age of twenty years.[18, 19] Lerch states he has seen it in one child.[66] We would agree with Cofield that this condition is confined to adults. Oppenheimer described an interesting case in which a bullet lodged in the second and third lumbar vertebrae and in the intervertebral disc between them.[79] The bullet lay anterolaterally in the vertebral bodies and a local ossification took place in the paravertebral ligaments adjacent to the bullet, but nowhere else.

CHANGES IN THE HEIGHT-WIDTH RATIO AND WEDGING OF THE INTERVERTEBRAL DISCS. In the days when tuberculosis of the spine was treated conservatively, attention was paid to producing what was called compensatory lordosis, both above and below the kyphosis in the growing child. Thus, some compensation for the kyphotic deformity was obtained.

This compensatory lordosis was produced by two changes in the spine: 1) reversal of the height-width ratio; and 2) wedging of the intervertebral disc.

Reversal of the Height-Width Ratio. Normal weight-bearing lumbar vertebrae in the human are wider than they are tall. In spinal tuberculosis with kyphosis in a growing child they become taller than they are broad. This shape is similar to the vertebrae of the quadruped, and the presumption is that the same reason obtains, that they are not weight-bearing and they grow according to Delpech's law, sometimes called the Heuter-Volkman law. Delpech recognized the inhibition of pressure

in epiphyseal growth and the stimulation of growth in release of pressure.

Wedging of the Intervertebral Discs. In addition to the changes in the vertebral bodies, the intervertebral discs become wedged and the nucleus pulposus migrates anteriorly.

X-ray Appearances

The x-ray appearances can be divided into two main categories: 1) soft tissue shadow; and 2) bony changes.

SOFT TISSUE SHADOW. This demonstrates the paravertebral abscess and is best seen in the thoracic spine, as there is good contrast between it and the lung. The shadow may take many forms; it may be fusiform (Fig. 12–10), globular, pyramidal, unilateral (Fig. 12–11), double or fusiform pointed to one side, indicating lung penetration.

In the soft tissue shadow of the paravertebral abscess may be seen sequestra and caseous pus.

BONY CHANGES. The vertebral bodies become osteoporotic at first, and this is followed by erosion most commonly found on each side of the intervertebral disc. Tomograms are very useful to demonstrate early disease within the vertebral body. Further destruction of the vertebral bodies occurs until one or more vertebral bodies are completely destroyed. The changes in the vertebra may appear as concertina collapse, aneurysmal syndrome, lateral deviation, bony bridging, reversal of the height-width ratio of the vertebral body and wedging of the intervertebral disc, calcification of the intervertebral disc, and changes in the ribs.

Special x-ray investigations which may be needed are tomography, myelography, venography, lymphangiography, arteriography, discography and intravenous pyelograms.

Further details may be obtained from Hodgson et al.[48-50, 52-56]

Differential Diagnosis

Usually, there is very little difficulty in diagnosing a case of tuberculosis of the spine. However, where the disease is uncommon it may be more difficult. We would emphasize that the best way of diagnosing the condition is by pathological and bacteriological methods and by fulfilling Koch's postulates.

Conditions which may be confused with

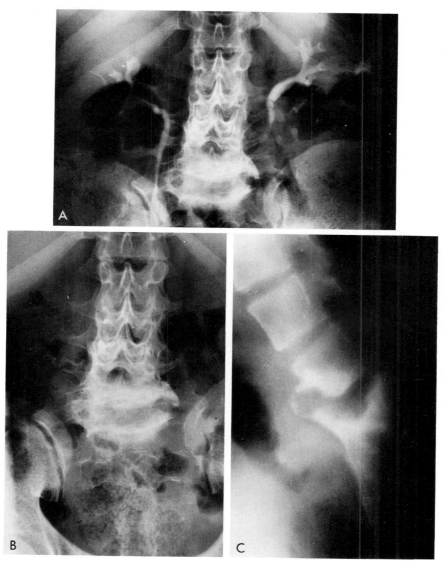

Figure 12–9. *A,* Intravenous pyelogram showing changes compatible with tuberculous infection of left kidney. Tuberculi bacilli were grown from catheter specimen of urine from left ureter. Note tuberculous infection of lumbosacral joint. *B,* Anteroposterior x-ray showing sclerosis and destruction of lumbosacral joint. Note attempt at bony bridging laterally. *C,* Lateral view, showing destruction and sclerosis of L5 and S7 vertebrae. Note bony bridging starting anteriorly.

Pott's disease are:
Low grade pyogenic infections of the spine
Brucellosis
Eosinophilic granuloma (Calvé's disease)
Typhoid fever
Other infections of the spine (Batty strain)
Congenital anomalies (Kyphoscoliosis (see
    Fig. 12–21)
Schmorl's nodes
Scheuerman's disease

Intervertebral disc lesions
Retrospondylolisthesis
Spondylosis
Neoplasms, primary and secondary malignant, innocent
Multiple myeloma
Hemangioma
Hodgkin's disease
Hydatid disease
Leukemia

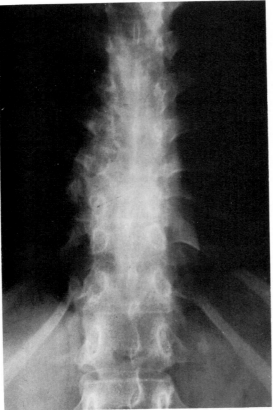

Figure 12–10. Anterior spine. Thoracic fusiform bilateral paravertebral abscess.

Treatment

The history of the treatment of tuberculosis has been varied over the past 2000 years, and falls into two groups: conservative and operative. Up till about 1870, the treatment has been mainly conservative with a few notable exceptions. Pott, and later Charcot, applied a red hot iron into the abscess in cases of paraplegia, to drain the abscess in an attempt to reduce pressure on the spinal cord. With the introduction of Lister's method of antiseptic and later aseptic surgery, operative attacks upon the lesion were carried out in the United Kingdom, United States, France and Germany. This became the first operative era. About 1900, a change in the treatment of tuberculosis occurred. The sanatorium regime was introduced, and this led to the movement of these cases into the country, geographically separated from the general hospitals in towns, and the treatment again became conservative,

possibly owing to the absence of surgeons at the sanatoria. As always, there were treatment exceptions in this era, which lasted into the 1940's. Erlacher of Vienna was a great advocate of surgical treatment during this period.

In 1944, Wilkinson became dissatisfied with the results of conservative treatment and taught himself to operate by way of a costotransversectomy to curet out the lesion in the spine. With the introduction of the antitubercular drugs, the operative era started again, and Orell and Kastert led the operative groups in their respective countries, using a costotransversectomy approach. In the United Kingdom, Capener, in 1932, introduced lateral rhachotomy, and later Dott and Alexander extended the costotransversectomy approach; later still, Griffiths, Roaf and Seddon extended the approach to an anterolateral approach.

These approaches were really all posterolateral approaches and, in 1955, the author, together with Professor F. E. Stock,[48] devised

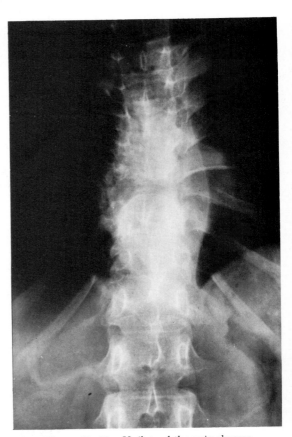

Figure 12–11. Unilateral thoracic abscess.

anterior approaches to the spine at various levels and postulated the principles of treatment of tuberculosis of the spine as:

1. Removal of all the avascular contents of the abscess, fluid or caseous pus, sequestra, sequestrated intervertebral discs, sloughs, avascular bone, and granulation tissue, so as to leave a raw, bleeding bed.
2. If this leaves an unstable spine, it should be stabilized. Because it is very difficult to stabilize the spine by posterior and lateral methods in the presence of an anterior defect, an anterior fusion is used.

It must be appreciated that certain cases of spinal tuberculosis will heal without treatment of any kind. A greater proportion will heal when antitubercular drugs are given. In order to have the largest percentage of healed cases in the shortest possible time, anterior debridement and fusion should be the treatment of choice.

There are three major defects in conservative treatment. The first is kyphosis and the second is paraplegia of healing, and sometimes both may be combined (Fig. 12–12). Kyphosis is a deformity in the thoracic spine which leads not only to loss of height but also to impairment of respiratory function from approximation of the ribs and absolution of chest expansion, leaving only the diaphragm to function; the pulmonary impairment of a 90 degree curve in the midthoracic spine is 50 per cent. Another disadvantage is that the diagnosis cannot be confirmed by pathological and bacteriological means and the sensitivity of the organism cannot be determined.

INDICATIONS FOR OPERATION

Operation is indicated in every case of tuberculosis of the spine, to establish the diagnosis. If a skilled bone pathologist is available, needle biopsy may be performed instead of operation. We prefer the surgical approach, for diagnosis can almost always be made on the operating table, and the operation can change from a biopsy to a formal anterior fusion procedure, thus saving a good deal of time. This may be regarded as a radical approach, as no doubt some cases will heal with antibiotic therapy and some will heal without treatment, but, as we have seen, these result in kyphosis and late paraplegia may develop. Kyphosis is not usually acceptable in the treatment of spinal tuberculosis. If any area of the spine is to be treated conservatively, it

would best be the cervical and lumbar spine. In the cervical region, severe kyphotic deformity is prevented by locking the lateral masses, while in the lumbar region, extensive destruction by stripping of the vertebral ligaments is prevented by the strong attachments of the origin of the psoas muscle.

Paraplegia or paraparesis is always an indication for immediate operation, as delay may result in penetration of the dura mater and involvement of the spinal cord in the tuberculous disease. This is an irreversible situation, while paraplegia caused by pressure upon the spinal cord by the contents of the abscess is rapidly reversed by evacuation of the abscess.

THE ANTERIOR FUSION OPERATION

It is usual to have the patient in hospital for about four weeks before operation. During this time the patient undergoes a full investigation and is put on antibacterial drugs. A thoracic physician is called in, because the tuberculosis of the spine is only a manifestation of general tuberculous disease. The only exception is the presence of paraparesis or paraplegia, which we think is an indication for emergency operation. In these cases, the antibacterial regime can only be a short one, perhaps a few hours, but this is not considered to be a drawback. The danger of operative intervention is that blood spread may occur and, as long as antibacterial drugs are circulating in sufficient concentrations in the blood at the time of the operation, this can usually be avoided. Details of the operation for anterior fusion at all levels of the spine will be found in previous articles by the author.[30, 48-50, 52-56] Only the transthoracic approach will be described here.

The patient is placed, left side uppermost; the rib selected is the one opposite the kyphosis in the mid-axillary line, or two ribs above the kyphosis at the junction of the ribs to the spine, usually the same rib; it is much safer to be too high than too low. The thoracotomy is performed, removing the whole of the selected rib back as far as possible, usually to the tubercle of the rib. Self-retaining rib retractors are used at this time to spread the ribs apart. The rib which has been removed is preserved in saline, as it will be used as an anterior strut graft later; it is simple to remove another rib if additional bone is required. The thoracotomy should expose the paravertebral

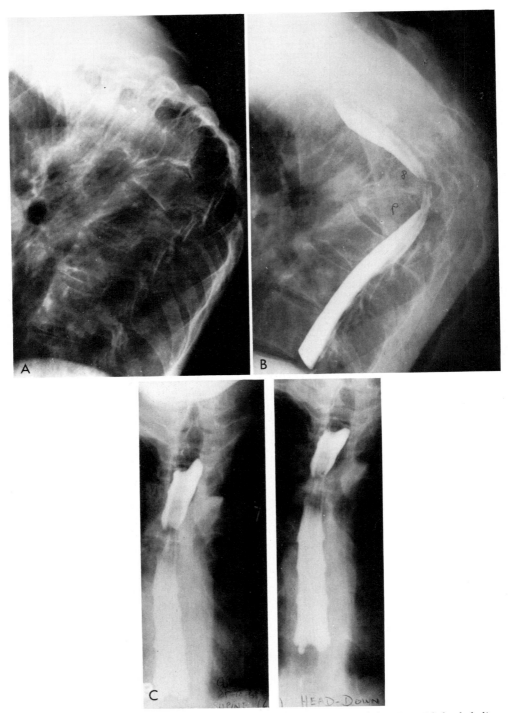

Figure 12–12. *A,* Result of conservative treatment (lateral view). Kyphotic deformity with healed disease. Early paraparesis. *B,* Pyelogram, lateral view. Note interruption of myelogram column at the apex of the kyphosis. *C,* Anteroposterior myelogram.

abscess, and the next step is to mobilize the aorta. The parietal pleura in the sulcus between the abscess and the aorta is divided along the length of the abscess, and the intercostal vessels are coagulated if small and ligated if large. A **T** incision is made in the abscess wall, the top stroke of the **T** is in the sulcus where the intercostals have been coagulated and the stem of the **T** across the middle of the abscess towards the ribs. If greater exposure is required, the **T** can be converted into an **I**. The flaps of the **T** or the **I** are stitched back to the parietal pleura and the contents of the abscess are evacuated. The contents consist of fluid or caseous pus, sequestra, sequestrated intervertebral disc, granulation tissue, especially on the abscess wall and in the spinal canal, sloughs and avascular bone, which is chiseled off to leave a straight surface of raw, bleeding bone. The abscess cavity should be a raw, bleeding bed to receive the graft and to allow the blood-borne antituberculotic drugs to diffuse through the abscess cavity. The vertebral bodies above and below have a mortise made in them to receive the strut rib graft, pressure is applied to the kyphosis to spring the vertebral bodies apart, and calipers are used to measure the distance between the mortise of the vertebral body above and the vertebral body below. One strut graft is cut to exactly this size and introduced into the respective mortises. This is the key graft, as it is under compression, and it should be possible to grasp it with the bone-holding forceps and shake the spine without dislodging the graft. (See Figs. 12–18 and 12–20.) It is only possible to lodge one graft in this fashion; further grafts are cut in the same way, to lie snugly between the vertebral bodies, and are fixed to the key graft with a double catgut tie around the grafts, in much the same way as a faggot of wood is fixed. Antitubercular drugs are instilled into the abscess cavity and the flaps sewn back into place. The thoracotomy is closed in a routine manner, and the chest drained with an underwater drain. For further details of this technique see pages 133 to 150.

The postoperative course is carefully charted and a blood transfusion given if necessary. With a diathermy coagulation technique, blood loss is minimal and a transfusion is not required. The drain is usually removed on the third postoperative day. The patient is nursed on a Lorenz plaster bed with an anterior turning cast, and turning is performed at least twice daily. The length of time on the plaster bed depends on the length of the graft and the age of the patient. A child with a short graft may be in the bed for four to eight weeks; adults with longer grafts will be on the beds longer. We use two tests to assess clinical union; one is the spring test, in which pressure is put on the kyphosis and the spine springs open; the other is the percussion test, in which the spinous process at one end of the graft is tapped by a finger while a stethoscope is applied to the spinous process at the other end of the graft; the quality of the note gives an idea of the stage of the union. Both these tests require some experience in interpretation. The great majority of the patients should be fully mobile in three months postoperatively.

CORRECTION OF KYPHOTIC SPINAL DEFORMITIES FOLLOWING TUBERCULOSIS OF THE SPINE

The author has been engaged in the correction of kyphotic spinal deformities since 1958. The results of conservative therapy in spinal tuberculosis have resulted in kyphosis to a greater or lesser extent, depending upon the number of vertebral bodies destroyed by the disease process. The site of the lesion has some part to play in the severity of the kyphosis; the worst deformities usually appear in the dorsolumbar junction, followed by mid-thoracic kyphosis, followed by cervicodorsal kyphosis; kyphotic deformity in the cervical and lumbar regions is the least severe.

Mid-thoracic kyphosis is always associated with impairment of pulmonary function, and a kyphosis of 90 degrees at this site reduces pulmonary function by 50 per cent.

The author was introduced to the halo method of skull traction during a visit to Rancho los Amigos in 1957, and returned to Hong Kong and designed a halopelvic distraction apparatus in 1958 for correction of tuberculous kyphosis (Fig. 12–13).[74, 81] A moderate amount of success was achieved with this method, but the large numbers of active cases requiring urgent operative treatment did not allow much time to treat many of the kyphotic cases, as the treatment was a lengthy one.

Three things have made it possible to tackle kyphotic tuberculous patients; a marked drop in the fresh cases of bone and joint tuberculosis, increased facilities, and the development of a halopelvic distraction apparatus by DeWald and Ray which allowed the patient to be ambulant.[23] This apparatus was

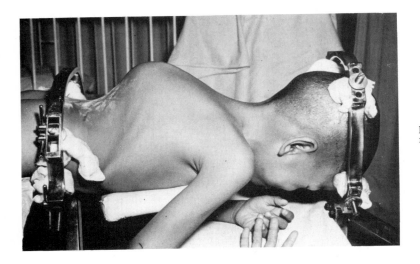

Figure 12–13. The original halopelvic distraction apparatus for correction of kyphotic deformities.

further developed in Hong Kong by constructing it of stainless steel, making it lighter, altering the connecting bars and, most important of all, measuring the forces we were putting through the upright bars of the apparatus. The apparatus is a very powerful one, and overdistraction may lead to complications.[15, 57, 76-78]

This apparatus is ideal for the correction of kyphosis resulting from tuberculous disease. However, the treatment is difficult and requires time, and it may be divided into stages.

1. Application of the halopelvic distraction apparatus.[15, 23, 78]
2. An anterior osteotomy, using an anterior approach is performed in cases with spontaneous fusion.[30, 50, 51] In active cases, a very extensive debridement is performed,

making sure that adequate release is obtained.

3. If there has been a spontaneous fusion posteriorly, a posterior osteotomy must be performed. It may be either a large osteotomy or several smaller, linear osteotomies, depending upon the extent of the fusion and the amount of the deformity.

Then follows the stage of correction during which the kyphosis is gradually corrected over a period of some weeks. Great care is taken that the forces put through the apparatus are measured and that distraction is not too forcible, usually below 40 lb., which is known through experience to be the maximum force that may be used without complications. The distraction varies with the age and weight of the patient and the extent of the deformity

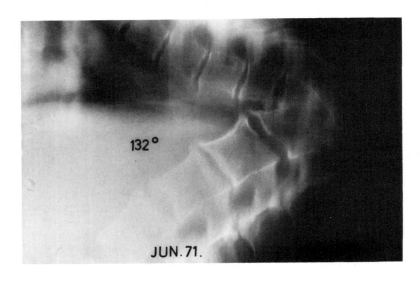

132°

JUN. 71.

Figure 12–14. Preoperative tomogram of patient with spinal tuberculosis treated conservatively. Note kyphosis and bony healing.

(Fig. 12–14). One rule we follow is that the distraction force must not be greater than the weight of the patient; usually it is between 50 and 75 per cent of the patient's body weight.

A force may be applied to the apex of the kyphosis, which will help in the correction (Fig. 12–15), particularly in the later stages of the correction, as the distraction force becomes less efficient as the angle of the kyphosis decreases.

When the maximum degree of correction is achieved—no further correction occurs or

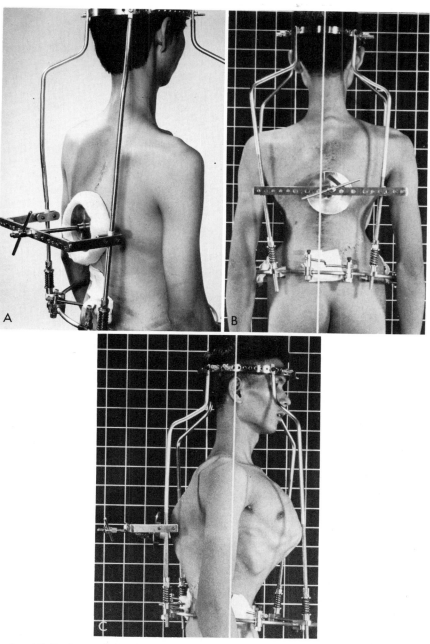

Figure 12–15. *A* and *B,* Pusher applying intermittent force into the apex of the kyphosis. *C,* The pusher attachment to the halopelvic distraction for correction of kyphosis, following conservative treatment of tuberculosis of spine.

the patient is unable to tolerate any more distraction—two further procedures are performed with the patient in the halopelvic distraction apparatus.

(1) An anterior approach is made, and strut rib grafts are introduced to bridge the gap in the spine produced by the correction.

(2) At an interval of two to four weeks, a posterior fusion is performed for a distance above and below the extent of the anterior rib grafts and into the compensatory lordosis.

Recently, the posterior osteotomy and fusion have been done at the same operation so as to cut down on the amount of surgery. Considerable thought has gone into the combination of anterior osteotomy and fusion, but a safe method has not yet been devised.

The patient remains in the halopelvic apparatus for six to eight weeks without distraction, using the device as a method of immobilizing the spine. The apparatus is then removed and an antigravity plaster jacket is applied for as long as is necessary for the anterior and posterior grafts to fuse.

Figure 12–16A and B show pre- and postoperative x-rays in a case of severe kyphosis and the result is what we would expect, an average correction.

Pott's Paraplegia

This may be the first sign of Pott's disease. Understanding of the cause of this condition has been poor, with some notable exceptions. The first to give a good description of the condition was Michaud, in 1871, who gave a masterly dissertation on the condition and who supported his views with histological findings.[72]

We have been very interested in this condition and have written on the subject.[48, 50] Our most important contribution has been a classification based on the living pathological findings.

CLASSIFICATION

It is easy to determine at operation whether the disease is active or healed, so we have divided the causes into two main groups: Group A, paraplegia of active disease; and Group B, paraplegia of healed disease.

GROUP A. This condition can be subdivided into two types: 1) paraplegia caused by external pressure on the spinal cord; and 2) paraplegia caused by penetration of the dura and involvement of the cord by the tuberculous infection.

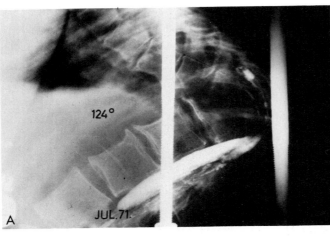
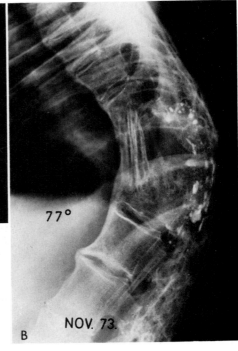

Figure 12–16. *A*, X-ray after anterior osteotomy; the patient is in halopelvic distraction apparatus and the uprights of the apparatus can be seen. *B*, X-ray following anterior and posterior fusion, showing an average degree of correction.

Pressure on the cord can be produced by pus, bony sequestra, sequestrated intervertebral disc, granulation tissue, concertina collapse, subluxations and dislocations of the spine and, occasionally, tuberculosis of the neural arch.

If a decompression is done promptly in these cases there is a rapid and immediate relief of symptoms; this is the most frequent cause of paraplegia in Pott's Disease and carries a good prognosis. This type of paraplegia can resolve spontaneously in some cases, but in others it can become a Group A2, with cord involvement, and when this happens the condition is irreversible. Clinically, the pure pressure paraplegia is of a mild nature and can be aggravated by sitting the patient up for a few minutes and relieved by placing the patient in a recumbent position for a few days. The paraplegia of cord penetration is very spastic; the patient has a withdrawal reflex, and passively moving one foot will cause spasm in the opposite buttock.

Penetration of the dura mater and involvement of the cord by the tuberculous disease was first described by Michaud, and he gives a very clear description of the condition.[72] He points out that all diseases involving the spinal cord in fibrosis and proliferation of the neuroglia, are characterized by marked spasticity. This may go hand in hand with a pure pressure paraplegia, both occurring together. It was found in 25 per cent of our cases, and was for the most part irreversible.

GROUP B. This disorder may be divided into two types: (1) transection of the spinal cord by a bony bridge; and (2) constriction of the cord by granulation and fibrous tissue.

Transection of the spinal cord was first described by Bouvier.[8] The method of production of the bony ridge we believe to be due to increasing kyphosis of the spine in the healing phase and retropulsion of the soft new bone across the canal, where it causes pressure on the spinal cord. The prognosis in these cases is not very good; some recovery may be expected after decompression but is slow and usually incomplete.

Paraplegia caused by constriction of the cord by granulation tissue, with, later in the disease process, the granulation tissue possibly becoming fibrous tissue, can co-exist with the bony ridge type. The granulation tissue appears to form around the Batson's veins and surrounds the cord, and can cause an indentation in the cord. When the granulation tissue becomes fibrous tissue, there is further shrinking and cord pressure.

TREATMENT

We should say that the prevention of Pott's paraplegia is the proper treatment of Pott's disease. This is the main indication for the early operative debridement of the disease process so that there may be no pressure upon the cord, and the dura and cord cannot be involved in the disease.

If paraplegia is present, it is of the greatest importance to expose the whole of the dura over the extent of the diseased spine and to remove any granulation from the surface of the dura (see Fig. 12–17). Usually it strips easily, but sometimes it has invaded the dura, and an attempt to remove it may produce a

(*Text continued on page 596.*)

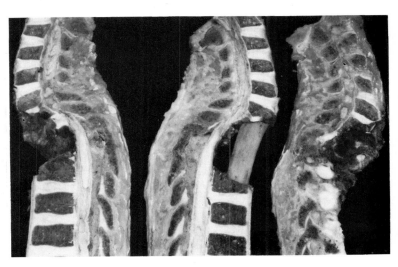

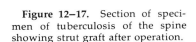

Figure 12–17. Section of specimen of tuberculosis of the spine showing strut graft after operation.

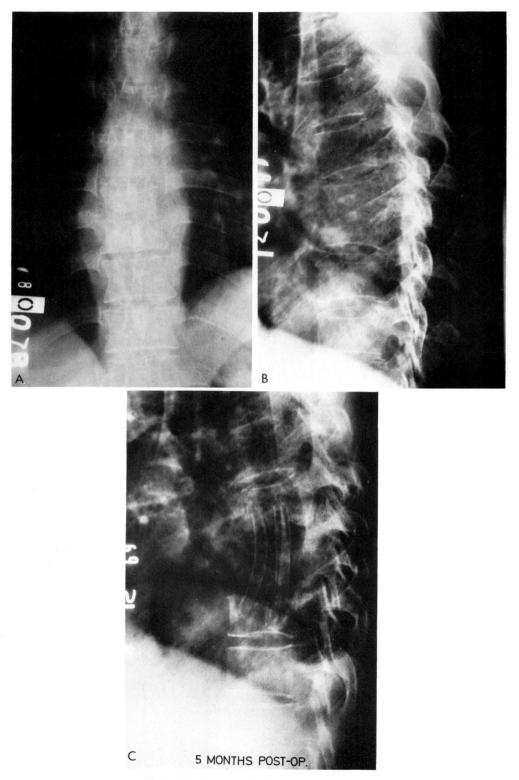

Figure 12–18.   *See opposite page for legend.*

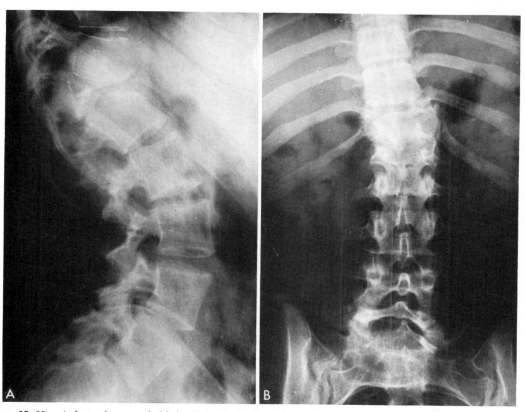

Figure 12–19. *A,* Lateral x-ray of old, healed spinal tuberculosis, after conservative treatment. The patient was 17 years old and had severe low back pain, possibly connected with the compensatory lumbar lordosis. *B,* Anteroposterior view, showing slight lateral deviation.

Figure 12–18. *A,* Preoperative anteroposterior x-ray, showing fusiform paravertebral abscess in the thoracic spine involving D8-D9. *B,* Preoperative lateral view, showing tuberculosis infection of D8-D9. Both vertebrae were riddled by the disease. *C,* Postoperative lateral view, showing three long grafts: the bodies of D8 and D9 had been excised. The anterior grafts were too scanty; five or more grafts should be the minimum number. If two or more vertebrae are excised, a posterior fusion operation should supplement the anterior procedure.

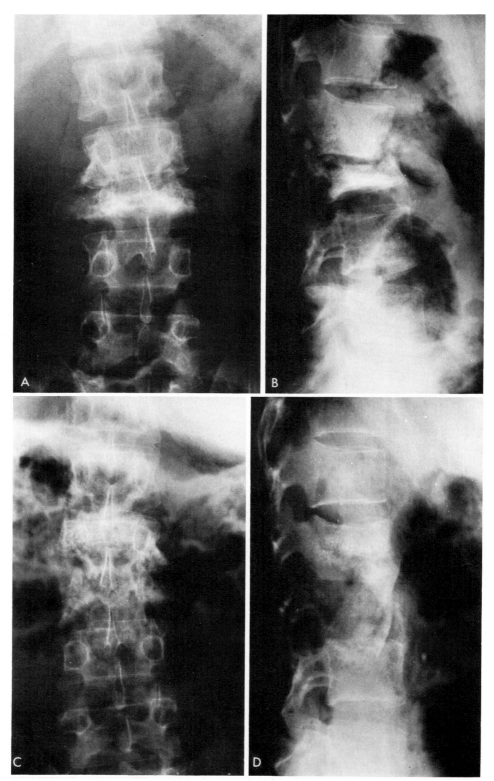

Figure 12–20. *A,* Preoperative anteroposterior view of lumbar spine, showing involvement of L3 by tuberculous infection. Note that L3 has collapsed. *B,* Preoperative lateral view, showing collapse of L3, involvement of L2 and narrowing of L2-L3 intervertebral disc space; the space between L3 and L4 is normal. *C,* Postoperative anteroposterior view after excision of disease and introduction of anterior strut graft. *D,* Postoperative lateral view showing that the intervertebral discs L2-L3 and L3-L4 and the diseased body of L3 and the partially diseased portion of L2 have been excised and replaced by a strut graft.

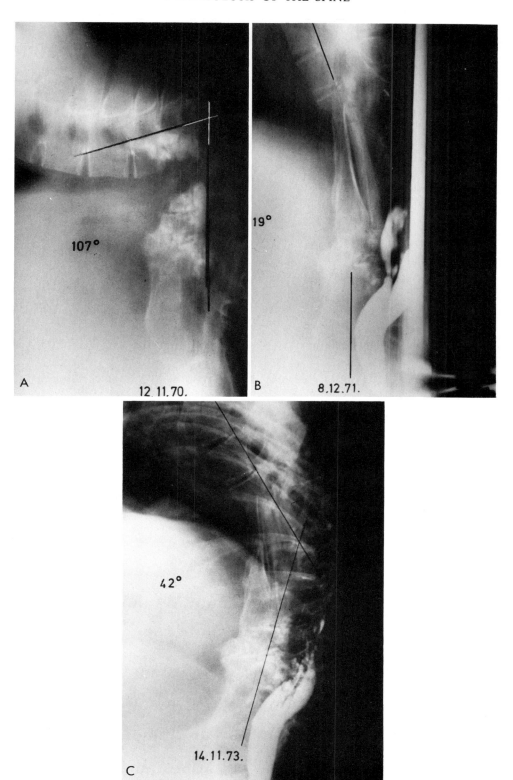

Figure 12–21. Correction of kyphosis.

cerebrospinal fluid fistula, with leakage of cerebrospinal fluid into the wound.

If the dura pulsates, all is well, and if it does not the dura should be opened and the cord inspected, as it is very probable that there will be a tuberculous meningomyelitis and even a tuberculoma in the cord itself. It is good procedure to remove the tuberculoma.

References

1. Abrahamson, L., McConnell, A. A., and Wilson, C. R.: Acute epidural spinal abscess. Brit. Med. J. *1*:1114, 1934.
2. Alderman, E. J., and Duff, J. P.: Osteomyelitis of cervical vertebrae as a complication of urinary tract disease. J.A.M.A. *148*:283–285, 1952.
3. Auerbach, O.: Tuberculosis of the skeletal system. Quart. Bull. Seaview Hosp. *6*:117–147, 1941.
4. Batson, O. V.: The function of the vertebral veins and their role in the spread of metastasis. Ann. Surg. *112*:138, 1940.
5. Batson, O. V.: The vertebral vein system. Caldwell Lecture 1956. Am. J. Roent. Rad. Ther. Nucl. Med. *78*(2):194–212, 1957.
6. Billington, R. W.: Spondylitis following cerebrospinal meningitis J.A.M.A. *83*:683, 1924.
7. Blacklock, J. W. S.: Injury as an etiological factor in tuberculosis. Proc. R.S.M. *50*(1):61–68, 1956.
8. Bouvier, H.: Lecons Cliniques sur les Maladies Chroniques de l'Appareil Locomoteur. Paris, Baillière, 1858.
9. Bremner, A. E., and Neligan, G. A.: Benign form of acute osteitis of the spine in young children. Brit. Med. J. *1*:856, 1953.
10. Breschet, G.: Recherches anatomiques, physiologiques et pathologiques sur le systeme veineux et specialement sue le cavaux veineux des os. Paris, Villaret, 1828–32.
11. Butler, E. C. B., Blusger, I. N., and Perry, K. M. A.: Staphylococcal osteomyelitis of the spine. Lancet *1*:480, 1941.
12. Butterworth, R. D., and Carpenter, E. B.: Pyogenic osteomyelitis of the cervical spine with quadriplegia secondary to cord pressure. South. Med. J. *42*:561–564, 1949.
13. Carson, W. H.: Acute osteomyelitis of the spine. Brit. J. Surg. *18*:400, 1930.
14. Charcot, J.-M.: Lecons sur les Maladies du Système Nerveux. Paris, Vol. *2*:88, 1880.
15. Clark, J. A., and Kesterton, L.: Halo-pelvic traction appliance for spinal J. Biomechanics Vol. 4: 589–595, 1971.
16. Clemens, H. J.: Die Venensysteme der menschlichen Wirbelsäule, Berlin, Gruyther, 1961.
17. Cleveland, M., and Bosworth, D. M.: The pathology of tuberculosis of the spine. J. Bone Joint Surg. *24*:527, 1942.
18. Cofield, R. B.: Hypertrophic bone changes in tuberculous spondylitis. J. Bone Joint Surg. *4*:332–342, 1922.
19. Cofield, R. B.: Bony bridging in tuberculosis of the spine. J.A.M.A., *70*(17):1391–1393, 1922.
20. Daverne, quoted by Lazarus, J. A.: Osteomyelitis of the vertebrae. Am. J. Surg. *15*:82–87, 1932.
21. DeFeo, E.: Osteomyelitis of the spine following prostatic surgery. Radiology *62*:396, 1954.
21a. Del Toro, R. A., Rullan, J. A., Torregroso, M., Freyre, J. L., and Lugo, A. L.: Serratia marcescens osteomyelitis of the cervical spine. Paper read at Am. Acad. Orth. Surg., May 2, 1973.
22. Derry, O. G.: Pott's disease in ancient Egypt. Med. Press Circ., July, 1938, pp. 196–200.
23. DeWald, R. L., and Ray, R. D.: Skeletal traction for the treatment of severe scoliosis. J. Bone Joint Surg. *52A*:233–238, 1970.
24. Donahue, C. D.: Osteitis of the spine. J. Urol. *61*:405, 1949.
25. Donati, quoted by Lazarus, J. A.: Osteomyelitis of the vertebrae. Am. J. Surg. *15*:82–87, 1932.
26. Eckenhoff, J. E.: Circulatory control in the surgical patient. Ann. Roy. Coll. Surg. Eng. *39*:67, 1966.
27. Elliot Smith, G., and Dawson, W. R.: Egyptian Mummies. London, 1924, p. 157.
28. Epstein, B. S.: The Spine. A Radiological Text and Atlas. 3rd Ed., Philadelphia, Lee & Febiger, 1969.
29. Ernst, J., and Ratjen, E.: Actinomycosis of the spine. Report of two cases. Acta Orthop. Scand. *42*:35–44, 1971.
30. Fang, H. S. Y., Ong, G. B., and Hodgson, A. R.: Anterior spinal fusion. The operative approaches. Clin. Orth. Rel. Res. *35*:16–33, 1964.
31. Finch, P. G.: Staphylococcic osteomyelitis of the spine in a baby aged three weeks. Lancet *2*:134, 1947.
32. Frank, T. J. F.: Osteomyelitis of the odontoid process of the axis (dens of the epistropheus). Aust. Med. J. *1*:198–201, 1944.
33. Garcia, A., Jr., and Grantham, S. A.: Haematogenous pyogenic vertebral osteomyelitis. J. Bone Joint Surg. *42A*:429, 1960.
34. Ghormley, R. K., and Bradley, J. I.: Prognostic signs in the x-rays of tuberculous spines in children. J. Bone Joint Surg. *10*:796–803, 1928.
35. Giaccai, L., and Idriss, H.: Osteomyelitis due to salmonella infection. J. Pediat. *41*:73, 1952.
36. Griffiths, H. E. D., and Jones, D. M.: Pyogenic infection of the spine. J. Bone Joint Surg. *53B*:383–391, 1971.
37. Guri, J. P.: Pyogenic osteomyelitis of the spine. J. Bone Joint Surg. *28*:29, 1946.
38. Hahn, O., quoted by Wilensky, A. O.: Osteomyelitis of the vertebrae. Ann. Surg. *89*:561, 1929.
39. Hall, J. E., and Silverstein, E. A.: Acute haematogenous osteomyelitis. Pediat. *31*:1033, 1963.
40. Harris, W. R., and Bobechko, W. P.: The radiographic density of avascular bone. J. Bone Joint Surg. *42B*:626–632, No. 3.
41. Hatch, E. S.: Acute osteomyelitis of the spine. A report of a case with recovery. Review of the literature. New Orleans Med. Surg. J. *83*:861–874, 1931.
42. Hellstadius, A.: Tuberculous necrosis of the whole vertebral body with negative x-ray findings. Acta Orthop. Scand. *16*:163, 1946.
43. Henriques, C. Q.: Osteomyelitis as a complication of urology. Brit. J. Surg. *46*:19–28, 1958 (July).
44. Henson, S. W., Jr., and Coventry, M. B.: Osteomyelitis of the vertebrae as a result of infection of the urinary tract. Surg. Gynec. Obstet. *102*:207, 1956.
45. Herlihy, W. F.: Revision of the venous system; the role of the vertebral veins. Aust. Med. J. *34*:661, 1947.
46. Herlihy, W. F.: Experimental studies in the internal

vertebral venous plexus. Essays in Biology, 151, 1948.

47. Hippocrates: The Genuine Works of Hippocrates. Translated by F. Adams. The Sydenham Society, London, 1849.

48. Hodgson, A. R., and Stock, F. E.: Anterior spinal fusion. A preliminary communication on the radical treatment of Pott's disease and Pott's paraplegia. Brit. J. Surg. 44185:266–275, 1956.

49. Hodgson, A. R., and Stock, F. E.: Anterior Spinal Fusion. In Rob, C., and Smith, R. (eds.): Operative Surgery. London, Butterworths, 1960.

50. Hodgson, A. R., Stock, F. E., Fang, H. S. Y., and Ong, G. B.: Anterior spinal fusion. The operative approach and pathological findings in 412 patients with Pott's disease of the spine. Brit. J. Surg. 48:172, 1960.

51. Hodgson, A. R.: Correction of fixed spinal curves. A preliminary communication. J. Bone Joint Surg. 47A,(6):1221, 1965.

52. Hodgson, A. R., Yau, A. C. M. C., Kwon, J. S., and Kim, D.: A clinical study of 100 consecutive cases of Pott's paraplegia. Paraplegia 5(1):1–16, May, 1967.

53. Hodgson, A. R., Skinsnes, O. K., and Leong, C. Y.: The pathogenesis of Pott's paraplegia. J. Bone Joint Surg. 49A:1147–1156, Sept. 1967.

54. Hodgson, A. R., and Yau, A. C. M. C.: Vordere Operative Zugänge sur Wirbelsäule. Stuttgart, Georg Thieme Verlag, 1969.

55. Hodgson, A. R., and Yau, A. C. M. C.: Anterior surgical approaches to the spinal column. In Recent Advances in Orthopaedics. London, Churchill, 1969.

56. Hodgson, A. R., Wong, W., and Yau, A. C. M. C.: X-ray appearances of Tuberculosis of the Spine. Springfield, C. C. Thomas, 1969.

57. Hodgson, A. R.: Correction of spinal deformities. Proc. LeRoy Abbott Soc. 2:9, May, 1972.

58. Jansey, F., and Anthony, J. E., Jr.: Staphylococcal spondylitis, with bilateral costotransversectomy. Northwest. Med. Bull. 31:114–119, 1957.

59. Klein, H. M.: Acute osteomyelitis of the vertebrae. Arch. Surg. 26:169, 1933.

60. Kulowski, J.: Pyogenic osteomyelitis of the spine. An analysis and discussion of 102 cases. J. Bone Joint Surg. 28:343–364, 1936.

61. Lame, E. L.: Pyogenic vertebral osteomyelitis following pelvic operation with special reference to preoperative infection. Presented at the Annual Meeting of the American Roentgen Ray Society, September, 1954.

62. Lame, E. L.: Vertebral osteomyelitis following operation on the urinary tract or sigmoid. Am. J. Roentgenol. 75:938, 1956.

63. Lazarus, J. A.: Osteomyelitis of the vertebrae with report of two cases simulating perinephric abscess. Am. J. Surg. 15:82–87, 1932.

64. Leach, R. E., Goldstein, H., and Younger, D.: Osteomyelitis of the odontoid process. J. Bone Joint Surg. 49A:369, 1967.

65. Leigh, T. F., Kelly, R. P., and Weens, H. S.: Spinal osteomyelitis associated with urinary tract infections. Radiology 65:334–342, 1955.

66. Lerch, Hanns: Uber die Bildung von Knochenspangen bei der Spondylitis Tuberculosa. Tuberkuloseazt 3:523–527, 1949.

67. Leri, A.: Les spondyloses. J. Mèdic Francais, p. 504, 1912.

68. Liming, R. W., and Youngs, F. G.: Metastatic vertebral osteomyelitis following prostatic surgery. Radiology 67:92, 1956.

69. Lovett, R. W.: Lateral deviation of the spine as a diagnostic symptom in Pott's disease. Trans. Amer. Orthop. Assn. 3:182–192, 1890.

70. Mankins, G. H., and Abbot, F. C.: An acute primary osteomyelitis of the vertebrae. Ann. Surg. 23:150–539, 1896.

71. Mayer, L. O.: Operations on the bodies of the vertebrae. J. Internat. Coll. Surg. 9:104–111, 1946.

72. Michaud, J.-A.: Sur le meningite de la myelite dans la mal vertébràle. Thèse de Paris, 1871.

73. Murray, R. A., and Jacobsen, H. G.: The radiology of skeletal disorders. In Exercises in Diagnosis, London, Churchill Livingstone, 1971.

74. Nickel, V. L., Perry, J., Garrett, R., and Heppenstall, M.: The halo. A spinal skeletal traction fixation device. J. Bone Joint Surg. 56A:1400–1409, 1968.

75. O'Brien, J. P.: The manifestation of arrested bone growth. The appearance of a vertebra within a vertebra. J. Bone Joint Surg. 51A:1376–1378, No. 7, 1969.

76. O'Brien, J. P., Yau, A. C. M. C., and Hodgson, A. R.: Halo-pelvic traction: a new method of external spinal instrumentation for the correction of kyphotic and scoliotic deformities. Far East. Med. J. 6:146–149, May, 1970.

77. O'Brien, J. P., Yau, A. C. M. C., and Hodgson, A. R.: Aparato de Traccion Craneo-Pelviano, (Halo Pelvic Traction). Rev. Orthop. Trauma. 15(3):223–226, Nov., 1970.

78. O'Brien, J. P., Yau, A. C. M. C., Smith, T. K. and Hodgson, A. R.: Halo pelvic traction. J. Bone Joint Surg. 53B:217–229, No. 2, May, 1971.

79. Oppenheimer, A.: Calcification and ossification of vertebral ligaments (spondylitis ossificans ligamentosa): Roentgen study of pathogenesis and clinical significance. Radiology 38:160–172, 1942.

80. Papathanassiou, B. T., Papachristou, G., and Hartofilakadis-Garofalidis, G.: Brucellar Spondylosis.

81. Perry, J., and Nickel, V. L.: Total cervical-spine fusion for neck paralysis. J. Bone Joint Surg. 41A:37–60, No. 1, 1959.

82. Pott, Percivall: Remarks on that kind of Palsy of the Lower Limbs Which is Frequently Found to Accompany a Curvature of the Spine. London, J. Johnson. 1779.

83. Pritchard, A. E., and Thompson, W. A. L.: Acute pyogenic infections of the spine in children. J. Bone Joint Surg. 42B:86, 1960.

84. Pritchard, A. E., and Robinson, M. P.: Staphylococcal infection of spine. Lancet 2:1165, 1961.

85. Robinson, B. H. B., and Lessof, M. H.: Osteomyelitis of the spine. Guy's Hosp. Rep. 110:303.

86. Schein, A. J.: Bacillus pyocyanus osteomyelitis of spine. Arch. Surg. 41:740, 1940.

87. Scott, W. W.: Blood stream infections in urology: Report of eighty-two cases. J. Urol. 21:527–576, 1929.

88. Selig, S.: Bacillus proteus osteomyelitis of the spine. J. Bone Joint Surg. 16:189, 1934.

89. Shehadi, W. H.: Primary pyogenic osteomyelitis of the articular processes of the vertebra. J. Bone Joint Surg. 34:343–364, 1936.

90. Sherman, M. S., and Schneider, G. T.: Vertebral os-

teomyelitis complicating postabortal and postpartum infection. South. Med. J. 48:333–338, 1955.

91. Smith, N. R.: The intervertebral discs. Brit. J. Surg. 18:358, 1931.

92. Souques, A., Lafourcade, and Terris: Vertèbre "d'Ivore" dans un cas de cancer metastatique de la colonne vertèbrale. Rev. Neurol. 32:3–10, 1925.

93. Stammers, F. A. R.: Spinal epidural suppuration, with special reference to osteomyelitis of the vertebrae. Brit. J. Surg. 26:366, 1938.

94. Stern, W. E., and Balch, R. E.: Surgical aspects of nonspecific inflammatory and suppurative disease of the vertebral column. Am. J. Surg. 112:314, 1966.

95. Stone, D. B., and Bonfiglio, M.: Pyogenic vertebral osteomyelitis. Arch. Int. Med. 112:491, 1963.

96. Sullivan, C. R., Bickel, W. H., and Svien, H. J.: Infection of the vertebral interspaces after operations on intervertebral disks. J.A.M.A. 166:173, 1958.

97. Swett, P. P., Bennett, G. E., and Street, D. M.: Pott's disease: The initial lesion, the relative infrequency of extension by contiguity, the nature and type of healing, the role of the abscess and the merits of operative and nonoperative treatment. J. Bone Joint Surg. 22:815–823, July, 1940.

98. Thibodeau, A. A., and Maloy, J. K.: Closed-space infection following removal of lumbar intervertebral disc. J. Bone Joint Surg. 40A:717, June, 1958.

99. Turner, P.: Acute infective osteomyelitis of the spine. Brit. J. Surg. 26:71, 1938.

100. Veal, J. R.: Typhoid and paratyphoid osteomyelitis. Am. J. Surg. 43:594, 1939.

101. Veal, J. R., and McFetridge, E.: Paratyphoid osteomyelitis. A report of two additional cases. J. Bone Joint Surg. 16:455, 1934.

102. Volkman, J.: Ueber die prim äre akute und subakute Osteomyelitis purulenta der Wirbel. Deutsche Zischr. f. Chir. 132:445, 1915.

103. Waisbren, B. A.: Pyogenic osteomyelitis and arthritis of the spine treated with combinations of antibiotics and gamma globulin. A preliminary report. J. Bone Joint Surg. 42A:414–429, 1960.

104. Wear, J. E., Baylin, G. J., and Martin, T. L.: Pyogenic osteomyelitis of spine. Am. J. Roentgenol. 69:90, 1952.

105. White, J. F.: Case of caries of the dorsal vertebrae with an abscess communicating with the lungs, and expectoration of Bone. Med. Exam. Phila. 4:213–214, 1841.

105. Wiessman, S. J., Wood, V. E., and Kroll, L.: Pseudomonas vertebral osteomyelitis in drug Addicts. Read at the American Academy of Orthopedic Surgeons, 5th February, 1973.

106. Wiltberger, B. R.: Resection of vertebral bodies and bone-grafting for chronic osteomyelitis of the spine. A case report. J. Bone Joint Surg. 34A:215–218, No. 1, 1952.

107. Wilensky, A. O.: Osteomyelitis of the vertebrae. Ann. Surg. 89:561, 1929.

108. Yau, A. C. M. C., and Hodgson, A. R.: Penetration of the lung by the paravertebral abscess. J. Bone Joint Surg. 50A:243–254, No. 2, 1968.

CHAPTER 13

Metabolic Bone Disease Affecting the Spine

A. M. PARFITT, B.A., M.B., B.Chir.
Henry Ford Hospital

H. DUNCAN, M.B., B.S.(Syd.)
Henry Ford Hospital

INTRODUCTION

The spine comprises a singular collection of bones whose response to disease processes may be quite distinctive when compared to the long, tubular bones which share a similar embryologic origin.

The boundaries of the spine are quite definite, both anatomically and conceptually, but the boundaries of metabolic bone disease are much less clear cut. Albright and Reifenstein in their classic monograph established the convention that metabolic bone disease, like Gaul, could be divided into three parts, namely osteoporosis, osteomalacia and osteitis fibrosa cystica.[6] They believed that all metabolic bone disease could be assigned to one of these categories, because each was uniquely linked to one of the three separate processes into which bone remodeling could be resolved. According to the views then current, bone formation comprised the two processes of matrix synthesis and mineralization, which were separable both in time and place, whereas bone resorption was a single process whereby both matrix and mineral were simultaneously removed. Osteoporosis was thought to result from a failure of matrix synthesis, osteomalacia from a failure of mineralization, and osteitis fibrosa from an acceleration of resorption, and the three disorders were defined in accordance with these unproved etiologic theories. This tripartite scheme of bone remodeling is still acceptable, but the etiologic theories based upon it are all, in varying degrees, incorrect or at least incomplete. Although these three classical forms of metabolic bone disease are still the most important, the door has been opened to the inclusion of many other disorders of bone, some of which result from a much more clearly defined metabolic or biochemical disturbance than has been detected in the great majority of patients with osteoporosis. Our decisions of what disorders to include and what to leave out of this discussion have been essentially subjective, but have been governed partly by the importance of the spinal manifestations, partly by the presence or absence of a suitable niche in some other chapter, and partly by our own interests and experiences.

A metabolic disease of bone, by definition, must affect other bones than the spine, and consideration of these other bones is frequently necessary for proper understanding of the disease, as well as for diagnosis and treatment of the patient. Accordingly, much of our discussion will center on bone as a tissue, regardless of its location. This book is intended primarily for orthopedic surgeons and neurosurgeons, and it could be argued that we should have included only the information needed to establish that a patient's problems are due to metabolic bone disease and not to some surgical condition of the spine. We have not taken this view because successful management of patients with metabolic bone disease often requires protracted collaboration between representatives of different disciplines. Many of the minutiae of diagnosis and treatment may be handled by an endocrinologist or internist, but we hope that this chapter will enable the interested surgeon to discuss these matters on equal terms with his colleagues, and to comprehend what is being done, and why, to the patients that he refers.

Bone as a Tissue

Here we will consider the chemical composition and structure of bone, its cells and their functions, the formation, growth and remodeling of bone, and its relationship to calcium homeostasis. The discussion will be quite general, but aspects of special relevance to the spine will be emphasized. The embryological development and anatomy of the spine are described in detail in Chapters 1 and 2, but certain points of particular importance in understanding metabolic bone disease will be reiterated.

Composition of Bone [399]

Mammalian bone is a specialized connective tissue which consists of a mineralized organic matrix in which living cells are dispersed. The matrix is composed of collagen fibers within a ground substance containing abundant protein-polysaccharide complexes. Fully hydrated young bone contains approximately 20 per cent by volume of tissue water (in vascular spaces, in cells and in ground substance), about 30 per cent of organic material, about 40 per cent of mineral and about 10 per cent of crystal-bound water; with increasing age, the amount of mineral increases at the expense of the crystal-bound water.

FIBERS. The fibrous protein collagen accounts for about 90 per cent by weight of bone matrix. Of total body collagen, which represents one third of total body protein, about 60 per cent is in bone and about 30 per cent in skin.

The basic unit of the collagen fibril is the tropocollagen macromolecule, a semirigid rod about 2800Å long and 15Å wide, composed of three helical polypeptide chains, each containing about 1000 amino acids, coiled around each other like a piece of rope. The exact way in which tropocollagen molecules are assembled into fibrils, with the typical cross bands at intervals of 640Å, is unknown.[89] The amino acid composition of collagen is unusual; glycine (32 per cent), alanine (13 per cent), proline (11 per cent) and hydroxyproline (11 per cent) are the most abundant, while tryptophan and cystine are completely lacking. Hydroxyproline and hydroxylysine (0.6 per cent) are found *only* in connective tissue.

GROUND SUBSTANCE. The ground substance of bone, as of other connective tissues, is a two-phase gel, one phase of low colloid high water content, the other of high colloid low water content.[162]

The high-water phase permits rapid diffusion of inorganic ions, but the low-water phase forms separate "domains" in which ions may be trapped.[193] The consistency of the gel depends on the degree of polymerization of carbohydrate-protein complexes, which are the main structural component. These complexes are of two main types, protein-polysaccharides and glycoproteins, both of which have a central protein core with carbohydrate side chains. In the protein-polysaccharides, these side chains are very long, and are composed of glycosaminoglycans (otherwise known as mucopolysaccharides), the commonest of which in bone is chondroitin sulfate. In the glycoproteins the side chains are much shorter and contain many different kinds of sugar. Many of both types of complex, but especially sialoprotein, have a high binding affinity for calcium, probably because of the large number of free acidic groups.

MINERAL. The mineral of bone contains mainly calcium, phosphate and carbonate in approximate molar ratio of 10:6:1. The mineral exists in two physical forms, amorphous and crystalline. The amorphous form (mainly tricalcium phosphate-Ca_3 $(PO_4)_2$) is most abundant when the mineral is first formed, and plays an important part in the process of mineralization (qv). The mineral becomes progressively more crystalline with time. The crystals are either thin, elongated hexagonal plates of length around 100 to 400Å, or thin needles of length around 400 to 1000Å; the size increases with age. Bound to the surface of each crystal is a layer of water (the hydration shell) containing ions in solution and ions adsorbed to the crystal surface.[285] The lattice structure of the crystals conforms to the empirical formula $3(Ca_3(PO_4)_2) \cdot Ca\ X_2$. According to the majority view, bone mineral consists mainly of hydroxyapatite ($X_2 = OH_2$), with traces of fluoroapatite ($X_2 = F_2$). [390] An alternative view is that carbonate-apatite ($X_2 = CO_3$) is the principal form. [47]

Structure of Bone[318]

The basic structure of all bone is similar, but two distinct anatomical forms can be discerned—cortical bone (or compacta), which is solid, and trabecular bone (or spongiosa), which is a network of plates and bars. [406, 411] Cortical bone constitutes 80 per cent of the total bone volume but provides only 30 per cent of the surface, whereas trabecular bone constitutes 20 per cent of the volume and provides 70 per cent of the surface. [169] This arrangement gives rise to four surfaces, which are covered with unmineralized fibrous connective tissue. These are periosteal, intracortical or Haversian, inner cortical or cortical endosteal, and trabecular endosteal (Fig. 13–1). These surfaces may be in one of three functional states: bone forming surfaces, which are covered by osteoid seams and osteoblasts; bone resorbing surfaces, which are scalloped by Howship's lacunae containing osteoclasts, and quiescent surfaces, which are covered by flattened cells of uncertain nature, which probably represent demodulation to osteoprogenitor cells. [297, 421] The somewhat ambiguous term "resting osteoblast" is also applied to these lining cells. The proportions of these different activities may be different on each of the four surfaces. The osteoblasts form a continuous cytoplasmic barrier, since their peripheral zones are in physical contact, with the formation of tight junctions or zonula occludens. [412] The cells adjacent to the quiescent surface are more widely spaced, without tight junctions, but the surfaces here are lined by an additional structure, an electron-dense layer termed the "lamina limitans." [349]

CORTICAL BONE. [244, 318] The basic unit of cortical bone is the Haversian system or osteon. This is a cylinder about 250 micrometers in diameter, with its long axis roughly parallel to that of the bone, containing concentric lamellae around a central Haversian canal about 80 microns in diameter, in which run nutrient vessels (usually only one), lymphatics, nerves and connective tissue. The vessels of adjacent osteons communicate via transverse Volk-

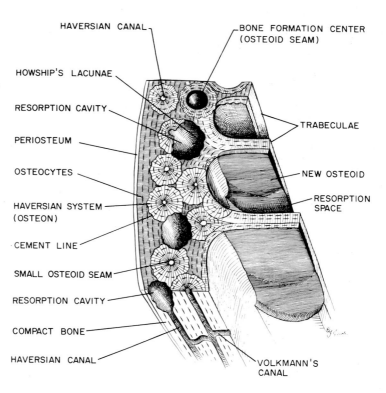

Figure 13–1. Cross and longitudinal section of bone showing the remodeling units in cortical bone and on endosteal surfaces.

HAVERSIAN CANAL

BONE FORMATION CENTER (OSTEOID SEAM)

HOWSHIP'S LACUNAE

RESORPTION CAVITY

PERIOSTEUM

OSTEOCYTES

HAVERSIAN SYSTEM (OSTEON)

CEMENT LINE

SMALL OSTEOID SEAM

RESORPTION CAVITY

COMPACT BONE

HAVERSIAN CANAL

TRABECULAE

NEW OSTEOID

RESORPTION SPACE

VOLKMANN'S CANAL

mann's canals (Fig. 13–1). Throughout the osteon are lacunae, with their long axes aligned circumferentially, containing osteocytes which communicate with one another via canaliculae which are oriented radially (Fig. 13–2). The lamellae are distinguishable because of alternation of the main direction along which the collagen fibers are oriented. With the scanning electron microscope, these changes appear less abrupt than they seem with conventional microscopy.[58] The boundary of the osteon is indicated by a cement line, a thin, clear layer of partly mineralized ground substance lacking collagen fibers, which separates pieces of bone made at different times. A cement line may be smooth (resting line), indicating deposition of new bone on a quiescent surface, or scalloped (reversal line), indicating

deposition on a previously resorbing surface.[344] Primary osteons are formed during development by infolding of the circumferential lamellae lying under the periosteum, while secondary osteons are made by the remodeling process (qv). Primary osteons are smaller, have an indistinct cement line, and may have several vessels in the central canal rather than just one. Between complete osteons are fragments of previously remodeled osteons which persist as interstitial lamellae. Around the outside of the bone are a few circumferential lamellae derived from the periosteum.

TRABECULAR BONE. Trabeculae are made primarily of layers of bone, as if an osteon were unrolled and spread over its surface. However, the lamellar structure, with osteocytes, canaliculae and cement lines, is essentially similar. Trabeculae are oriented in relation to the direction of mechanical stress, and are in close relation to the bone marrow.

APPLICATION TO THE SPINE. The vertebral body is composed almost entirely of trabecular bone, whereas the vertebral appendages — the transverse process, spinous process and neural arch — are, like the ribs, composed mainly of cortical bone.

Loss of cortical bone owing to metabolic bone disease is manifested primarily by fracture. The vertebral appendages, being well protected by muscles, are rarely subject to fracture except with severe trauma or metastatic disease. Consequently, in metabolic bone disease, both clinical and radiographic manifestations are due primarily to changes in the vertebral body. The high proportion of trabecular bone, with the high surface-to-volume ratio which this entails, is one of the factors which modify the expression of metabolic bone disease in the spine.

The cortex of the vertebral body, in the lateral walls and on the upper and lower surfaces where contact is made with the periphery of an intervertebral disc, is only about 0.5 to 1 mm thick, or about 5 to 10 times the thickness of an average trabecula, which is about 100μ. Nevertheless, the cortex may contribute half of the total compressive strength of the vertebrae.[336] The center of the upper and lower surfaces may be virtually devoid of cortex. The radiographically dense region, several millimeters thick, which is identifiable as the end plate, is composed primarily of dense trabecular bone in which the horizontal trabeculae are not only much more

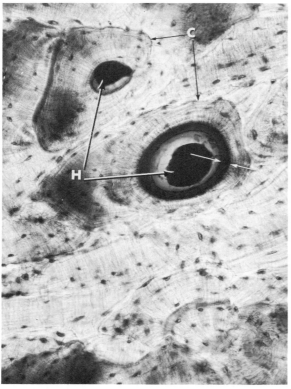

Figure 13–2. Photomicrograph of a fresh-cut, fully mineralized section of lamellar bone stained with basic fuchsin. Note the cement lines (C) surrounding one completed and one active osteon. The Haversian canals (H) contain remnants of blood vessels and some debris from the preparation of the section. The canal is lined by a homogenously stained osteoid seam (between arrows), at the outer edge of which is the zone of mineralization. Note also the osteocytic lacunae and radially arranged canaliculae.

numerous but also slightly thicker than in the centrum. The trabeculae form a network of vertical pillars and horizontal plates with smooth junctions,[411] perforated by round openings of varying size.[12] Anteriorly, the trabeculae have a radial distribution. Some larger vertebral trabeculae contain complete osteons.

Bone Cells and their Function

The principal cells of bone are the osteoblast, which makes bone, the osteocyte, which maintains the integrity of bone, and the osteoclast, which removes bone. Osteoblasts and osteoclasts are only found on bone surfaces, whereas osteocytes are completely surrounded by mineralized bone. All these develop from undifferentiated mesenchymal cells which are abundant in the vascular channels (Haversian and Volkmann's canals) and lining bone surfaces.

OSTEOBLASTS.[319] These are plump cells, ovoid or rectangular, with their long axis usually perpendicular to the surface, the nucleus lying at the farthest end. Normally, they form only a single layer. Osteoblasts are fully differentiated cells which do not divide. They originate from precursor cells known as preosteoblasts or, less specifically, as osteoprogenitor cells, since the type of differentiated cell to which a precursor cell will give rise cannot be predicted from its appearance. These precursor cells may form an additional layer behind the osteoblast and are derived, in turn, from undifferentiated mesenchymal cells.[297]

The function of osteoblasts is to make bone, that is, to make bone matrix by the synthesis of collagen and ground substance, and to preside over its mineralization.

Matrix Synthesis. The biosynthesis of collagen involves the uptake of precursor amino acids by the ribosomes of the endoplasmic reticulum, their assembly into polypeptide chains of protocollagen, and the extrusion of immature forms of collagen to enter the extracellular soluble collagen pool. Most of this is used to assemble tropocollagen molecules and collagen fibrils, but part is degraded to smaller molecular weight peptides containing hydroxyproline, some of which are recoverable in the urine.[241] An indication of the speed of this process is that tritiated proline can be demonstrated by autoradiography in osteoid within six hours of its administration.

Osteoid Seams. The osteoblasts are unique among protein-synthesizing cells in that their product is not removed to other parts of the body, but remains in situ. Consequently, measurement of the rate of matrix apposition enables the protein-synthetic capacity of individual cells to be estimated.[146] At surfaces where bone formation is occurring is a layer of as yet unmineralized matrix adjacent to the osteoblasts, the osteoid seam (Fig. 13–3). The junction of the osteoid seam with mineralized bone is a zone about 3 to 4 μm wide

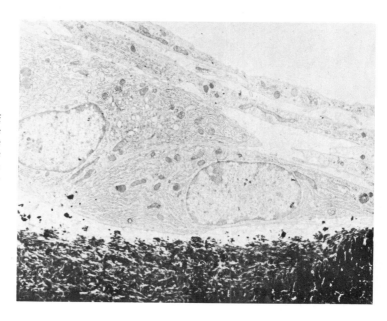

Figure 13–3. Electron micrograph of normal trabecular surface. The pale zone lying between the osteoblasts and the mineralized bone (dark shaded, at the bottom of the figure) is an osteoid seam. Above the osteoblasts is a blood vessel. (Courtesy of D. A. Cameron.)

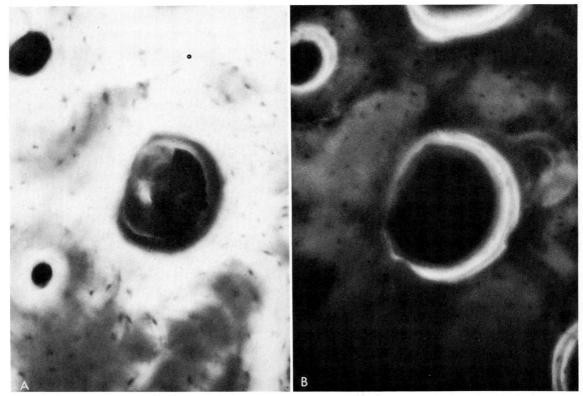

Figure 13–4. A photomicrograph of an active formation site with an osteoid seam covering the right side of the Haversian canal seen *(A)* with bright field illumination and *(B)* with ultraviolet/blue illumination. The latter reveals the yellow fluorescence of two bands of tetracycline, deposited with the calcium at the sites of mineralization, which were active at the time the tetracycline markers were given. The mean distance between these bands divided by the number of days between the administration of the markers gives the appositional rates. (Mineralized section, 70 microns thick, Osteochrome stain × 300.)

and having special staining properties where tetracyclines are taken up, the so-called mineralization front or line of demarcation. Measurement of the distance between two bands produced by tetracycline given at known times enables the rate of apposition of new matrix to be estimated (Fig. 13–4). On the average, this rate is about 1μ daily, so that the average seam thickness of about 10μ represents a delay between the synthesis of matrix and its mineralization (mineralization lag time) of about 10 days. During this period, changes occur in the maturation of both collagen fibers and ground substance, which prepare the matrix for mineralization.

Mineralization. Investigation of the physical density of bone by microradiography suggests that approximately 75 per cent of the mineral which a given volume of matrix can accept is laid down in the first few days.[145]

This process is referred to as primary mineralization, and is under the control of the osteoblast. Primary mineralization may be divided into an initial phase when seam thickness remains constant, and a terminal phase when the seam gets progressively narrower and mineralization proceeds more slowly. The distinction between these phases depends on the rate at which the mineralization front is advancing, not the rate at which an individual moiety of bone becomes mineralized. In the succeeding three to six months mineralization continues at a slower rate until about 90 per cent of the maximal level is reached. This is known as secondary mineralization and is unrelated to osteoblastic function. Primary mineralization involves the movement of ions through the preosseous matrix and the deposition of new crystals, whereas secondary mineralization involves the movement of ions through the tissue and crystal-bound water of bone and the growth of existing crystals.

Although the chemical basis of mineralization is still uncertain, a plausible sequence of events has been suggested (Table 13–1).[326] The initial step is formation of an amorphous solid phase, which is transformed to an initial crystalline form, most likely octocalcium phosphate, which in turn is transformed to a second crystalline form, hydroxyapatite. Once this has occurred, further formation of hydroxyapatite is possible directly from the solution and from the amorphous phase without the intervention of octocalcium phosphate. The most important point about these chemical reactions is the need to remove hydrogen ions to enable them to proceed.[345]

According to the traditional view, bone crystals are thought to be in direct equilibrium with the plasma, or with some local extracellular fluid (ECF) phase of similar composition to a plasma ultrafiltrate. However, if the concentrations of calcium and phosphorus are related to true thermodynamic ion activities, it is found that although plasma is supersaturated with respect to hydroxyapatite, it is too unsaturated to permit the direct precipitation of either $CaHPO_4$ or $Ca_3(PO_4)_2$.[285] These relationships have two important consequences. First, some mechanism in addition to the plasma levels of calcium and phosphate is needed to achieve the initiation of mineralization, and second, there must be some way of restraining the unbridled growth of hydroxyapatite crystals once formed.

The site of initial deposition of calcium is also debated. The widely accepted view that crystals form along the fibers of collagen has been challenged by recent evidence from electron microscopic studies suggesting that the earliest detectable clusters of mineral appear *between* rather than on or in the collagen fibers.[54, 58, 70]

Calcium ions destined for mineral deposition are actively taken up by cells, sequestered within mitochondria, and subsequently extruded from the cell.[260] Calcium and phosphate are pumped into and concentrated within the mitochondria, with the precipitation of granules of insoluble amorphous tricalcium phosphate within the mitochondrial matrix. These granules are probably stabilized in colloidal form by some mineralization inhibitor and represent the smallest transportable form of solid calcium phosphate.[248]

The fluid phase lying between the cells and the bone or cartilage surface differs in composition from the ECF, and the differences are maintained by cellular activity. In calcifying cartilage, this fluid can be aspirated directly by micropuncture. It contains protein-polysaccharides capable of both nucleating and inhibiting mineralization and has a high pH maintained by carbonic anhydrase activity, probably for neutralization of the hydrogen ion produced during mineralization.[91, 313]

A variety of complex particles, variously described as calcifying globules and matrix vesicles, containing mineral within a membrane, have been isolated from calcifying cartilage and bone.[9, 54] These particles originate from cells from which they are probably extruded by reversed pinocytosis; the cytoplasmic extensions of the osteoblast apparently infiltrating the osteoid may represent a similar phenomenon. It seems likely that they represent the extracellular form of the mitochondrial granules previously described. In some way these vesicles carry their cargo of mineral and unload it at sites of mineralization, where accumulation of their membranes probably accounts for the very high local levels of phospholipid.[88]

TABLE 13–1.   CHEMICAL REACTIONS INVOLVED IN POSSIBLE SCHEME OF MINERALIZATION*

Overall: $10\ Ca^{++} + 6\ HPO_4^{=} + 2\ H_2O \rightleftharpoons Ca_{10}(PO_4)_6(OH)_2 + 8\ H^+$		Hydroxyapatite
Possible steps:		
1.	$4\ Ca^{++} + 4\ HPO_4^{=} \rightleftharpoons 4\ CaHPO_4$	Secondary calcium phosphate
2.	$4\ CaHPO_4 + 2\ Ca^{++} \rightleftharpoons 2\ Ca_3(PO_4)_2 + 4\ H^+$	Tertiary calcium phosphate
3.	$2\ Ca_3(PO_4)_2 + 2\ Ca^{++} + 2\ HPO_4^{=} \rightleftharpoons Ca_8(PO_4)_4(HPO_4)_2$	Octocalcium phosphate
4.	$Ca_8(PO_4)_4(HPO_4)_2 + 2\ Ca^{++} + 2\ H_2O \rightleftharpoons Ca_{10}(PO_4)_6(OH)_2 + 4\ H^+$	Hydroxyapatite

*Note especially the generation of H^+ ions at Steps 2 and 4; the reactions will be halted if these are not neutralized or removed.

Inhibitors. Inhibitors of mineralization are needed not only to prevent crystal overgrowth, as already mentioned, but also at several other points in this scheme. The possible role of protein-polysaccharides in binding and sequestering calcium has already been mentioned. Calcium ions may also be bound by phospholipid and ATP. Many more specific inhibitors of mineralization have been identified, but only for inorganic pyrophosphate has a plausible case been made for a normal function in bone. Pyrophosphate ($O_3P-O-PO_3$) is present in blood and in bone, where it represents about 0.5 per cent of total phosphorus. It can replace $HPO_4^=$ in the apatite crystal lattice, and such crystals do not grow in solutions with physiologic calcium and phosphorus levels. Pyrophosphate is formed as a byproduct of many reactions involving organic phosphate esters, including the formation of cyclic AMP from ATP, and is rapidly metabolized by many naturally occurring pyrophosphatases which include both alkaline and acid phosphatase. The major effect of pyrophosphate is to prevent the conversion of amorphous calcium phosphate to a crystalline form. The function of pyrophosphate has been conceived as guarding bone mineral at quiescent surfaces and being removed by pyrophosphatase to permit either mineralization or bone dissolution.[343]

THE OSTEOCYTE.[32, 318, 344] Within the substance of the bone is a network of cells lying within lacunae, together with their interconnecting processes (up to 50 for each cell) within canaliculae (Fig. 13–2). Approximately 10 per cent of osteoblasts remain viable and become buried under successive layers of new bone, and persist as osteocytes.

Most illustrations of osteocytes show a space around the body and processes of the cell which is presumed to permit the movement of water and ions between the bone substance and the Haversian canal or trabecular surface. This space may be an artifact; the cell and its processes probably completely fill the lacunae and canaliculae, the movement of water and ions occurring along microtubules within the cell and its processes.[200] The perilacunar and pericanalicular bone is less fully mineralized and is more permeable to permanganate (but not to fuchsin stain) than is more distant bone; the permanganate-permeable zone has been termed halo volume.[151] Mineral in this region is also more soluble, and the electron microscopic appearances suggest that the crystals and collagen fibers are less densely packed.[399] The precise functions of the osteocyte are still controversial, but can be considered under three headings — maintenance of structural integrity, local tissue turnover, and mineral homeostasis.

The Osteocyte and Structural Integrity of Bone. Bone has the ability to detect and repair microfractures which otherwise would accumulate into overt fatigue fractures, normally a rare event.[148] It seems likely that both the protection and repair mechanism depend in some manner on living osteocytes. As bone ages, some osteocytes wither and die.[149] When this happens, the bone around the lacuna becomes hypermineralized, a phenomenon referred to as micropetrosis;[150] presumably one function of the osteocyte is to prevent this by holding the level of mineralization at approximately 10 per cent less than the maximum possible. Micropetrosis is accompanied by increased brittleness, decreased mechanical strength, and increased susceptibility to fatigue microfracture. All these changes are more evident in extra Haversian bone than in Haversian systems.

Local Tissue Turnover. The osteocyte is able to enlarge its lacuna by removal of bone mineral and matrix, a process known as periosteocytic osteolysis, and also retains a limited capacity to make new bone.[32, 38] The cyclical removal and replacement of the perilacunar bone is of small magnitude but serves to maintain the characteristic low density and increased permeability of the bone in this region.[35]

Mineral Homeostasis. The enormous area of the lacunar-canalicular system, which is about 2000 times as great as the normal Howship's lacunar surface,[35] and the intimate relationship to the bone mineral, such that no crystal is farther than 5μ away, both suggest that the osteocyte may be involved in mineral homeostasis and specifically in plasma calcium regulation. There is abundant evidence for rapid exchange between the ECF and the bone and this probably depends on a dynamic equilibrium between calcium ions in the ECF and in the hydration shell, and in surface positions in the crystal lattice. The plasma level at which this dynamic equilibrium is set could be regulated by a local change in pH produced by the osteocytes and consequent change in the apparent solubility of the bone mineral. In addition, the osteocyte may function as a pump to maintain a high rate of water flow, both through the lacunar-canalicular system[352] and percolating through the bone substance,[15] and calcium homeostasis may be regulated by the resting osteoblasts lining quiescent trabecular surfaces.[385].

THE OSTEOCLAST.[175]   This is a giant, multinucleated cell seen at bone surfaces undergoing resorption. In contrast to bone formation, which takes place in two stages, bone resorption is a single process in which separation and degradation of the mineral, collagen fibers and ground substance takes place, if not simultaneously, at least in rapid succession. The osteoclast has an extensive ruffled border, with many cytoplasmic extensions which actively infiltrate the disintegrating bone surface (Fig. 13–5). Within and between these processes, crystals and fragments of collagen fibrils from partly resorbed bone can be seen. Cine films show that the osteoclast is extremely mobile, its domain covering a much larger area than itself, and produces rapid disappearance of the bone in contact with the ruffled border.

Osteoclasts make a large variety of hydrolytic enzymes active at both acid and neutral pH ranges.[108] These are packaged into membrane-bound cytoplasmic particles known as lysosomes, which are released in a controlled manner through the ruffled border. Osteoclasts also make a variety of collagenases, both lysosomal and non-lysosomal. Apart from periosteocytic osteolysis, osteoclasts are responsible for all bone resorption, normal and abnormal.[119] Osteolytic metastases induce recruitment of osteoclasts around them, but foreign cells do not themselves directly resorb bone.

Osteoclasts probably originate by fusion of cells belonging to a distinct subpopulation of osteoprogenitor cells.[297, 421] Preosteoclasts can be differentiated from preosteoblasts by electron microscopy but not by light microscopy. Osteoclasts may also develop from wandering macrophages or histiocytes which also have phagocytic properties, especially where resorption occurs in situations other than normal bone remodeling. There is no direct evidence for the suggestion that osteoclasts might arise by fusion of osteoblasts or osteocytes. The life span of the osteoclast is only a few hours or days, during which it resorbs as much bone as osteoblasts can make in a month.

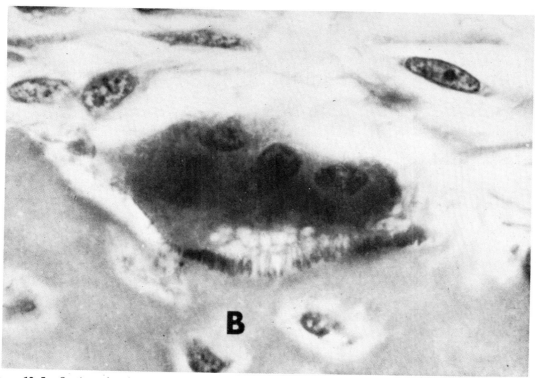

Figure 13–5.   Section of embryonic jaw bone. Note multinucleated osteoclast in center of field with ruffled brush border applied to the bone surface. (Courtesy of N. A. Hancox.)

Some osteoclasts are able to demodulate back to osteoprogenitor cells.[421]

Formation and Growth of Bone

The vertebrae share with the long bones and the base of the skull an osseous development from a cartilaginous model of the bone (endochondral ossification), whereas the vault of the skull, mandible, scapulae and pelvic brim develop directly in condensations of connective tissue (intramembranous ossification). Both of these processes cease at the time of skeletal maturity. All normal bone formation in adult life (and much during the growth period) is appositional, bone being laid down on an existing surface. Bone formation during growth will be described now, and appositional bone formation later in relation to bone remodeling.

INTRAMEMBRANOUS OSSIFICATION.[145, 175] Within a local condensation of fibrous tissue (membrane) precursor cells differentiate into osteoblasts which directly form bone matrix. The bone formed is fibrous or woven bone, which lacks the orderly arrangement of collagen fibers that characterizes lamellar bone. Woven bone is structurally weaker and has fewer canaliculi and more, osteocytes than lamellar bone, and responds differently to many humoral agents.[145] The distinction between woven and lamellar bone is of fundamental importance and will be referred to at several points in subsequent discussion. Woven bone is rapidly formed, rapidly mineralized and usually short-lived, being progressively replaced by lamellar bone.[145, 344] In intramembranous bone formation some of the newly formed woven bone is resorbed by osteoclasts and within the space created, and on the surface of as yet unresorbed woven bone, lamellar bone is laid down by a new batch of osteoblasts.

ENDOCHONDRAL OSSIFICATION. The development of a typical long bone is a result of three separate but coordinated bone-forming processes located at the periosteal collar, the growth plates and the epiphyses. Osteoblasts differentiate from precursor cells in the inner layer of the perichondrium (now periosteum), and a circumferential collar is formed around the cartilaginous model by intramembranous ossification.

At the growth plate the sequence of events is more complex. The chondrocytes are arranged in columns perpendicular to the epiphyseal plate, each column containing cells in successive stages of development as they move away from the germinal layer adjacent to the plate. As they mature, these cells become progressively rounder and larger as they pass through the so-called proliferative, hypertrophic and provisional calcification zones. The hypertrophic cells appear to degenerate at the onset of cartilage calcification but many of them survive and eventually become transformed into bone cells.[201] Calcification occurs mainly in the longitudinal cartilaginous septa between the columns of cells rather than in the transverse septa. The spaces between the bars of calcified cartilage are now invaded by capillaries, carrying with them primitive mesenchymal cells from the diaphyseal side of the growth plate. These cells, and perhaps the capillary endothelial cells also, differentiate first into chondroclasts which partially resorb the calcified cartilage bars, and second into osteoblasts which lay down woven bone on their surfaces. The trabeculae of scalloped calcified cartilage surrounded by woven bone constitute the chondro-osseous complex or primary spongiosa. This in turn is subjected to piecemeal resorption by successive waves of osteoclasts followed by osteoblasts and hematopoietic stem cells, which produce replacement, partly by lamellar bone and partly by bone marrow, to form the secondary spongiosa. In the third location, in the epiphysis itself, osteogenesis in general resembles that of the epiphyseal plate, but differs in detail, primarily in relation to the development of articular cartilage and its subjacent layer of persistent mineralized cartilage.[230]

WOVEN BONE AND LAMELLAR BONE FORMATION. The two types of growth-related bone formation we have discussed differ only in the presence or absence of a prior stage of calcified cartilage, and have in common the formation of woven bone followed by its resorption and replacement by lamellar bone. These two steps are representative of two fundamental processes, which together account for almost all bone formation, normal or abnormal, during or after growth, inside or outside the skeleton. These processes are firstly the *formation de novo* of woven bone where no bone existed, and secondly the *replacement* of existing bone, either woven or lamellar, by lamellar bone. De novo formation of woven bone is an important component of both intramembranous and endochondral bone formation. These are the only ways in which new trabeculae can be made, and they normally cease when skeletal maturity is attained. However, the potential for woven bone formation remains dormant and is reactivated in response to fracture, osteomyelitis, osteogenic sarcoma, severe hyperparathyroidism, Paget's disease, and other pathologic processes. The far-reaching significance of the fact that lamellar bone formation occurs primarily as replacement, and hence is normally preceded by resorption, will become apparent when the processes of remodeling are considered. An exception to this generalization is the apposition of bone at the periosteal surface during growth, a subject which leads naturally to the concepts of modeling and remodeling.

MODELING AND REMODELING. A typical long bone retains the shape of its metaphyses as it grows in length, by resorption of the surplus bone at the periosteal surface. More complex changes, involving drifts or movements of surfaces through tissue space as in the growing ribs, are likewise produced by excess resorption or formation at different surfaces. Such processes, which alter the shape and amount of growing bones, and which involve either resorption without succeeding formation, or formation without preceding resorption are referred to as *modeling*.[342] This is to contrast them with processes which replace old bone with new throughout life, but which do not alter the shape or (by very much) the amount of bone, which are referred to as *remodeling*. Modeling changes brought about by periosteal or endosteal apposition without preceding resorption constitute the exception to the general rule that lamellar bone formation is essentially a replacement mechanism.

APPLICATION TO THE SPINE. Endochondral ossification begins at the center of the vertebral bodies by the thirteenth intrauterine week, and by birth osseous replacement of the cartilage model is largely complete (see Chapter 1). Cartilage growth plates continue to separate the transverse processes from the body, and hyaline plates lie at the caudal and cephalic ends of each vertebra—these are the equivalent of the epiphyseal growth plates of the long bones. The major difference is that in vertebrae transverse growth is much more important and growth in length much less important than in long bones. As lateral expansion occurs, osteoclasts remodel the endosteal surface of the vertebral walls to produce vertical trabeculae and extend the existing horizontal

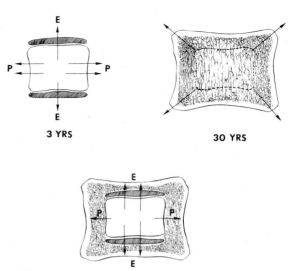

Figure 13–6. These diagrams depict the expansion of a vertebra from three years to thirty years. Vertical epiphyseal growth (E) is produced by endochondral ossification, and periosteal expansion (P) increases the width of the vertebra.

trabeculae (Fig. 13–6). In the mature vertebra the central trabeculae are of earliest origin and result from endochondral ossification, whereas peripheral trabeculae result from intramembranous ossification which occurred during transverse expansion of the vertebral walls. After completion of growth, there is a minute increase in the circumference of the vertebrae but not in their height, analogous to the continued periosteal bone deposition which has been documented in many other bones.[372]

Remodeling of Bone

It is obvious that any individual moiety of bone must be formed before it can be resorbed. This truism, and a preoccupation with growth-related processes, have together suggested that bone *formation* should be considered the primary event. Unfortunately, attempts to make some sense of the sequence of formation followed by resorption have uniformly failed. The interval of time between them varies from a few weeks to many decades and is quite unpredictable. Many have concluded that formation and resorption are unrelated processes, randomly dispersed throughout the skeleton, a view still widely held. However, if we stop thinking of the life history of an individual moiety of bone and consider instead the significance of remodeling for bone tissue as a whole, an entirely different pattern emerges. As we have seen, even from the first primary spongiosa, lamellar bone formation is primarily a replacement mechanism. An equally obvious truism is that bone must be removed before it can be replaced, suggesting that *resorption* is the primary event. It is clear that this must be so within the cortex, since there is simply no room for new bone to be formed until a space has been made. No such physical constraint dictates the primacy of resorption on trabecular surfaces, but there is strong evidence, based on the frequency of reversal lines and the rarity of resting cement lines, that the same sequence normally holds.[182] We can conclude that in trabecular bone also, remodeling involves an unchanging sequence of cellular events, as can be seen for cortical bone by examination of an osteon in longitudinal section (Fig. 13–7).

Since osteocyte death is associated with decreased structural integrity, one function of remodeling is to ensure that aging bone is removed before or soon after it dies. This serves to maintain skeletal age at less than the chronological age of the individual. Also, since old bone becomes more densely mineralized and diffusion locked, remodeling ensures a constant supply of young, metabolically active bone which can subserve mineral homeostasis by diffusion of water and ions.

The formation of an osteon begins with the appearance of a new group of osteoclasts which arise by proliferation of osteoprogenitor cells, which line the vascular channels. The signal that initiates precursor cell proliferation (or activation) is unknown, but the frequency with which this occurs is partly under hormonal control, being increased by parathyroid hormone and decreased by calcitonin and estrogens. The new osteoclasts arrange themselves as at the point of a drill or "cutting cone."[219] This cutting cone advances longitudinally in the cortex, producing a resorption tunnel (Fig. 13–7), either along the existing osteon or more usually beginning at an angle and then running parallel to it, giving rise to the characteristic branching structure.[83, 87]

Behind the advancing osteoclasts is a zone of undifferentiated spindle-shaped cells with many mitotic figures, from which successive groups of new osteoclasts will proliferate, and behind these cells are the blood vessels which will eventually traverse the mature Haversian canal. Some way behind the advancing front, refilling of the hole ("closing cone") begins from the circumference toward the center by surface apposition of new bone laid down by osteoblasts, and this continues until a normal canal diameter has been attained. Cross sections through different levels indicate the successive changes of this process (Fig. 13–7).

In man, the length of the cutting cone is about 400μ and the width about 200μ. Indi-

OLD BONE   NEW BONE   OSTEOID

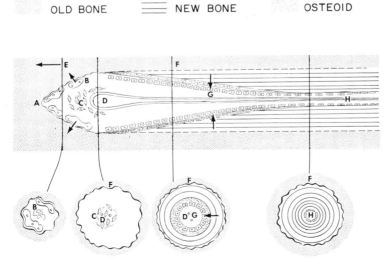

Figure 13–7. Diagram showing longitudinal (above) and transverse (below) sections through a cortical remodelling focus (active osteon). A, Point of advancing osteoclastic front ("cutting cone"). B, Osteoclasts with arrow showing possible direction of movement. C, Spindle-shaped mitotically active mesenchymal cells. D, Capillary loop. E, Direction of movement of entire system through the bone. F, Cement lines separating new bone from old. G, Osteoblasts applied to osteoid seams, showing centripetal direction of movement producing "closing cone." H, Canal of completed Haversian system with flattened lining cells.

rect estimates based on the relative prevalence of resorption and formation spaces in cross sections and the directly measured apposition rate suggest that this cutting cone represents about 20 days' work, with a longitudinal resorption rate of 20μ per day and a radial resorption rate of 5μ per day; these compare with directly measured rates in the dog of 40μ per day and 7μ per day, respectively.[215] The total length of the remodeling unit is about 2000μ or 2 mm. The time taken for the entire sequence of events to unfold at any point (known conventionally as sigma) is about 100 days,[153] comprising 20 days of resorption (sigma$_R$) and 80 days of formation (sigma$_F$). The total length of the tunnel, and so the length of time for which one unit remains in existence as a discrete anatomical structure, is unknown.

In trabecular bone, the osteoclasts of a remodeling focus are spread out over a front up to 800μ wide, as if the cutting cone had been cut open longitudinally and unfolded. They advance across the surface, gouging out a shallow groove 10 to 100μ deep and about 1000μ long, which in cross section corresponds to a Howship's lacuna.[216] Whether the time relationships are the same for trabecular remodeling as for cortical remodeling is unknown. The dynamics of remodeling may differ markedly on different types of surfaces (periosteal, Haversian, endosteal or trabecular) even though the basic sequence is the same.

The predictable evolution of each remodeling cycle in time and space has some important implications. A steady-state equilibrium between total formation and total resorption exists in normal adults over an extended period of time. In considering this equilibrium, each focus of resorption should be balanced against a focus of formation occurring at a different (later) time in the same place, rather than one occurring at the same time at a different place. Clearly, any alteration in the frequency with which new remodeling cycles are initiated (the activation frequency) will introduce an immediate disequilibrium between resorption and formation which will persist until the time of completion on one remodeling cycle (sigma) has elapsed, after which equilibrium will be reattained. Since the activation frequency is the main determinant of the total rate of bone turnover, it can be seen why changes in turnover over a wide range are not accompanied by any substantial change in bone or calcium balance, a conclusion which has been confirmed also by kinetic studies with radiocalcium.[176]

It is important always to consider whether any agent which has effects on bone does so by altering the activation frequency, the duration of resorption or formation within individual remodeling cycles (sigma$_R$ and sigma$_F$), or by altering the balance between resorption and formation within each cycle — normally the amount of bone replaced is almost, but not quite, equal to that resorbed.

Changes in sigma$_R$ and sigma$_F$ reflect the time taken to perform a given amount of metabolic work, an indication of individual cell vigor, and so define remodeling at the cellular level. Remodeling at the tissue level depends on the number of remodeling cycles present in a unit volume of bone tissue. This, in turn, results from the number of new cycles created in unit time (the activation frequency) and the length of each cycle. Using an epidemiological analogy, the *prevalence* (number of cases present at any one time) is a function of the *incidence* (number of new episodes of disease which begin in a given time) and the mean *duration* of the disease. Finally, it is possible to define a third level of remodeling, the organ level, which depends on the total amount of bone in the body, so that a given amount of total body bone remodeling could be the same in two individuals, one of whom had a low bone mass and a high tissue level turnover and the other a high bone mass and a low tissue turnover.[153]

PHYSIOLOGY OF BONE AND ITS CONSTITUENTS AND OF THE AGENTS WHICH ACT UPON THEM

Here we will consider the extraosseous metabolism of calcium and phosphorus, hydrogen ion control as it relates to bone disease, the physiology of vitamin D, parathyroid hormone and calcitonin, and the mechanisms of calcium homeostasis.

Calcium

The main pathways of calcium metabolism involve ingestion and absorption from the gut, carriage in the blood, deposition in and removal from bone, and excretion in the urine and feces. Excretion from the skin is negligible except with copious sweating, but may need to be taken into account in accurate balance studies.

NUTRITIONAL CONSIDERATIONS. In developed, Western-type countries, most dietary calcium comes from milk and milk products. Other foods high in calcium such as chocolate, nuts, beans, canned fish and caviar, are normally eaten in insufficient quantities to be nutritionally significant. In underdeveloped countries, vegetable sources of calcium are more important. The calcium in drinking water (mainly as bicarbonate) varies considerably, and hard water may contain 10 to 15 mg per 100 ml, but this is unlikely to be important unless other sources are defective or consumption of water is unusually high. Utilization of calcium varies with different foods. In spinach, the calcium is mostly present as insoluble oxalate, while the lactose in milk enhances absorption. It also may be important to consider the timing of ingestion. If the whole day's allotment of milk is taken at one sitting, less calcium is absorbed than if the same amount of milk is taken in smaller amounts throughout the day. With these provisos, nutritional assessment can be based on the total daily intake, or more simply, on the total consumption of dairy foods.

The other components of the diet are relatively unimportant so far as their effect on calcium is concerned, except for the presence in unrefined flour of phytic acid (inositol hexaphosphoric acid) which forms an insoluble unabsorbable complex with calcium and magnesium.

ABSORPTION AND FECAL EXCRETION.[22] Calcium absorption occurs mainly in the upper small bowel. Absorption is most efficient in the duodenum and is an active, carrier mediated, energy dependent process, but most calcium is absorbed in the jejunum and ileum, primarily by passive or facilitated diffusion. A small amount of calcium is absorbed from the colon. Calcium absorption throughout the gastrointestinal tract is increased by vitamin D, which is much the most important regulatory factor. The degree of dependence on vitamin D and the exact mechanisms of vitamin D action probably differ at different sites.

It is important to distinguish between *net* absorption, which is the difference between dietary intake and fecal excretion, and *true* absorption. Net absorption, which is measured by calcium balance studies, represents the difference between true absorption and endogenous secretion in bile, pancreatic juices, and other digestive juices entering the gastrointestinal tract. Of this digestive fluid calcium, the bulk mixes with dietary calcium and is absorbed in the same manner. True calcium absorption expressed as a percentage of the combined dietary and secreted calcium pool is a measure of absorptive efficiency and is normally about 40 per cent. For example, with a dietary intake of 800 mg daily and endogenous secretion of 200 mg, net absorption would be 200 mg and fecal excretion 600 mg. Net absorption would thus be 25 per cent of the intake, compared to 40 per cent for true absorption.

The most important fact concerning calcium absorption is that it is regulated homeostatically in response to bodily need. The efficiency of absorption is high in growing children, in pregnancy, and after exposure to a low calcium diet. These adaptations require the presence of vitamin D. The efficiency of calcium absorption and probably also the ability to adapt to a low calcium diet diminish in old age;[20, 64] whether this is due to vitamin D deficiency or to old age per se is unknown.

TRANSPORT IN BLOOD. The total plasma calcium is about 9.5 mg per 100 ml; the exact values for mean and range depend on the method of analysis. Of this, about 4.5 mg per 100 ml is free ionized calcium and about 5.0 mg per 100 ml is diffusible or ultrafiltrable, comprising about 4.5 mg per 100 ml bound to protein and about 0.5 mg per 100 ml complexed with organic acid, such as citrate. The ionized calcium is maintained at a fairly constant level despite changes in the concentration of protein and protein-bound calcium, so that the percentage ionized or percentage ultrafiltrable varies with the protein concentration. Of the proteins which bind calcium, albumin is the most important, accounting for about 75 per cent of the total binding, the remainder being due to as yet unidentified globulins. Protein binding increases with increasing pH, and vice versa.

EXCRETION IN THE URINE.[120, 292] Urinary excretion of calcium represents a balance between the processes of glomerular filtration and tubular reabsorption. The filtered load of calcium is approximately equal to the product of the ultrafiltrable calcium concentration and glomerular filtration rate (GFR), and is normally about 10 gm daily. The urinary excretion of calcium is normally about 200 mg daily, so that about 98 per cent of the filtered load is reabsorbed in the tubules. In the proximal convoluted tubule, and in the ascending limb of the loop of Henle, the fraction of the filtered load of calcium which is reabsorbed is approximately the same as for sodium, so that from 70 to 80 per cent of the tubular reabsorption of calcium is linked to sodium reabsorption. The dependence of calcium on sodium probably differs at different sites in the nephron.

The dependence of the bulk of calcium reabsorption on sodium reabsorption has two important practical consequences. First, urinary calcium measurements cannot be interpreted without reference to sodium excretion and sodium balance. Second, the dependence of urinary calcium on small changes in plasma calcium is markedly attenuated, so that a 1.0 mg per 100 ml change in plasma calcium would correspond to a change in 24-hour urine calcium of about 250 mg rather than about 1000 mg.

The remaining 20 to 30 per cent of the filtered load of calcium is subject to reabsorption by transport mechanism(s) which subserve calcium rather than sodium homeostasis. This homeostatic calcium reabsorption is increased by parathyroid hormone (which is the most important regulatory factor), phosphate loading, magnesium depletion, carbohydrate administration and metabolic alkalosis.

As with calcium absorption and fecal excretion, urinary calcium shows adaptive changes in response to bodily need. Urinary calcium excretion is decreased during growth, during pregnancy, and in response to dietary calcium deprivation. The mechanism of calcium conservation during growth is obscure, but in the other situations it probably depends in part on increased secretion of parathyroid hormone and in part on a very small decrease in plasma calcium.

ADAPTATION AND CALCIUM REQUIREMENTS. The ability of normal individuals to conserve calcium in time of need, by increasing the efficiency of absorption and reducing the rate of loss in the urine, increases the difficulty of defining the normal calcium requirement. When calcium balance is studied in normal individuals at different levels of intake, the minimum level at which calcium equilibrium is attained, which is the classical way of defining the nutritional requirement, reflects primarily the intake prevailing before the experiment began. Most normal individuals can eventually adapt to substantially lower dietary calcium levels, but in people whose intake is customarily high, conservation may never become as efficient as in those who have been exposed to a lower intake throughout their lives.

The levels of calcium intake suggested for the United States (800 to 1000 mg daily) are in an absolute sense probably too high, and if the entire community grew up with lower levels, most likely no harm would result.[407] However, an individual patient whose intake has been high since childhood may no longer be able to adapt to a low intake and, therefore, may need calcium supplements.

Phosphorus

Apart from the skeleton, most phosphorus in the body is inside cells as organic esters of phosphoric acid and as phosphoproteins. However, the main pathways of inorganic phosphorus metabolism are similar to those of calcium. In contrast to calcium, absorption has been studied much less intensively than urinary excretion.

NUTRITION, ABSORPTION AND TRANSPORT. In the developed Western countries, dairy products and meat each provide about half the total daily intake of about 1000 to 1200 mg of phosphorus, other sources such as grains and vegetables being much less important. These priorities are reversed in underdeveloped countries. Phosphorus is absorbed by two pathways, one linked to calcium, the other not.[280] In vitamin D deficiency, there is an approximately equimolar depression of both calcium and phosphorus absorption, and the administration of vitamin D produces an apparently equimolar increase. Normally, net absorption is about 70 per cent of the dietary intake, or about 25 mM compared to about 5 mM for calcium, so that the bulk of phosphorus must be absorbed by an additional mechanism unrelated to calcium. Because of differences in the pH of the intestinal contents, dietary phosphorus is absorbed in the distal part of the small bowel, whereas calcium is mainly absorbed more proximally.

RENAL EXCRETION OF INORGANIC PHOSPHATE.[46] Phosphate is probably excreted only by glomerular filtration and tubular reabsorption, although the existence of a tubular secretory mechanism has not yet been completely ruled out. The filtered load is approximately equal to glomerular filtration rate (GFR) × plasma phosphate. Reabsorption occurs mainly in the proximal convoluted tubule, but probably in more distal sites also. Tubular reabsorption of phosphate resembles that of glucose in that, provided the ECF volume and GFR remain stable, as the blood level and filtered load rise, reabsorption increases to a maximal rate known as the tubular maximum or Tm. The Tm varies with renal tissue mass, and so with body size, but the mean threshold (Tm per GFR × 100) is less variable. The Tm also varies with sodium balance and ECF volume, because changes in the proximal tubular reabsorption of sodium are accompanied by proportional changes in many other components of the glomerular filtrate including glucose, phosphate, bicarbonate, urate, and amino acids as well as calcium.

A decrease in the Tm or mean threshold for phosphate causes a fall in the blood level of phosphate, but only a temporary increase in urinary phosphate, which soon returns to its previous level. This is because the kidney itself is primarily responsible for controlling the blood level, which automatically adjusts so that absorption and excretion of phosphate come into equilibrium. In a steady state, urinary phosphate is approximately 60 to 80 per cent of the dietary intake, regardless of the Tm or the blood level of phosphorus.

Phosphorus excretion is affected by all three of the main regulatory factors for bone and calcium, and also by almost every other hormone, but parathyroid hormone (PTH) is still probably the most important. PTH increases phosphorus excretion by inhibiting tubular reabsorption in the proximal tubule and probably also at some more distal site.

Hydrogen (H⁺) Regulation

The importance of the skeleton as a buffer source, and the effect of chronic acidosis on bone have been debated for many years. More recently, important interactions between PTH and H^+ balance have been described.[31]

The generation of H^+ ions other than by CO_2 accumulation depends mainly on the protein content of the diet, with a small quantity resulting from fecal excretion of bicarbonate. In Western, developed countries, the resultant H^+ load is about 50 to 100 mEq daily, all of which must be excreted in the urine to maintain H^+ balance. This is accomplished by the secretion of H^+ ions into the urine in exchange for Na^+ ions. H^+ ion secretion in the proximal tubule effects the reabsorption of filtered HCO_2 ions, and H^+ secretion in the distal tubule effects net H^+ ion excretion as titratable acidity and ammonia.

An acute change in body content of H^+ ions, whether due to a change in H^+ generation or excretion, equilibrates not only with the extracellular bicarbonate-carbonic acid system, but also with intracellular buffers such as hemoglobin in red cells and other proteins and phosphates in soft tissues. Chronic accumulation of H^+ ions is also buffered by the dissolution of bone mineral. Athough conveniently measured by the amount of calcium liberated, it is the phosphate, hydroxyl and carbonate ions in bone which are actually responsible for the buffering. Soft tissue buffers are rapidly available, accessible by simple diffusion of H^+ ions across vascular walls and cell membranes, but of small capacity. Some buffer anions in bone are accessible to the osteocyte regulated percolation of water, but the bulk of bone buffers require dissolution of bone, and so are only slowly available and require the active intervention of cells, but are of much greater magnitude than soft tissue buffers.

How bone resorbing cells are stimulated by H^+ ion accumulation is unknown, but it is probably a direct effect not mediated by parathyroid hormone.

Vitamin D[21]

The naturally occurring form of vitamin D in the animal kingdom is cholecalciferol or vitamin D_3; vitamin D_2 and dihydrotachysterol (DHT) are synthetic substances which are antirachitic in man but will be considered mainly in relation to treatment.

SOURCES, ABSORPTION AND TRANSPORT. Vitamin D is produced in the skin by ultraviolet irradiation of the precursor 7-dehydrocholesterol (Fig. 13–8); this occurs mainly in the stratum germination, and so is regulated by the melanin content of the overlying stratum corneum; this p.gmentation may have been an evolutionary adaptation to prevent vitamin D intoxication.[253]

Dietary vitamin D from fortified milk products, animal liver and fish oils is absorbed by the jejunal mucosa and the intestinal lym-

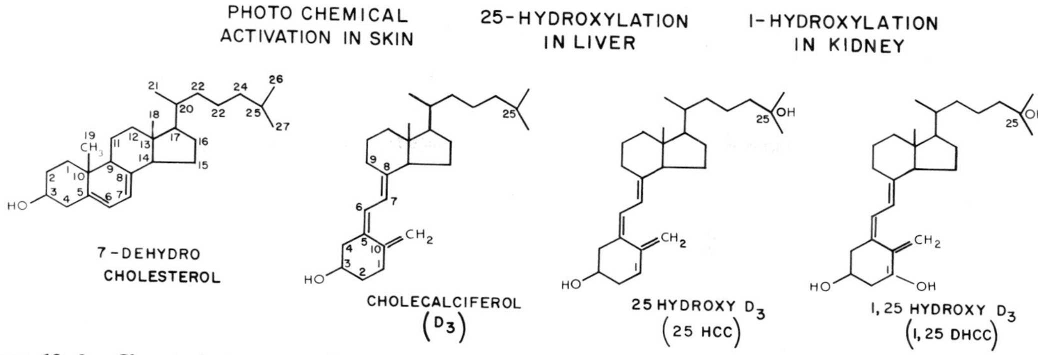

Figure 13–8. Chemical structures of vitamin D and its metabolites. Photochemical activation of 7 dehydrocholesterol opens the steroid ring at the 9–10 bond. Successive hydroxylation in positions of 25 and 1 produces 1,25 DHCC, the probable metabolically active form of vitamin D.

phatics into chylomicrons in the blood. Absorption is enhanced by bile salts, fatty acids and monoglyceride. After dispersion of the chylomicrons, vitamin D is carried in the blood bound to a specific globulin.

METABOLISM AND METABOLITES. Vitamin D_3 is hydroxylated in position 25 in the liver (Fig. 13–8) to form 25 hydroxy D_3 (25 HCC); this compound has some biologic activity but acts mainly as a transport form of vitamin D. Twenty-five HCC inhibits the enzyme responsible for 25 hydroxylation, so that variation in the supply of vitamin D has less effect on the formation of the metabolite. Any surplus vitamin D which is not metabolized is stored in muscle and adipose tissue. Twenty-five HCC is further metabolized in the kidney by an additional hydroxylation in position 1, to form 1,25 dihydroxy cholecalciferol (1,25 DHCC), which is the principal biologically active metabolite (Fig. 13–8).

Hydroxylation in position 1 is regulated indirectly by the plasma calcium level. In rats, dietary calcium depletion enhances the formation of 1,25 DHCC, whereas dietary calcium excess inhibits its formation. This effect of diet is probably mediated by hormonal changes since 1-hydroxylation is enhanced by small doses of parathyroid hormone and inhibited by calcitonin.

ACTIONS OF VITAMIN D. In a Vitamin D-depleted subject, as little as 2.5 μg (100 IU) daily will decrease fecal calcium excretion and increase calcium retention. This physiological effect contrasts with the pharmalogical effect of a much higher dose. In a Vitamin D-replete subject, a dose 100 times as large will have no discernible effect, but a dose 1000 times as large (2.5 mg or 100,000 IU per day)

will decrease fecal calcium and increase urinary calcium to the same extent, with no change in external balance.[300] These physiologic and pharmacologic effects are due to actions on target cells in gut, kidney and bone.

Effect on Gut. Vitamin D probably increases calcium absorption by both active transport and facilitated diffusion. These effects probably depend on increasing the synthesis of two proteins, a calcium-stimulated, magnesium dependent ATPase, which also acts as an alkaline phosphatase and which is produced in the brush border, and a calcium-binding protein secreted into the intestinal lumen.

Effect on the Kidney. Both 25 HCC and 1,25 DHCC have a direct effect on the renal tubule to enhance the reabsorption of phosphate. This is directly opposite to the effect of parathyroid hormone and appears to be a true physiologic antagonism, since the action cannot be demonstrated in the absence of parathyroid hormone. Thus the renal tubular reabsorption of phosphate seems to reflect a balance between the opposing influences of physiologic levels of PTH and vitamin D metabolites.

Effects on Bone. Vitamin D has effects on all three main cell types in bone.[300] In pharmacological doses, both osteoclastic resorption and periosteocytic osteolysis are enhanced by mechanisms independent of parathyroid hormone. These effects probably underlie the demonstration that vitamin D can raise the plasma calcium independently of any effect on calcium absorption, and may be concerned in the effects of vitamin D intoxication. In physiologic doses, vitamin D also raises the plasma calcium by increasing calcium release from bone, an effect which requires the presence of parathyroid hormone. Conversely, the effect of PTH on calcium release from bone requires vitamin D. This interaction of physiological levels of vitamin D and PTH which subserves calcium homeostasis is probably mediated by the osteocyte and its control of the blood bone equilibrium. A deficiency of either PTH or vitamin D can be overcome by a sufficiently large dose of the other.

In accordance with the traditional theory of cartilage and osteoid mineralization, promotion of these by vitamin D is ascribed solely to its effect on the calcium and phosphorus levels in blood. The recognition that the fluid in contact with bone is of different composition from the plasma, and of the other roles of the cell in mineralization has made this belief much less plausible. In vitamin D deficiency, there is a marked slowing of matrix synthesis as well as of mineralization, indicating a general depression of osteoblastic function.[324] This could be a direct consequence of vitamin D lack or it could result from intracellular phosphorus depletion. It seems likely that vitamin D may act on the transfer of calcium by bone cells, as well as by cells in the intestinal mucosa.

Parathyroid Hormone (PTH)[14, 315]

Normally, there are four parathyroid glands, which in the adult weigh about 30 mg. each. They are derived embryologically from cells of the neural crest via the branchial arch. The various cell types probably represent different stages of a cyclic process and so are interrelated; the basic cell is the chief cell. The ultrastructure suggests a secretory cycle similar to that of other peptide hormone secreting cells. The parathyroids are unique among endocrine glands in not being under pituitary control and in only secreting a single hormone.

STRUCTURE, SYNTHESIS, SECRETION AND METABOLISM OF PTH. Bovine, porcine and human PTH molecules are all polypeptides with a molecular weight of approximately 9500, containing 84 amino acids. The exact sequence of bovine PTH has been determined, and progress is being made with the human hormone. In both bovine and human glands, there is a prohormone (with a molecular weight of around 11,500 to 12,500) containing approximately 120 amino acids. This prohormone acts as a short term storage form which is cleaved to the smaller molecule prior to secretion. The secreted hormone has a short half-life, and a further cleavage to a still smaller molecule of molecular weight around 7000 takes place soon after the hormone enters the circulation. This has a long half-life, and probably represents the major immunoassayable form of PTH present in the circulation, but may be biologically inert. The lack of purified human hormone and the consequent inability to prepare antihuman PTH sera, together with the multiple forms of PTH present in the blood, have seriously hampered the development of reliable radioimmunoassay methods for human PTH. However, the solution to these problems is in sight and probably will have been achieved by the time this appears in print. The availability of purified bovine hormone, and homeostatic problems resulting from massive lactation have combined to make the cow an especially fruitful object of study which has provided much of the presently available information concerning the control of PTH secretion.

The most important factors so far identified which produce acute changes in hormone secretion are the divalent cations calcium and magnesium. A fall in the concentration of either in the blood perfusing the gland increases the release of PTH, and, conversely, a rise of either inhibits release. The secretion of PTH is also increased by acute metabolic alkalosis, by phosphate loading and by intravenous hydrocortisone, all of which may cause a transient depression of plasma-ionized calcium. Whether these effects can be sustained is not known. Acute and chronic effects are not always the same since chronic metabolic acidosis increases PTH secretion, probably by increasing urinary calcium excretion.

There is some evidence that calcitonin increases PTH secretion directly as well by inducing hypocalcemia, possibly be decreasing the calcium content of the parathyroid cell. A calcium-binding protein has been extracted from the gland, raising the question of whether vitamin D may also have a direct effect on PTH secretion.

The kidney has been identified as a major site of metabolic degradation of PTH; the enzymes responsible are probably located in microsomes of renal cortical cells. Some bioassayable PTH is normally excreted in the urine.

ACTIONS OF PTH ON BONE. There is no

doubt that PTH increases the plasma calcium by some action on bone, and there is a large body of experimental work directed to understanding the cellular basis of this process. In considering the application of this work to clinical medicine, certain reservations must be borne in mind. Firstly, most in vitro work with isolated bone preparations, and all work with organ and tissue culture have of necessity concerned woven bone rather than lamellar bone. Since these two tissues may respond quite differently to the same stimulus, the relevance of such work to lamellar bone and to human physiology and disease is uncertain. Secondly, most experiments have considered only the acute effects of single doses rather than the long-term effects of continued administration. This preoccupation reflects, but also reinforces, the widespread confusion between two entirely different aspects of plasma calcium homeostasis. Restoration of the prevailing steady state level by correction of deviations, and determination of a particular steady state level (high, normal, or low) both depend on PTH, but conceptually they are as different as are steering a course and deciding what course to steer. Finally, partly from the short duration and partly from inappropriate choice of experimental animal,[146] there is little definite information concerning the effect of PTH on the basic remodeling parameters defined in the previous section. In the rat, which has been most commonly used, the epiphyses never close, and bone cell activity throughout life is related to growth and modeling. Consequently, most of the voluminous literature concerning the rat is inapplicable to the remodeling of mature human bone. With these provisos, some of the data can now be considered.

PARATHYROID HORMONE AND OSTEO-CLASTS.[306, 399] In acute studies, PTH increases the resorptive activity of existing osteoclasts and also stimulates the proliferation of precursor cells into new osteoclasts. The effects on existing osteoclasts are shown by increases in both nuclear and especially cytoplasmic RNA synthesis within a few hours, and subsequent stimulation of all the metabolic machinery of the cells that is concerned with resorption. There is no evidence that these effects can be sustained. The increase in the number of osteoblasts is not evident for about 24 hours, and is preceded by an increase in nuclear but not cytoplasmic RNA synthesis in the preosteoclast segment of the osteo-

progenitor cell population. The precursor cells presumably undergo cell division and proliferation, followed by fusion into multinucleated cells. Increased numbers of osteoclasts occur within Haversian systems and within the bone marrow, but not on the endosteal surface.

PARATHYROID HORMONE AND OSTEO-BLASTS.[306, 399] There is a complex biphasic effect of PTH on osteoblasts. In tissue culture, PTH causes disappearance of osteoblasts preceded by loss of basophilic staining in the cytoplasm and of the endoplasmic reticulum, but continued PTH administration in rats is followed by a decrease in the number of osteoclasts and an increase in the number of osteoblasts, associated with increased formation of woven bone within a few weeks.[231] Parathyroid hormone also leads to increased osteoblastic activity in man by a different mechanism. In most patients with primary hyperparathyroidism, there is an increase in precursor cell activation and formation of new remodeling foci.[146] According to the scheme of lamellar bone remodeling described earlier, this would inevitably lead to an increase in osteoblastic activity.

PARATHYROID HORMONE AND PLASMA CALCIUM. The hypercalcemic response to PTH is a complex phenomenon which is affected by many factors.[306] These include species differences, the effectiveness of the homeostatic defense against hypercalcemia, the initial level of plasma calcium, the extent of osteoid covering bone surfaces, the plasma phosphorus level, the blood pH and the bone blood flow. The onset of the hypercalcemic response is very rapid and is preceded by an even earlier *fall* in plasma calcium which begins within a few minutes. This is due to increased uptake of calcium by bone cells associated with depolarization of the membrane potential.[306] This occurs at the same time as increased uptake by the cell of cyclic AMP, and both calcium and cyclic AMP uptake result from binding of the hormone to the cell membrane and activation of the membrane-bound enzyme adenylcyclase.

ACTIONS OF PTH ON THE KIDNEY.[306] An increase in urinary phosphorus is one of the earliest effects of PTH administration and may be apparent within minutes after PTH is injected directly into the renal artery. As explained earlier, while the acute effects are most clearly seen in the urine, the long-term effects of continued administration are best seen in the blood. The phosphaturic effect of

PTH is closely linked with the activation of adenylcyclase. The administration of PTH, both to rats and to normal human subjects, produces a short-lived increase in the excretion of cyclic AMP, which precedes the increase in urinary phosphorus.

Paratyphoid hormone has an important effect to increase calcium reabsorption in the distal nephron, so that at any filtered load of calcium, urinary calcium is higher than normal in hypoparathyroid states and lower than normal in hyperparathyroid states. This action plays an important role in the regulation of plasma calcium.[289]

Acutely, PTH also increases the excretion of sodium, potassium, bicarbonate, amino acids and water, as well as phosphate, by inhibiting their reabsorption in the proximal convoluted tubule. The effect on bicarbonate reabsorption lowers the threshold for bicarbonate excretion, and so hyperparathyroidism, both primary and secondary, is associated with a low plasma bicarbonate, and hypoparathyroidism with a high plasma bicarbonate. The effect on amino acid reabsorption accounts for the finding of aminoaciduria in states of secondary hyperparathyroidism and occasionally in primary hyperparathyroidism.

Calcitonin[131]

This hypocalcemic hormone is secreted by the parafollicular or C cells of the thyroid. These have a different embryological origin from the other cells of the thyroid, migrating from the neural crest via the branchial arch. In non-mammalian vertebrates, these cells retain separate anatomical identity as the ultimobranchial body, but in mammals they are incorporated into the substance of the thyroid.

STRUCTURE, SECRETION AND METABOLISM. In all species, calcitonin is a 32 amino acid polypeptide, but there are important differences in the amino acid sequence between different species. Human calcitonin exists in two forms, a dimer and a monomer (calcitonin M). Synthesis is not closely linked to secretion, so that, in contrast to PTH, large quantities of calcitonin may accumulate in the thyroid if the secretion rate is low.

One important factor controlling calcitonin secretion is the level of calcium in the blood perfusing the gland, high levels stimulating and low levels inhibiting secretion, the opposite relationship to PTH. Magnesium in high concentration also stimulates calcitonin release, but is much less effective than an equimolar amount of calcium. Calcitonin secretion is also stimulated by several gastrointestinal hormones, such as glucagon, and especially gastrin. In the rat, both human and salmon calcitonin is metabolized by microsomal enzymes in the kidney, although porcine calcitonin is metabolized mainly by the liver. The fate of calcitonin in man is unknown.

ACTIONS OF CALCITONIN. Calcitonin inhibits bone resorption both by reducing the activity of existing osteoclasts and by inhibiting the proliferation of precursor cells into new osteoclasts, effects opposite to those of PTH but not dependent on its presence. This produces an increased accumulation of trabecular bone during growth,[132] but not after skeletal maturity. Assuming a constant effect on the activity of each osteoclast, the magnitude of the acute fall in plasma calcium induced by calcitonin depends on the total number of osteoclasts, and hence correlates with prevailing rates of total bone resorption determined kinetically. In accordance with the scheme of normal bone remodeling, suppression of precursor cell proliferation (activation) leads eventually to a reduction in osteoblastic, as well as osteoclastic, activity. In patients with medullary carcinoma of the thyroid, a calcitonin-secreting neoplasm of the parafollicular cells, very high plasma levels of calcitonin are associated with almost total suppression of remodeling, the bone being virtually acellular.[274] It is of interest that the plasma calcium in these patients is usually normal and that they do not have osteosclerosis.

Calcitonin increases the renal excretion of calcium, sodium, potassium, inorganic phosphorus, magnesium and water. The effect on calcium is thus the opposite to that of parathyroid hormone, whereas the effect on the other ions is in the same direction.

FUNCTIONS OF CALCITONIN. The normal physiological function of calcitonin is still obscure. It acts jointly with parathyroid hormone to counteract deviations from the normal plasma calcium levels; for example, patients who lack calcitonin because of thyroidectomy show an increased rise in plasma calcium in response to calcium infusion. Calcitonin may participate in a specialized feedback mechanism to minimize the hypercalcemic response to dietary calcium ingestion. Calcitonin may also function to preserve bone mass in the face of situations (such as pregnancy) in which there would otherwise be increased bone loss to supply calcium.

The fundamental action of calcitonin on bone cells is possibly opposite to that of parathyroid hormone. The initial effect may be a small rise with release of labeled calcium from the skeleton, and this may be associated with polarization of the bone cells and movement of calcium out of them into the circulation.[73]

Plasma Calcium Homeostasis

For many years it has been widely believed and taught that variation in the rate of bone resorption was the primary method of determining the plasma calcium level. This belief has persisted in the face of an impressive body of evidence with which it is totally inconsistent. Bone resorption may be increased as much as tenfold in Paget's disease and decreased tenfold in hypothyroidism, so that normal levels of plasma calcium can be sustained in the face of a hundredfold change in the process on which the plasma calcium level is supposed to depend. This dissociation is supported by the usual normocalcemia in medullary carcinoma of the thyroid. Consideration of the normal remodeling cycle makes it clear why this is so. An increase in bone resorption can only produce a temporary increase in plasma calcium, since, within a period of one sigma (from 3 to 4 months) there will inevitably be an almost equivalent increase in bone formation. In fact, any steady state level of plasma calcium can coexist with any level — high, normal or low — of remodeling rate. This is most strikingly illustrated by the occurrence of hypocalcemia in patients with simultaneous Paget's disease and hypoparathyroidism. The undoubted relationship between steady state plasma calcium level and parathyroid status may reflect the effects of PTH on gut and kidney, or some effect of PTH on bone in addition to the control of bone remodeling. Alteration in the blood-bone equilibrium brought about by some action of PTH on the osteocyte-resting osteoblast system could account for continued hypercalcemia which did not depend on continued removal of calcium from the periosteocytic and perilacunar bone. A combination of increased intestinal calcium absorption and increased renal tubular reabsorption could also account for continued hypercalcemia in primary hyperparathyroidism,[289] but it seems to us merely perverse to suppose that the 1000 gm of calcium in the skeleton are unrelated to plasma calcium homeostasis simply because the bone resorption theory has been disproved.

Changes in bone resorption brought about by PTH and calcitonin are thought to constitute a second line of defense against a hypo- or hypercalcemic challenge, if this is too large or of too long duration to be met by the osteocyte-resting osteoblast system. Just as the mechanism whereby steering errors are corrected is the same whatever course is being steered, so the method of correcting deviations in plasma calcium from the prevailing level is essentially the same at widely different plasma calcium levels, albeit at a different rate.

MORPHOLOGIC DEFINITION OF THE MAJOR CATEGORIES OF METABOLIC BONE DISEASE

Morphologic definition of metabolic bone disease is needed to insure agreement on the use of diagnostic terms and to provide a standard against which the validity and accuracy of other diagnostic techniques can be assessed. Bone biopsy has been a standard procedure in Europe for many years, but it has been seriously neglected in the United States until quite recently. Not every patient with metabolic bone disease needs a bone biopsy; it is most useful for the confirmation or exclusion of osteomalacia and least useful in osteoporosis. Before considering the definitions, it is convenient to describe certain technical and methodological aspects of bone biopsy.

Bone Biopsy as a Diagnostic Tool — the Quantitative Approach to Bone Morphology[55]

Bone is most commonly taken from the ilium, which is easily accessible and consists predominantly of trabecular bone. A full-thickness sample with cortex at both ends should be taken from a few cm below the iliac crest, so that fragmentation of the trabeculae is minimized. Only a local anesthetic is needed and the patient can walk the following day. The sample is embedded in plastic (which takes several weeks), and suitably stained undecalcified sections are prepared by grinding or cutting with a sledge microtome or other suitable instrument. Because of varied orientation of trabeculae to the plane of section, the dynamic parameters of bone remodeling cannot be determined, and to circumvent these difficulties, bone is taken by open biopsy from the eleventh rib, after suitable labeling. A general anesthetic may be needed, but the morbidity is little more than with iliac biopsy, although occasionally a pneumothorax is induced. A suitable labeling schedule is to give Declomycin (or equivalent tetracycline) 300–600 mg b.d. for four days, followed by a 10 day break and then a further 6 day period of Declomycin. Bone biopsy is then taken 7 to 10 days later. The solidity of the predominantly cortical bone enables undecalcified sections to be made by simple abrasion under running water, without plastic embedding, but for cytological details additional decalcified sections must be prepared.

Use of these techniques in patients with metabolic bone diseases affecting the spine rests on the assumption that the effects of such diseases are generalized, even though different bones may be affected to different extents. Vertebral biopsy is unsuitable for routine diagnostic use because of its increased difficulty and danger, but it may be very helpful in distinguishing between metabolic and nonmetabolic, especially neoplastic, disease.[197]

From either type of sample, ilium or rib, static measurements can be made of the volumes of mineralized, unmineralized and total bone as fractions of the total volume of the sample, of the areas of different types of surface as fractions of the total surface and as absolute areas per unit volume, and of thicknesses, lacunar dimensions and other lengths of interest. The theoretical basis of the methods is discussed elsewhere.[304, 348]

Sites of resorption are easily identified as Howship's lacunae, but in trabecular bone, only about 5 per cent of such lacunae contain an osteoclast to indicate that resorption was actually in progress at the time the biopsy was taken. Because osteoclasts are mobile, their domain of influence is larger than the area of bone with which they are in contact at any moment, but, even so, it is unlikely that more than 15 per cent of the lacunar surface is undergoing active resorption. At the remaining 85 per cent, resorption has ceased, either temporarily or permanently. It is claimed that active and inactive resorption can also be distin-

guished by microradiography,[225] but the validity of this method is open to serious question. Values for active resorption surface determined by microradiography are of the same order of magnitude as values for active formation surface. Since the linear resorption rate is at least five times as rapid as the appositional rate,[215] preservation of skeletal balance requires that the active resorption surface be only about one fifth of the formation surface. Values obtained by microradiography are probably equivalent to total resorptive surface, active and inactive, determined by more direct methods. An increase in this surface could result from an increase in the extent of active resorption or from a delay in the commencement of formation on surfaces where resorption has been completed. It should be noted that this conclusion casts some doubt on inferences drawn from microradiography concerning pathogenesis, but it does not reduce the diagnostic value of any empirical correlations which have been established between total resorption surface and various disease states.

Sites of bone formation are identified by the presence both of matrix synthesis and of mineralization. Matrix synthesis is indicated by an osteoid seam and mineralization by the uptake of tetracycline (recognized by fluorescence),[153] by special stains for the mineralization front, such as toluidine blue,[55] or by low density bone revealed by microradiography.[225] All three methods indicate that normally about 85 to 90 per cent of the total osteoid seam surface is associated with mineralization.

Seams can be further subdivided according to the morphology of the osteoblast so that four types of normal seam can be defined (Fig. 13–9).[348] At the onset of seam formation, matrix synthesis proceeds for about ten days, until the seam widens to full thickness and primary mineralization begins; this may be called a nascent seam. During the rest of the active life of the osteoblast, the seam thickness remains constant, the mineralization front advancing at the same rate as the apposition of new matrix; this may be called a growing seam. After a time, matrix synthesis slows down or ceases, the morphology of the osteoblast changes from active to inactive, and primary mineralization continues at a slower rate, while the seam (which may now be called a maturing seam) gets progressively thinner, until eventually the osteoid is completely re-

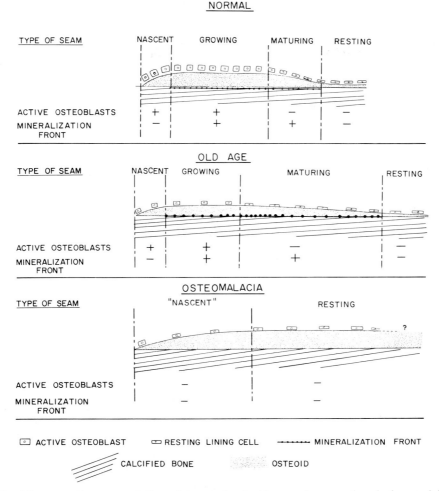

Figure 13–9. Diagrammatic representation of types of osteoid seam in normal and abnormal bone showing postulated temporal progression from left to right. Upper panel shows four normal types which can be distinguished according to the presence or absence of active osteoblasts and of a mineralization front. Center panel shows prolongation of seam maturation due to slowing of osteoblast function with increasing age. Bottom panel shows accumulation of abnormal seams characteristic of osteomalacia.

placed by mineralized bone. Finally, there may be a small number of resting seams at which matrix synthesis and primary mineralization have both ceased. Most resting seams eventually complete their mineralization, but the manner in which they do this is unknown.

Criteria for recognizing these four types and their relative abundance in trabecular and cortical bone are given in Table 13–2, together with the other three types of surface which can be recognized by a combination of the surface configuration, presence or absence of a mineralization front, and morphology of the cells.

Although surface-based measurements

are of great value in diagnosis, they all suffer from the disadvantage that rates cannot be determined from surface areas. The fraction of the total surface occupied by a particular type is equal to the fraction of the total turnover time for which the corresponding stage of remodeling activity persists. Since the volume of bone turned over by one remodeling cycle is approximately constant, a decrease in the linear resorption or appositional rate will inevitably lead to an increase in the time taken to resorb (or form) a given volume of bone. This in turn would lead to an increase in the per cent of surface occupied by resorption (or formation). Thus, an increase in per cent of sur-

TABLE 13–2.   MORPHOLOGIC TYPES OF BONE SURFACE AND THEIR CHARACTERISTICS

State	Surface	Cell Morphology	Seam Thickness	Mineralization Front
1. Quiescent	Smooth	Flat lining cells	—	—
2. Active resorption	Scalloped	Osteoclasts	—	—
3. Post resorption	Scalloped	None or as 1	—	—
4. Nascent seam	Smooth	Active osteoblasts	Reduced	—
5. Growing seam	Smooth	Active osteoblasts	Normal	+
6. Maturing seam	Smooth	Inactive osteoblasts	Reduced	+
7. Resting seam	Smooth	Flat lining cells	Variable	—

face of resorption (or formation) may indicate a decrease in cellular activity as well as an increase in remodeling rate.

We will now consider the definitions of the different types of metabolic bone disease, and how the information from bone biopsy may be used for diagnosis.

Osteoporosis

Strictly interpreted, osteoporosis means increased porosity of bone, but this usage is now universally disregarded, the term osteoporotic being applied to many patients whose bones are thin, but not porous. The usual definition of osteoporosis is a reduction in the amount of bone tissue, the remaining bone being apparently normal. The amount of bone is best defined by volume rather than by weight, since alterations in density reflect changes in mineralization which should be excluded from the definition. Absolute bone volume, which is the volume of whole bone less the volume of its various holes—marrow space, Haversian and Volkmann's canals, lacunae and canaliculae—is the best expression of the amount of bone.[152] To characterize this quantity as low, normal, or high requires comparison with a standard, and for reasons discussed later, two standards are needed. One is derived from sex-matched, healthy adults at skeletal maturity and the other from controls matched for age as well as sex. The definition of osteoporosis as an absolute bone volume which is reduced in relation to one of these standards still leaves certain difficulties. Some people use the term osteoporosis to refer to a process, as well as a state; this ambiguity can be resolved by referring to the process which may lead to the state of osteoporosis as bone loss. The stipulation that osteoporotic bone is normal except in amount is intended merely to exclude osteitis fibrosa and osteomalacia; it should not be taken to exclude other physical and chemical changes which may affect osteoporotic bone and which are described later. The recognition of osteoporosis as an additional and separate abnormality which may coexist with osteitis fibrosa or osteomalacia is best accomplished by excluding woven bone and considering only normal lamellar bone, both mineralized and unmineralized, in the determination of absolute bone volume. A final problem is the relationship of osteoporosis as defined to clinical disability. There is considerable evidence that structural failure of bone depends on changes in quality as well as in amount. Whether this is so or not, it is clearly important to refer separately to the state of the bones and to the clinical disability, if any, resulting from that state.[47] One approach is to restrict the term osteoporosis to patients with a clinical disability, and to refer to a reduced absolute bone volume, with or without symptoms, as osteopenia. This is unambiguous, but the use of osteoporosis in both senses is too well entrenched to be dislodged. Another approach is to distinguish between an osteoporotic patient and an osteoporotic skeleton, whose owner may or may not be disabled.[146] We will refer, when necessary, to symptomatic and asymptomatic osteoporosis.

The diagnosis of osteoporosis on bone biopsy rests on demonstrating that the total volume of bone (both mineralized and unmineralized) expressed as a fraction of the total sample volume, is less than the appropriate standard (ideal or age matched). Such measurements are of value in epidemiologic and population studies, but there is some question of their accuracy in a small volume of trabecular bone. Histologic methods are consequently not very useful in the positive diagnosis of osteoporosis in an individual patient, but serve to exclude osteomalacia and osteitis fibrosa cystica. They also enable different anatomical patterns of bone loss to be determined.

Osteomalacia

The classic histological hallmark of osteomalacia is an increase in the accumulation of osteoid, considered as evidence of a specific impairment of mineralization. In recent years, the nature of this defect has been much clarified and it has been recognized that osteoid may accumulate for other reasons, so that the histologic definition of osteomalacia must be re-examined. The most accurate assessment of the amount of osteoid is given by the osteoid volume expressed either as a fraction of the total tissue volume or of the total bone volume. However, this does not take into account the characteristics of individual seams. Most of the difference between normal and abnormal values is given by the area, or, in cortical bone, by the number of seams (Fig. 13–10). The mean seam thickness may be only slightly increased or not at all. This is because there is a reduction in the rate of matrix synthesis as well as in mineralization. Only in advanced osteomalacia is there a significant increase in osteoid seam thickness, which is more evident in trabecular than in cortical bone.[55, 146] Unless seam thickness is markedly increased, the definition of osteomalacia simply in terms of number of seams or the extent of seam surface is unsatisfactory because increased osteoid can arise from an acceleration of bone turnover and is also found in elderly people in the absence of a mineralization defect. These problems can be resolved by considering the four types of normal seam (Table 13–2). With a high rate of bone turnover, nascent, growing and maturing seam surfaces are all increased in the same portion, with no change or fall in the resting seam surface. In the aged, both maturing and resting seam surfaces are increased with a decrease in nascent and growing seams. This results from a combination of reduced activation and turnover and a slowing down in the terminal phase of primary mineralization leading to accumulation of more slowly maturing seams (Fig. 13–9B). In osteomalacia there is an increase in resting seams and a decrease in all other kinds (Fig. 13–9C). This results from partial or complete arrest of both matrix synthesis and of the initial phase of primary mineralization, leading to accumulation of abnormal seams (Fig. 13–10). In cortical bone, resting seams may be increased in some osteoporotic patients,[400] but they are much thinner than normal and of smaller circumference, indicating that they are at the end of the remodeling cycle. In osteomalacia, the resting seams are of normal or increased thickness and of normal circumference (Fig. 13–9C).

The simplest way to define the severity of osteomalacia is to measure the mineral content after ashing, expressing the result per unit

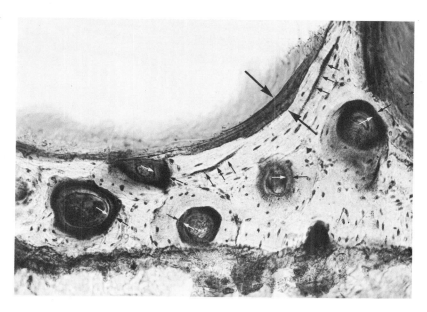

Figure 13–10. Mineralized, unembedded, cross section of a human eighth rib biopsy showing osteomalacia. All the Haversian canals are lined with osteoid seams as indicated by the dark and light circular bands bracketed by the small white and black arrows. At the extreme upper right is a trabecula showing a microfracture as a dark line running downward (small arrows). A light-stained osteoid seam lines the endosteal surface (large arrows) at the middle right portion of the picture. The zone of demarcation, which is seen in normal osteoid seams, is missing. Note the scalloped edges at the periosteal surface (bottom portion of the picture). The darkly stained nuclei in the Haversian and extrahaversian bone are osteocytes. Tetrachrome bone stain, 175×. (Courtesy of A. R. Villanueva.)

volume or weight of dry, fat-free bone, or per gram of nitrogen.[304] This avoids the difficulties of quantitative microscopy but does not permit the identification of the specific mineralization defect of osteomalacia.

Osteitis Fibrosa and Hyperparathyroidism

The traditional full name for the bone disease of primary hyperparathyroidism is osteitis fibrosa cystica generalisata. Since the process is not inflammatory, some authors have abandoned the term, but for clarity of thought and exposition, it is necessary to refer separately to hyperparathyroidism and to its effects, if any, on the bones, and no suitable alternative to osteitis fibrosa is available.

Historically, the recognition of primary hyperparathyroidism as a disease entity resulted entirely from its striking osseous manifestations, but it was soon realized that in most patients with hyperparathyroidism the bones were clinically and radiographically normal. It has repeatedly been suggested that patients with and without bone disease could be clearly separated.[6, 101] However, increasing use of bone biopsy has blurred this distinction, since histologic abnormalities can be found in almost all patients. We think that the distinction should be preserved, since the bone involvement in the two groups of patients show qualitative as well as quantitative differences. The classical histological sign of hyperparathyroidism is an increase in the extent of osteoclastic resorption. In most patients without overt bone disease, this reflects an increase in normal remodeling, as in hyperthyroidism, with increased numbers of resorption spaces of normal size in the cortex and increased extent of resorption surface in the trabeculae, and increase in osteoblasts and seams. We refer to this as high turnover osteoporosis, not osteitis fibrosa, since the resorbed bone is replaced by normal lamellar bone. In severe hyperparathyroidism, resorption spaces in cortical bone may become confluent, producing osteoclast-lined cavities which are larger than normal Haversian systems (Fig. 13–11), and in cancellous bone the osteoclasts may burrow deep into the substance of the trabeculae instead of remaining on the surface (Fig. 13–12). The resorbed bone is replaced, not by normal lamellar bone, but by fibrous tissue and woven bone; this is

the distinctive morphologic feature of osteitis fibrosa, and is seen both within the marrow and within Haversian canals (Figs. 13–11 and 13–12). Increased fibrosis is also common in the lesions of fibrous dysplasia (osteitis fibrosa disseminata), but these also contain islands of cartilage. Replacement of lamellar bone by woven bone also occurs in Paget's disease (q.v.), but in osteitis fibrosa the architecture of the bone is better preserved and the extreme irregularity of the cement lines characteristic of Paget's disease is only rarely seen. In osteitis fibrosa woven bone is first laid down in condensations of fibrous tissue within the space created by resorption of lamellar bone.[94] In extreme cases the entire skeleton may consist of abnormal bone formed since the beginning of the disease.[204]

Sometimes more woven bone is formed than lamellar bone removed, leading to more

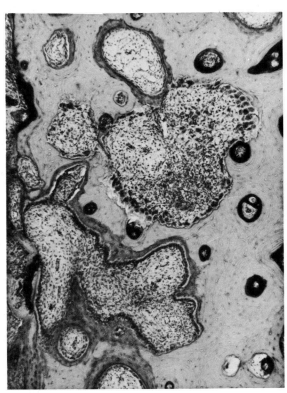

Figure 13–11. Section through cortical bone from a patient with osteitis fibrosa due to primary hyperparathyroidism. *In the upper half* of the figure is a large resorption space which is much larger than a normal Haversian system, lined with osteoclasts. *In the lower half* is shown another resorption space which is now lined with osteoblasts. Note fibroblastic proliferation within both spaces.

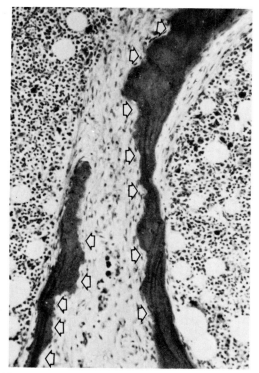

Figure 13–12. Section through vertebral bone from a patient with osteitis fibrosa due to secondary hyperparathyroidism. Note multiple Howship's lacunae (white arrows) and erosions deep into the trabeculae. (Courtesy of N. A. Hancox.)

densely packed trabeculae, partial obliteration of the marrow space and osteosclerosis. This is especially common in secondary hyperparathyroidism due to uremia but can also occur in primary hyperparathyroidism even without significant renal failure.[121, 413]

Cysts of osteitis fibrosa are of two kinds: true cysts, which consist of unusually large resorption cavities filled with fluid; and pseudocysts, which consist of masses of osteoclasts and fibrous tissue (Table 13–3) and incompletely mineralized bone, the classical brown tumor, which resembles the osteoclastoma or giant cell tumor. Both types may expand the outline of the bone, producing bizarre deformities. Osteoclastomas may sometimes occur in hyperparathyroidism in the absence of other evidence of osteitis fibrosa, suggesting that a moderate increase in PTH secretion has triggered the proliferation of a mitotically unstable group of mesenchymal cells.

An important diagnostic feature of bone in hyperparathyroidism is an increase in the size of osteocytic lacunae caused by periosteocytic osteolysis even when other histologic features are minimal or even absent. The osteocytic lacunae are, on the other hand, of normal size in hyperthyroidism.[276]

Some features of hyperthyroid and hyperparathyroid bone disease are compared in Table 13–3 in order to emphasize the distinction between an increase in remodeling rate alone and the additional features of osteitis fibrosa. The mild histologic lesion of hyperparathyroidism closely resembles that of hyperthyroidism, with the addition of periosteocytic osteolysis. There is an increased remodeling rate and either no clinical or radiographic abnormalities at all—bone involvement rather than bone disease—or the clinical and radiographic features (described later) of high turnover osteoporosis. By contrast, the severe histologic abnormalities of hyperparathyroidism, comprising the distinctive features of osteitis fibrosa are associated with the classic clinical and radiographic findings.

It will be evident that the diagnostic value

TABLE 13–3. MORPHOLOGIC CHARACTERISTICS OF HYPERTHYROIDISM, MILD HYPERPARATHYROIDISM (HIGH TURNOVER OSTEOPOROSIS), AND SEVERE HYPERPARATHYROIDISM (OSTEITIS FIBROSA CYSTICA)

	Hyper-thyroidism	Mild Hyper-parathyroidism	Severe Hyper-parathyroidism
Number of cortical resorption spaces	Increased	Increased	Increased
Size of cortical resorption spaces	Normal	Normal	Confluent
Surface area of trabecular resorption	Increased	Increased	Increased
Morphology of trabecular resorption	Lacunar	Lacunar	Dissecting
Fibrous tissue replacement	Absent	Absent	Present
Woven bone replacement	Absent	Absent	Present
Cysts (true or false)	Absent	Absent	Present
Periosteocytic osteolysis	Absent	Present	Present

of bone biopsy will be much greater in the mild form than in the severe, and most quantitative measurements relate to the high turnover osteoporosis rather than to the classical lesions of osteitis fibrosa. However, even here, bone biopsy may provide some surprises by revealing evidence of osteomalacia as well as osteitis fibrosa; not only an increased number of seams due to increased remodeling but also an unequivocal mineralization defect. This osteomalacia may significantly modify the clinical, radiographic and biochemical manifestations of hyperparathyroidism, and awareness of it may be important in management.

Thus, in primary hyperparathyroidism, the bones may be clinically and radiographically normal, or may show high turnover osteoporosis, or varying degrees of osteomalacia and osteosclerosis as well as osteitis fibrosa.

OTHER METHODS OF STUDY

In this section, we describe the clinical, radiographic and laboratory procedures which may help firstly in confirming or excluding metabolic bone disease in a patient with a spinal abnormality and secondly in establishing a diagnosis.

Clinical Assessment

Points of special importance in the history, family history, nutritional assessment, and physical examination which must be considered in every patient, but which relate primarily to one distinct type of metabolic disease are described later; however, some presenting manifestations common to each type can conveniently be considered here. Often, the patient will be asymptomatic, an abnormality having been found incidental to some unrelated radiographic examination, but if there is a presenting symptom, it is likely to be pain, deformity, fracture, or difficulty in walking.

PAIN IN METABOLIC BONE DISEASE. The innervation of bone consists primarily of small unmyelinated and a few myelinated fibers. These enter the nutrient foramina in association with blood vessels,[354] extend along the Haversian canals,[87] and arborize over the trabeculae from the endosteum. These fibers may be autonomic, since no nerve endings have been found within the bone,[87] and it has been

suggested that all bone pain comes from the periosteum,[354] in which there are both free and complex unencapsulated nerve endings.[211] However, inserting a needle into bone produces an unpleasant sensation of pressure which can be distinguished from that of periosteal irritation,[235] and expanding lesions within the bone, such as metastases, produce pain long before there is any periosteal involvement. The injection of saline under subcutaneous periosteum produces severe pain well localized to the site of injection, but with less superficial periosteum pain is poorly localized and is referred segmentally.[235] Nonmyelinated nerve fibers are also found in connective tissue structures around the spine, such as the anterior and posterior longitudinal ligaments, anulus fibrosus and capsules of interspinous joints.[211] The injection of saline into interspinous ligaments produces segmentally referred pain similar to that for the periosteum.[235]

These anatomical facts provide a basis for the usual characterization of bone pain as a dull ache which may be throbbing, poorly localized and subject to referral,[137] since these are the characteristics of slow pain transmitted by nonmyelinated fibers.[154] Periosteal involvement may explain pain from vertebral collapse with cortical buckling, or from expansion of the cortex by a cyst or by Paget's disease and the localized tenderness of bone to percussion. Both local and referred pain from ligaments and muscles subjected to abnormal strain may result from the mechanical effects of vertebral deformity. Root pain may arise from direct pressure, but more commonly by referral from periosteum or spinal ligaments.[137] Deep pain, possibly related to raised intramedullary pressure (as in osteoarthritis), may occur in vascular lesions such as in Paget's disease and osteitis fibrosa. It is less easy to explain the severe acute and lancinating pain which may follow vertebral collapse, why osteomalacic bone is in general so much more painful than osteoporotic bone, and why some patients with osteoporosis may have bone pain and tenderness resembling osteomalacia, whereas others with apparently similar bones may be asymptomatic.

In general, pain is most prominent in osteomalacia and least in osteoporosis, except with recent fracture. Complete absence of pain is possible in both osteitis fibrosa and osteoporosis, but not in osteomalacia. Pain is usually worse with walking and weight-bearing, and is usually worse in the hips and legs than in the shoulders and arms. Often the pain is bilateral, a fact which may help differentiate it from other causes of root pain such as disc disease.

All subcutaneous bones, the malleoli, tibiae, iliac crest, pubic rami, ribs, sternum, clavicles, and acromion processes, as well as the spinous processes, should be tested for tenderness to percussion.

DEFORMITY IN METABOLIC BONE DISEASE. In children, the historical pattern of growth and present skeletal development should be noted. At any age, the time of onset and rate of progression of deformity should be determined if possible, although only rarely will previous serial height observations be available. Measurements should be made of the total height, upper segment (crown-pubic symphysis) and lower segment (pubic symphysis—heels). Normally, in adults the upper and lower segments should be equal and the height should equal the span of the outstretched arms from fingertip to fingertip. Except in hypogonadism, and before epiphyseal closure when the limbs are disproportionately long, these measurements will detect shortening of the spine of more than about one inch.

Deformity of the spine will most commonly be a regular kyphosis which can occur in all three types of metabolic bone disease. There may be a local increase in curvature and slight angulation, but true gibbous formation is rare. Severe kyphosis and shortening may cause the ribs to rub painfully on the iliac crest, and there will often be a transverse crease across the abdominal wall.[100] Scoliosis is not usually a feature of the three main types of bone disease, but occasionally it may have a metabolic or biochemical cause.

FRACTURES IN METABOLIC BONE DISEASE. Although most information about fractures is gained from x-rays, it is convenient to consider them at this point. Excluding greenstick fractures in children, fractures are of three main types—traumatic, pathologic and stress. Classically, a traumatic fracture is one which occurs in a normal bone exposed to excessive stress, but fractures in bone mechanically weakened by osteoporosis in the absence of any localized abnormality are also included. Pathologic fractures occur through a localized weakness resulting from disease, classically a metastasis, but fractures in osteitis fibrosa through a cyst or a zone of gross osteoclastic resorption are also correctly described as

pathologic. Strictly speaking, a stress fracture occurs in normal bone with abnormal use, but the concept has been usefully extended to include any fracture without gross displacement caused by the cumulative effect of repeated nonviolent subthreshold trauma.[308] In this sense, stress fractures comprise *fatigue* fractures in bone with normal elastic resistance subjected to abnormal stress, and *insufficiency* fractures in bone with subnormal elastic resistance subjected to normal stress. Stress fractures as defined may occur in osteoporosis, and the characteristic radiographic lesion of osteomalacia, the Looser zone, is a special variety of stress fracture. Looser zones are sometimes called pseudofractures, a term best avoided because it has often been used in a wider sense to comprise all stress fractures, and because a Looser zone, like any other stress fracture, may, with slight additional trauma, become complete, with separation and displacement of the bone fragments.[76] We emphasize these distinctions because the fracture pattern is different in each type of metabolic bone disease, but the information needed to determine the type of fracture is frequently omitted from published reports.

In the clinical evaluation of patients with respect to suspected metabolic bone disease, any previous fracture should be carefully characterized with respect to the circumstances in which it occurred, the degree of trauma, the presence and amount of pain, the need for surgical intervention, the type and duration of immobilization, the duration of healing, and any residual deformity.

MUSCLE WEAKNESS IN METABOLIC BONE DISEASE.[317, 365] The gait should always receive special attention. Difficulty in walking may be due to pain and limitation of movement, but another component may be true muscle weakness. This may sometimes conform to the pattern of a proximal myopathy with muscle wasting, hypotonia, and normal reflexes. The patient may have difficulty in walking up stairs without using his arms to lift the legs, or may even resort to crawling. There may be difficulty in getting up from a bending or stooping position. The EMG may show a myopathic pattern, with random loss of muscle fibers, or evidence of denervation. The clinical feature may resemble polymyositis or carcinomatous neuromyopathy, and the relationship to the underlying metabolic bone disease may be overlooked. This type of muscle weakness may occur in both osteomalacia and osteitis fibrosa, but in osteoporosis muscle weakness is more likely a result of poor nutrition, immobilization, and the muscle atrophy of old age.

The etiology of this metabolic myopathy is uncertain. Vitamin D seems to be stored in muscle and conceivably could affect the uptake of calcium by the sarcoplasmic reticulum, an important factor in muscular contraction. Another possibility is that muscle weakness may result from intracellular phosphate depletion, presumably the lack of some organic phosphate compound concerned in the production of energy. Both abnormal vitamin D metabolism and phosphate depletion may occur in both osteomalacia and hyperparathyroidism.

NEUROSURGICAL ASPECTS OF METABOLIC BONE DISEASE.   Very occasionally the integrity of the central nervous system is compromised to a degree sufficient to require neurosurgical intervention. These situations will be considered in relation to individual diseases, but it may be useful to summarize the information here.

Basilar Impression.   If caused by bone disease, this results from changes in the skull rather than in the spine, but frequently the spinal cord is involved as well as the brain. Basilar impression, in which the vertebral column is invaginated into the base of the skull, owing to softening of the basiocciput, must be distinguished from platybasia, an abnormality in the shape of the floor of the skull, of interest to physical anthropologists but of no medical significance. Basilar impression can occur in osteogenesis imperfecta, Paget's disease, fibrous dysplasia, osteomalacia, and osteitis fibrosa cystica.[205, 206] In some cases, the bone disease may be prolonged and subclinical,[205] so that all patients with apparent primary basilar impression should be vigorously investigated to rule out metabolic bone disease.

Cord and Root Compression.   Although segmentally referred pain is common in metabolic bone disease, actual compression of neural structures is rare. Cord and root compression occasionally may develop because of an expanding lesion within the vertebra, such as an osteoclastoma of hyperparathyroidism or fibrous dysplasia, or from an enlargement of the whole vertebra, as in Paget's disease, or from exostosis and ossification of paraspinal ligaments, as in osteofluorosis and in adults with familial hypophosphatemia.

Vertebral compression fractures due to

metabolic bone disease do not cause spinal cord compression unless there is substantial trauma and vertebral displacement, except in Paget's disease. If the amount of bone is reduced, as in osteoporosis, vertebral compression does not cause any horizontal expansion of the lateral walls of the vertebral body. In Paget's disease, however, the abnormal bone is structurally weak and vertebral compression may occur even though the amount of bone is increased, so that bone may be squeezed out horizontally, expanding the vertebral circumference.

Radiographic Assessment

The most useful films differ somewhat from those best for the detection of osseous metastases, the other circumstance in which a skeletal survey may be requested. In the spine, lateral views are more informative. Anteroposterior and oblique films help in the initial exclusion of degenerative, arthritic and neoplastic causes of backache, but often do not distinguish one type of metabolic bone disease from another. Isolated changes in L5, as in Paget's disease, may be seen most clearly in the PA film, since this vertebra may be obscured by the pelvic brim, and increased bone density from various causes may be more easily seen in this view. Once a diagnosis is established, only lateral views are needed to assess progress. Of the other bones, the hands are the most important although they are only rarely involved by osseous metastases. If further information is needed, views of the pelvis and upper femora, lateral skull, chest, including the outer ends of the clavicles and outer borders of the scapulae, AP of knees and upper tibiae, feet, and renal areas will encompass almost all the pertinent abnormalities in adults. In children, views of the whole length of the femora and tibiae in two planes may be needed to detect bowing.

THE SPINE.   Radiographic abnormalities in the spine can be considered under three headings—alterations in radiolucency, in shape of the vertebral bodies, and in trabecular structure. Changes in cortical structure are of minor importance.

Changes in Radiolucency.   In all three types of metabolic bone disease there may be a reduction in the amount of calcium in a unit volume of bone. The terms used to describe the resultant change in x-ray appearance have given rise to much confusion. "Osteoporosis" was at one time commonly used, until this term was given its present more precise and restricted meaning.[6] "Decalcification" or "demineralization," although in frequent current use, are appropriate to what happens to bone in vitro but not in vivo. If reference is made to changes in "density," this must be understood as optical density (which depends on the absorption of light of particular wavelength) and not as the physical density of mass per unit volume. The relationship between optical and physical density is discussed in the section on densitometric measurement. The most neutral noncommital terms are "rarefaction" or "radiolucency."

Standard x-rays are rather insensitive to changes in mineral content. In general, at least 30 per cent of the bone tissue must be lost before a change is readily discerned. Holes up to three fourths inch in diameter drilled in vertebral bodies may completely escape detection.[11]

There are several pitfalls in the radiographic assessment of vertebral density. The apparent density is decreased by inspiration and increased by expiration, and is affected by many other technical factors in film preparation.[109] After vertebral collapse, compression of the same amount of bone tissue into a smaller volume may increase density even in a porotic vertebra. In some forms of osteosclerosis, the centra may be mistakenly regarded as less dense than normal in relation to the increased density of the end plates.[302] Even accurate assessments of vertebral density are of little help in differential diagnosis.

Changes in Shape. These can be resolved into three separate components—increased concavity, wedging, and compression (Fig. 13–13). Increased concavity is due to ballooning of the intervertebral disc into the center of the vertebral body, with preservation of the walls. If it affects both ends equally, it produces the so-called codfish vertebra (Fig. 13–13). It is easy to get a false impression of ballooning of the disc in vertebrae which are not centered accurately in the x-ray beam, so that the end plates are seen in oblique view (Fig. 13–14).[66, 74, 207] For this reason, the severity of changes in concavity is most accurately assessed by laminograms. A numerical expression of this severity is given by the shortest vertical distance between the end plates as a fraction of the height of the posterior vertebral wall.[28]

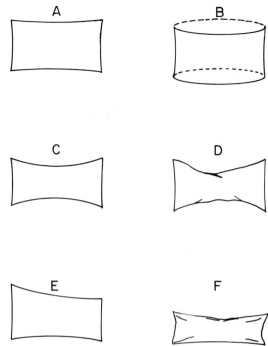

Figure 13–13. Diagrammatic representation of various alterations of vertebral shapes seen in lateral radiographs. *A,* Normal. *B,* False biconcavity due to oblique direction of x-ray beam. *C,* Osteomalacic biconcavity (codfish vertebra) which is smooth and symmetrical about the horizontal plane through the center. *D,* Osteoporotic biconcavity which is irregular and asymmetrical about the horizontal plane (should not be called codfish vertebra). *E,* Wedging with reduced anterior border but normal posterior border. *F,* Compression with reduction of both anterior and posterior borders.

Another type of encroachment of the intervertebral disc on the space normally occupied by bone is the Schmorl's node. This represents herniation of the nucleus pulposus through a localized defect in the cartilaginous or bony end plate. Schmorl's nodes have been described in association with both osteoporosis and osteitis fibrosa,[6] but statistical evidence that they occur more commonly in these conditions than in the absence of metabolic bone disease is still lacking.

Wedging refers to a reduction in the vertical height of the anterior border of a vertebral body compared to the posterior border (Figs. 13–13 and 13–15). Normally, the upper and lower borders are parallel, and minor degrees of wedging are best detected by demonstrating that lines projected from these borders converge at some point. Wedging can arise during development, with unequal

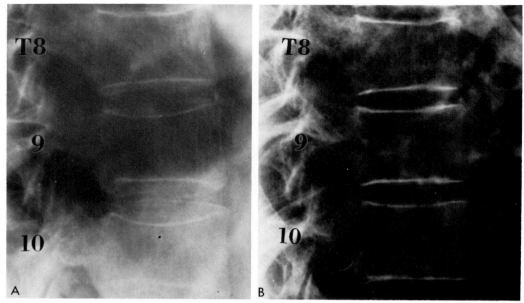

Figure 13–14. Spine of the same patient x-rayed two days apart, showing illusion of biconcavity in a normally shaped vertebra. *A,* Effect of obliquely directed x-ray beam showing end plates of T-10 as ellipses. *B,* Correctly aligned film showing normal shape.

growth of the vertebral body, especially with early or delayed closure of the epiphyses or so-called epiphysitis (Fig. 13–16).[6, 133] However, if wedging occurs after normal size has been

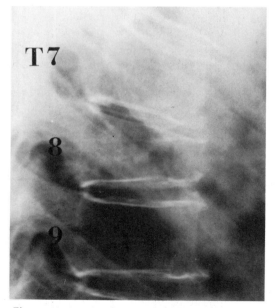

Figure 13–15. Wedging of T8 in a 62-year-old woman with involutional osteoporosis. Note that height of posterior border is unchanged.

attained, it signifies partial collapse of the vertebral body. Because the vertebra is strengthened posteriorly by the neural arch and the paravertebral muscles, such partial collapse is usually more severe anteriorly. Wedging is much the most common vertebral deformity.

Compression is recognized by a reduction in the vertical height of the posterior border of the vertebral body (Figs. 13–13, 13–17 and 13–18). It may occur without, but more commonly with, associated wedging, depending on whether the anterior border is affected to the same or to a greater extent. Similar changes in shape may occur during growth; however, compression signifies a more severe degree of collapse than does wedging. Minor degrees of compression may be detected by comparing the shape of adjacent vertebrae, or, if many vertebrae are affected, by comparison with normal standards for shape.[60] With severe compression the neural arches telescope together, and adjacent spinous processes may come into contact and pseudoarthroses may even develop between them.[66]

The vertebral collapse underlying both wedging and compression results from fracture, although radiologists are frequently reluctant to make this diagnosis. It must be emphasized that in metabolic bone disease there may be no radiographic evidence of

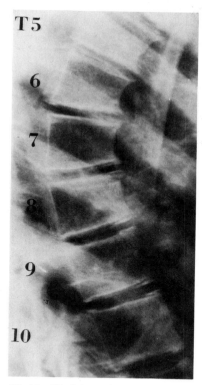

Figure 13–16. Wedging of T6 and T7 in a girl aged 17 with kyphosis due to severe bronchial asthma. Note unfused vertebral epiphyses.

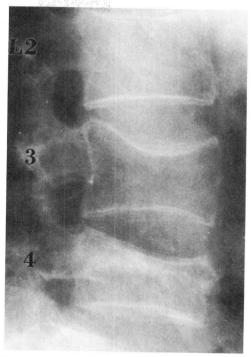

Figure 13–17. Compression of L4 due to traumatic fracture in a man aged 44 with idiopathic osteoporosis. Note sclerosis of upper half of body with bulging of the anterior border.

gross or macrofracture other than the changes in shape just described.

Recognition of these three components of change in shape is of some value in differential diagnosis. In general, in osteomalacia increased concavity is the most common finding. The curvature is smooth, and both upper and lower ends are affected to the same extent (codfish vertebra) (Fig. 13–19). This reflects the fact that in osteomalacia the bone may be softer than normal but not brittle. Wedging is usually of minor degree and compression is rare, except in the adult onset nonfamilial form of vitamin D refractory hypophosphatemic osteomalacia. In osteoporosis, both wedging and compression are common and are often severe. Increased biconcavity is less characteristic,[100] notwithstanding many statements to the contrary.[6, 28] Several random surveys have shown that the degree of biconcavity correlates very poorly with the amount of bone in the vertebrae.[69, 403] If biconcavity occurs, the curvature is likely to be irregular and the upper and lower margins are usually not affected to the same extent (Fig. 13–20).

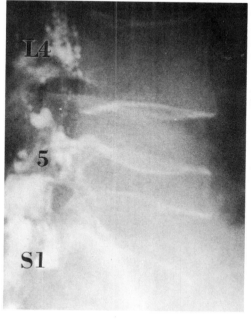

Figure 13–18. Compression of L5 due to spontaneous fracture in a man aged 37 with idiopathic osteoporosis. Note absence of sclerosis and anterior bulging. The opaque dye is from a previous myelogram.

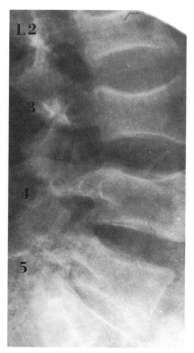

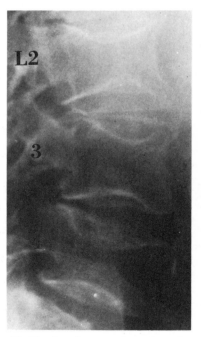

Figure 13–19. Lumbar vertebrae in a patient with osteomalacia. Note that biconcavity is symmetrical and of approximately equal degree in each (codfish vertebrae). L2 shows slight convexity of the end plates indicating some obliquity of the x-ray beam, but in remaining vertebrae the end plates are seen in true lateral view.

Figure 13–20. Lumbar vertebrae in a 76-year-old woman with involutional osteoporosis. Note that biconcavity is asymmetrical and of unequal severity in each; such vertebrae should not be described as codfish.

This reflects the fact that osteoporotic bone is often brittle and fractures easily, but is not soft. In osteitis fibrosa, shape changes of any kind are less common, and virtually any combination of increased concavity, wedging and compression may be seen.

As well as differences in the characteristic type of deformity, there are differences in the distribution of changes among different vertebrae. In osteomalacia, adjacent vertebrae are affected to the same extent and, although the lumbar vertebrae may be affected more severely than the thoracic, this difference progresses smoothly throughout the length of the spine (Fig. 13–21).[76, 100] In osteoporosis, by contrast, shape changes are characteristically quite unevenly distributed. Severely affected vertebrae may be separated by one of normal shape, and usually no two affected vertebrae are alike (Fig. 13–22). In osteitis fibrosa, the distribution is intermediate, more regular than in osteoporosis, less regular than in osteomalacia.

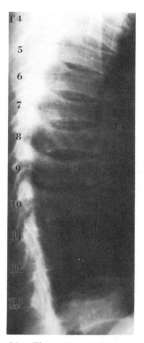

Figure 13–21. Thoracic vertebrae in a patient with osteomalacia. The degree of biconcavity is slightly more in L1 than in the upper thoracic region, but adjacent vertebrae show little difference in shape.

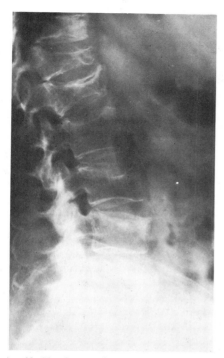

Figure 13–22. Lower thoracic and lumbar vertebrae in a patient aged 56 years with steroid induced osteoporosis. Varying combinations of concavity wedging and compression are seen. All vertebrae are asymmetrical and no two are alike.

especially so in adults who had familial hypophosphatemic rickets in childhood. The osteosclerosis of osteomalacia tends to affect the whole vertebral body evenly, rather than affecting the end plates disproportionately, as in the osteosclerosis of hyperparathyroidism and renal osteodystrophy. If the osteoid which accumulates is completely unmineralized rather than partly mineralized, the increased trabecular width will not be apparent on the x-ray, individual trabeculae will appear thinner than normal, and the density of the bones will be reduced. However, even in severe osteomalacia some trabecular structure is usually visible.

In osteoporosis, the individual trabeculae are thinner than normal, and many of them disappear completely. Horizontal trabeculae (which are plates) tend to be lost before vertical trabeculae (which are bars). The reason for this is unknown but it may reflect the biomechanical or bioelectric effect of loading in compression. Consequently, accentuation of vertical trabeculation is a relatively early radiographic sign (Figs. 13–24 and 13–25). In advanced osteoporosis, no trabecular pattern may be visible at all, in contrast to osteomala-

All these distinctions are less clear cut in growing children, in whom the vertebral changes in osteoporosis may be similar to those described for adults with osteomalacia. In this situation, the presence or absence of the epiphyseal signs of rickets is of cardinal importance.

Changes in Trabecular Structure. Although the pattern is blurred by the superimposition of structures at different depths, the individual lines do broadly correspond in size and configuration with individual trabeculae.[335] In osteomalacia, accumulation of osteoid may lead to an increase in total trabecular width. If the osteoid is partly mineralized rather than completely unmineralized, this increase in width will be apparent on the x-ray, even if the amount of fully calcified bone is reduced. However, the edges of the trabeculae will be fuzzy and indistinct; the resultant radiographic appearance is often described as "coarsening of the trabecular pattern" (Fig. 13–23). Sometimes the accumulation of partly mineralized osteoid is so great that the density of the bones is actually increased.[295] This is

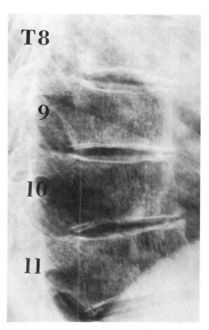

Figure 13–23. Thoracic vertebrae in a patient aged 59 with osteomalacia due to gluten enteropathy. Note preservation of normal trabecular orientation with only minimal vertical accentuation, but the trabeculae are wider ("coarser") than normal.

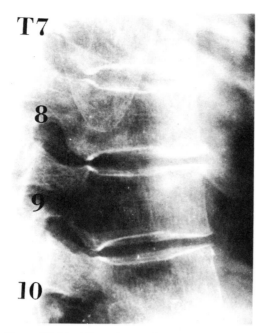

Figure 13–24. Thoracic vertebrae in a 65-year-old woman with involutional osteoporosis. Compared to Figure 13–23 there is a greater degree of vertical accentuation, and individual trabeculae are thinner, but the differences are small and are not a reliable basis for differential diagnosis. In both this and the previous case, the nature of the bone disease was confirmed histologically.

cia. Small focal condensations of bone representing healing or healed trabecular microfractures may be seen in laminograms but are not usually visible in standard films. It is important to note that the trabecular pattern is a much less accurate basis for the differentiation between osteomalacia and osteoporosis than the shape changes mentioned earlier. If these changes are absent, the trabecular pattern should not be relied on (Figs. 13–23 and 13–24).

In osteitis fibrosa, formation of woven bone within the fibrous tissue laid down adjacent to the eroded trabeculae may give the appearance of widened trabeculae with hazy margins ("coarsened trabecular pattern"), similar to that seen in osteomalacia but with a greater degree of irregularity (Fig. 13–20). Small foci of sclerosis on a background of diminished density may impart a mottled appearance but this is much less evident than in the skull.[71] End-plate sclerosis may occur, similar to that seen in renal osteodystrophy with secondary hyperparathyroidism, usually

(but not only) in patients with significant renal insufficiency (Fig. 13–26). There may or may not be associated reduction of density in the centra; in either case the alternating bands of increased density are often referred to as the "Rugger Jersey Spine," after the horizontal stripes of the jerseys of British Rugby football players (Fig. 13–27). In some patients the appearance may be indistinguishable from that of osteoporosis, but the number in whom the severity of such change is greater than expected for the patient's age and sex is small.

Other important findings in the spinal x-rays are osteophytosis and other signs of osteoarthritis, since these may be responsible for backache incorrectly attributed to osteoporosis. There is evidence that osteoarthritis in the hip and osteoporosis of the femoral neck do not occur together and that patients with osteoarthritis in the hip may have above-normal metacarpal density.[130] In patients with osteoporosis of the spine, the incidence of degenerative spinal changes and osteophytosis has variously been found to be less than,[369] and the same as,[209] in age- and sex-matched controls. In elderly patients, ankylos-

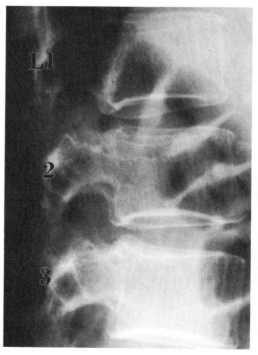

Figure 13–25. Lumbar vertebrae in a 59-year-old woman with involutional osteoporosis. Vertical trabeculation is accentuated by the overlying gas-filled colon.

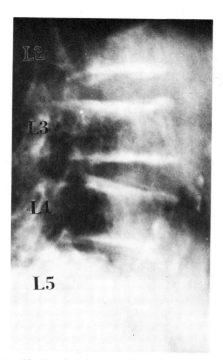

Figure 13–26. Lumbar vertebrae in a 62-year-old woman with osteitis fibrosa due to primary hyperparathyroidism. The trabeculae are coarsely thickened and indistinct. Note characteristic end-plate sclerosis although renal function is unimpaired in this patient.

correlates poorly with the mineral content of the radius determined by photon absorptiometry,[242] but this probably reflects the inadequacy of cortical bone in the extremities as a guide to trabecular bone in the spine.[105, 361]

THE HANDS. Views of the hands on fine-grain industrial film should be obtained in *every* patient with suspected metabolic bone disease. Apart from being the most sensitive site for the detection of hyperparathyroidism, hand films lend themselves to several specialized techniques. Because of the large number of epiphyses and ossification centers, hand films are also very useful in the assessment of growth and development.

Subperiosteal Erosion. This consists of a serrated indentation of the cortex immediately under the periosteum, caused by the centripetal advance of osteoclasts. It is best seen in the phalanges, especially the radial side. In normal periosteal remodeling shallow resorption spaces occupy a small fraction of the circumference and completely refill. In osteitis fibrosa, the refilling by lamellar bone is aborted, so that resorption spaces slowly accumulate

ing vertebral hyperostosis,[227] with fusion of osteophytes arising from adjacent joints, may produce a bamboo spine resembling ankylosing spondylitis (Fig. 13–28), and may lead to wedging and kyphosis with minimal osteoporosis (Fig. 13–29). Finally, there is an unexplained association between vertebral osteoporosis and calcification of the abdominal aorta.[57]

TRABECULAR PATTERN IN THE FEMUR. The cancellous bone in the upper end of the femur is arranged in arches corresponding to compression and tension stresses and can be subdivided into five anatomical groups.[360] Involutional bone loss is associated with a predictable sequence, beginning with loss of the secondary compressive trabeculae and finally leaving only the primary compressive trabeculae. Based on this, a semiquantitative seven point scale has been devised. This index correlates well with the amount of trabecular bone in the vertebrae and with the incidence of compression fractures of the spine,[361] although fractures can develop with no change in the index (Figs. 13–30 to 13–33). The index

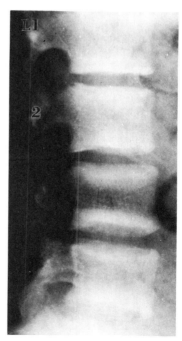

Figure 13–27. End plate sclerosis of lumbar vertebrae in a 14-year-old patient with renal osteodystrophy, showing alternating horizontal bands with greater and lesser density ("rugger jersey spine"). Note that centra are less dense than the end plates but not less dense than normal.

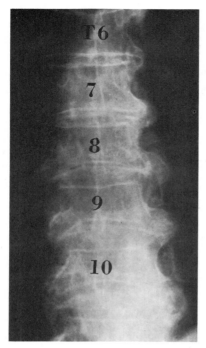

Figure 13–28. Bamboo spine due to fusion of osteocytes of adjacent vertebrae in an 81-year-old woman with ankylosing vertebral hyperostosis. There were no symptoms referable to the spine.

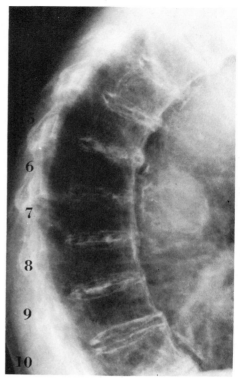

Figure 13–29. Increased kyphosis and wedging of thoracic vertebrae in a 90-year-old woman with ankylosing vertebral hyperostosis. There were no symptoms referable to the spine.

and may become continuous around the periosteal circumference, and periodically advance farther into the cortex. There is no evidence for the widespread presumption that the linear resorption rate (that is, the rate of advance of the osteoclastic front) is increased, and some evidence (mentioned earlier) to the contrary.

As in osteitis fibrosa elsewhere, the space left by the erosion process may be filled with fibrous tissue, in which case there will be a ghost of the original periosteal outline in the same place (Fig. 13–34), or by woven bone, in which case the original periosteal outline may be expanded by an irregular lacework pattern of trabeculae (Fig. 13–35).

Endosteal Erosion. The normal, slow expansion with age does not greatly alter the endosteal surface, which is generally smooth with a few rounded indentations, but if endosteal resorption increases in extent, the surface may become visibly scalloped. A large increase in the number of resorption tunnels arising from the endosteum may coalesce and convert the inner cortex into trabecular bone, and obliterate the normal clear inner margin of

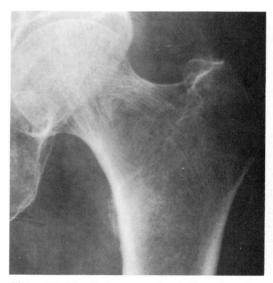

Figure 13–30. Trabecular pattern of left upper femur in a 68-year-old woman with involutional osteoporosis. This falls into Grade 4 on the Singh scale. (Figures 13–30 to 13–34 are same patient.)

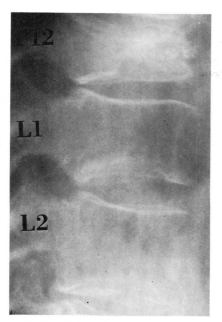

Figure 13–31. Spine of patient, taken at the same time, showing compression of T12 only.

Magnification Radioscopy. A fine-grain film contains more detail than is visible to the naked eye, and with a suitable optical system, up to tenfold magnification may be used to bring out this additional information.[271] In this way the subperiosteal erosion of hyperparathyroidism may be detected at an earlier stage and linear striations may be seen within the cortex, representing intracortical porosity. This is usually due to an increase in Haversian remodeling, with an increase in the number of unfilled resorption spaces in the bone, so that magnification radioscopy is a valuable means for detecting high turnover osteoporosis (q.v.) (Fig. 13–36). Like endosteal tunneling, intracortical striation may occur with or without subperiosteal erosion (Fig. 13–37).

Radiographic Morphometry. This procedure consists of measuring cortical dimensions on an x-ray film with a suitable caliper. Although applicable in principle to many bones, the hands are most suitable since the distance of the bones from the x-ray film is

the cortex seen on x-ray. Irregular endosteal resorption may occur with subperiosteal erosion in hyperparathyroidism, and without subperiosteal erosion in other high turnover states.

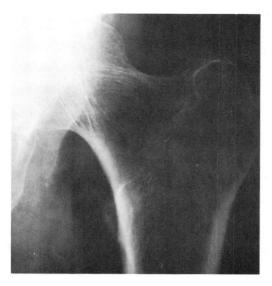

Figure 13–32. Trabecular pattern of left upper femur in the patient three years later. There is no change in the grading on the Singh scale.

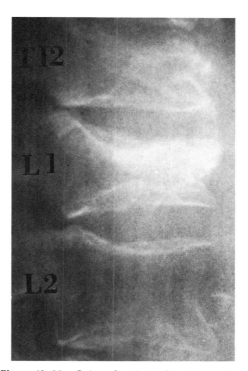

Figure 13–33. Spine of patient taken at same time as Figure 13–32, showing compression of L1 as well as T12.

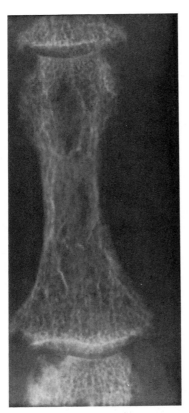

Figure 13–34. Middle phalanx of right middle finger of woman aged 61 with osteitis fibrosa due to primary hyperparathyroidism. Note severe subperiosteal resorption along the ulna (right hand) border of the shaft, with the original periosteal outline still visible as a fine shadow, and also erosion in the juxta-articular region of the metaphyses.

Measurement of Bone Mineral Content

Because of the inaccuracy of the visual estimation of the optical density of an x-ray film, several alternative methods have been devised for obtaining information on the bone mineral content. It should be noted that none of these methods measures bone density, and it is incorrect to refer to them as densitometric methods. Estimates of the mineral density of both bone tissue and whole bone can be made by combining bone mineral and morphometric measurements.[268, 363]

In the ensuing discussion, it is important to keep in mind the distinction between the volume of a bone as an organ, which is the volume of space enclosed in the periosteal envelope, and the volume of bone as a tissue, which excludes marrow and other spaces.

Another general point about bone mineral measurements is that they obviously tell one nothing about the pathological basis for any lack of mineral. In epidemiologic and population studies, because osteoporosis is so overwhelmingly more common than either osteomalacia or osteitis fibrosa, a reduction in bone

less variable, so that if the tube distance is long enough, parallax error is negligible. The basic measurements, usually made at the midpoint of the third left metacarpal (Fig. 13–38) are total diameter and medullary diameter.[105, 158] The latter measurement is less accurate because the endosteal margin of the cortex is less clearly defined than the periosteal margin. From these measurements can be derived several other quantities of interest, such as the cortical thickness, cortical area and cortical area/total area ratio.[105]

Since osteoporosis is best defined in terms of bone volume, these radiogrammetric measurements provide valuable estimates of the presence and severity of osteoporosis, although they do not give any data on intracortical porosity. The cortical area/total area ratio is also an estimate of the physical density of the whole bone. Cortical thinning may also occur in osteomalacia.[82]

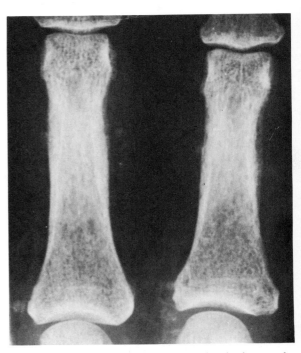

Figure 13–35. Middle phalanges of right fore- and middle fingers of patient aged 34 with osteitis fibrosa due to secondary hyperparathyroidism. The space eroded under the periosteum is filled with a lacework of new bone. Note soft tissue calcification.

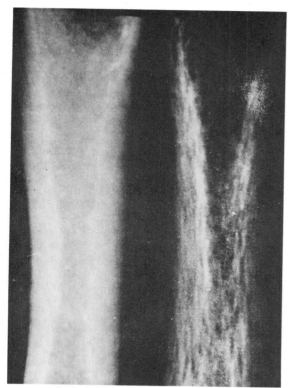

Figure 13–36. Severe intracortical porosity in a metacarpal shown by magnification radioscopy in a patient with hyperthyroidism, compared to normal on left. The longitudinal striation represents increased numbers of remodeling foci (active osteons). (Courtesy of H. E. and S. Meema.)

box is more accurate, since the absorption coefficient is closer to that of apatite.[269] Ivory or suitably prepared human bone can also be used. The main barrier to accuracy is the varying absorption by the soft tissues and the varying wavelength of x-rays. A wide range of bones can be examined, including the phalanges, metacarpals and both bones in the forearm, but in these locations photon absorptiometry may be more convenient and more accurate. In the spine, photon absorptiometry is so far inapplicable and radiographic photodensitometry is the present method of choice.[209, 291, 335]

PHOTON ABSORPTIOMETRY.[220, 264] The principle of this method is that photons emitted from a monochromatic source, usually [125]I (odine) or [247]Am(ericium), are focused onto the bone to be examined, and the absorption of energy by the bone is determined by a detector on the other side. This principle has now been incorporated into a commercially available instrument by means of which the electronic processing of the data is automatically

mineral content can be assumed to result only from a reduction in absolute bone volume, with little chance of error in any conclusions drawn from the data. However, in clinical medicine, such an assumption is clearly out of the question, and the finding of a reduced bone mineral content is an indication for further study and not an end in itself. Finally, measurements of bone mineral content may be seriously misleading in renal osteodystrophy, since the combination of osteosclerosis and osteomalacia at different sites may give a normal reading.

RADIOGRAPHIC PHOTODENSITOMETRY. The principle of this method is to x-ray a standard on the same film as each bone to be examined, and to measure the optical density on the film of both the standard and the unknown with a recording densitometer. The most commonly used standard is an aluminum step wedge, but a solution of K_2HPO_4 in a plastic

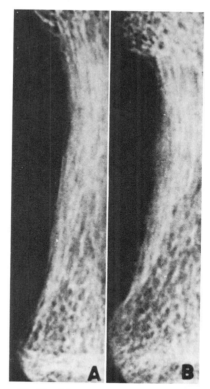

Figure 13–37. Metacarpal striation indicating intracortical porosity (A) without subperiosteal resorption in hyperthyroidism, and (B) with subperiosteal resorption in hyperparathyroidism. (Courtesy of H. E. and S. Meema.)

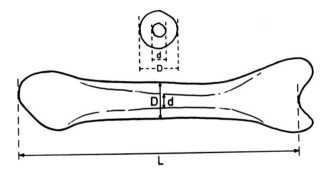

Figure 13–38. Diagram of metacarpal showing measurements used for radiographic morphometry. D = external (periosteal) diameter. d = internal (endosteal) diameter. L = length. (Courtesy of J. Dequeker.)

performed and the bone mineral content in grams per centimeter of the bone is displayed. The instrument also measures the width of the bone. The procedure involves scanning across the bone after determination of the soft tissue absorption. The main disadvantage of this procedure at present is that only the radius can be examined. The relatively poor correlation between bone mineral content of the radius and the degree of vertebral osteoporosis has already been mentioned. Many other bones have been used for photon absorptiometry but the equipment has to be built and assembled individually.[167, 363] In order to permit comparison between bones of different size, the bone mineral content is usually expressed as a ratio to the bone width. It is more accurate, although somewhat more troublesome, to measure the cortical thickness in the line of the photon beam, that is, perpendicular to the direction of the scan, and obtain estimates of the mineral density of bone tissue and of whole bone.[271]

COMPTON SCATTERING. Recently, a new method, dependent on the Compton effect, that is the scattering of electrons by an incident photon, has been devised. It has several advantages over photon absorptiometry and may become the method of choice for measuring bone mineral content. Because two beams are used, the results are independent of soft tissue absorption, and accurate focusing of the intersection between the two beams enables the mineral content of cortical and trabecular bone to be measured separately.[161]

NEUTRON ACTIVATION AND TOTAL BODY CALCIUM. The patient's body is bombarded with neutrons and, subsequently, the radiation emitted by the patient at different energies is assessed in a whole-body counter. The method does not permit distinction between calcium in bone and in soft tissues. The method is cumbersome and unsuitable for rou-

tine diagnostic use, but it has permitted formulation of the useful generalization for estimating the mineral content of the body at skeletal maturity from the height: total body calcium $(Kg) = \frac{1}{5} (ht(m))$.[3, 78]

Laboratory Studies in the Evaluation of Metabolic Bone Disease

Much of the interpretation of biochemical tests is implicit in the previous discussion on normal physiology. It would be ideal to measure the concentrations of each of the three main hormones acting on bone, but in practice we still have to rely to a large extent on indirect assessments of the effect of hormone excess or deficiency.

HORMONE ASSAYS. Bioassays have in the past been useful in research, but have always been too cumbersome for diagnostic use. Present-day methods of hormone assays depend on the principle of saturation analysis and competitive protein binding. In principle, the unlabeled hormone in the sample to be analyzed is incubated with a known quantity of radioactive labeled hormone, and a protein which binds the hormone in some manner. The labeled and unlabeled hormone compete for binding sites on the protein and, by measuring the amounts of labeled hormone which are bound and the amounts which are free, the concentration of unlabeled hormone can be estimated. If the binding protein is an antibody, the procedure is a radioimmunoassay.

Parathyroid Hormone. Although much useful information has been garnished, this radioimmunoassay is still unsuitable for routine use in the investigation of spinal disease. The assays available at present are useful mainly in the investigation of patients with kidney stones and other nonosseous manifestations of primary hyperparathyroidism. They do not differentiate between primary and secondary hyperparathyroidism in patients with osteitis fibrosa, with or without osteomalacia, but may be helpful in detecting secondary hyperparathyroidism as a result of depletion or impaired action of vitamin D.

Calcitonin. At present, the only proven value of this radioimmunoassay in clinical diagnosis is in the recognition of medullary carcinoma of the thyroid, but spinal complications other than metastases do not usually occur in this condition. In bulls, nutritional calcitonin excess induced by the high calcium diet appropriate for lactating cows is associated with osteosclerosis, but no clear relationship has yet emerged between elevated calcitonin levels and the various human forms of osteosclerosis.

Vitamin D.[21] Here the binding protein is not an antibody but either the normal vitamin D binding protein present in the blood or a local tissue-binding protein extracted from the kidney. The assays which have been developed measure the 25 hydroxy derivatives of both D_2 and D_3, but cannot distinguish between them. Any 25 hydroxy compound derived may, therefore, have been derived either from vitamin D_2 in the diet or from vitamin D_3 made in the spine. A low level of 25 hydroxy D_3 equivalent in the blood is the most certain and direct way of detecting vitamin D deficiency, and suggests, but does not, of course, prove, that the patient has osteomalacia. An analogy may be drawn with the relationship between low plasma vitamin B_{12} levels and megaloblastic anemia. Demonstration of vitamin B_{12} deficiency does not establish that the patient is anemic, but if anemia is present it is more likely to be megaloblastic than of some other kind. Even if there is no anemia, a low B_{12} level is an indication for replacement therapy. In just the same way, a low vitamin D level does not establish that the patient has any disease of the bones, but if there is such a disease it is likely to be osteomalacia rather than some other. Also, even if no bone disease is present, a low vitamin D level is an indication for replacement therapy. The diagnostic value of the vitamin D assays is especially great in elderly patients, who may have osteomalacia as well as osteoporosis.

PLASMA AND URINARY LEVELS OF THE INORGANIC CONSTITUENTS OF BONE. In the present context, the main function of these is to seek indirect evidence for abnormalities in PTH or vitamin D (Table 13–4).

Plasma Total Calcium. The blood for this test should, as far as possible, be drawn without venous stasis and in the fasting state. In order to allow for the contribution of changes in protein-bound calcium to changes in total calcium, some correction for protein binding must be applied, so that total protein or albumin must be measured with each calcium determination. Most of the frequent laboratory errors in the measurement of total calcium result from the introduction of contamination at some point,[168] so that if several results are discrepant, the lowest is most likely to be correct. Since only the ionized fraction is of physiologic importance, direct measurement of this fraction would be ideal, but is attended by many problems.

In the present context, a low plasma calcium is likely to be due to vitamin D deficiency, intestinal malabsorption, or chronic renal failure, and to be associated with osteomalacia. Transient hypocalcemia may be due to acute pancreatitis. A high plasma calcium suggests primary hyperparathyroidism, mye-

TABLE 13–4. EFFECTS OF CHANGES IN ACTIVITY OF VITAMIN D AND PARATHYROID HORMONE WHICH MAY BE FOUND IN METABOLIC BONE DISEASE*

	Deficiency of Vitamin D action	Excess of Parathyroid hormone action
Plasma calcium	↓	↑
Plasma phosphorus	↓	↓
Plasma alkaline phosphatase	↑	↓
Tubular reabsorption of calcium	?	↑
Urinary excretion of calcium	↓	↑
Tubular reabsorption of phosphorus	↓	↓
Urinary excretion of phosphorus	↓	↑

*Note that urinary excretion reflects changes in filtered load as well as tubular reabsorption. In secondary hyperparathyroidism, where vitamin D action and increase in parathyroid hormone are found, changes in the opposite direction, as in plasma calcium, may cancel out.

lomatosis, osseous metastases or immobilization.

Urinary Calcium. Urinary calcium usually changes in the same direction as plasma calcium, but the magnitude of this change depends also on tubular reabsorption. The contribution of this is best assessed by comparing the relationship between calcium excretion per 100 ml creatinine clearance (Ca_E) and plasma total calcium, with the normal relationship determined by calcium infusion.[289]

In the context of spinal disease, urinary calcium determination is of value in four situations. First, in osteomalacia, because of secondary hyperparathyroidism and possibly also because of lack of some vitamin D action on the kidney, urinary calcium is usually low, even when plasma calcium is normal. This may help to select those patients with nonspecific vertebral rarefaction who need more detailed study, but, unfortunately, the difference in urinary calcium between osteoporosis and osteomalacia diminishes with age. Second, in a patient with definite osteomalacia, the urinary calcium may occasionally be unexpectedly high, either before or as a result of treatment. This suggests the presence of some renal tubular dysfunction, phosphate depletion or need for phosphate supplements, or unrecognized primary hyperparathyroidism. Third, in a patient with spinal disease and hypercalcemia, increased tubular reabsorption of calcium favors primary hyperparathyroidism rather than neoplastic disease, whereas decreased tubular reabsorption of calcium has the opposite significance. Fourth, in osteoporosis, the 24-hour urinary calcium is usually normal and a high level suggests either very rapid bone loss or some type of high turnover osteoporosis.

In general, the patient should be on a normal, *not* a low calcium, diet when urinary calcium is first measured, although this injunction is more important in the investigation of renal stones than of bone disease. The reason for this is that the effect of lowering calcium intake varies between diseases. For example, in a hypercalcemic patient dietary calcium restriction may produce no change in urinary calcium in malignancy, a moderate fall in primary hyperparathyroidism, and a pronounced fall in sarcoidosis or vitamin D intoxication.

Plasma and Urinary Inorganic Phosphate. As with calcium, it is important to measure plasma inorganic phosphorus in the fasting state. Food intake produces complex changes—high phosphate foods tending to raise the plasma phosphate and carbohydrate tending to lower it by promoting movement into cells.

Plasma phosphate tends to be low in primary hyperparathyroidism and in the secondary hyperparathyroidism of osteomalacia, but is usually normal, or even slightly increased, in osteoporosis. Plasma phosphate may also be low because of a low dietary phosphorus intake or consumption of aluminum-containing antacids (which form insoluble aluminum phosphate), and in genetically determined disorders of renal tubular function. Plasma phosphate may be high in renal failure and in hypoparathyroidism. An increased phosphate load may follow increased dietary phosphorus, increased bone resorption, or increased mobilization of intracellular phosphorus because of starvation. The rise in plasma phosphate in the last three situations is minimal unless renal function is depressed, since the normal kidney can markedly increase urinary phosphate with little change in blood level.

In situations in which the load of phosphate presented to the kidney may be abnormally low or high, it is useful to measure the urinary phosphate. In conjunction with estimates of dietary intake, this permits evaluation of the various extrarenal factors which may affect plasma phosphate, and also allows the renal tubular reabsorption of phosphate to be assessed directly. In the present context, the most important use of measurement of tubular phosphate reabsorption is in the indirect assessment of parathyroid function in the study of osteomalacia. There are many other factors which affect phosphate reabsorption, but, in general, decreased reabsorption suggests increased parathyroid function.[46] This may be useful in the investigation of hypercalcemia in a patient with a spinal lesion, and may help select patients who need to be studied further for osteomalacia from among the large number with nonspecific spinal rarefaction, although a normal value certainly does not rule out osteomalacia.[391]

ALKALINE PHOSPHATASE.[314] This is the name for a family of enzymes of different structure which can split inorganic phosphate from a variety of organic phosphate substrates at alkaline pH. Structurally and immunologically different alkaline phosphatases are produced by the placenta, the hepatobiliary system, the intestinal mucosa, and bone. A high alkaline phosphatase may thus result from pregnancy or from disease of liver or gut, as well as bone, or may result from the infusion of albumin or other plasma protein derivatives which may contain placental alkaline phosphatase. Often the clinical context may clearly indicate which organ is involved, but if there is doubt the enzymes can be separated by various techniques. The simplest for routine use is heat inactivation.[314] This consists of repeating the measurement of total alkaline phosphatase after incubation at 56°C for 30 minutes, and can be performed in any laboratory which is able to measure alkaline phosphatase. Bone alkaline phosphatase is much more heat labile than hepatobiliary phosphatase and so the degree of heat inactivation permits a rough estimate of the relative proportions of these two forms.

Skeletal alkaline phosphatase is made by osteoblasts, but the level cannot be directly equated with osteoblastic function since in many high bone-turnover situations such as hyperthyroidism the alkaline phosphatase may be normal or only marginally increased. In a wide variety of diseases no correlation was found between the alkaline phosphatase and the extent of lamellar bone formation.[355] In general, high bone alkaline phosphatase comes from two sources. In vitamin D deficiency the enzyme escapes from lamellar osteoblasts, whose function is disturbed in so many other ways; this accounts for the high alkaline phosphatase of rickets and osteomalacia. Secondly, in the absence of vitamin D deficiency, woven bone osteoblasts release much more alkaline phosphatase than lamellar bone osteoblasts, so that alkaline phosphatase is increased in all situations in which woven bone formation is increased, as in normal growth, or extensive fractures, Paget's disease and osteitis fibrosa, and in the reparative phase of osseous metastases.

In the interpretation of alkaline phosphatase levels it is essential to refer to the appropriate normal range for age and sex. The levels fall progressively during early childhood, increase during the adolescent growth spurt, fall again with the completion of skeletal maturity, and then rise slowly and progressively.[104, 168] Both in childhood and early adult life, levels are lower in females than in males, but this difference becomes insignificant after 40 to 50 years. A final source of confusion is that at least five systems of units are in use, so that it is essential that the practice in a particular laboratory be known. For convenience, some normal ranges for adults are given in Table 13–5 and the conversion factors for different units in Table 13–6.

The most important practical point is that a high skeletal alkaline phosphatase is incompatible with uncomplicated osteoporosis, and, therefore, is an indication for more detailed study. Also serial measurements of alkaline phosphatase may be valuable in following the response to treatment.

URINARY TOTAL HYDROXYPROLINE. Hydroxyproline is an imino acid found only in collagen and formed by hydroxylation of proline after it has been incorporated into the collagen molecule. Hydroxyproline released from bone cannot be reutilized, and so urinary hydroxyproline is widely used as an index of bone turnover. This use is subject to four qualifications. First, the dietary intake of gelatine (denatured collagen) must be standardized by eliminating such foods as Jello and ice cream 24 to 48 hours before urine collection is begun. Second, the skin contains a substantial amount of collagen, and there may be in-

TABLE 13–5. NORMAL SERUM ALKALINE PHOSPHATASE VALUES IN ADULTS BY AGE AND SEX*

Age (Yr.)	M	F
20	18–74	12–63
30	19–75	14–67
40	20–77	16–71
50	21–78	18–75
60	21–79	20–79
70	22–81	22–83

*Expressed in international units shown as 2.5 to 97.5 percentiles (95% confidence limits). (Quoted from Goldsmith,[168] with permission.)

TABLE 13–6. ALKALINE PHOSPHATASE CONVERSION FACTORS TO INTERNATIONAL UNITS[*]

Method	Factor
King-Armstrong	3.53
Bodansky	5.37
Shinowara-Jones-Reinhart	5.37
Kind-King	7.06
Auto-Analyzer (Technicon)	7.06
Bessey-Lowry-Brock	16.66

[*] 1.U./liter = μ moles PO_4 released/min./liter. (Reprinted from Goldsmith,[168] with permission.)

creased collagen turnover in burns, psoriasis and other dermatoses, and in adrenocortical overactivity; in all of these situations urinary total hydroxyproline may be increased in the absence of bone disease. Third, of the hydroxyproline formed by the breakdown of collagen, only about one fifth appears in the urine; the remainder is oxidized to carbon dioxide and water, so that the carbon atoms are excreted in the lungs. Almost nothing is known of the factors which determine the fraction which escapes oxidation, but, clearly, urinary hydroxyproline may change for reasons other than alterations in bone collagen breakdown. Fourth, only a very small fraction of total hydroxyproline is normally excreted as the free imino acid, the bulk being in the form of hydroxyproline-containing peptides of varying size. A large number of such compounds can be identified, but for practical purposes separation into dialyzable and nondialyzable fractions is sufficient.[241] In general, the nondialyzable fraction is made up of large molecular weight peptides derived from the breakdown of recently formed soluble immature collagen, and so reflects bone matrix formation. The dialyzable fraction comprises the small amount of free imino acid, together with small-molecular-weight peptides derived from the breakdown of mature insoluble collagen, and so reflects bone matrix resorption. Normally, the dialyzable fraction is about 80 per cent of the total, so that changes in total hydroxyproline mostly reflect changes in bone resorption. Obviously, however, this does not permit differentiation between an increase in normal resorption, as when mesenchymal cell activation and consequent remodeling is increased, and an increase in abnormal resorption, as in metastatic malignancy or myeloma. In certain situations, such as healing osteitis fibrosa and chronic renal failure, the nondialyzable fraction is relatively much larger, and values for total hydroxyproline may then be misleading.

URINARY CYCLIC AMP. Urinary cyclic AMP, which reflects primarily the activation of adenylcyclase at renal tubule cell membranes by PTH and by antidiuretic hormone, tends to be elevated in primary hyperparathyroidism and to be depressed in nonparathyroid hypercalcemia, and it may change acutely in response to changes in PTH resulting from raising or lowering the ionized calcium. The most well established diagnostic use of cyclic AMP is in the recognition of renal tubular resistance to PTH in pseudohypoparathyroidism.

METABOLIC BALANCE STUDIES. Normally, 99 per cent of the total body calcium is in bone, so that the external balance of calcium is an accurate reflection of the skeletal balance of calcium. If the degree of mineralization is not disturbed, this is equivalent to the skeletal bone balance, but in osteomalacia changes in calcium balance do not reflect changes in absolute bone volume but changes in osteoid mineralization. Even in the absence of osteomalacia, short term changes may reflect movement of calcium in relation to homeostasis, rather than bone remodeling.

Interpretation of balance studies is subject to several pitfalls. First, there are many technical difficulties in the accurate measurement of dietary intake and all pathways of excretion over a sufficiently long time; dermal losses are especially difficult to measure and so are usually ignored. In particular, it is not possible to detect daily losses of much less than about 100 mg daily, so that in most patients with osteoporosis in whom the daily loss is of the order of 20 to 50 mg daily, the calcium balance cannot be distinguished from equilibrium. Second, most changes in calcium balance, especially in response to treatment, are short-term, transient effects which can only be interpreted in relation to the concepts of bone remodeling outlined earlier.[144] For example, suppression of activation of new remodeling cycles will promptly lead to a positive calcium balance which will continue while existing cycles complete their formative phases, but the balance will inevitably return to pretreatment levels within the period needed for completion of one remodeling cycle (sigma).

Calcium balances are too cumbersome and expensive for routine use and, except in one situation, the information they provide, while invaluable for research, is not needed for diagnosis and treatment. The exception is in the treatment of rickets and osteomalacia, in which changes in calcium balance give an accurate indication of response to treatment which can otherwise only be obtained by frequently repeated bone biopsy.

CALCIUM INFUSION. This consists of raising the plasma calcium by intravenous infusion of calcium, usually 15 mg per kg of body weight over a four hour period, and observing various effects. The test has many uses, but only two are relevant to the problem of spinal disease. First, the amount of calcium retained on the day of infusion, that is, the difference between the amount infused and the amount excreted in the urine, has been proposed as a means of distinguishing osteoporosis and osteomalacia, and so avoiding the necessity for bone biopsy, but it is much too inaccurate for this purpose. Second, the extent to which parathyroid hormone secretion is suppressible can be assessed indirectly by measuring changes in phosphate reabsorption or cyclic AMP excretion, or directly by measuring the PTH in blood. This test may have some value in the recognition of normocalcemic hyperparathyroidism (q.v.).[30]

CALCIUM RADIOKINETICS. *Accretion Rate and Pool Size.* If radioactive calcium (^{45}Ca or ^{47}Ca) is administered and serial observations made of plasma, urinary, and fecal radioactivity, it is possible on the basis of a number of reasonable assumptions to calculate two quantities, the size of the exchangeable calcium pool and the accretion rate. Similar measurements can be made using either stable or radioactive strontium. In general, the pool size reflects plasma calcium levels, the amount of soft tissue calcium and the turnover rate. The accretion rate is the rate of calcium entry into the nonexchangeable fraction of bone calcium, excluding both short and long term exchange processes, and regardless of the anatomical location or morphological concomitant of this entry. The accretion rate includes primary mineralization (calcium deposited in newly formed matrix), secondary mineralization (growth of existing crystals) and periosteocytic mineral deposition. The accuracy with which accretion rates can be determined is limited by the difficulty of assessing the contributions of exchange processes.[186] Exchange is a function primarily of mean skeletal age which determines the fraction of well hydrated bone through which calcium ions can freely diffuse.[181] There is the additional possibility of recycling calcium by resorption of some newly formed bone during the study.

The accretion rate corresponds approximately to organ-level bone formation determined morphologically, and values for the two methods are in good agreement—about 200 to 400 mg daily. The apparent discrepancy between kinetic and morphologic methods in osteomalacia reflects, primarily, the difference between cell level formation and organ level bone formation, so that in osteomalacia cell level bone formation (appositional rate) is markedly depressed but organ level bone formation, which corresponds with kinetic measurement of accretion rate, may be low, normal or high, depending on the number of bone-forming sites. An increased pool size is a sensitive indication of osteomalacia, but, in general, kinetic studies of turnover are research tools rather than clinical methods.

Absorption. Radio calcium studies are most useful in the determination of calcium absorption. Balance methods may detect net absorption, that is, diet minus fecal excretion, but true absorption and endogenous fecal secretion are of more significance. A measurement of endogenous fecal calcium secretion is possible, using two isotopes, one given orally and the other intravenously. This method is accurate, but the analysis of the data is mathematically formidable and several simpler methods have been proposed, measuring only the blood level at a single time after oral ingestion of a single isotope, or measuring the activity by external counting over the forearm.

Isotopic tests of calcium absorption give low values in osteomalacia, low or normal values in osteoporosis, and high values in hyperparathyroidism. They are of most use in osteomalacia associated with intestinal malabsorption, both in diagnosis and in following the response to vitamin D therapy.

OTHER DYNAMIC STUDIES. Because of persistent difficulties with parathyroid hormone radioimmunoassay, and the possible importance of recognizing normocalcemic hyperparathyroidism in patients with osteoporosis, several other procedures have a small place. These include EDTA infusion, phosphate deprivation, phosphate loading, and thiazide challenge.

OSTEOPOROSIS

We come now to a consideration of the individual forms of metabolic bone disease, and give pride of place to osteoporosis, since not only is it much the most common, but it most characteristically involves the spine.

From the time of skeletal maturity, most people lose bone progressively with increasing age. This is such a common occurrence that it must be regarded at least in some sense as normal. This age-related bone loss is a constant background to any discussion of any aspect of osteoporosis, and its existence immediately raises a number of basic questions. Is it possible or even desirable to separate normal (physiologic) bone loss from abnormal (pathologic) bone loss?[394] If it is not possible, should osteoporosis be regarded as a disease at all, or just as a nonspecific manifestation of senescence?[286] If the latter, does it make sense to seek to prevent or treat osteoporosis except in the context of fundamental research into the aging process? There are at this moment no certain or even generally agreed answers to these questions. The reader is urged to remember this in case the presentation of our own views should appear overly dogmatic.

Age Changes in Bone in Relation to Age Dependent (Involutional) Osteoporosis

Some general aspects of bone growth were mentioned earlier, but the upward curve of bone accumulation must now be considered in more detail before coming to the downward curve of bone loss. Before this, two general points must be made. First, almost all studies have been cross sectional rather than longitudinal. Cross-sectional studies give no infor-

mation on the sequential changes in individuals, and are also subject to bias because subjects compared differ not only in age but also in year of birth. If mean bone volume in a population tended to increase with time because of (for example) improved nutrition, then of two individuals examined at the same time, one might have less bone than the other because of an earlier birth, rather than because of increased age.[111] Fortunately, any such secular trend is of smaller magnitude than the age-dependent changes to be described. Second, most studies are based on limited sampling, either with respect to number of bones or number of sites within a bone, and even collectively the data are not necessarily representative of the skeleton as a whole.

CHANGES DURING BONE GROWTH. Most data have been obtained with radiographic morphometry of the second metacarpal.[105, 158] Although significantly less accurate than photon absorptiometry during the growth period, this technique permits separate measurement of the subperiosteal and endosteal diameters.[263]

Subperiosteal apposition follows a pattern similar to that of growth in height—a steady increase with accelerations of small magnitude in early infancy and again in adolescence, a few years earlier in girls than in boys. The total increase during the growth period is about 40 mm² in the area enclosed by the periosteum. The changes at the endosteal surface are more complex (Fig. 13–39). There is net resorption during the first two years of life, followed by net apposition from the second to the sixth year, a second net resorptive phase from the sixth to the twelfth year, and a second net appositional phase from the twelfth to the twentieth year. Although these changes are difficult to detect in an individual subject, their existence is important, since they establish the capacity of the endosteal surface to gain bone. It seems likely, although impossible at present to prove, that individual trabeculae also enlarge during these appositional phases. Endosteal gain may occur in all bones, but the appropriate measurements to establish this cannot be made with sufficient accuracy in the vertebrae, and only external changes can be readily shown (Fig. 13–40).

In boys, the adolescent net endosteal apposition begins about three years later and is of smaller magnitude than in girls. In both sexes, endosteal apposition begins a bit later

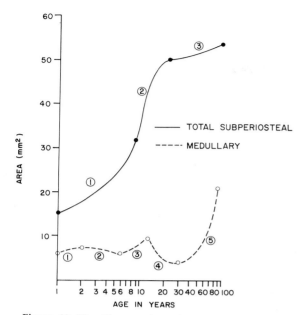

Figure 13–39. Changes in subperiosteal diameter (solid line) and medullary (endosteal) diameter (dotted line) throughout life. Subperiosteal diameter shows progressive increase divided into three phases of childhood (1), adolescence (2) and adult (3). Medullary diameter shows an initial resorptive phase in infancy (1), an appositional phase in early childhood (2), a second resorptive phase in prepuberty (3), a second appositional phase in adolescence and early adult life (4) and, finally, a third resorptive phase which continues until death (5). (Redrawn from Garn, S. M.)

than the adolescent growth spurt. The sex differences at this age suggest that net periosteal apposition is relatively more sensitive to androgens and net endosteal apposition relatively more sensitive to estrogens.[159]

The accumulation of bone during growth, both trabecular bone resulting from endochondral ossification, and cortical bone resulting from net periosteal and endosteal apposition together determine the amount of bone present in the body at the time of skeletal maturity. Differences in this amount between persons are clearly of the utmost importance in respect to future bone status, regardless of what answer is given to the questions posed earlier. Assuming the same rate of bone loss with age, the less bone that is present at the completion of growth, the earlier will the amount of bone be reduced to the critical level where structural failure and fractures occur. Conversely, if sufficient bone is accumulated during growth, this critical level may never be reached during a normal life span (Fig. 13–41). On this basis, it has been proposed that osteoporosis can be divided into three main groups — congenital, growth related, and acquired.[146] Congenital osteoporosis results from a failure to accumulate bone during intrauterine growth as in osteogenesis imperfecta, growth related osteoporosis from failure to accumulate a normal amount of bone by en-

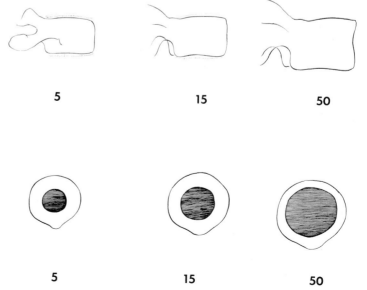

Figure 13–40. Diagrammatic change of size of a vertebra viewed from the lateral aspect at ages 5, 15 and 50 years. Below is the corresponding change in appearance of cross sections of the mid-femur at the same ages. Note the increasing diameter of bone marrow cavity, increasing periosteal diameter and diminishing cortical thickness.

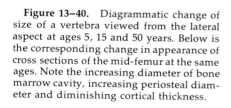

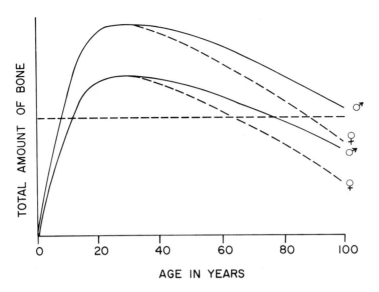

Figure 13–41. Diagrammatic representation of the course of bone gain and loss throughout life. Horizontal dotted line represents critical level below which structural failure and fractures are much more likely. This level is reached earlier in women (♀) than in men (♂), because of differences in the timing and magnitude of age-dependent bone loss, and this level is also reached earlier in both sexes in those who accumulate less bone during growth (lower set of lines) than in those who accumulate more bone (upper set of lines).

dochondral bone formation and subperiosteal apposition, and acquired osteoporosis from an increased net loss of bone after attainment of skeletal maturity.

Little is known about the control of bone accumulation during growth. Genetic factors are probably concerned, since Americans of African descent acquire more bone than Caucasians.[52, 369] Muscular work is undoubtedly important, and there is a high correlation between muscle weight and amount of bone;[110] this could be a factor in the apparent racial differences. Epidemiologic studies suggest a role for the fluoride content of the natural water supply, less bone being present at skeletal maturity in areas where fluoride is lacking, leading to a higher incidence of osteoporosis in later life.[41] Apart from isolated cases of extreme calcium deficiency, there is no good evidence that the dietary calcium level is critical during the growth period,[100] since calcium conservation is extremely efficient in growing children.[407] Hormonal factors are undoubtedly important. The correlation between the amount of bone and both height and weight may reflect the action of growth hormone.[347] The sex differences already mentioned, and the increasing bone volume during growth, undoubtedly depend in part on normal gonadal function. The importance of this is further indicated by the positive relationship between parity and bone volume, shown by several different techniques.[158, 287] Despite the calcium drain of pregnancy and lactation, the net effect

of pregnancy in young women is to increase the amount of bone.

CHANGES AFTER SKELETAL MATURITY. Bone volume shows only a minor decline until the fifth decade, when the rate of loss increases more markedly in women than in men.[279]

Net Periosteal Apposition. After completion of the adolescent appositional spurt, periosteal expansion continues slowly throughout life (Figs. 13–39 and 13–40). This phenomenon is not confined to the bones of the hand—it was first recognized in the femur,[372] and has also been shown in the rib and in the skull. In the second metacarpal the periosteal diameter gains about 0.4 mm between the ages of 20 and 80 years, so that the change is difficult to demonstrate in an individual. In prospective longitudinal studies, an increase of about 0.1 mm was found in women but not in men during an 11 year period,[1] but no change was found in either sex over only a five year period.[105]

Net Endosteal Resorption. Beginning at about age 40 in women and at about 45 to 50 in men, there is progressive expansion of medullary width and cross-sectional area (Fig. 13–40). In the metacarpal, the magnitude of change is greater than at the periosteal surface, the medullary canal increasing by about 1.8 mm in width by 80 years, while the subperiosteal diameter increases only by 0.4 mm (Fig. 13–39). The net result is a reduction in the cortical cross-sectional area of about 25 per cent. A similar loss of trabecular bone has been shown by morphologic measurement in iliac biopsy samples,[55] and in vertebral bone at autopsy.[16, 62] The loss of trabecular bone in the vertebrae explains the progressive loss of height with age.[105]

Intracortical Porosity. In the femur there is increasing accumulation of large resorption spaces in the inner half of the cortex,[19, 224] which results from longitudinal tunneling resorption from the endosteal surface. Increased intracortical porosity may also be due to accumulation of small, unfilled resorption spaces due to abortive remodeling cycles,[214] prolongation of the interval between completion of resorption and commencement of formation within each cycle, or to the crumbling away of dead bone around the Haversian canal,[244] and its presumed removal by normal phagocytic action, all of which contribute to the small increase in mean Haversian canal diameter which occurs with age.

In the upper extremity, direct measurement of porosity is lacking, but indirect estimates of mineral density from combined radiographic photodensitometry and morphometry suggest that the increase in intracortical porosity is slight in the metacarpal,[363] but significant in the radius.[268] However, taking the skeleton as a whole, an increase in intracortical porosity makes only a modest contribution to the total loss of bone with age.

Qualitative Changes in Bone with Age. There is a progressive increase in the amount of "dead" bone, especially in the cortex This is characterized by death of osteocytes leaving empty lacunae, plugging of the lacunae and canaliculae with partly mineralized connective tissue debris,[224] hypermineralization of bone or micropetrosis,[150] and increased accumulation of microfractures through extra Haversian bone, presumably indicating increased brittleness.[148] Identical changes are produced by radium poisoning.[341] There are also changes with age in bone collagen, which loses its structure on decalcification and becomes more soluble after alkaline denaturization.[105, 252] These changes in bone collagen with age are associated also with a reduction in skin collagen, the skin becoming thinner and more transparent,[265] a change which correlates with the degree of osteoporosis.[270] These changes shed no light on the question of whether pathologic osteoporosis is more than just bone senescence, but they do establish that age changes are qualitative as well as quantitative.

Changes in the Distribution and Arrangement of Trabecular Bone with Age. The changes are complex and three main patterns occur in different bones and in different individuals. First, the trabeculae become thinner but their number does not change. Second, some trabeculae disappear completely but those that remain are of normal size.[406] Third, some trabeculae disappear completely and some of those that remain become thicker than normal.[75, 381] These differences are important in relation to the possible reversibility of osteoporosis. As long as a trabeculum remains, then, however thin it has become, there is a possibility that it may regenerate, but once a trabeculum has disappeared completely, there is no way in which it can be replaced except by reactivation of woven bone formation.

In the vertebrae there is disproportionate loss of horizontal trabeculae, which accounts for a reduction in strength disproportionate to the loss of total bone tissue.[39] Both in the iliac crest and in vertebrae a bimodal population of trabeculae develops, some becoming thinner than normal and some thicker.[275] The extent of this compensatory thickening of remaining trabeculae determines in large part the mechanical strength of the bone and the liability to fracture.

Relationship of Thin Bones to Fractures. It seems obvious that the amount of bone tissue must have some bearing on bone strength and on the liability to fracture, but proof of this has been elusive. Such a relationship has been doubted because with age the incidence of fracture rises much more steeply than the amount of bone falls. But if the proportion of the population in which the amount of bone falls below some critical level is related to age, the curves closely match the incidence of fracture.[286] The fracture rate in the lower forearm is inversely related to the amount of bone in the radius and ulna, estimated by radiographic photodensitometry,[290] and femoral neck fractures seem to reflect loss of cortical bone throughout the body.[383] Patients with vertebral compression fractures have significantly less bone in the spine than age and sex matched controls and also significantly less bone in the hands and in the forearms.[290] There no longer is any need to doubt that the amount of bone is an important determinant of fracture,[279] but it is still possible that other factors besides the amount of bone and the degree of trauma are important. Apart from the qualitative changes already mentioned, in the vertebrae one such factor may be size; increased anteroposterior diameter increases the risk of fracture, probably because the stress on the anterior part of the vertebral body during flexion is increased.[368]

Biological Significance of Age-Related Bone Loss. Net loss of bone has been confirmed by radiographic photodensitometry,[270, 291] by photon absorptiometry,[167, 363] and by quantitative morphometry in biopsy and autopsy samples,[55, 62] and has been shown in all bones amenable to study. Bone loss has been found in all populations so far examined, and at first sight appears to be a universal and inevitable human characteristic.[158] A rise in blood pressure with age has also been regarded as inevitable, but in some parts of the world, such as New Guinea, this rise does not occur, and comparable exceptions may exist for bone loss. There are, for example, significant differences in the amount and rate of loss between different peoples. South African Bantu women lose significantly less bone with age than Caucasian women,[96, 407] and similar ethnic differences are apparent in the United States.[52, 369] Bone loss begins earlier and is greater in women than in men, a difference which is temporally more clearly related to the menopause than to age.[291] The mean rate of loss in a population is about the same for different bones and for cortical and trabecular bone, and continues at about the same rate with increasing age, but there are significant differences in the pattern and distribution of loss between different individuals, and in prospective studies some individuals have been shown to lose no bone at all (at least in certain sites) for periods of up to ten years.[1] Age-related bone loss does however seem to be a more nearly universal human characteristic than is a rise in blood pressure.

BONE REMODELING IN AGE-DEPENDENT BONE LOSS. The occurrence of bone loss at the endosteum does not indicate that this loss occurs because of an increase in resorption, as is often held. Neither does periosteal bone gain indicate an increase in bone formation. At both surfaces, the type of remodeling is the same, but the balance of bone within each remodeling cycle is not constant. The striking difference in behavior between the inner and outer sides of the cortex is thus in degree rather than in kind.[419] At the periosteal surface each remodeling cycle puts back slightly more bone than is removed, but at the endosteal surface each cycle puts back only about 70 per cent of the bone removed. This reflects both an increase in the amount of bone resorbed and a reduction in the amount formed within each remodeling cycle on the endosteal surface compared to the periosteal and Haversian surfaces. There is thus a gradient in bone loss, the bone balance per remodeling cycle becoming increasingly negative from the periosteal to the endosteal surface. It is evident that, given a constant mean net loss per remodeling cycle, the average rate of loss depends on the remodeling rate; that is, on the number of remodeling cycles initiated in unit time. When this rate is accelerated as in hyperparathyroidism, both net endosteal resorption and net periosteal apposition are increased and cortical cross sectional areas reduced in relation to age.[105, 202] Conversely, when this rate is diminished as in hypoparathyroidism, net endosteal resorption is diminished and cortical cross sectional area is increased in relation to age.[202] These changes are at present only detectable after the menopause, when the negative bone balance per remodeling cycle becomes most evident.

NATURE OF AGE-DEPENDENT BONE LOSS. In the light of the foregoing information, we will now attempt to answer the three questions posed earlier:

Is There any Difference Between "Physiologic" and "Pathologic" Osteoporosis? We will rephrase this question in a more rigorous manner: Do persons who have had a vertebral fracture differ from other individuals in any way except in the amount of bone they have? As mentioned earlier, such patients as a group have less bone in the spine than do patients without fracture; on the other hand, many patients with the same amount of, or even less, bone have sustained no fracture.[370] This difference could be related to differences in the severity of the stresses of everyday life or might reflect differences in the quality of bone. Two types of evidence suggest that patients with vertebral fracture may comprise a different population. First, the accumulation of dead bone and other consequent changes which characterize senescence seem to occur at a younger age. In other words, in such patients, the bones have aged disproportionately to the rest of the body.[394] Second, patients who have had a vertebral fracture differ markedly in their dynamics of bone remodeling in the rib from persons of the same age and sex and amount of bone who have not sustained such a fracture. There is a reduced activation frequency and remodeling rate, a substantial reduction in the appositional rate, with a consequent prolongation of the formative phase within each remodeling cycle,[418] and an increase in the number of very thin, mostly inactive osteoid seams, indicating that completion of normal mineralization has been prematurely arrested.[400] The reduced remodeling rate may explain the increased accumulation of dead bone, and suggests that, in contrast to hyperparathyroidism, increased net endosteal resorption is due to an even greater depression of bone formation than resorption within each remodeling cycle, and consequently a greater net bone loss per cycle.

Is Osteoporosis a Disease? On the grounds that no criteria have been devised which would enable a person with osteoporosis to be distinguished from healthy persons of the same age and sex, and that something which occurs to everybody cannot be a disease, it has been suggested that osteoporosis is merely the inevitable osseous manifestation of senescence.[279, 286] In other words, because of its universality and inevitability osteoporosis is regarded as normal.

The different senses of the word "normal" require careful definition.[283] Two in particular which are easily confused, and which are relevant to the present discussion, are ideal normality and statistical normality. The difference between these concepts can be brought out by consideration of obesity. A spread of gluttony in an affluent society would make it entirely possible for every member of such a society to become obese. Obesity would then be statistically normal. The harmful effects of obesity in an individual would, however, in no way be reduced by the increased prevalence of obesity in the population, so that, from the point of view of ideal health, obesity would continue to be abnormal. These harmful effects are documented by life insurance statistics which enable us to formulate standards of ideal weight. Obesity is defined as a sufficiently larger departure from this ideal standard, and the definition is quite independent of the prevalence of obesity in any particular community, which may vary from 0 to 100 per cent. Thus the universality of a phenomenon is not sufficient grounds for denying that it is a disease, provided that some standard of ideal normality is available. For the bones, this standard is provided by the amount of bone normally present at skeletal

maturity. It may be true that there is no criterion for separating obese from healthy subjects of the same age and sex except the amount of adipose tissue, and that any dividing line between normal and abnormal is arbitrary, but it remains true that in some patients the excess weight is causing harm and that some benefit follows from treatment designed to reduce this weight. In much the same way, even if we accept that no criterion exists for separating healthy from osteoporotic subjects except the amount of bone present, it remains true that bone loss of sufficient magnitude is harmful and thus causes a disease, in the sense of a constellation of features which together induce a patient to seek medical advice.[347]

Is It Worth Trying To Prevent or Treat Osteoporosis? One of the arguments leading to the view that osteoporosis is not a disease is that the variance of the amount of bone among different individuals remains the same with increasing age, suggesting that no large number can be separated from the remainder of the population. However, longitudinal studies have shown that while most people lose bone, some do not, and even among those who do the rate of loss is quite variable. It would seem sensible to attempt to find reasons for these individual differences and to hope that this knowledge would enable excessive bone loss to be prevented.

Conclusions. We will assume, henceforth, that age-dependent bone loss does lead, in some individuals, to the disease involutional osteoporosis, characterized by fractures, bone pain, and loss of height. This clinical state depends on a reduction mainly in the amount of bone, but also in its quality. The former is, like obesity and hypertension, a quantitative departure from normality; the amount of bone present at the onset of clinical disability is a function of the amount present at the time of skeletal maturity, as well as of the rate of bone loss with age. Qualitative changes in bone which may increase the risk of clinical effects include alterations in shape, reduction in mechanical strength due to redistribution of trabecular bone, and retarded healing of microfractures.

Clinical Features of Involutional Osteoporosis, Postmenopausal and Senile[50, 86]

The use of the terms postmenopausal osteoporosis and senile osteoporosis must first be clarified. Since bone loss begins earlier in women than in men, proceeds more rapdily, and is clearly related in time to the menopause, we use the term postmenopausal osteoporosis to identify that component of involutional osteoporosis which represents the difference between men and women. We use the term senile osteoporosis to identify that component of involutional osteoporosis which remains after eliminating any difference between the sexes.

The usual mode of presentation is with a vertebral compression fracture, but the patient may have noticed increasing roundness of the shoulders due to dorsal kyphosis for several years previously, together with varying degrees of ill-defined pain, which is heightened by coughing, sneezing and other sudden movement.[394] The incidence of symptomatic osteoporosis is six times greater in women than in men, probably because a relatively small decrement in bone mass may increase considerably the proportion who fall below a particular level; there is no evidence that women are more likely to have symptoms for the same degree of bone loss. In both sexes, only about one third of those with osteoporosis severe enough to be detectable on routine x-rays will have symptoms.[370]

A vertebral fracture may be precipitated by minor stress such as may be caused by bending forward and straining to open a stiff sash window. Pain is severe and of sudden onset, and may be incapacitating. It is usually well localized but may be felt only in the back, or there may be segmental radiation. Vertebral compression fractures are most common in T12 and L1 (Fig. 13–42), but if higher thoracic vertebrae are involved, the pain may resemble that of myocardial ischemia or pleurisy.[105, 164] The most important fact about the pain of vertebral fracture is that, however severe it may be, it will eventually subside spontaneously as the fracture heals, usually in two to three months. Subsequently, there may develop pain in the low back from increased lumbar lordosis as compensation for the increased curvature at the fracture site. This pain in turn usually subsides in three to six months.[147] In patients with many fractures, chronic low and mid back pain may remain and seems to be related to continued stress on ligaments, muscles and apophyseal joints, resulting from the altered vertebral mechanics.

The strong tendency for both of the first two types of pain to improve spontaneously with time makes interpretation of the results of treatment especially difficult, since any treatment begun within a few weeks or months of a vertebral fracture is likely to be given the

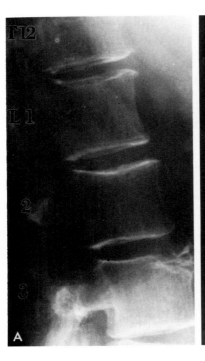
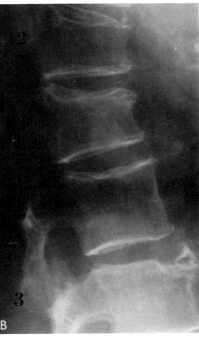

Figure 13–42. Vertebrae from woman with involutional osteoporosis showing A, wedging of T12 with normal shape of L1 at age 63 and B, wedging of L1 with no further change in T-12 at age 67.

credit for any improvement, even though this would have occurred in the absence of any treatment.

A fourth type of pain, that is true bone pain, often associated with tenderness to percussion, may occur in some patients. The character of the pain is suggestive of osteomalacia but is confined to the spine, whereas in osteomalacia the pain and tenderness are equally severe in ribs, pelvis and lower limbs. The patient with osteoporosis is obviously not immune to other causes of backache, and statistical confirmation that pain of this kind in the absence of vertebral deformity occurs more commonly in patients with osteoporosis than without is still lacking, but we think that it is a genuine phenomenon. Conceivably, it might be related to repeated microscopic fracture or trabecular microfracture of insufficient extent to cause detectable change in vertebral shape.

Vertebral fractures may be completely painless,[284] and many surveys have revealed a surprisingly high incidence of such asymptomatic vertebral compressions.[163] It is possible that in these cases the compression developed gradually rather than suddenly.[66] Such asymptomatic fractures may be peculiar to the very old, and so to senile rather than to postmenopausal osteoporosis as we have defined these terms.

The subsequent clinical course of patients with vertebral fracture depends on whether the fracture resulted primarily from decreased mechnical strength of the bone or from increased stress; if caused by increased stress in circumstances whose recurrence can be prevented, no more fractures may occur. In such patients, who sustain only a single fracture even after many years, serial measurements of height show a very slow decline or no change. In other patients, in whom the fracture resulted from a critical reduction in bone mass, continued fractures may occur, either by further compression of the same vertebra or by involvement of a different (often adjacent) vertebra (Fig. 13–42). In such patients, there may be a stepwise decrease in height, each sudden loss resulting from a fracture, with little change in between. This process may cease at any time or may continue until finally the ribs come to rest on the pelvic brim.[394] Sometimes compression fractures seem to cluster in groups of two or three within a few months, with many years of freedom between clusters. The episodic clinical course naturally does not imply that the progression of the underlying bone loss is constant; according to Urist this may progress to a certain critical level and then cease.[394]

An important difference between vertebral fractures due to osteoporosis and those which occur in the normal individual due to trauma is the complete absence of any risk of spinal cord involvement. Traumatic factors may be associated with instability and displacement,. but osteoporotic fractures are purely compressive. There are only two published cases of spinal cord compression in patients with vertebral collapse ostensibly due to osteoporosis,[236] and in neither case were spinal metastases ruled out. The occurrence of signs of cord compression in the elderly patient with vertebral collapse almost certainly indicates some more serious pathological process in addition to any osteoporosis which may be present. Spinal nerve root compression in a patient with a collapsed vertebra may be due to coincidental disc disease. Degenerative changes in the spine and osteoarthritis may result from altered pressure on intervertebral articular facets because of increasing dorsal kyphosis, thus it may be difficult to decide whether this or the osteoporosis is the principal cause of symptoms.

Pathogenesis of Involutional Osteoporosis

The pathogenesis of involutional osteoporosis is unknown, but several plausible theories have been suggested which indicate hopeful lines of investigation. First, estrogen deficiency is at least part of the explanation for postmenopausal osteoporosis as we have defined it—that is, for that component of involutional osteoporosis which represents the difference between men and women. Although the onset of involutional osteoporosis in women is several years before the menopause, ovarian failure may be a gradual process which begins several years earlier than the cessation of menstruation. The mechanism whereby estrogen deficiency enhances bone loss is unknown, but it has been proposed that the bone is rendered more sensitive to the resorbing action of parathyroid hormone.[157, 202] The experimental work indicating that estrogen inhibits resorption of the primary spongiosa in rats and increases medullary bone during egg formation in birds involves actions on woven and not lamellar bone and is of no relevance to human disease, but the evidence in man stands on its own merits.

Second, it is reasonably certain that some patients with involutional osteoporosis fail to accumulate enough bone during growth.[220] The detection of such patients who are especially liable to develop symptomatic osteoporosis can provide a group in whom the prophylactic value of various treatments can be assessed. Third, the high meat diet of developed countries generates a greater load of hydrogen ion for urinary excretion than does a vegetarian diet, and it is possible that this is partly buffered at the expense of bone.[404] Chronic metabolic acidosis is known to lead to bone loss in rats,[31] and may contribute to osteoporosis in chronic renal failure.[307] However, the disproportionate loss of bone carbonate characteristic of metabolic acidosis is not found in involutional osteoporosis; in fact, bone carbonate seems to increase with age relative to apatite.[273]

Fourth, there is considerable evidence relating involutional osteoporosis to calcium deficiency. The mechanism whereby calcium deficiency is thought to lead to osteoporosis is often not stated explicitly by proponents of this theory. The most popular idea involves a form of secondary hyperparathyroidism with consequent increase in bone resorption. The original concept of Nordin, who did so much to popularize this theory,[293] was that calcium was withdrawn from bone under the influence of the osteocyte-regulated blood-bone equilibrium, and did not necessarily involve parathyroid stimulation. The basis for this view was that calcium deprivation regularly failed to induce changes in the renal tubular reabsorption of phosphate, which at that time was the only simple index of parathyroid function. However, failure of phosphate reabsorption to change probably reflects the fact that dietary calcium deprivation causes inhibition of calcitonin secretion as well as stimulation of PTH, since these hormones have the same effect on phosphate excretion. There is now good evidence that dietary calcium depletion does indeed lead to parathyroid stimulation.[309] The evidence for the calcium deficiency theory is as follows: 1) Most,[256,290] but not all,[371] dietary surveys have shown that calcium intake is significantly less in patients with symptomatic osteoporosis than in age- and sex-matched controls;[372] 2) There is a significant, although small, correlation between the intake of calcium and the amount of vertebral bone, determined by a radiographic photodensitometric procedure.[208] 3) There is a decline in calcium absorption with increasing age,[20, 64] and in patients with osteoporosis.[375] It is possible, although not yet proved, that this is due to vitamin D deficiency of insufficient magnitude to cause osteomalacia.[367] This conclusion rests on the assumption that vitamin D has some direct effect in the promotion of normal mineralization, independent of its effect on intestinal calcium absorption, the evidence for which belief was reviewed earlier (q.v.). If this is correct, then it is conceivable that more vitamin D is necessary to promote optimal absorption in the elderly than is necessary to maintain normal osteoblastic function, and, therefore, a moderate deficiency of vitamin D might lead to significant impairment of calcium absorption without the production of osteomalacia. 4) There is a significant incidence of lactose intolerance among patients with symptomatic osteoporosis.[48] Lactose intolerance is a disorder in which the enzyme lactase is deficient in the intestinal mucosa, so that dietary lactose is not split into its constituent monosaccharides. This leads to the development of a characteristic set of symptoms after the ingestion of milk, so that patients with this disorder voluntarily limit their consumption of milk and milk products. 5) A significant number of patients with osteoporosis have high urinary calcium excretion and fail to show a normal reduction in urinary calcium in response to dietary calcium restrictions.[44, 327] This is not a very cogent argument, since a high urinary calcium may be a feature of osteoporosis for several different reasons. A more significant observation is the presence of *fasting* hypercalciuria in postmenopausal women, reversible by estrogen administration; this may provide a link between the hormonal and nutritional theories.[290] 6) There is a moderate amount of circumstantial evidence linking involutional osteoporosis to parathyroid hormone.[185] In addition, some patients with osteoporosis have increased levels of immunoreactive parathyroid hormone,[14, 155] but it is unclear whether this is due to secondary hyperparathyroidism or to normocalcemic primary hyperparathyroidism.

Although this evidence taken together is persuasive, there are some grounds for disbelief. 1) Epidemiologic studies comparing the incidence of osteoporosis with calcium consumption in many different parts of the world have shown very little relationship.[288] The only positive ·finding in keeping with the theory is that in Finland the incidence of osteoporosis is the least and the intake of calcium is the most of all the countries examined. There is no relationship between dietary calcium and the amount of cortical bone,[158] but this is not necessarily relevant because calcium deficiency may lead to preferential loss of trabecular rather than cortical bone. In the South African Bantu, in whom dietary calcium intake is low throughout life, the incidence of osteoporosis is less and the mean bone volume greater than in Caucasian South Africans, whose intake of calcium is much higher.[96, 407] However, the fact that the South African Bantu is able to adapt very efficiently to a low calcium intake does not necessarily mean that this is a universal human characteristic. Also, there is an important difference between a low calcium intake which is present throughout life and a low intake which occurs after becoming accustomed to a high intake. Conceivably, the continuation of an unnecessarily high calcium intake beyond infancy throughout the growth period, and into adolescence and early adult life, which characterizes the United States and other developed countries, may lead to irreversible atrophy of the mechanisms for calcium conservation. Such people may, in effect, have become addicted to calcium and, consequently, need a continued high intake for the remainder of their lives, and if this high intake is for any reason curtailed, or if they becomes less able to absorb calcium they will suffer from the effects of calcium deficiency. 2) Balance studies, using an inert marker to prevent overestimation of calcium retention through loss of small amounts of fecal material containing a lot of calcium, show that the retention of calcium after increasing the intake is short-lived and does not usually persist beyond one sigma (the length of the remodeling cycle).[338] 3) No improvement in x-ray appearances or in bone mineral content has been demonstrated from high calcium feeding. This is disappointing but hardly surprising, since a modest increase in bone turnover continued for a long time would lead to a dominance of irreversible as opposed to reversible bone loss (see p. 656). For example, a twofold increase continued for 20 years would result in 90 per cent of the bone loss being irreversible and only 10 per cent reversible. The best that can be hoped for from high calcium feeding in

someone with established osteoporosis is a reduction in the rate of loss to a normal value. For a twofold increase in remodeling rate, this maximum effect would be a reduction in the annual rate of bone loss from 2 per cent to 1 per cent per year. It is likely that a minimum of ten years of observation would be necessary to confirm or exclude such a possibility. 4) The most telling evidence against the calcium deficiency theory is that, as explained above, it requires that bone turnover be modestly increased, whereas bone remodeling dynamics studied with tetracycline uniformly show a reduction in bone turnover in patients with symptomatic osteoporosis.[400, 418] Contrary evidence that bone resorption is increased in involutional osteoporosis is insecurely based. The first suggestion came from kinetic studies in patients who were immobilized. However, traumatic osteodystrophy is a high turnover state, and the findings cannot be transposed to other situations. The increased extent of resorbing surface found by microradiography results from a depression in the resorption rate,[330] rather than an acceleration of remodeling. The endosteal expansion which characterizes involutional osteoporosis reflects a net but·not an absolute increase in endosteal resorption. In order to reconcile the calcium deficiency theory with the dynamics of bone remodeling actually present in patients with symptoms, it is necessary to postulate that dietary calcium depletion is one factor contributing to involutional loss of bone which remains asymptomatic, and that some additional factor or factors leads to a change in remodeling dynamics and bone quality in someone whose bone mass has already been critically reduced, leading to structural failure and symptomatic osteoporosis.

Finally, we come back to the striking fact that in involutional osteoporosis the loss is almost exclusively of bone which was in physical contact with the bone marrow; that is, on trabecular and cortical endosteal surfaces.[141] The relevance of this juxtaposition is shown by several lines of evidence.[138] Erythroid hyperplasia, as in sickle-cell anemia, leads to thinning of the cortex, owing to increased net endosteal resorption. The pattern of this loss is to affect the extremities in infancy, the skull in later childhood, and the ribs, spine and pelvis in adults.[233] In involutional osteoporosis there is progressive replacement of cellular marrow by fat, so that fat accumulation occurs at the expense of both marrow cells and bone tissue.[277] Increased numbers of mast cells are found in marrow patients with osteoporosis, and mast cells release heparin, a known bone-resorbing cofactor for parathyroid hormone. Further work on the relationship of bone marrow cells to endosteal and trabecular bone loss is clearly indicated.

High and Low Turnover Osteoporosis

In involutional and most other types of symptomatic osteoporosis, bone turnover is reduced, but in a few conditions it is increased. Increased bone turnover primarily reflects an increase in the initiation of new remodeling cycles (the activation frequency) and this can only be measured by means of double tetracycline labeling. However, bone turnover may be estimated indirectly with sufficient accuracy for the purpose of this classification, and certain common features of high turnover osteoporosis can be defined.

Bone loss from increased bone turnover has two components, one of which is reversible and the other irreversible. The reversible component is bone which has been removed during remodeling and not yet replaced, and so is a direct consequence of the number of remodeling cycles present at one time; the average volume of bone missing during the formation of one osteon is about 0.02 cubic mm. The irreversible component is the bone lost because of the small deficit of bone in each normal remodeling cycle multiplied by a larger factor, so that the number of bites taken out in unit time is increased. The relative magnitude of these two components depends on the duration of the increased remodeling rate. The reversible component remains unchanged for as long as a given increase in the level of turnover persists, since it depends on the number of *uncompleted* remodeling cycles present at one time. By contrast, the irreversible component increases progressively with time, since it depends on the number of *completed* remodeling cycles which have accumulated since the onset of the increased turnover. For example, a fivefold increase in activation frequency and in bone turnover will increase the reversible bone loss from about three per cent of total bone volume to about 15 per cent, and will increase the irreversible loss from about one per cent per year to about five. If this increased remodeling rate persists for only one year, then 75 per cent of the bone

loss is reversible and about 25 per cent is irreversible. However, if this increase persists for five years, then only 40 per cent of the bone loss is reversible and 60 per cent is irreversible. It is evident that this places a high premium on early diagnosis in those cases of high bone turnover which are amenable to treatment. The typical course of bone loss and recovery in high turnover osteoporosis is shown diagrammatically in Figure 13–43. For comparison, the typical course of bone loss in chronic low turnover osteoporosis, such as in Cushing's syndrome, is shown in Figure 13–44.

The increased bone loss due to increased remodeling cannot be recognized directly in trabeculae, but in cortical bone it is evident as unfilled resorption spaces. The radiographic hallmark of high turnover osteoporosis is, therefore, an increase in intracortical porosity, best shown by magnification radioscopy (q.v.). The irreversible loss due to accelerated net endosteal and trabecular resorption differs in no way from that occurring in involutional osteoporosis. The static morphologic hallmark is an increase in the same proportion in the number of resorption spaces and seams in cortical bone, and in the fraction of surface occupied by resorption and formation in trabecular bone, but such an increase also may occur with normal or reduced bone turnover if both

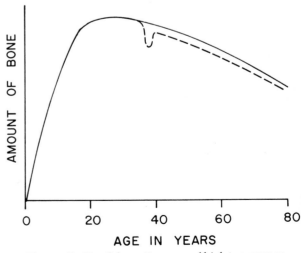

Figure 13–43. Schematic course of high turnover osteoporosis. Solid line represents normal gain and loss of bone throughout life. Dotted line shows rapid loss followed by rapid but incomplete recovery with a permanent deficit, and subsequent age-dependent loss at a normal rate.

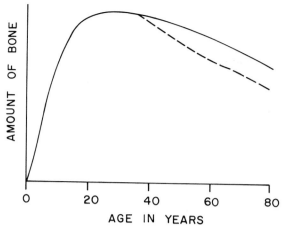

Figure 13–44. Schematic course of chronic low turnover osteoporosis, such as in Cushing's syndrome. Solid line represents normal gain and loss of bone throughout life. Dotted line shows a moderate increase in the rate of bone loss, eventually accumulating to a larger bone deficit than shown in Figure 13–42, but over a much longer period of time, lack of recovery when the cause of the increase is removed, and subsequent bone loss continuing at a normal rate.

resorption and formation are slowed, and thus the period of time occupied by these activities is prolonged. Some authors describe the histologic findings of high turnover osteoporosis as osteitis fibrosa,[30] but the fibrous tissue and woven bone replacement which characterize the latter condition are not seen. An increase in bone turnover alone does not alter the thickness of osteoid seams, but if the appositional rate is increased as in hyperthyroidism,[276] and the mineralization lag time remains the same, the osteoid seam thickness may increase and cause confusion with osteomalacia.[127]

The increase in organ-level bone resorption and formation which characterizes a high turnover state may be shown by an increase in radiokinetically determined accretion, by an increase in total and in both nondialyzable and dialyzable hydroxyproline in the urine, and by an increase in urinary and sometimes in plasma calcium. The increase in urinary calcium is the least accurate guide, since a sudden and almost complete cessation of formation, as may occur in some patients with idiopathic osteoporosis, may also produce a substantial increase in urinary calcium. Clinically, *generalized* high turnover osteoporosis may be completely asymptomatic, except when of long duration, whereas *localized* high turnover osteoporosis may be associated with severe local pain and disability. These several characteristics of high turnover osteoporosis are shown in Table 13–7.

Generalized high bone turnover osteoporosis may be caused by hyperthyroidism, primary hyperparathyroidism and active acromegaly (Table 13–8), all of which may affect the spine, and is also a feature of osteogenesis imperfecta (q.v.). It is possible, as mentioned earlier, that nutritional secondary hyperparathyroidism due to dietary calcium depletion or prolonged lactation also leads to high turnover osteoporosis. Secondary hyperparathyroidism also occurs in pregnancy, but any adverse effect which this may have on the bones seems to be overcome by the other endocrine changes.[407] Localized high turnover osteoporosis occurs in traumatic osteodystrophy and in regional migratory osteolysis.[17] There is no convincing evidence that either of these conditions affects the spine, but the distinction between traumatic osteodystrophy and immobilization osteoporosis (which may affect the spine) is of some importance.[146] Since trauma with its complications is the most common reason for prolonged immobilization, these two conditions commonly occur together and so are still frequently confused. Traumatic osteodystrophy develops soon after the injury, which in this context is interpreted rather broadly to include other noxious agents such as denervation and trauma, and is associated with radiographic and histo-

TABLE 13–7.   CHARACTERISTICS OF HIGH AND LOW TURNOVER OSTEOPOROSIS

Characteristics	High	Low
Dynamic morphologic — activation frequency	↑	↓
Static morphologic — specific surface	↑	N or ↓
Radiographic — intracortical porosity	↑	N or ↓
Kinetic — accretion rate and pool size	↑	N or ↓
Biochemical — urinary total hydroxyproline	↑	N or ↓
Biochemical — urinary total calcium	↑	N or ↓

TABLE 13–8. CAUSES OF HIGH TURNOVER OSTEOPOROSIS

Hyperthyroidism
Primary hyperparathyroidism
Nutritional secondary hyperparathyroidism
Acromegaly
Osteogenesis imperfecta
Traumatic osteodystrophy
Regional migratory osteolysis
Idiopathic

logic evidence of high turnover, sometimes with periosteal involvement resembling the subperiosteal resorption of osteitis fibrosa.[223, 338] This may be accompanied by circulatory and sudomotor evidence of autonomic dysfunction. The reversibility of traumatic osteodystrophy which characterizes all high turnover states is responsible for the reports of healing in immobilization osteoporosis.[338] True immobilization or disuse osteoporosis is not seen until many months later, is characterized by low turnover and is, at least in the present state of knowledge, irreversible.

Finally, in a few cases of high turnover osteoporosis none of the previously mentioned factors can be found. Such patients may have greater disability than is usual with high turnover osteoporosis, and the prognosis is less favorable. The possible relationship of this idiopathic high turnover osteoporosis to normocalcemic hyperparathyroidism is discussed later.

In two remarkable cases in middle-aged men, severe osteoporosis was associated with striking hypercalciuria (600 to 760 mg per 24 hours), hypercalcemia, and extensive osteocyte necrosis.[344]

Osteoporosis Due to Other Identifiable Etiologic Factors

Some textbooks contain long lists of alleged causes of osteoporosis, many of which were first proposed before the near universality of age-related bone loss was appreciated and which have been unthinkingly perpetuated by subsequent authors. For example, uncontrolled diabetes was given as a cause of osteoporosis by Albright and Reifenstein in 1948,[6] and despite continued lack of evidence,[100] this idea still lingers. In order to identify a factor as of etiologic importance, it is necessary to demonstrate that the amount of bone in a sufficiently large number of persons with the factor is significantly less than in persons of the same age and sex without the factor. A list of reasonably well documented causes is given in Table 13–9. Two additional points must be mentioned: First, the situations before and after skeletal maturity are so different that an etiological factor established in growing children cannot be assumed without additional evidence to operate in adults, and vice versa. Second, any etiologic factor identified by appropriate epidemiologic study cannot be assumed to act directly on bone, since the effect may be mediated by normal endocrine or metabolic influences. Some genuine etiologic factors which cause localized osteoporosis not involving the spine will be mentioned only very briefly.

OSTEOPOROSIS DUE TO GENETIC ABNORMALITY. *Osteogenesis Imperfecta.*[267] This is a genetically determined disorder of connective tissue characterized by abnormally thin bones of increased fragility. Most cases show dominant inheritance, but it is likely that several genetically distinct conditions are grouped together because of similarity in their clinical effects. Two main forms are described: osteogenesis imperfecta congenita, in which multiple fractures cause death in utero or soon

TABLE 13–9. IDENTIFIABLE CAUSES OF OSTEOPOROSIS

Genetic:	Osteogenesis imperfecta
	Homocystinuria
Endocrine:	Hypogonadism
	Hyperadrenocorticism
	Hyperthyroidism
	Hyperparathyroidism
	Acromegaly
Nutritional:	Calcium deficiency
	Protein deficiency
	Ascorbic acid deficiency
	Intestinal malabsorption
Drug Induced:	Heparin
	Anticonvulsants
	Methotrexate
	Ethanol
Miscellaneous:	Metabolic acidosis
	Rheumatoid arthritis
	Trauma
	Disuse

after birth, and osteogenesis imperfecta tarda, in which fractures only develop after birth.

The spinal manifestations may be indistinguishable from other varieties of osteoporosis. The vertebrae show increased lucency, with multiple wedging or compression; or there may be diffuse symmetrical biconcavity of vertebrae, which is more characteristic of osteoporosis in children than in adults (Fig. 13–45). Sometimes there may be extreme flattening of the vertebrae, known as platyspondylosis. Many patients have scoliosis, most likely from laxity of spinal ligaments. In other bones there is extreme cortical thinness and narrowing of the shafts of the long bones with metaphyseal flaring. Fractures may heal normally with abundant callus, but lack of normal remodeling of multiple fractures may lead to diffuse curvature of the long bones, an apparent exception to the rule that bending of bone is a feature of osteomalacia rather than osteoporosis.

Frequently associated features are blue sclerae, lax ligaments, as in other heritable disorders of connective tissue, basilar impression, with a so-called tam-o-shanter deformity of the skull, abnormal transparency of the teeth due to odontogenesis imperfecta, an increased number of Wormian bones in the skull, and deafness due to otosclerosis in adult life. Often there is clinical evidence of hypermetabolism, with increased body temperature, tachycardia, tachypnea, sweating, lack of subcutaneous fat, and small body size. This may be accompanied by increased basal metabolic rate and chemical evidence of mild hyperthyroidism.[90]

In the milder forms of the disease no abnormality may be noted during early childhood. The patient may present with symptoms that may at first appear indistinguishable from those of idiopathic osteoporosis—(q.v.) in adolescence, or even, in adult life, osteogenesis imperfecta tardissima.[100] The family history, blue sclera, and lax ligaments are the most useful clues in this situation.

The basic defect is most likely to be the formation of an abnormal and immature form of collagen, an abnormality which may be widespread throughout the body. The amount of collagen in a unit area of skin is reduced.[384] Collagen fibers in the cornea show a reduction in diameter of about 30 per cent, and cross striations are rare. Histochemical investigations of corneal collagen have also been consistent with a disorder of tropocollagen synthesis or of the extracellular aggregation of collagen. In bone, collagen fibers are abnormal, not only in structure but also in their spatial orientation in bundles.[251]

Bone remodeling dynamics have indicated an increase in bone turnover, with normal or only slightly depressed cell level bone formation and considerably increased tissue level bone formation, indicating that there is no fundamental defect in the amount of collagen synthesized by osteoblasts.[402] By inference, the failure to maintain a normal amount of bone must arise from a greater increase in bone resorption. There is also a failure to maintain the periosteal drift which is necessary to increase transverse bone diameter during growth and thus to produce normal remodeling of fractures. It is possible that both the increased bone turnover and the failure of

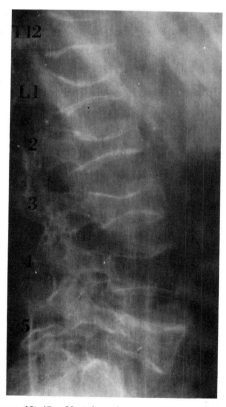

Figure 13–45. Vertebrae from a patient aged 12 with osteogenesis imperfecta. Note that biconcavity is symmetrical in T12, L3 and L5, and only slightly asymmetrical in L1, L2 and L4. In this respect, the shape changes resemble those of osteomalacia, as is usual with osteoporosis in this age group, but the degree of abnormality is different in each vertebra, as is usual in adult osteoporosis.

periosteal drift are consequences of the basic defect in collagen structure, causing a substantial weakness of bone and increased liability to fracture. The increase in turnover represents an attempt to remove bone of poor physical quality, an attempt which continues indefinitely because the bone which replaces it has the same abnormal structure.

No treatment is available, although fluoride has given encouraging but inconclusive results, including a suggestive reduction in fracture rate.[7]

Homocystinuria.[267] This is a heritable disorder of connective tissue having some clinical features resembling Marfan's syndrome. There may be a generalized osteoporosis, particularly affecting the spine, with biconcavity and wedging of vertebrae. The skull also may be involved. An unusual feature is that posterior wedging may occur in all the lumbar vertebrae; this is normally only seen in L5 and occasionally in L4. The age of onset of these osteoporotic changes is uncertain, but they have been found in the early twenties. Associated features comprise disproportionately long legs, genu valgum, kyphoscoliosis, ectopia lentis, mental retardation, and multiple arterial and venous thrombi, often leading to death from early ischemic heart disease. The diagnosis is confirmed by demonstrating the presence of homocystine in the urine.

ENDOCRINE CAUSES OF OSTEOPOROSIS. Although rare, the endocrinopathies causing osteoporosis are important because they are all treatable and, therefore, bone loss should be preventable even if not reversible.

Hypogonadism. Since the normal pubertal changes in gonadal function are important determinants of the accumulation of bone during the adolescent growth spurt, it appears obvious that gonadal failure during growth must have some harmful effect on bone. Some workers have denied this by drawing an improper analogy between the adult and the child. Albright and Reifenstein originally argued that because postmenopausal osteoporosis was due to estrogen deficiency, estrogen deficiency during growth must cause osteoporosis.[6] Those who do not accept the premise of this argument feel constrained to deny the conclusion, but both the original syllogism and its contrary are equally fallacious because the situations during growth and in late adult life are so different. Even so, the relationship between hypogonadism in

childhood and osteoporosis is by no means simple. The osteoporosis of gonadal dysgenesis may be in part one of the associated constellation of congenital abnormalities, including webbing of the neck and cubitus valgus, collectively known as Turner's syndrome. Osteoporosis may occur in Turner's syndrome even in the absence of gonadal insufficiency.[133] Also, many of the reports of osteoporosis have been based on misinterpreted x-rays. There may be hypoplasia of cervical vertebrae as a developmental abnormality.[125] Delayed epiphyseal fusion may lead to vertebral wedging and anteroposterior elongation of the vertebral bodies associated with backache.[4, 133] The changes may resemble those of Scheuermann's disease,[125] and have been referred to as epiphysitis. Despite these reservations it seems reasonably certain that both male and female hypogonadism during growth leads to osteoporosis because of failure to accumulate a normal complement of bone. Similar observations apply to the secondary hypogonadism due to hypopituitarism in children. In patients with the X-O chromosome pattern, regardless of the presence or absence of the associated features comprising Turner's syndrome, there are both reduced net subperiosteal apposition and increased net endosteal resorption, shown by radiographic morphometry of the hands.[160]

Hyperadrenocorticism. Osteoporosis, compression fractures of the vertebrae, and kyphosis are well known features of Cushing's syndrome. Although in mild cases the spinal changes may be indistinguishable from involutional osteoporosis, there are some points of difference. Cushing's syndrome affects the axial skeleton relatively more than the appendicular skeleton. The skull may show patchy rarefaction in the absence of evidence of raised intracranial pressure, and the ribs are affected much more than in involutional osteoporosis, and are frequently fractured. These fractures heal slowly but with abundant callus formation, like stress fractures elsewhere,[146] another instance of the dissociation between lamellar bone and woven bone. Involvement of the pelvis may be shown by protrusio acetabuli. The other features of Cushing's syndrome consist of a moon-shaped face, truncal obesity, purple-colored striae, hypertension, hirsutism, muscle weakness and wasting, thinness of the skin and diabetes. In mild forms, it may be impossible to differentiate Cushing's syndrome clinically from the obesity and hirsutism which are quite commonly seen in middle-aged women.

The pathogenesis of bone loss in Cushing's syndrome is controversial. Studies with microradiography indicate an increase in resorption surface and decrease in formation surface.[329] The pitfalls in the interpretation of surface-based measurements in general and microradiography in particular have been described earlier. The dynamics of remodeling indicate that in the chronic steady state situation Cushing's syndrome is characterized by a reduced activation frequency and bone turnover, there is a marked reduction in cellular and tissue level bone resorption and bone formation, especially the former, and the balance per remodeling cycle is more negative due to a disproportionate reduction in bone formation.[400] In other words, the changes are similar to those in symptomatic involutional osteoporosis, with the addition of a greater depression of bone resorption rate which leads to accumulation of the indolent resorptive surfaces found by microradiography. The typical natural history of the bone loss was shown in Fig. 13–44.

Osteoporosis, vertebral compression and kyphosis may also occur with exogenous corticosteroid therapy.[92] In general, the situation here is similar, but with a number of important differences. The underlying disease may itself predispose to osteoporosis, as does rheumatoid arthritis, in which there may be not only porosis at the ends of the bones in relation to the inflamed joints but also an increased incidence of spinal porosis. Other treatment given concurrently, such as salicylates, may also affect the bone.[114] The dose schedule used may be of particular importance and there may be differences both in the type of steroid and the method of administration.[114] Experiments in rabbits with corticosteroid administration have revealed an additional early phase of increased activation and markedly accelerated endosteal and trabecular resorption which is not followed by formation. This subsides after a few months but is responsible for a large part of the total loss of bone. This increased phase of accelerated resorption is probably dose-dependent, and may not occur in spontaneous Cushing's syndrome, but may be important in exogenous hypercortisonism when an initial high dose is used.[114] Finally, endogenous Cushing's syndrome may be associated with increased androgen secretion, whereas exogenous hypercortisonism may be

associated with decreased androgen, estrogen and growth hormone, because there is some spillover from the depressant effect on pituitary ACTH secretion to other pituitary hormones. In growing children, the associated depression of gonadal and growth hormones probably contributes to the growth depressant effect of corticosteroid therapy and may be the reason why ACTH in equal anti-inflammatory doses has less adverse effect, both on growth and on the accumulation of bone.

Hyperthyroidism. This produces a high turnover osteoporosis as defined and described earlier, with the additional special characteristic that cortical bone is involved with disproportionate severity compared to trabecular bone. The appositional rate, which is a measure of osteoblastic activity, may be increased up to twofold, so that osteoid seams may be wider as well as more numerous. This has led previous authors to describe osteomalacia in hyperthyroidism.[127] Tunneling or dissecting resorption may be seen in severe cases, when the tissue is extremely vascular,[127] but replacement by fibrous tissue and woven bone does not occur. In young people, specific osseous manifestations are not usually added to the clinical features of hyperthyroidism but they nevertheless will occur if the disease is left untreated long enough. Von Recklinghausen described severe kyphoscoliosis in a 23-year-old woman who had been hyperthyroid for five years; at autopsy the bones were all extremely soft. There may also be fractures of ribs, vertebral bodies and long bones,[140] with increasingly severe bone pain.[276] Symptomatic hyperthyroid osteoporosis is more likely in older persons, in whom the process of bone loss has already begun. The increase in net bone loss in each endosteal remodeling cycle which characterizes involutional osteoporosis is magnified by the increase in turnover, so that the total rate of bone loss is accelerated. The predilection for the middle-aged and elderly reflects also the fact that hyperthyroidism in the elderly may lack the classical features of Graves' disease, and so may escape detection for a much longer period. The recurrence of hyperthyroidism after surgical treatment is especially likely to be undiagnosed for a long time and to lead to thyrotoxic osteopathy.

Hyperparathyroidism. A high turnover osteoporosis, usually asymptomatic, is a common occurrence in this disease, as in hyperthyroidism. For the same reasons, the magnitude of the resultant bone loss is much greater after the menopause than before. As in other high bone turnover states, an increase in bone mineral content may occur after successful treatment in the absence of osteitis fibrosa cystica.[129] In most such cases the diagnosis of primary hyperparathyroidism was made because of other manifestations, the osseous features being incidental. More recently, it has been suggested that in some patients primary hyperparathyroidism may cause a clinically significant, apparently idiopathic osteoporosis in the absence of an elevated plasma calcium.[30, 189] This situation (if it exists) must be distinguished from primary hyperparathyroidism with osteitis fibrosa and associated vitamin D deficiency, with normal or even reduced level of plasma calcium.[237]

Soon after the discovery of primary hyperparathyroidism as a disease entity, a large number of parathyroid operations were carried out for many different reasons, including osteoporosis, and many remarkable symptomatic improvements were reported.[26, 156] These claims were finally disposed of at a historic meeting of the American Orthopaedic Association in Toronto in 1932,[33] and we think it important that there should be no recurrence of this epidemic of unnecessary parathyroid operations. So far, only two cases have been reported in which a plausible argument has been made that apparent idiopathic osteoporosis may be produced by normocalcemic primary hyperparathyroidism.[30]

Acromegaly. Although there is some dispute about whether the metabolic bone disease of acromegaly should be classified as osteoporosis, it is convenient to consider it here. Early reports of increased radiolucency of vertebral bone failed to take into account the relationship to age-dependent bone loss, and more recent work has indicated that compression fractures of the vertebrae and other manifestations of symptomatic osteoporosis are extremely uncommon. The radiographic findings in the spine are of exaggerated osteophytosis and narrowing of disc spaces with increased posterior concavity of the vertebral bodies, rather than osteoporosis.[380] In the active stage of the disease, there is histologic,[323] radiographic,[271] and kinetic[184] evidence of a high turnover osteoporosis of moderate degree. The mineral content of the forearm bones is usually normal for the patient's age,[112] and may even be slightly increased.[328] However, because of increased periosteal apposition

during the active stage, the external diameter of the bone is increased and the ratio of the cortical cross-sectional area to the total cross-sectional area may be reduced.[160] Thus, the total volume of cortical bone may be increased in absolute terms, but decreased in relation to the increased size of the bone. Clearly, whether or not one chooses to call this osteoporosis is a matter of definition. When the disease is burned out, continued endosteal bone loss may lead to thinning of the cortex and an unequivocally subnormal amount of bone. There is loss of trabecular bone in the upper femur, shown by semiquantitative estimation.[328] Similar loss in the vertebrae may be obscured by the increased amount of soft tissue. The enlarging of the remaining trabeculae, which occurs to some extent in involutional osteoporosis, is even more evident in acromegaly.[328] The relative freedom from vertebral collapse has been attributed to the increase in anteroposterior diameter of the vertebrae (Fig. 13–46).[405] However, such an increase may in fact be associated with a greater liability to fracture![368]

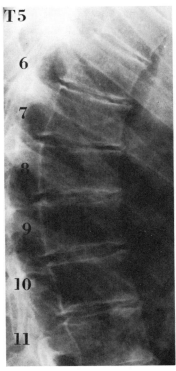

Figure 13–46. Vertebrae from a patient aged 42 with mild acromegaly. Note the increase in AP diameter in the midthoracic region. The disc spaces are somewhat reduced for the patient's age.

NUTRITIONAL CAUSES OF OSTEOPOROSIS. *Calcium Deficiency.* This undoubtedly causes osteoporosis in growing animals,[100] and has been widely promulgated as a cause of osteoporosis in adult humans. The accumulation of a normal amount of bone during growth represents an average retention of calcium of about 150 mg per day for the first 20 years of life, but the extreme degree of reduction in calcium intake needed to prevent this is very uncommon and has only been documented in one case.[100] The epidemiologic evidence that calcium deficiency is an important factor in the common involutional, osteoporosis was reviewed earlier. Similar evidence might show a relationship between normal variation in dietary calcium in children and bone accumulation during growth, but this remains to be established. Probably, there are individuals in whom calcium deficiency is of major importance, particularly those whose calcium intake or absorption is reduced as a result of disease and in whom renal conservation may be inefficient.

Protein Deficiency. Protein malnutrition in growing children causes osteoporosis owing to accelerated net endosteal resorption.[158] Hypoproteinemia may be responsible for the high incidence of osteoporosis in children with the nephrotic syndrome (increased renal loss),[133] and in children with chronic liver disease (impaired synthesis).[133, 393] The effects in adults are less well established.

Scurvy. Ascorbic acid deficiency impairs collagen synthesis in bone as in other tissues, and osteoporosis is a well known feature of scurvy in children. In the South African Bantu male, scurvy may also cause osteoporosis in adults,[218] but the etiological relationship is obscured by the frequent coexistence of hemosiderosis.[351] Stiffness, pain, tenderness and muscle spasm in the back are common, and x-rays show varying degrees of vertebral compression and collapse, progressing occasionally to vertebra plana.[218]

Intestinal Malabsorption. Although usually considered in the context of osteomalacia, intestinal malabsorption may also cause osteoporosis, especially in children. Multiple deficiencies of calcium, protein and possibly vitamin D may be involved. Osteoporosis is an important component of the bone disease after partial gastrectomy, and in association with pancreatic disease, both in children and adults.

MISCELLANEOUS CAUSES OF OSTEO-POROSIS. Chronic metabolic acidosis as a result of renal tubular disease or glycogen storage disease is frequently associated with osteoporosis in children. Metabolic acidosis may lead to preferential loss of bone carbonate and may contribute to the osteoporosis of chronic renal failure,[307] but the effects of acidosis are otherwise less well documented in adults. Recently, it has been suggested that chronic respiratory acidosis may be associated with osteoporosis,[100, 212] but this is so far unconfirmed.

In patients with ischemic heart disease given large doses of heparin, vertebral collapse has been observed in several instances.[172] Heparin is known to potentiate the bone resorbing actions of parathyroid hormone in tissue culture. With diminishing emphasis on this form of treatment and a reduction in dose, this is now rarely seen.

Chronic anticonvulsant administration may lead to metaphyseal osteoporosis,[374] as well as osteomalacia (q.v.). Spinal osteoporosis has not been described specifically in this context, but, conceivably, this may account for the reported association of epilepsy with vertebral collapse.[100] Another drug-induced form of osteoporosis is caused by methotrexate therapy for leukemia in children.[321]

Excess alcohol consumption predisposes to osteoporosis,[100, 347] probably in several different ways. Malnutrition, malabsorption and cirrhosis of the liver may all lead to hypoproteinemia, and impaired metabolism of cortisol may also be important.

Rheumatoid arthritis may be associated with osteoporosis, not only locally in relation to involved joints but also in the spine, even in the absence of corticosteroid therapy.[114]

Chronic disuse or immobilization may lead to severe osteoporosis with extreme cortical and trabecular thinning. This is usually localized to the involved part, but may affect the spine of patients who are totally incapacitated and bedridden. The important distinction between traumatic osteodystrophy and disuse osteoporosis was made earlier.

Idiopathic Osteoporosis

The term idiopathic osteoporosis was introduced by Albright to describe patients whose osteoporosis was neither postmenopausal nor senile, and in whom all other known causes were excluded. Unfortunately, the usage of the term has become less precise, and it is often used indiscriminately to include involutional osteoporosis. This trend should be reversed since it has delayed wider recognition of the existence of osteoporosis in young people which is undoubtedly not involutional. We will redefine idiopathic osteoporosis in a manner which conforms to the spirit if not the letter of Albright's concept. Idiopathic osteoporosis refers to patients in whom the amount of bone is so far below the normal range for their age and sex that they clearly constitute a separate population, but in whom none of the conditions described in the previous section are present. This definition does not include any reference to age, but in practice almost all patients falling into this category will be well below the age of involutional osteoporosis.

As in any situation defined by exclusion, it is likely that we are dealing with a number of different conditions that we do not yet know how to distinguish. Since the clinical features and diagnostic problems of patients with idiopathic osteoporosis depend more on age than on any other factor, it is convenient to classify them according to the age of presentation, without implying either that all patients presenting at the same age have the same disease or, alternatively, that patients presenting at different ages have different diseases. Before considering the features at different ages, two general characteristics which distinguish idiopathic from other varieties of osteoporosis deserve mention. The onset is usually more acute with respect to symptoms and loss of height and more clearly identified in time than is usual in involutional osteoporosis, although an asymptomatic prodromal phase cannot be excluded. The loss of bone, vertebral collapse,

severe symptoms, and loss of height tend to be compressed into a few years rather than spread out over decades. (Note that in relation to bone disease the word "acute" refers to a much longer time scale than usual.) Eventually, the disease seems to burn out and, as judged by serial height measurement, either ceases to progress or progresses much more slowly than before (Fig. 13–47). The patient is then left with the mechanical effects of whatever bone loss occurred during the acute phase. If the disease occurs in childhood and a sufficiently long growth period remains, then enough normal bone may develop to offset the effects of the disease and the radiographic appearance of the bones may return almost to normal, as seen in successfully treated Cushing's syndrome in children. If growth has ceased, there is no longer this possibility of improvement (Fig. 13–48). A second general point is that, despite the severity of the vertebral changes of idiopathic osteoporosis, there is characteristically a much more varied and much more severe involvement of the extremities with respect to both the symptoms and the x-ray appearances (Fig. 13–49). This is especially true in children, in whom the presenting symptom is frequently unrelated to the spine.

IDIOPATHIC JUVENILE OSTEOPOROSIS.[103] This comprises all patients in whom idiopathic osteoporosis begins before skeletal maturity. The usual age of onset is from eight to 12 years, with extremes of about three and 15 years. The initial symptoms are usually related on one or more fractures after trivial trauma, with or without displacement. In younger children, there may be limping or other abnormality of the gait and refusal to

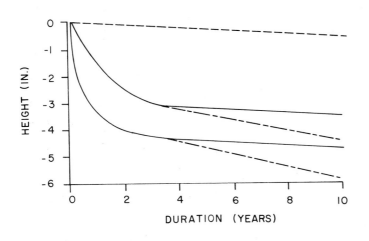

Figure 13–47. Schematic illustration of height loss in idiopathic osteoporosis. Upper dotted line represents normal slow height loss with age. Curved lines show accelerated height loss for one or two years, followed by either loss at a rate which is much less than in the acute phase, but greater than normal (dotted lines) or return to a normal rate of height loss (solid lines).

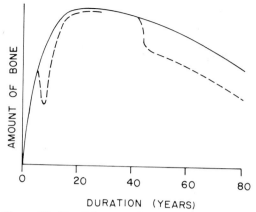

Figure 13–48. Schematic illustration of bone loss in idiopathic osteoporosis. Solid line represents normal gain and loss of bone throughout life. If onset is sufficiently far before skeletal maturity (left-hand dotted line) almost complete recovery is possible. If onset is in adult life (right-hand dotted line) the same degree of bone loss leaves a permanent deficit even when the disease becomes inactive. Note rapid rate of initial loss as in high turnover osteoporosis, but no recovery.

walk, with pain in the heels, ankles, knees or ribs. If the fractures are of the stress type without overt displacement, the earliest radiographic abnormality may be a hairline of increased density, which may not be evident at the onset of symptoms, so that a misdiagnosis of arthritis or malingering is common. The vertebral changes consist of severe compression with symmetrical biconcavity; there may be a slight degree of wedging equally distributed throughout the spine; the appearances resemble those of osteogenesis imperfecta (Fig. 13–45). These changes may develop to an extreme degree in as little as one year, associated with rapid loss of height due to shortening of the trunk. X-ray of other bones shows metaphyseal osteoporosis, indicating that the most recently formed bone is abnormal, whereas older bone may still have a normal appearance ("neo-osseous osteoporosis"). The fractures in the cortex of the abnormal bone may progress with impaction and compression of the weakened metaphysis, especially in the distal femora and tibiae. True fractures with separation of the bone ends are also common and usually heal well with normal callus.

Usually, there are no biochemical abnormalities, although these children are susceptible to hypercalcemia with immobilization, and

this may lead to exploration of normal parathyroid glands.[103] No characteristic change in urinary hydroxyproline has been found. Calcium balance studies show a high fecal calcium excretion which may fall with vitamin D,[103, 282] but this does not produce long-term calcium retention.

Bone histology may show accumulation of unfilled resorption surfaces,[81, 239] and absence of osteoblasts, indicating arrest of the formative phase of the remodeling cycle. In one case, the remodeling rate was reduced to about half of normal and the appositional rate to about one third of normal.[170]

No treatment is known to influence the course of the disease, but spontaneous improvement usually occurs within two to five years, with cessation of bone loss and resumption of normal bone growth. If enough time is left before the epiphyses fuse, the bones may return to almost normal. Kooh and colleagues, whose patients have been younger than most others described, used the term transient osteoporosis of childhood,[239] but in severe cases in whom the disease activity does not subside until close to skeletal maturity there may be permanent severe disability due to the deformity resulting from repeated fractures. Even in the most severe cases, some improvement usually takes place in the vertebral changes.[103]

The disease is frequently confused with osteogenesis imperfecta tarda, but the complete normality before the onset of the disease, the suddenness of onset and rapidity of progression, the x-ray changes showing that only the most recently formed bone is abnormal, the spontaneous healing, the absence of blue sclera, lax ligaments, dental abnormalities and family history, clearly identify this as a different condition.

Other diseases which may give rise to severe osteoporosis in childhood, such as metabolic acidosis associated with renal tubular dysfunction or with glycogen storage disease, the nephrotic syndrome, and chronic liver disease should give little difficulty in diagnosis.[133] The clinical and radiographic features of idiopathic juvenile osteoporosis may be mimicked exactly by acute leukemia; in one case this diagnosis did not declare itself until many months after the onset of osseous symptoms, repeated peripheral blood and two bone marrow examinations having been normal in that period.[103]

IDIOPATHIC OSTEOPOROSIS IN ADULTS. In contrast to both idiopathic juvenile osteo-

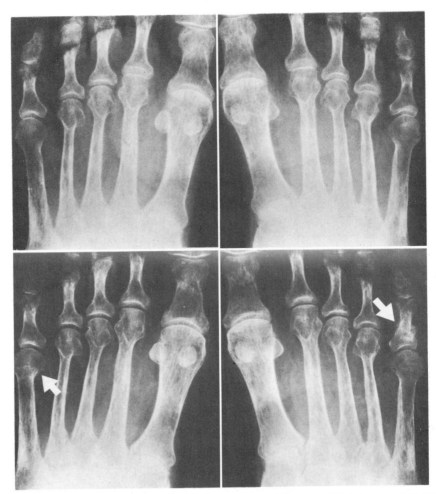

Figure 13–49.   Feet from a patient with idiopathic osteoporosis. *Above,* aged 24; *below,* aged 25. Note markedly abnormal bone structure and, in later film, fractures of the neck of the left fifth metatarsal and right fifth proximal phalanx. (From Parfitt, A. M., Massry, S. G., Winfield, A. C., Depalma, J., and Gordon, A.: Clin Orthop. *87*:287–302, 1972.)

porosis and involutional osteoporosis, idiopathic osteoporosis in adults is more common in men than in women. In the largest published series,[212] there were 27 men and 11 women, and in our own experience there have been 12 men and 6 women. There is a significant difference in the usual age of onset between the two sexes, about a decade later in men than in women, but whether this indicates a difference in pathogenesis is uncertain. In women, the age of onset is most commonly between 25 and 30 years, with extremes of about 16 and 40 years. It may be difficult to decide whether younger patients belong to the juvenile or adult groups. Frequently, the earliest symptoms occur during or soon after pregnancy,[282,]

[294] but the significance of this association is doubtful, since pregnancy is common in this age group and the association may be fortuitous. Also, pregnancy is liable to worsen the symptoms in any type of back disorder, including that due to osteoporosis. Normal pregnancy increases the accumulation of endosteal bone,[158, 287] and subsequent pregnancies in women with idiopathic osteoporosis are uneventful and do not lead to worsening of their bone disease.[100] The initial symptom is related to the spine in about two thirds of cases, a higher proportion than in idiopathic juvenile osteoporosis and a lower proportion than in involutional osteoporosis. There may be pain in the back from a compression fracture

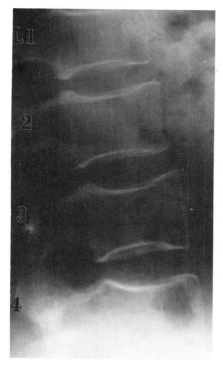

Figure 13–50. Lumbar vertebrae of a woman aged 32 with idiopathic osteoporosis. Note symmetrical biconcavity of moderate degree with widening of intravertebral disc spaces.

caused by trivial trauma such as sneezing.[212] Symptoms may also begin suddenly because of fractures in the ribs and extremities, although this is less common than in idiopathic juvenile osteoporosis. In these fractures, callus may be slow to appear and even slower to disappear. In about half the cases, whether the first symptoms are related to the spine or not, the onset is gradual, with progressive and increasingly severe skeletal pain, especially on walking, sometimes with evidence of systemic ill health as weight loss, tiredness and elevated sedimentation rate. In some cases, striking height loss may occur in the absence of any pain in the back.[100] Radiographic findings in a spine are intermediate between those of juvenile and those of involutional osteoporosis; in younger patients, symmetrical biconcavity is the rule (Fig. 13–50). Severe compression without wedging is more common than in involutional osteoporosis (Fig. 13–51). In the extremities, there may be irregular endosteal resorption and focal trabecular osteoporosis, similar to that which is sometimes seen with corticosteroid therapy (Fig. 13–52).[302] Jackson described a characteristic appearance on chest x-ray, a downward sloping of the upper ribs resembling an isosceles triangle. The course of idiopathic osteoporosis in adults is

Figure 13–51. Thoracic spine of man with idiopathic osteoporosis. *A,* In 1960 (aged 37) and *B,* in 1970 (aged 47). Note severe vertebral compression with no wedging, and no change 10 years later.

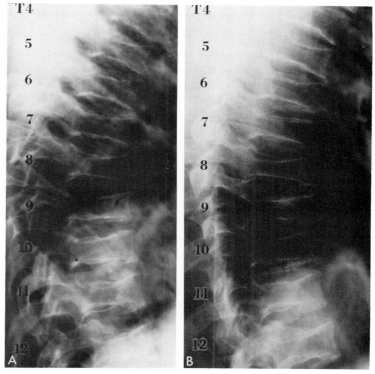

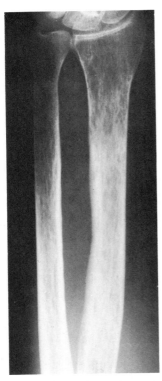

Figure 13–52. Right forearm of man aged 43 with idiopathic osteoporosis. Note extreme thinning of cortex and irregular mottled and striated appearance.

usually similar to that of idiopathic juvenile osteoporosis but over a longer time scale, the initial "acute" phase of bone and height loss extending for about two to five years rather than one to two years, and then slower progression and eventual arrest of the disease after a further five to 10 years.[51] In a small minority of patients, there is relentless progression of vertebral collapse and kyphosis leading eventually to death from cor pulmonale,[100] as in severe kyphoscoliosis.[40]

Treatment of Osteoporosis

There are many difficulties in the evaluation of any treatment for osteoporosis. The inevitable symptomatic improvement consequent on the healing of a fracture is easily attributed to treatment given concurrently. Symptomatic relief is as great with an inert placebo as with estrogen or androgen.[373] In idiopathic osteoporosis, the natural history is toward spontaneous cessation of accelerated bone loss in a few years, and a similar phenomenon may occur over a longer time scale in some patients with involutional osteoporosis. The symptoms of osteoporosis tend to be episodic and bear no clear relationship to the severity of the underlying disease. Once a critical reduction of bone mass has been reached, further fractures might continue to occur even if treatment were successful in arresting the progress of the disease. The only certain way of proving the effectiveness of treatment is to demonstrate a significant reduction in the frequency of the specific morbid event of osteoporosis; that is, of fractures.[325] Apart from the treatment of an identifiable cause, there is at the time of writing no unequivocal evidence that any form of medical treatment is of value in any form of osteoporosis. Because of this, and in reaction to the uncritical enthusiasm of earlier generations, it is easy to take a completely nihilistic approach. It is important to recognize the inevitable limitations of therapy. Except for the natural improvement in the reversible component of high turnover osteoporosis, there is no instance of actual replacement of bone which has been lost, so that the best that can be hoped for is to arrest the progress of the disease and to minimize future loss. The apparent improvement in the osteoporosis of Cushing's syndrome in children after adrenalectomy reflects the growth of normal bone around the abnormal bone which remains porotic.[6, 362] Except where the loss is very rapid, it is likely that a minimum of five years of followup would be needed to demonstrate with certainty the difference between continued slow loss and maintenance of the same bone mass. This situation will continue until the exaggerated bone deficit in each remodeling cycle which characterizes the trabecular and endosteal surface can be reversed, which is unlikely to occur until the cause is found. For this reason, all therapy at present is essentially preventive, whether it is begun at the time of first development of symptoms or at some earlier time in patients thought to be especially susceptible to later complications.

We will now describe the various current medications and the rationale underlying their use, and then consider briefly each type of osteoporosis in turn.

PREVENTION DURING THE GROWTH PERIOD. Any measure which increases the accumulation of bone during growth will minimize the effects of the inevitable subsequent loss of bone. It is possible that the benefits of fluoridation programs may be greater for the bones than for the teeth, which can be replaced, though bones cannot. Vigorous physical activity should be encouraged from an early age, and any unnecessary immobilization avoided at any age. The value of vitamin and mineral supplementation of the diet is probably negligible. The possible advantage of deliberate restriction of calcium intake in order to stimulate calcium-conserving mechanisms is worthy of further exploration.

TREATMENT. *Estrogen Therapy.* There is reasonably secure, although not absolutely certain, evidence that with estrogen administration to all women from the time of the menopause, postmenopausal osteoporosis as we have defined it would be prevented; that is, that the difference between men and women with respect to bone loss would be abolished. The remaining component of involutional bone loss common to both sexes would be unaffected. In prospective studies, estrogen administration significantly reduces the amount of height lost in the first five years after the menopause,[192] and diminishes the rate of bone loss as measured by radiographic photodensitometry and photonabsorptiometry.[93, 272] In all three studies controls were used but they were not carefully matched with the treated patients, and the subjects were not randomly allocated to treatment and control groups, so the possibility remains that some medical or socioeconomic factor determining selection for estrogen replacement accounted also for the subsequent difference in the rate of bone loss. Even if not started at the time of the menopause but at the time of onset of symptoms, there is some evidence of benefit. Henneman and Wallach found that subsequent height loss was arrested,[190] and Gordan in a very large series found that the incidence of fracture and vertebral collapse was considerably reduced after the institution of treatment.[226] Although Gordan's series did not include controls, the magnitude of change probably exceeded the limits of spontaneous arrest, which in the absence of treatment is less characteristic of involutional than of idiopathic osteoporosis (Fig. 13–53). Although increased risk of neoplasm was feared by many, this has not been borne out; in fact, in Gordan's series the incidence of genital and breast malignancy was significantly reduced. The usual technique of therapy is cyclical administration to reproduce the menstrual cycle, e.g., Premarin 1 to 3 mg daily for four weeks out of five. It has been found that a longer cycle than the normal menstrual cycle of four weeks is necessary, otherwise there may be failure of withdrawal bleeding, followed by breakthrough bleeding in subsequent cycles. The addition of a progestational agent also may permit a more regular bleeding schedule.[191] The main disadvantage of therapy is that some additional work is created for gynecologists. Some women dislike the perpetuation of regular withdrawal bleeding but this is not a medical problem. If bleeding is intermittent or intermenstrual, uterine curettage is advisable to rule out underlying neoplasia, but if bleeding is regular it would seem from Gordan's results that a normal annual Papanicolaou smear would provide sufficient assurance. An alternative is to give the estrogen continuously, but unpredictable breakthrough bleeding will occur in some pa-

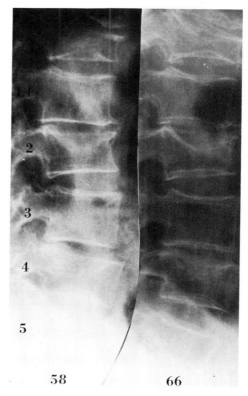

Figure 13–53. Effect of estrogen therapy in a woman with postmenopausal osteoporosis. Note no change in shape of any vertebra or (allowing for exposure differences) in mineral content. It is probable, although not yet certain, that such arrest of the disease is less likely in the absence of treatment, but this is the most that can be expected.

tients, creating a greater need for gynecologic investigation.

The mechanism whereby estrogens reduce bone loss is probably inhibition of activation, that is, reducing the number of new remodeling cycles initiated in unit time. For this reason, the initial effect of estrogen is deceptive. The calcium balance becomes positive, and morphometric study of bone shows a reduction of resorptive surface, but after one generation of new remodeling cycles has passed (one sigma time period) bone formation inevitably falls by about the same amount,[245, 330] and calcium balance reverts to its previous level. However, in view of the small deficit of bone per remodeling cycle, diminishing the activation frequency must lead to some diminution in the rate of bone loss. It seems more sensible to give estrogens from the time of menopause rather than to wait for vertebral collapse to occur, since in such patients bone remodeling is already subnormal.[146] There is some evidence for an additional action of estrogens in directly antagonizing the action of parathyroid hormone on bone.[202] Estrogen administration leads to a significant fall in both plasma and urinary calcium in patients with primary hyperparathyroidism,[157] and also improves calcium absorption in postmenopausal women.[72] In terms of the concepts presented earlier, such effects are not explicable simply in terms of reducing the activation frequency and suggest a more direct interaction between parathyroid hormone and estrogens in calcium homeostasis.

Androgens and Anabolic Steroids. The most widely quoted evidence that these are of value in involutional osteoporosis derives from a balance study in only one patient;[6] the limitations of balance studies in evaluating the long-term effect of treatment in osteoporosis have already been indicated. Androgens may have an effect similar to estrogen, since the extent of resorbing surface is reduced.[245, 330] There is also limited evidence based on serial bone biopsies that nortestosterone (Durabolin) increases the number of both seams and active osteoblasts lining the trabecular surfaces, indicating new bone formation,[113, 250] but these conclusions were based on qualitative impressions rather than on measurement, and there is no evidence that the amount of bone was increased as a result. Many patients seem to get symptomatic relief, but this may be related to an increase in muscle strength

rather than to any effect on the bone. There is slightly stronger evidence that androgens may be beneficial in corticosteroid induced osteoporosis. Balance studies in Cushing's syndrome were more impressive than those in senile osteoporosis,[6] and there is some evidence for a long-term effect in patients on corticosteroid therapy, but the weight of evidence is against this. Androgens are probably indicated concurrently with corticosteroid therapy in growing children in order to help restore a normal hormonal milieu during growth.

In males, the normally occurring androgen testosterone is probably the most effective. It is convenient to give methyltestosterone, which can be administered sublingually rather than by intramuscular injection. Anabolic steroids are a group of synthetic agents claimed to preserve the anabolic effect of testosterone but not its androgenic effects, a separation well established in rats but much less certainly in man.[100] Of the allegedly nonvirilizing anabolic agents, we normally recommend Durabolin, simply because there is marginally more evidence that it has a beneficial effect on the bones, but it has the disadvantage of needing intramuscular injection. There is probably little to choose between the various oral preparations.

CALCIUM AND VITAMIN D. The early claims of striking beneficial effects with calcium supplements were based on technically inadequate balance studies which demonstrated an apparent calcium retention which would have led to easily detectable increases in bone mineral or in soft tissue calcification.[245, 338] However, in light of the evidence reviewed earlier concerning the possible role of calcium, it would seem wise to ensure a dietary intake of at least one gram daily, especially in patients whose self-chosen intake of dairy foods is low. Also, in view of the evidence of mild vitamin D deficiency in the elderly, small vitamin D supplements should probably be given routinely. These measures are harmless and may produce a modest benefit. One practical point of importance when giving both calcium and vitamin D is that they should never be combined into a single preparation, since vitamin D preparations containing calcium deteriorate very quickly.[300] Thus, if a calcium preparation containing vitamin D is given, the small amount of vitamin D should be disregarded and additional vitamin D given separately. Any striking benefit from this treatment probably indicates that the patient had undiagnosed nutritional osteomalacia. Vitamin D in conjunction with estrogen may produce a temporary improvement in calcium balance in patients with idiopathic osteoporosis, but no long term benefit has been demonstrated.

Intravenous calcium given as a series of infusions of 15 mg per kg of body weight has also been tried.[299] This produces temporary suppression of parathyroid hormone and stimulation of calcitonin, and the expected consequences of a depression of activation of new remodeling cycles. No long-term benefit has been established.

FLUORIDE.[331] The dense bones characteristic of endemic fluorosis have long suggested a possible place for fluoride in the treatment of osteoporosis.[278] We have already mentioned the epidemiologic evidence for a relationship between fluoride deficiency during the growth period and the incidence of involutional osteoporosis. Fluoride administration alone produces a dramatic increase in the number of osteoblasts and, in a few cases, large doses have induced radiographically evident osteofluorosis. There is a great increase in the osteoid surface area and a moderate reduction in apposition rate of about 50 per cent. With small doses, some studies have shown no significant improvement in calcium balance, probably because the duration of treatment was too short. In some patients there may be a worsening of osteoarthritic symptoms, accumulation of unmineralized osteoid, and possibly secondary hyperparathyroidism.

More promising is a combination of fluoride with vitamin D and calcium. The rationale for this is that the increased amounts of osteoid formed on the endosteal surface under the influence of fluoride may not mineralize normally unless vitamin D and calcium supplements are given as well. Vitamin D may also enhance the osteoblastic response to fluoride. This treatment is potentially important because it is the only one for which the claim has been made that the negative bone balance at the endosteal surface may be reversed and that an actual increase in the amount of bone is possible. However, extensive long-term results are still awaited, and enthusiasm must be tempered with the realization that the new bone formed is of abnormal structure and that it is possible that any beneficial effect on the bones may be outweighed by the development of exostoses and ligamentous calcification which cause such crippling disability in endemic osteofluorosis (q.v.).

There is some experimental work in rabbits which indicates that fluoride may reduce the adverse effect of corticosteroids on bones.[118] The use of fluoride in osteogenesis imperfecta was mentioned earlier.

PHOSPHATE. Evidence from in vitro experiments suggests that phosphate may inhibit resorption in tissue culture, so phosphate supplements have been advocated in the treatment of osteoporosis. There is no evidence that they are beneficial, and they may induce a harmful degree of secondary hyperparathyroidism. It is possible that phosphate may have some use in conjunction with other measures. Some patients develop an exaggerated fall in serum phosphate with estrogen therapy and might conceivably benefit from extra phosphate.

CALCITONIN. In view of the known action of this hormone, and in view of the prevailing theories of increased bone resorption in osteoporosis, it was natural that this agent should be tried. The evidence to date is not very encouraging.[408] Since the major action of calcitonin on bone remodeling is to depress activation of new remodeling cycles, it is likely that the long-term effects will be much the same as those of estrogen, with the disadvantages of intramuscular injection. Calcitonin would be a logical treatment in idiopathic high-turnover osteoporosis, but experience so far is inconclusive. Calcitonin might also be beneficial if given during the first three months of high dose corticosteroid therapy, in the hope of preventing the initial phase of accelerated resorption, during which much of the bone loss occurs.

ALBUMIN INFUSIONS. Albright advocated albumin infusions in the treatment of idiopathic osteoporosis, and apparent success was achieved in one case but no response was elicited in three other cases.[100] Its use has been generally abandoned.

DIPHOSPHONATES. These also are alleged to inhibit bone resorption and may be beneficial in Paget's disease. Too little is known of their action on normal bone to recommend their use in osteoporosis at present.

GROWTH HORMONE. In dogs this agent apparently increases endosteal bone formation.[177] There are no data available in human osteoporosis, and the bone changes in acromegaly suggest that this mode of treatment would probably not be of much value.

FUTURE PROSPECTS. The foregoing long list of ineffective modes of therapy must make depressing reading — the only realistic hope at present is to offset the disadvantage which women suffer with respect to men. A more promising approach may be to exploit the relationship of the endosteal surface to the bone marrow.[141] One of the reasons osteoporosis tends to be irreversible is that the mechanism of making new bone ceases with epiphyseal fusion. From this point, new trabeculae can only be made by reactivation of woven bone formation. This occurs in Paget's disease, fracture, and osteogenic sarcoma, none of which would constitute an acceptable treatment for involutional osteoporosis, even if they could be produced at will. A more promising condition may be myelosclerosis, in which dense bone is formed by reactivation of woven bone formation, but at the expense of a leukoerythroblastic anemia.[249] For the hematologist caring for these patients, the increased amount of bone is simply a nuisance, since it makes it more difficult to obtain a bone marrow sample, but from the point of view of preventing bone loss there may be something to be learned.

SUMMARY OF THERAPEUTIC RECOMMENDATIONS IN DIFFERENT SITUATIONS. *Involutional Osteoporosis.* Any established nutritional deficiency should be corrected, and it is probably reasonable to give enough calcium to make up the total intake to 1 to 2 gm daily, and enough vitamin D to provide a total intake of 0.1 mg daily (4000 units). In postmenopausal osteoporosis we recommend the cyclical administration of estrogens as described. For patients with severe symptoms brought about by senile osteoporosis, oral or intramuscular anabolic steroids may be worth a trial. In the most severely affected patients, the use of fluoride combined with vitamin D and calcium should be considered, although fluoride is not yet approved by the FDA for this purpose.

Idiopathic Osteoporosis. In children, no treatment other than physiotherapy to maintain mobility is indicated. In adults with idiopathic osteoporosis, at present only the fluoride, vitamin D and calcium regimen offers any prospect of success, but with serious reservations about the long-term complications.

Corticosteroid Therapy. We suggest a trial of calcitonin during the first three months of high dosage therapy, and the use of ACTH in equal anti-inflammatory doses, where possible. In growing children, androgen and estrogen replacement is indicated.

Disuse Osteoporosis. In contrast to traumatic osteodystrophy, true disuse osteoporosis is irreversible, but is partly preventable by early mobilization and weight-bearing. In permanently bedfast children, sodium fluoride, supplemental phosphate and oxymetholone all increased bone mineral in the os calcis when given for about nine months, but the increase was lost in the year after discontinuation of therapy.[232] In adults, diphosphonates may have a prophylactic effect on bone, but treatment is designed primarily to protect the kidneys.[17]

Treatment of Spontaneous Compression Fractures in Osteoporotic Patients. Since these are never complicated by spinal cord compression, there is no indication for a greater degree of immobilization than that dictated by the patient's symptoms.[45] Analgesics should be given as indicated and early mobilization encouraged. The dangers of a brace or corset in terms of immobilization have probably been exaggerated,[332] and such support may help the patient to resume normal activity more quickly, but the patient should be encouraged to discard either after a few months. Exercise to strengthen the back muscles may reduce the likelihood of continuing back pain.

OSTEOMALACIA AND RICKETS

Osteomalacia is the osseous disorder characterized by accumulation of increased amounts of osteoid as the result of slowing or arrest in the initial phase of primary mineralization. Rickets is a disease in which there is impaired mineralization of cartilage, leading to arrest in the formation of the primary spongiosa during endochondral ossification. Rickets, by definition, can no longer be present after epiphyseal fusion, while osteomalacia can exist as soon as significant amounts of lamellar bone have been formed in replacement of woven bone. Children, therefore, usually have both rickets and osteomalacia, whereas adults have only osteomalacia. The clinical and radiographic manifestations of a mineralization defect in childhood are dominated by the epiphyseal changes in infancy, but the balance slowly shifts in favor of osteomalacia as skeletal maturity advances.

Pathogenesis of Rickets and Osteomalacia

We can consider this under two headings — first, the abnormalities in chondroblast and osteoblast function which underlie the morphologic changes and second, the cause of this defective cellular function.

BONE REMODELING DYNAMICS AND OSTEOBLASTIC FUNCTION. Investigation of the dynamics of remodeling depends on measuring the appositional rate by the thickness of bone deposited between two tetracycline markers. This measurement can be made only on lamellar bone, and so remodeling dynamics can be studied in osteomalacia but not in rickets. However, the available evidence suggests that essentially the same disturbances affect the chondroblasts during endochondral ossification.

The conventional explanation for the increased thickness of osteoid seams in advanced osteomalacia is that matrix synthesis continues at a normal or even accelerated rate while mineralization is slowed down. Such an uncoupling would lead to a progressive increase in osteoid seam thickness far in excess of that actually observed. In fact, the rate of matrix synthesis by osteoblasts is very markedly slowed, to less than 5 per cent in very severe cases. Mineralization may be slowed down to the same or to an even greater extent, so that the seam thickness may remain unchanged or may increase very slowly. However, the degree of uncoupling of matrix synthesis and mineralization rate is far less than the degree of reduction in both.[146, 324] The mineralization lag time, that is, the mean seam thickness divided by the appositional rate, is markedly increased both in man and in the rat.[18, 36, 324] Possible exceptions to this generalization are rare forms of osteomalacia resulting from specific inhibition of mineralization by fluoride and by diphosphonates in which matrix synthesis may proceed at a normal rate.

The slowing down of mineralization characteristic of osteomalacia is a qualitative as well as a quantitative change. The evidence suggests that, at least in Haversian remodeling, most osteons are eventually completed, and so must eventually mineralize completely, but that this mineralization is abnormal. First, it may proceed in the absence of tetracycline uptake or of a mineralization front, and second,

patchy clusters of mineral appear within the osteoid seam. This partly mineralized osteoid is characteristic of osteomalacia.[55, 229]

As explained during the discussion of surface-based measurements, the slowing of any surface activity inevitably leads to an increase in the extent of surface occupied by that activity. Consequently, a slowing down of the rate of osteoid seam maturation leads to accumulation of seams.

Normally, newly formed osteoid changes during the 10-day period between matrix synthesis and its mineralization. The changes comprise progressive intra- and extrafibrillar cross-linking of the collagen fibers and chemical changes in the distribution of glycosaminoglycans, which together are described rather vaguely as maturation. In osteomalacia this maturation is defective. Osteoid from vitamin D-deprived animals does not mineralize normally when placed in solutions of physiological calcium and phosphorus concentration,[410] and differs from normal preosseous matrix in staining characteristics of ground substance and in the arrangement and ultrastructure of the collagen fibers.[53, 229]

Thus, in osteomalacia all functions of the osteoblast — the synthesis, maturation and mineralization of matrix — are defective.

CAUSE OF DEFECTIVE OSTEOBLAST FUNCTION IN OSTEOMALACIA. There are many different clinical types and causes of osteomalacia, and a unifying concept applicable to all types is still not possible. Nevertheless, there are two factors, either or both of which are of central importance in almost all patients — deficiency of the active metabolites of vitamin D and deficiency of phosphorus.

Phosphorus deficiency in the blood has played a central role in the chemical theories of osteomalacia for many years. According to this view, lack of vitamin D leads to impaired calcium absorption, impaired release of calcium from bone, hypocalcemia, parathyroid stimulation, reduced renal tubular reabsorption of phosphate, and hypophosphatemia, which finally produces impairment of mineralization because of undersaturation of plasma with respect to calcium phosphate. The complexities of the mineralization process which were reviewed earlier (p. 604) and the abnormalities of cell function in osteomalacia are both inconsistent with this simple concept, but there is a considerable amount of evidence that phosphorus deficiency may in some manner impair the function of the osteoblast.[300] In rats, phosphorus deficiency induces enzyme changes in the growing cartilage, and impaired matrix synthesis characteristic of osteomalacia, all of which are reversed by phosphorus administration. Phosphorus depletion also impairs the formation of organic phosphate compounds which bind to collagen and may play a role in mineralization. The relationship of hypophosphatemia and intracellular phosphate is complex, but it is likely that at least some patients with hypophosphatemia have intracellular as well as extracellular deficits of phosphorus, as shown for example by reduction in the activity of 2-3 diphosphoglycerate.[300] Intracellular phosphate depletion may also be concerned in the muscle weakness which occurs in severe osteomalacia and hyperparathyroidism.

Phosphate depletion in osteomalacia may result from dietary deficiency, intestinal malabsorption, lack of vitamin D action on the gut, metabolic acidosis, or a low renal threshold for phosphate from intrinsic renal tubular defect, lack of Vitamin D action on the renal tubule, or secondary hyperparathyroidism.

The role of vitamin D in the pathogenesis of the mineralization defect in osteomalacia is more complex. Impaired intestinal absorption of calcium is a universal finding, but lack of calcium absorption is not the main cause of osteomalacia. Since calcium malabsorption is found in rickets and osteomalacia due to phosphorus deficiency as well as vitamin D deficiency, it has been speculated that bone cells send some messenger to the gut to inhibit calcium absorption when the mineral cannot be deposited. The main point at issue is whether vitamin D deficiency leads to impaired osteoblast function as a result of intracellular phosphate depletion or in some more direct manner. The accumulation of vitamin D metabolites in the growing ends of bone, and the speed with which mineralization of cartilage and maturation of chondrocytes is resumed after vitamin D administration both suggest a direct action, possibly related to the synthesis of a protein concerned in calcium transport, as in the intestinal mucosa.

Clinical Features of Rickets and Osteomalacia

Although the overall clinical picture depends in large part on the underlying disease there are certain common features regardless of etiology. It is convenient to consider rickets and osteomalacia separately.

RICKETS. Although the vertebrae are affected by the same disturbance in endochondral bone formation as are the long bones, the rate of longitudinal growth in the vertebrae is so much less that clinical findings related to the spine are not so striking.

In mild rickets, there may be a long, shallow, smooth and reducible curvature of the whole spine, usually apparent only on sitting up and caused primarily by muscle weakness and ligamentous laxity. Later, this curvature worsens because of involvement of the vertebral bodies, and in severe cases, the epiphyseal development of the vertebrae becomes irregular, leading to kyphorotoscoliosis, sometimes of extreme degree.[366] Spinal tenderness may occur, but is unusual.[195] In metabolic rickets, the severity of the disease depends on delay in diagnosis, but in nutritional rickets, the worst deformities, sometimes known as Glissonian rickets,[234] occur only where some socioeconomic, climatic, ethnic or genetic factor prevents the normal seasonal remission which otherwise occurs in vitamin D depletion, so that the effects of the disease are cumulative.

The other clinical features of rickets depend on the age of onset and are described fully elsewhere.[303, 305, 366]

OSTEOMALACIA. The spinal manifestations of osteomalacia are of generalized pain and tenderness beginning in the low back, initially without deformity, but later with slowly progressive kyphosis and shortening of the spine. In severe cases, various combinations of rotation and scoliosis may occur as well as kyphosis. The spine may bend almost at a right angle, leading to apposition to the xyphisternum and the pubic symphysis.[262] Severe spinal deformity is often accompanied by pigeon chest, owing to buckling of the sternum. Another characteristic finding is abrupt angulation of the sacrum. In one large series of cases of nutritional osteomalacia, backache was present in every case and spinal tenderness in 90 per cent.[389] Abrupt changes in height due to vertebral compression fractures such as occur in osteoporosis do not occur in osteomalacia unless the patient has osteoporosis as well. It has been suggested that the presence of concomitant osteomalacia protects the vertebrae to some extent against fracture, perhaps by increasing the elasticity of the bones so that the stress is more easily dissipated.[100] Although the spinal manifestations of osteomalacia and osteoporosis may be similar, there are some differences in the quality and pattern of the pain. In both, the pain is made worse by activity, but with osteomalacia it is muscular strain, weight bearing or pressure which is painful, rather than movement per se. Some movements are painless if carefully performed, and complete immobility in certain postures may also bring relief. Another major difference is that in osteomalacia pain and tenderness are almost always found in bones other than the spine, notably in the ribs, pelvis and extremities. Characteristically, the pain begins in the low back and hips and later involves the extremities and the upper reaches of the spine.[137, 337] Initially, the pain may be confused with arthritis or other locomotor condition. Muscle weakness is a common feature, often associated with a waddling gait because of proximal limb girdle myopathy. Some patients present with malunion of a traumatic fracture. There may be bowing of the legs and other severe deformities of the extremities. In advanced cases, deformities occur in the pelvis with severe protrusio acetabuli and narrowing of the birth canal leading to obstructed labor. This tends to occur only in areas where vitamin D deficiency is endemic, since, even with a high level of medical suspicion, some patients escape detection until late in the course of the disease.

Occasionally, kyphosis and shortening of the spine may develop with little pain and few or no symptoms in other bones. These conditions are especially difficult to differentiate from osteoporosis. Usually, the problem is to separate pure osteoporosis from osteoporosis combined with osteomalacia.

Radiographic Features of Rickets and Osteomalacia

RICKETS. Diffuse radiolucency is the earliest change in the spine. In severe cases, there may be very little visible bone structure.[296] In mild cases, there may be globular areas of rarefaction related to the distribution of blood vessels within the medullary space. These changes in density are accompanied by flattening and loss of normal biconcavity of the vertebral body and widening of the intravertebral disc spaces.[296] In severe cases, biconcavity and compression of the vertebrae

occur, as in osteomalacia. Although the vertebrae have epiphyses, widening of the epiphyseal plate as in the long bones, is not seen. A double density may develop during the course of treatment.[68]

The characteristic radiographic changes of rickets are at the ends of the long bones. The zone of provisional calcification is absent, the growth plate is widened and indistinct, and the ends of the metaphyses are cupped, widened and irregular in outline.[68, 254] The shafts of the long bones may show cortical striation, periosteal thickening, and irregularity and fractures (Fig. 13–54).

Metaphyseal dysostosis and Morquio's disease are both accompanied by changes in the growth plate which resemble those of mild rickets, and hypophosphatasia (q.v.) produces definite changes of severe rickets.

OSTEOMALACIA.[98] The characteristic changes in the spine have already been described. In other bones, the most important feature of osteomalacia is the Looser zone.

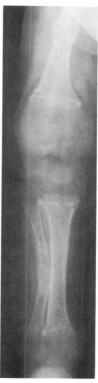

Figure 13–54. Extremities in a two-year-old boy with severe rickets. Note very wide zone of unmineralized cartilage, fraying of metaphases, striation and irregularity of the shaft and fractures of the femur and fibula.

This is a band of radiolucency which abuts on the cortex perpendicular to the long axis of the bone and is usually symmetrical (Fig. 13–55). Looser zones occur most commonly in ribs, pubic rami, outer edges of the scapulae and near the ends of long bones, especially on the lateral sides,[106] and 80 per cent will be detected by a penetrated chest film and a view of the pelvis and upper femora.[76] Somewhat similar lesions may occur in Paget's disease, fibrous dysplasia, Cushing's syndrome, and osteogenesis imperfecta, but in these conditions the lesions are usually not symmetrical, and they occur in zones of obviously abnormal bone, whereas Looser zones occur in bone which may appear otherwise normal, and there may be signs indicating cartilaginous union rather than uncalcified callus.[6] Looser zones begin as a stress fracture but do not develop the line of increased density which normally occurs during healing. In some cases, presumably because of fluctuation in the metabolic state, Looser zones may show partial healing with adjacent sclerosis and limited callus formation, but more usually they remain unchanged until treatment is given. The precipitating cause of the initial stress fracture is unknown; there is suggestive evidence that some are related to blood vessels coursing over the bone,[382] but this mechanism does not apply to all cases.

In the various forms of metabolic osteomalacia, the presence of Looser zones has been held to indicate a relatively acute onset.[98] Looser zones were found in 100 per cent of a large series of patients with nutritional osteomalacia.[389]

Another common radiographic finding is phalangeal subperiosteal erosion as a result of associated secondary hyperparathyroidism. In patients who lack Looser zones, this may be the most tangible radiographic finding, even though osteomalacia, rather than osteitis fibrosa, is the dominant lesion in the bones.

In the extremities, thinning of the cortex occurs in osteomalacia as well as in osteoporosis.[68] The coarse trabeculation described for the vertebrae also may be seen in the extremities. Occasionally, greenstick-type fractures may occur, as in rickets.[76]

Laboratory Findings in Rickets and Osteomalacia

The changes depend to some extent on the underlying cause, but certain findings are characteristic. The alkaline phosphatase is usually raised, sometimes considerably so, not because osteoblastic function is increased[6] but because the enzyme escapes in some manner when osteoblastic function is defective. In nutritional osteomalacia, the plasma calcium is usually moderately reduced and the plasma phosphate distinctly reduced. Tests of renal tubular phosphate reabsorption show inhibition, due partly to secondary hyperparathyroidism and partly to lack of vitamin D action on the nephron. However, such changes are too inconstant to be certain of identifying osteomalacia in patients with nonspecific vertebral rarefaction.[391] Other signs of secondary hyperparathyroidism such as aminoaciduria and low plasma bicarbonate are also commonly found. In some patients the bones become more than usually refractory to the action of parathyroid hormone, and the plasma calcium may become very low, leading to tetany and other

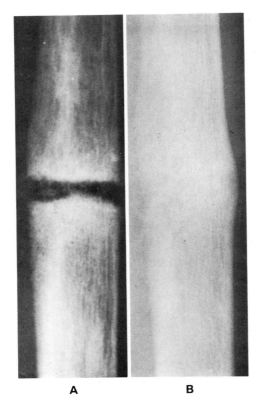

A   **B**

Figure 13–55. Ulna of patient with sporadic hypophosphatemia, before (A) and after (B) Vitamin D and phosphate treatment, showing healing of a Looser zone. Radiolucent band is unusually wide and contains some partly mineralized osteoid. Adjacent bone is slightly sclerotic.

related symptoms. This has been attributed to the covering of all available trabecular surface with osteoid which is refractory to osteoclastic resorption. Since regulation of plasma calcium does not depend on osteoclasts, a more likely explanation is that severe vitamin D deficiency impairs the action of parathyroid hormone on the osteocyte. It is noteworthy that in hypophosphatemic vitamin D refractory rickets and osteomalacia the plasma calcium is never reduced, however severe the bone disease. The urinary calcium is usually low in osteomalacia. This results from both secondary hyperparathyroidism and reduced filtered load due to hypocalcemia, and possibly may also reflect skeletal need for calcium signaled to the kidney by some as yet unidentified mechanism. A high urinary calcium may be found in renal tubular acidosis, in various forms of multiple renal tubular disease, such as the Fanconi syndrome, and the oculocerebrorenal syndrome, and in primary hyperparathyroidism. In the presence of severe phosphate depletion, urinary calcium may be low before treatment is initiated but may rise disproportionately with vitamin D therapy until the phosphate depletion is overcome. Urinary hydroxyproline may be markedly elevated in all forms of rickets and osteomalacia.

Rarely, there may be no laboratory abnormalities in patients with unequivocal osteomalacia shown by bone biopsy.

Specific Etiological Categories of Rickets and Osteomalacia[18]

Knowledge of the many diseases in which rickets and osteomalacia may occur is important in two contexts. First, in any of these conditions is encountered for reasons other than the osseous manifestations, some screening procedure may be needed to detect occult or incipient osteomalacia. Second, and more important in the present context, in the patient whose presenting manifestation is an osseous abnormality found to be due to osteomalacia, the exact etiology must be determined as a basis for long-term management. The most important varieties are given in Table 13–10, but a detailed discussion of all these would be out of place. We will consider nutritional osteomalacia in some detail because an understanding of this is fundamental to understanding all the other varieties, and because of its global importance. Other diseases we select on the

basis of special features in their spinal manifestations.

VITAMIN D DEFICIENCY. Vitamin D deficiency is rare in the United States,[6] but undoubtedly it is still seen in the nutritionally disadvantaged.[409] From the global viewpoint, however, vitamin D deficiency is still by far the most common and most important cause of rickets and osteomalacia.

In Great Britain, where vitamin D supplementation of dairy products is not routine, many adults hover on the verge of vitamin D deficiency, and osteomalacia is not uncommon in the elderly. In one orthopedic clinic, 93 cases were seen in six years; the mean age was 70 in females and 62 in males and two thirds were over 60.[76] In making the diagnosis of osteomalacia in elderly patients, it is important to remember that increased numbers and extent of osteoid seams may result from slowing of seam maturation and the terminal phase of primary mineralization. Judged by the response to treatment, the vitamin D requirement appears to increase sharply with age. Nutritional osteomalacia is also common in food faddists.

In the period between 1920 and 1940, osteomalacia was extremely common in China, and it was estimated that over 100,000 cases were present at any one time.[262] Much of our knowledge of the consequences of human vitamin D deficiency stems from the work carried out in the Peiping Union Medical College during this period. Accurate information on the prevalence of osteomalacia in China at present is lacking, but it is likely that some of the socioeconomic circumstances which contributed to its frequency have changed.

At present, nutritional osteomalacia seems to be most common in northern India, and in some centers new cases are seen on an average of once a day; one series comprised 3200 cases accumulated over a period of 10 years.[389] It is predominantly a disease of young women in the reproductive years, as was found previously in China. In one series, the peak age of onset was 20 to 25 years and the initial presenting manifestation occurred in relation to pregnancy or lactation in 88 per cent of the cases. In another large series, all the cases were in women, less than 10 per cent of whom were postmenopausal.

Sixty years ago, osteomalacia in India was stated to occur primarily in upper class women who were constrained to remain indoors for religious reasons, whereas their poor

TABLE 13–10. CAUSES OF RICKETS AND OSTEOMALACIA AND USUAL RANGE OF THERAPEUTIC DOSES OF VITAMIN D

Disease	Vitamin D dose (mg)
1. Vitamin D deficiency	0.05–0.1*
2. Vitamin D dependency	
genetic	0.5–1.5
drug induced	0.1–0.5
liver disease	0.05–0.25
primary hyperparathyroidism	0.05–0.1
3. Vitamin D malabsorption**	
post gastric surgery	0.1–0.2
intestinal mucosal disease	1.0–10.0
hepatobiliary disease	0.25–1.0
pancreatic disease	0.25–1.0
4. Phosphorus depletion	
dietary	–
prolonged antacid use	–
malabsorption	–
5. Hyperchloremic acidosis	
renal tubular acidosis	0.25–1.0
ureterosigmoidostomy	0.25–1.0
6. Chronic renal failure	0.5–5.0
7. Hypophosphatemic vitamin D refractory	
familial	1.0–2.0
sporadic	
idiopathic	1.0–5.0
neurofibromatosis	1.0–5.0
tumor dependent	–
8. Multiple renal tubular defects (including 5 and 7)	
Fanconi syndrome, genetic or acquired	1.0–2.5
Oculocerebrorenal syndrome	0.05–0.25
9. Mineralization inhibition	
fluoride	?
diphosphonates	?

*This is the range of doses usually given for treatment, not the vitamin D *requirement*.
**Dose of vitamin D much less if given parenterally.

sisters who worked in the sun escaped the condition. Today, osteomalacia seems to occur in all classes of Indian society.

Although a poor intake of vitamin D is adequately documented, the apparent need to give large doses of vitamin D,[395] and the frequency of rickets and osteomalacia in Indian and Pakistanian migrants to the United Kingdom has suggested that there may be a genetic predisposition;[300] a hereditary factor which influences the liability to nutritional rickets seems well established.[246] However, other factors may be more important in the migrant population. In most people, skin synthesis is a more important source of vitamin D than the diet,[253] and exposure to ultraviolet light is poor in the United Kingdom.[255] The Indian migrants have the additional burden of skin pigmentation adapted to a much greater degree of sun exposure. However, this cannot be

the whole explanation, since nutritional osteomalacia is encountered less frequently in migrants from the West Indies, who have a comparable degree of skin pigmentation.[379] The customary diet in North India provides a high intake of whole meal flour with high phytate content in the form of chappatties.[128] Sodium phytate impairs the absorption of calcium and magnesium from the gut, as already described; by addition, possibly some of this material is absorbed and inhibits the hydroxylation of 25-HCC to 1,25 DHCC in the kidney, and thus prevents the formation of the active metabolite of vitamin D.[198] Continuation of a high phytate intake, and the reduced skin exposure to ultraviolet light, probably account for the high incidence of vitamin D deficiency in the migrant population and for its occurrence in adolescent and adult males, normally an uncommon event. It seems unnecessary to invoke genetic abnormalities in vitamin D metabolism, a theory for which there is at present no evidence.[261]

VITAMIN D DEPENDENCY. This term identifies a situation in which the clinical, radiographic and biochemical findings are the same as in vitamin D deficiency, but in which the amount of vitamin D needed for treatment and subsequent prevention is much greater than normal; in other words, the vitamin D requirement is raised. It is probable that vitamin D dependency, as defined, always results from some abnormality in the intermediary metabolism of vitamin D. Vitamin D dependency may be genetic, or acquired as a result of anticonvulsant therapy,[377] liver disease,[422] and increased parathyroid hormone secretion.[416]

The genetic form of dependency probably comprises a group of diseases in which different patterns of enzyme deficiency are present.[340] The clinical features of genetic vitamin D dependency are the development of rickets in childhood which resembles severe vitamin D deficiency.[366] The chemical changes are variable,[49] but hypocalcemia and signs of secondary hyperparathyroidism are usual.[13] If the diagnosis is missed or if treatment is given with small amounts of vitamin D appropriate to Vitamin D deficiency, severe and crippling deformities of the spine and the extremities may ultimately develop;[366] the vertebrae may show anterior beaking resembling Morquio's disease.[366] The hallmark of the disease is that all manifestations respond completely to adequate vitamin D therapy, with the exception of residual deformity (Table 13–11).

The bone changes associated with anticonvulsant therapy are complex. Although hypocalcemia is common and rickets and osteomalacia resulting from altered Vitamin D metabolism are well documented, significant osteoporosis may also occur.[374] In children, this affects the juxtaepiphyseal bone in the metaphyses, as in idiopathic juvenile osteoporosis. In adults, the trabeculae at the proximal end of the femur, assessed by the method of Singh, show an increased rate of disappearance in anticonvulsant-treated patients compared to normal subjects of the same age and sex. Whether these osteoporotic changes are also caused by altered vitamin D metabolism is unknown. Conceivably, they might result from alterations in folate metabolism, since the folate antagonist methotrexate is known to induce osteoporosis when given to children for the treatment of leukemia. The exact disturbance in vitamin D metabolism is still not completely elucidated, but probably depends on induction of hepatic microsomal enzymes.

Some patients with liver disease, both children and adults, have impaired 25 hydroxylation leading to a special form of vitamin D dependency. This has been found in neonatal hepatitis, in which rickets can be prevented by the administration of 0.1 mg of vitamin D daily.[422] In other types of hepatic disease, the situation may be complicated by the coexistence of impaired vitamin D absorption from bile salt deficiency.

TABLE 13–11.   DIFFERENCES BETWEEN THE MAIN KINDS OF HYPOPHOSPHATEMIC RICKETS AND OSTEOMALACIA*

	Vitamin D Deficient	Vitamin D Dependent	Vitamin D Refractory	Fanconi Syndrome
Plasma Ca (untreated)	Low or normal	Low or normal	Normal	Normal[1]
Plasma Ca (treated)	Normal	Normal	Normal	Normal
Plasma P (untreated)	Low or normal	Low or normal	Low	Low
Plasma P (treated)	Normal	Normal	Low	Low
Plasma HCO_3^- (untreated)	Low	Low	Normal	Low
Plasma HCO_3^- (treated)	Normal	Normal	Normal	Low
Urinary AA[2] (untreated)	Present	Present	Absent[3]	Present
Urinary AA (treated)	Absent	Absent	Absent	Present
Dose of vitamin D	0.01–0.1 mg.	0.5–2.0 mg.	0.75–3.0 mg.	0.5–5.0 mg.[4]

*Modified from Parfitt.[303]
[1]May be low if renal failure present
[2]AA = Amino acids
[3]Except for isolated increase in glycine in sporadic nonfamilial cases
[4]Varies with extent of renal failure

The occurrence of osteomalacia and rickets in primary hyperparathyroidism is of particular interest. Vitamin D deficiency superimposed on primary hyperparathyroidism may produce a normal or even reduced plasma calcium, worsening of bone pain, exacerbation of the clinical and radiographic manifestations of bone disease and histologic evidence of true osteomalacia. This combination may result when primary hyperparathyroidism occurs in regions where vitamin D deficiency is endemic;[396] also, both vitamin D deficiency and parathyroid adenoma may be complications of intestinal malabsorption.[364] In other cases it seems likely that an increased vitamin D requirement may result from some action of PTH on vitamin D metabolism.[416]

Whatever the cause of this association, its recognition is important for two reasons. First, a small dose of vitamin D may lead to a significant rise in plasma calcium, so the unexpected development of hypercalcemia in a patient who seems to have pure osteomalacia suggests the possibility that primary hyperparathyroidism is the underlying cause. Second, in patients with primary hyperparathyroidism the presence of osteomalacia due to associated vitamin D deficiency suggests the need for treatment with vitamin D or 25-HCC before parathyroid surgery in order to minimize the severity of tetany in the postoperative period.

VITAMIN D MALABSORPTION. This can arise from one of four different mechanisms (Table 13–10). In each case there is likely to be osteoporosis as well as osteomalacia, and other complicating factors such as a low vitamin D intake. In general, malabsorption of vitamin D is associated with steatorrhoea, but malabsorption due to gluten enteropathy may occur with normal fat absorption,[281] and even if chemical steatorrhoea is present, the intestinal disease may be clinically silent.[316]

HYPOPHOSPHATEMIC VITAMIN D REFRACTORY RICKETS AND OSTEOMALACIA. This term identifies patients who are refractory to vitamin D therapy and in whom the cardinal abnormality is persistent hypophosphatemia with a normal plasma calcium (Table 13–11). This group is made up of at least two different diseases, one familial and the other sporadic. The familial form is of great interest to orthopedic surgeons, but spinal manifestations are relatively minor in children, so only a brief description will be given.

Familial.[303] Familial hypophosphatemic vitamin D refractory rickets and osteomalacia is genetically determined, with a sex-linked dominant mode of transmission. The onset is usually in early infancy, and there are lifelong hypophosphatemia and impaired longitudinal growth as well as rickets. Differentiation from other forms of rickets is shown in Table 13–11. At cessation of growth, the rickets may heal, and osteosclerosis, ligamentous calcification and osteomalacia may cause symptoms in middle age.

In children, the spine is usually uninvolved; the vertebral radiolucency and spinal curvature of nutritional vitamin D deficiency or vitamin D dependency are not seen. In fact, even at an early age, the bones look more dense than normal, with coarse trabeculation. In adult life, this increased density is accentuated, so that quite severe osteosclerosis may occur even in the presence of active osteomalacia. The recurrence of active disease may be associated with a normal alkaline phosphatase and elevation of urinary hydroxyproline, but can only be proved by bone biopsy.

The vertebrae involved by osteosclerosis may be larger, harder and more dense (Fig. 13–56), and there may also be ectopic calcification and ossification of muscle attachments, tendons and ligaments. In the spine, the annulus fibrosus, apophyseal joint capsules, interosseous and interspinous ligaments, and ligamenta flava may all be involved. These changes are associated with pain and stiffness and restricted mobility of the back, even in the absence of active osteomalacia. The most serious manifestation of the disease in adults is spinal cord compression, owing to a combination of expansion of the vertebrae and neural arches and ligamentous calcification. This has been reported in six patients, in both the cervical and thoracic regions. The response to early surgical decompression has been good.[196]

The serious spinal manifestations in adults with familial hypophosphatemia may be the presenting symptom. In such patients the stigmata of childhood rickets are likely to be present, with short stature, primarily involving the legs, and bowing of the tibia with genu valgum. In some patients, these stigmata may be minimal and easily overlooked, the rickets never having been diagnosed. The differential diagnosis will be between other causes of a stiff, aching back and radiographic evidence of ligamentous calcification,[178] such as ankylosing spondylitis, ankylosing vertebral hyperos-

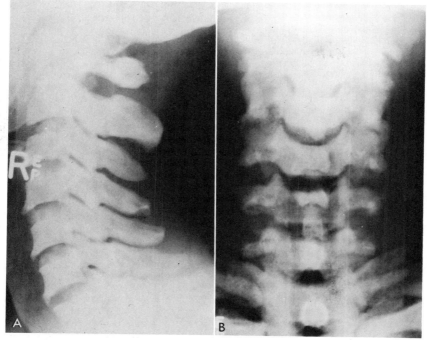

Figure 13–56. Lateral and AP views of the cervical spine in a man aged 47 with familial hypophosphatemia. Note uniform increase in density. The patient had histologically proven osteomalacia at the time these films were taken.

tosis, familial paravertebral calcification, Reiter's syndrome, fluorosis, hypoparathyroid spondylosis, Wilson's disease and hypophosphatasia. In the last condition, there also may be the stigmata of rickets.

Sporadic.[102] The sporadic nonfamilial form of hypophosphatemic osteomalacia usually begins in adolescence or early adult life, with absence of rickets and retarded growth during childhood, and with a negative family history. It merits separate description because the spinal manifestations are quite different from those of familial hypophosphatemia. The onset is most frequently between ages 20 and 40. The symptoms are typical of osteomalacia—pain in the back and legs, and severe muscle weakness. The spine is severely involved. Usually, a few years after the onset of the other symptoms there is a rapid loss of trunk height with severe kyphosis. The radiographic findings in the spine are similar to those described for osteomalacia in general (p. 628), but are often disproportionately severe, with generalized wedging and compression, as well as biconcavity (Fig. 13–57). In the other bones, there is a generalized reduc-tion of bone density, usually associated with Looser zones. Ligamentous calcification and osteosclerosis do not occur.

The biochemical features are similar to those of familial hypophosphatemia, but are of greater severity, the serum phosphorus usually being well below 2 mg per 100 ml. The urine calcium may be raised before treatment is begun, and rises excessively if treatment is mistakenly given with vitamin D alone. There is also increased excretion of glycine in the urine. The differences between the familial and sporadic form of hypophosphatemia are summarized in Table 13–12.

An identical syndrome may occur in association with various mesenchymal tumors which have been referred to as hemangiopericytomas, and in association with neurofibromatosis.[27] Hypophosphatemia and osteomalacia may disappear after excision of such a tumor. The cases in association with neurofibromatosis may begin in early childhood, but the other features of the disease resemble the adolescent onset, nonfamilial type rather than the familial hyperphosphatemia, which is the usual cause in children.[303]

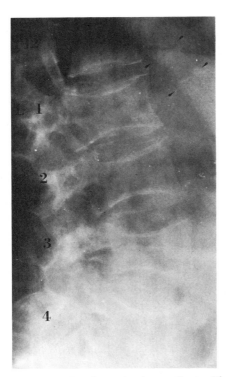

Figure 13–57. Lumbar spine in a patient with sporadic hypophosphatemia. Note reduced density, typical osteomalacic biconcavity and two Looser zones in a rib (shown by arrows). The changes in shape were more marked in the thoracic spine, but the bones were too radiolucent for satisfactory reproduction.

MULTIPLE RENAL TUBULE DEFECTS.[18, 99] As originally described, the Fanconi syndrome is characterized by impaired renal tubular reabsorption of phosphate, glucose, amino acids, bicarbonate and sometimes uric acid due to cystinosis, a condition in which cystine is deposited in many organs of the body, including the bone marrow and the kidneys. The term is also used somewhat loosely to denote the occurrence of multiple defects of renal tubular function of varied etiology. The rickets associated with the Fanconi syndrome resembles that of familial hypophosphatemia, with the extra features of renal tubular acidosis, and eventually chronic renal failure and early death (Table 13–11). The Fanconi syndrome in adults involves a heterogeneous collection of diseases having in common acquired injury to the renal tubes, such as Wilson's disease, cadmium poisoning, myelomatosis, administration of out-dated tetracycline and amphotericin therapy. There is also an idiopathic adult form of Fanconi syndrome in which none of these conditions can be found; the prognosis is much better than in childhood.

The spinal manifestations of the adult Fanconi syndrome resemble those of sporadic nonfamilial hypophosphatemic osteomalacia, but are generally less severe.

DRUG AND OTHER CHEMICALLY INDUCED OSTEOMALACIA. It is convenient to consider together the various drugs and other compounds which may induce osteomalacia by different mechanisms.

Anticonvulsants. Phenobarbital and Dilantin may both lead to osteomalacia by interfering in some way with vitamin D metabolism.

Cholestyramine. This bile-sequestering agent, used in the treatment of pruritus in obstructive jaundice, and in chronic diarrhea, may impair vitamin D absorption because of bile salt deficiency in the gut.[187]

Laxatives. Laxatives containing phenolphthalein, such as Ex-Lax, may cause chronic diarrhea and impair vitamin D absorption.[135]

Antacids. Chronic administration, especially with aluminum-containing compounds, but also those containing magnesium trisilicate may form insoluble compounds with dietary phosphate, thus causing osteomalacia from phosphate depletion.[300]

Chronic Cadmium Poisoning. This may induce osteomalacia by two mechanisms—renal tubular damage of the Fanconi

TABLE 13–12. DIFFERENCES BETWEEN FAMILIAL AND NONFAMILIAL FORMS OF HYPOPHOSPHATEMIA[*,**]

	Familial	Nonfamilial
Vertebral collapse	No	Yes
Loss of trunk height	No	Yes
Muscle weakness	No	Yes
Fractures[1]	No	Yes
Osteosclerosis	Yes	No
Ligamentous calcification	Yes	No
Increased glycinuria	No	Yes
Perilacunar low density bone	Yes	No[2]
Phosphate depletion[2]	No	Yes
Stigmata of rickets	Yes	No

   [*]Those dependent only on the age of onset are not included.
   [**]Modified from Parfitt.[303]
   [1]Looser zones (pseudofractures) occur in both.
   [2]Evidence inconclusive.

type and interference with vitamin D metabolism.

Outdated Tetracycline and Amphotericin. Both induce a Fanconi type of renal tubular damage with disproportionately severe renal tubular acidosis.

Fluorides and Diphosphonates. Both induce osteomalacia by inhibition of mineralization.

Treatment of Rickets and Osteomalacia

MEDICAL TREATMENT. The cornerstone of treatment is vitamin D. Cases due to phosphate depletion may only need supplemental phosphorus, and if some correctable etiologic factor is found, mild cases may need no other treatment. In all other cases, vitamin D will be needed, but the dose and duration of treatment differ markedly according to the etiology. Only the general principles of vitamin D therapy can be given here; the reader is referred elsewhere for more extensive discussion.[300, 303] The total duration of healing consists of two phases; the first extends from the start of treatment until renewal of normal mineralization, the second continues until normal bone structure is restored. During the first phase optimal levels of vitamin D metabolites are established and normal chondroblastic and osteoblastic function is resumed. During the second phase complex reparative processes occur in bone, hyperplastic parathyroids may involute, and vitamin D stores become repleted. In vitamin D depletion, the first phase may take only a few days, but in patients needing pharmacologic doses, this phase may take many weeks or months. The duration of the second phase lasts for a few weeks to many months, depending on the severity of the osseous changes rather than on the underlying cause.

In the use of physiologic doses of vitamin D to correct deficiency, it is invariable practice to begin with a larger dose than the expected maintenance or prophylactic dose, and to continue this until healing begins. The onset of healing will be expedited, and the risk of intoxication is negligible. However, with pharmacologic doses of vitamin D, this initial high dose regimen may be extremely hazardous.

The pharmacologic use of vitamin D is in some ways analogous to the use of digitalis. During the first phase of treatment, body stores of vitamin D and its metabolites in blood, liver, fat and muscle must be filled to a particular level; this level varies between diseases, between different patients with the same disease, and between the same patient at different times. If this is attempted too rapidly, then, as with digitalis, the risk of intoxication is much increased. It is, therefore, best to begin with a dose of vitamin D somewhat less than the expected maintenance dose shown in Table 13–9 and to increase this infrequently and by small amounts. On a constant daily dose of vitamin D it takes four to six weeks to attain vitamin D equilibrium, at which point the rate of degradation and excretion equals the rate of administration, and the levels of metabolites will thereafter remain stable. From this point, it takes at least four further weeks before the effect of this dose may be adequately assessed by clinical, radiographic and biochemical study. Normally, therefore, the interval between successive increments should be no less than eight weeks. When in this way an effective level is found, it should be maintained until healing is fairly advanced, then the dose may be reduced until the lowest effective dose is found. Usually, if the foregoing policy has been adopted, the maintenance dose will be only slightly less or even the same as the dose which produces healing.

When the various metabolites of vitamin D are more widely available for clinical use it may be possible to shorten the first phase, and it will probably be safer to expedite healing by starting with a higher dose than the expected maintenance dose, because the action of the metabolites will be much more short-lived than the action of the parent vitamin.

Certain varieties of rickets and osteomalacia may require the administration of supplemental phosphate as well as vitamin D;[165] this is especially true in the sporadic nonfamilial form of hyperphosphatemic vitamin D refractory rickets and osteomalacia.[102]

ORTHOPEDIC TREATMENT. As a general rule, it is not feasible to attempt surgical correction of the spinal deformities of rickets and osteomalacia. However, occasionally mechanical correction has been attempted with worthwhile results. In one case of sporadic nonfamilial hypophosphatemia with severe kyphoscoliosis, traction to the spine followed by plaster fixation was performed 12 times in succession at weekly intervals, with significant improvement in the degree of kyphosis and increase in total height of 5.5 cm.[56] Similarly, traction to the legs and pelvis improved femoral and tibial angulation in a patient with neurofibromatosis.[27] These mechanical maneuvers should be initiated immediately while the bones are still soft. Operative treatment such as osteotomy should be deferred until vitamin D treatment has become fully effective. The need for operative intervention in adults with familial hypophosphatemia and spinal cord compression due to ectopic ossification was mentioned earlier.

OSTEITIS FIBROSA AND HYPERPARATHYROIDISM

Osteitis fibrosa signifies the osseous abnormality resulting from a considerable excess of parathyroid hormone, sufficient to produce the special features which differ from a simple increase in bone turnover.

Etiology of Osteitis Fibrosa

As defined, osteitis fibrosa can be due to primary, ectopic or secondary hyperparathyroidism (Table 13–13). Primary hyperparathyroidism is due either to hyperplasia, adenoma or carcinoma of the parathyroid. In general, osteitis fibrosa develops in patients with more rapidly progressive disease who are more likely to have an adenoma or carcinoma than hyperplasia. Most patients with primary hyperparathyroidism never get osteitis fibrosa because the disease is too slowly progressive. Such patients may have bone involvement with the radiographic and histologic features of high turnover osteoporosis, as described earlier. The patients come to medical attention

because of kidney stones or because of accidental diagnosis, and they are either diagnosed or treated, or die from renal failure or hypertension before osteitis fibrosa develops. Conversely, patients with the most rapidly progressive disease may get so sick from hypercalcemia that they either die or are cured by surgery before the osseous manifestations of osteitis fibrosa have had time to develop. Thus, osteitis fibrosa tends to occur in patients with primary hyperparathyroidism of an intermediate degree of severity and speed of progression.

Ectopic hyperparathyroidism signifies the production of some form of parathyroid hormone by a nonparathyroid neoplasm. In general, such patients present with the effects of hypercalcemia, but histologic and, occasionally, radiologic evidence of osteitis fibrosa may be observed. Severe spinal abnormalities are unlikely to be encountered in such patients, except as a result of vertebral metastases.

Secondary hyperparathyroidism signifies an increase in parathyroid hormone secretion which is compensatory, in the sense that it represents an attempt to correct hypocalcemia or hyperphosphatemia. Osteitis fibrosa as a result of secondary hyperparathyroidism is a frequent concomitant of some kinds of osteomalacia, as already mentioned, but although often more easily detected than osteomalacia on hand x-rays, it is not usually the dominant abnormality in the bones and does not usually contribute to the spinal manifestations of osteomalacia, except through the production of osteosclerosis, as described earlier. Secondary hyperparathyroidism also may occur in patients with pseudohypoparathyroidism, in which there is target-cell resistance to the action of parathyroid hormone at the osteocyte and in the renal tubule, which leads to hypocalcemia and hyperphosphatemia, as in hypoparathyroidism. In some patients the osteoclasts may also be resistant to parathyroid hormone, in which case the bones may become more dense than normal. In others, the osteoclast remains responsive to parathyroid hormone, with the production of osteitis fibrosa. The extremities are characteristically involved most severely, and severe spinal manifestations are unlikely. The secondary hyperparathyroidism of chronic renal failure is described later.

The etiologic distinction between primary and secondary hyperparathyroidism was until

TABLE 13–13.   VARIETIES OF HYPERPARATHYROIDISM

Type	Pathology	Liability to Osteitis Fibrosa
Primary	Hyperplasia	Low
	Adenoma	Intermediate
	Carcinoma	High
Ectopic	Any neoplasm	Low
Secondary	Nutritional	Low[1]
	Intestinal malabsorption	Low
	Chronic renal failure	High
	Pseudohypoparathyroidism	Low

[1]In man; high in some other species.

recently thought to correspond exactly to a structural and histologic difference (adenoma vs. hyperplasia) and to a functional difference (autonomy of hormone secretion vs. normal secretory control), but it is increasingly evident that there is no simple correspondence between these three methods of classification—etiologic, structural, and functional. This is well illustrated by so-called tertiary hyperparathyroidism. This confusing term is applied to patients who develop persistent hypercalcemia in the context of long-standing secondary hyperparathyroidism.[301] Sometimes the term is restricted to patients in whom the parathyroid pathology is of one or more adenomas, rather than hyperplasia, a usage which serves to call attention to the fact that some patients who develop hypercalcemia may not need more than one parathyroid gland removed. In intestinal malabsorption there is evidence that parathyroid adenomas may develop without evidence of an intervening stage of secondary parathyroid hyperplasia,[364] which may explain the occasional patient in whom severe osteitis fibrosa is the dominant abnormality in the bones.[65] In chronic renal failure there is no correlation between the parathyroid histology and the extent of parathyroid autonomy judged by hypercalcemia.

Thus, for practical purposes, severe spinal manifestations are confined to patients with primary hyperparathyroidism and we will say no more about the various forms of secondary hyperparathyroidism except in the context of renal osteodystrophy described later.

Histopathogenesis of Osteitis Fibrosa

Although this is always due to a substantial increase in parathyroid hormone secretion, the mechanism whereby the bone cells respond to this increase to produce osteitis fibrosa is not completely clear. Since the osteoclast is a relatively short-lived cell, a substantial increase in the number of osteoclasts can only arise by increased proliferation of osteoclast precursors. This is one basic abnormality in osteitis fibrosa which leads to increased activation of new remodeling cycles and increase in bone turnover. Since the acute effect of parathyroid hormone administration is to stimulate the cellular chemistry of resorption, it is widely assumed that the individual

osteoclasts are overactive in hyperparathyroidism. There is no direct evidence for this assumption and good evidence that in some cases the linear resorption rate, which is related to the activity of individual osteoclasts, is actually reduced.[401] This reduction in resorption rate inevitably leads to a prolongation of the time taken to resorb a given volume of bone, and this prolongation will, according to the principles discussed earlier, lead to accumulation of resorption spaces and to an increased fraction of trabecular surface occupied by resorption. Sometimes a substantial delay in the changeover from resorption to formation within each remodeling cycle leads to further accumulation of unfilled resorption spaces. In severe cases, there may also be a partial or complete suppression of normal lamellar bone formation. This may possibly represent a reactivation of growth-related modeling, which could explain two otherwise puzzling facts about osteitis fibrosa—the preferential involvement of the subperiosteal rather than the endosteal surface, and the preferential location of subperiosteal resorption at the metaphyses of the long bones. Normal periosteal remodeling leads to continued slow expansion, but during growth the maintenance of metaphyseal flaring requires net resorption of surface subperiosteal bone. Finally, in the spaces created by these unfilled resorption spaces there is increased formation of fibrous tissue and of woven bone. In summary, the histodynamic abnormalities of osteitis fibrosa consist of: 1) increased proliferation of osteoclast precursors; 2) slowing down of osteoclastic resorption, with prolongation of the resorption phase and further accumulation of active resorption spaces; 3) prolongation of the switchover of resorption to formation and increased accumulation of inactive resorption spaces; 4) reactivation of modeling, leading to resorption which is not followed by formation, especially on the subperiosteal surface and at the metaphyses of the long bones; and 5) replacement of lamellar bone by fibrous tissue and woven bone.

Clinical Features of Osteitis Fibrosa

THE SPINE. The spinal manifestations of osteitis fibrosa may be quite mild, even with severe disease elsewhere. Alternatively, the spinal manifestations may dominate the clinical picture. However, most patients with clinically significant osteitis fibrosa will have some degree of spinal involvement. For example, of the first 17 patients with hyperparathyroidism at the Massachusetts General Hospital, all five who had osteitis fibrosa had kyphosis and pain in the back.[3] A good example of the spinal manifestations was provided by Captain Charles Martell, the first patient to undergo parathyroid surgery in the United States.[5] There may be loss of height and increasing kyphosis due to vertebral collapse. This occurs in all three types of metabolic bone disease affecting the spine, but the height loss of osteitis fibrosa is distinctive in several respects (Table 13–14). First, it is usually continuous in time and distributed regularly throughout the spine as in osteomalacia, rather than being episodic in time and irregularly distributed throughout the spine as in osteoporosis (but see Fig. 13–58). Second, it is more rapidly progressive than in osteomalacia, approaching in rate the acute phase of bone loss in idiopathic osteoporosis, but extending over a longer time. Captain Martell, for example, lost seven inches in height in eight years.[5] Third, it may involve the cervical spine as well as the dorsal and lumbar spine, with severe shortening of the neck.[5] Finally, although bone pain and tenderness in the vertebrae are common, severe height loss can occur in osteitis fibrosa with complete absence of pain, a combination which occurs only rarely in osteoporosis and never in osteomalacia. The regular kyphosis of osteitis fibrosa does not cause any neurologic disturbance, but there is one case on record of an osteoclastoma due to primary hyperparathyroidism causing spinal cord compression.[353] Another spinal manifestation is fracture of the spinous processes producing sudden severe pain in the neck as a presenting symptom.[266]

OTHER OSSEOUS MANIFESTATIONS. Often, even with obvious radiographic evidence of osteitis fibrosa, there may be no bone symptoms at all. There may be ill-defined pain in the extremities similar to that occurring in os-

teomalacia and also ascribed to arthritis or other locomotor disorder. The bones may be tender, but this is less prominent than in osteomalacia. The known occurrence of osteomalacia in primary hyperparathyroidism, the resemblance between the clinical manifestations of osteomalacia and osteitis fibrosa, and the occurrence of quite severe osteitis fibrosa in the complete absence of pain, raise the interesting speculation that symptomatic bone disease in osteitis fibrosa is due partly to coexistent osteomalacia.

Pathologic fractures may occur in advanced disease, usually through a cyst or osteoclastoma, or through a zone of gross osteoclastic resorption, as in the femoral neck. Traumatic fractures through bone uninvolved by serious localized disease may nevertheless fail to unite until the hyperparathyroidism is treated. Malunion of a fracture may be the presenting feature in patients who lack any other clinical or radiographic evidence of osteitis fibrosa.[146, 210]

Cysts and osteoclastomas may cause symptoms by expansion, either producing visible deformity as in the jaw or pressing on adjacent structures. Apparent clubbing of the fingers is caused by severe erosion of the terminal phalanges, with collapse of the soft tissues of the pulp.

There are at least three causes of arthritis in patients with primary hyperparathyroidism: classical gout, pseudogout associated with chondrocalcinosis, and a more-specific arthropathy caused by severe erosion of subchondral bone and consequent deformity of the articular cartilage.[67]

OTHER CLINICAL MANIFESTATIONS OF PRIMARY HYPERPARATHYROIDISM. Taking the disease as a whole, fatigue caused by muscle weakness is probably the commonest symptom, and nephrolithiasis the commonest objective manifestation, occurring in from 60 to 80 per cent of patients, usually those with a more slowly progressive disease. Nephrolithiasis is present in only 10 to 20 per cent of pa-

TABLE 13–14. VERTEBRAL INVOLVEMENT AND HEIGHT LOSS IN METABOLIC BONE DISEASE

	Temporal Distribution	Spatial Distribution	Rate
Involutional osteoporosis	Episodic	Irregular	Slow
Idiopathic osteoporosis	Episodic	Irregular	Rapid
Osteomalacia	Continuous	Regular	Slow
Osteitis fibrosa	Continuous	Regular	Rapid

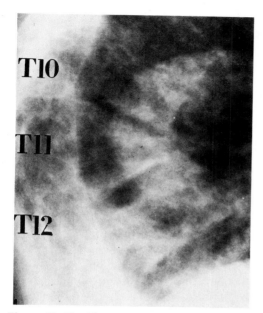

Figure 13–58. Thoracic vertebrae in a 61-year-old woman with severe osteitis fibrosa due to primary hyperparathyroidism. Note extreme coarseness and irregularity which made it impossible to obtain satisfactory radiographs. Nevertheless, the extreme wedging of T11 with angulation can be discerned. This is an unusual finding.

tients presenting with bone disease. Nephrocalcinosis is much more common and even if not visible radiographically, probably occurs in most patients whose disease is undiagnosed for more than a few years. Although severe osteitis fibrosa is possible with completely normal renal function[266] patients with bone disease usually have a more severe degree of renal insufficiency, owing to hypercalcemic nephropathy, than patients who present with kidney stones. The reason for the relative freedom from stones in patients with osteitis fibrosa is unknown. Possibly, some peptide fragment from collagen excreted in the urine may exercise a protective effect on mineral precipitation, since few patients with hyperthyroidism get stones despite considerable hypercalciuria.

Hypercalcemia, as well as causing renal insufficiency, has its own train of symptoms. Mild hypercalcemia may produce polyuria and thirst, owing to impaired renal concentration, in the absence of renal failure. More severe hypercalcemia may lead to anorexia, nausea and vomiting, and extreme hypercalcemia produces impairment of consciousness progressing to stupor and coma.

An extensive discussion of the many other aspects of this protean disease would be inappropriate for the scope of this chapter, and the reader is referred elsewhere.[101, 210, 320, 386]

Radiographic Abnormalities

Changes in the spine and hands have already been described. In severe spinal osteitis fibrosa, the vertebrae are all compressed and slightly wedged, with coarse trabeculations and moderate endplate sclerosis,[71] but occasionally severe wedging with angulation may occur (Fig. 13–58). Cysts and giant cell tumors may have similar radiographic appearances and the difference may only become apparent after surgical treatment; true cysts tend to remain unfilled indefinitely, whereas osteoclastomas may be replaced by more dense bone than normal.

Laboratory Abnormalities in Primary Hyperparathyroidism

The most constant abnormality in osteitis fibrosa is elevation of the serum alkaline phosphatase associated with increased formation of woven bone. If the alkaline phosphatase is normal, osseous abnormalities are unlikely to be due to osteitis fibrosa. The plasma calcium is usually raised, but occasionally is normal if there is associated vitamin D deficiency, as already described. Other explanations for the occasional finding of normocalcemia in patients with osteitis fibrosa have been advanced[259] but not confirmed. The serum phosphorus is commonly reduced, but this may be obscured by renal insufficiency. Findings of high turnover osteoporosis, as described earlier, will also be found in patients with osteitis fibrosa.

Differential Diagnosis

In a patient with spinal disease due to osteitis fibrosa there always will be subperiosteal erosion in the phalanges and a high alkaline phosphatase. These findings establish that there is excess parathyroid hormone but do not distinguish between primary, ectopic and secondary hyperparathyroidism. In one extraordinary case in a patient who apparently presented with spinal manifestations resem-

TABLE 13–15.　DIFFERENTIAL DIAGNOSIS OF HYPERCALCEMIA IN
PRESENCE OF A SPINAL LESION*

Disease	X-Ray of Hands	Alkaline Phosphatase	PTH Assay
Primary hyperparathyroidism	OFC	Increased	Increased
Ectopic hyperparathyroidism	OFC	Increased	Increased
Other humoral hypercalcemia	Normal	Normal or increased	Normal
Metastatic disease	Normal	Increased	Normal
Lymphoma	Normal	Increased	Normal
Myeloma	Normal	Normal	Normal
Immobilization	Metacarpal striation	Normal	Normal or increased

*Note that the response to corticosteroid suppression is of little value in differentiating between these conditions.
OFC = osteitis fibrosa cystica.

bling osteoporosis, the hand x-rays were normal and the only indication of the presence of osteitis fibrosa was a raised alkaline phosphatase.[134] In this rare situation a bone biopsy may be necessary to make the diagnosis.

The differential diagnosis in a patient with a spinal lesion and hypercalcemia includes primary hyperparathyroidism, ectopic hyperparathyroidism, humoral hypercalcemia of malignancy due to other compounds, myelomatosis, secondary carcinomatosis, lymphoma, and immobilization. It is evident from Table 13–15 that the x-ray of the hands is the most important simple way of excluding all conditions other than ectopic hyperparathyroidism. In some patients the osteitis fibrosa is likely to be asymptomatic and detected only on x-ray of the hands or biopsy. There are immunologic differences between the hormone secreted in primary and in ectopic hyperparathyroidism, in which a higher molecular weight polypeptide, possibly the pro-hormone, may be released into the circulation. The common sites of origin for ectopic PTH secretion are the kidney and bronchus. If both IVP and bronchoscopy are negative, neck exploration may be necessary to establish this diagnosis by finding four normal parathyroid glands.

Summary of the Osseous Manifestations of Primary Hyperparathyroidism

HIGH TURNOVER OSTEOPOROSIS.　This is usually asymptomatic and accounts for bone involvement and not bone disease in most patients with primary hyperparathyroidism, regardless of the presenting manifestations.

OSTEITIS FIBROSA.　This represents a more severe disease with higher blood levels of parathyroid hormone, and has the additional features of reactivation of modeling, slowing of linear resorption rate and replacement of lamellar bone by woven bone and fibrous tissue.

OSTEOSCLEROSIS.　Vertebral osteosclerosis with end-plate thickening (rugger-jersey spine) is a common finding in osteitis fibrosa, especially in renal failure.[2] Occasionally, generalized osteosclerosis may develop.

OSTEOMALACIA RESULTING FROM ASSOCIATED VITAMIN D DEFICIENCY.　This condition is either nutritional or caused by intestinal malabsorption, or is due to an effect of PTH on the intermediary metabolism of vitamin D.

UNUNITED FRACTURE.　In the absence of overt osteitis fibrosa, this may be the presenting feature.

"IDIOPATHIC" OSTEOPOROSIS.　The arguments for and against this concept have been discussed earlier.

Note that all of these, with the exception of ununited fracture, may affect the spine. Since vertebral fractures are always impacted, malunion in the ordinary sense is not a problem.

Treatment

The only curative treatment is surgical. Various maneuvers are available to aid the preoperative localization of the tumor. These are most useful in patients needing reoperation because the first operation was negative; the details of the surgical procedure are described elsewhere.[386] The main point of contention is whether all parathyroid glands should be identified histologically or simply by inspection. Visual identification minimizes the risk of postoperative hypoparathyroidism but increases the risk of recurrence with need for reoperation in patients with hyperplasia. This latter risk probably is less serious in patients presenting with bone disease than in patients presenting with stones. In patients with bone disease there is a much greater likelihood of tetany in the postoperative period. This is a potentially catastrophic complication in a patient with severe osteitis fibrosa, since convulsive seizures may lead to bilateral femoral neck fracture. The severity of postoperative tetany can be minimized by preoperative correction of vitamin D depletion[416] and magnesium depletion, and by bringing the plasma calcium down close to normal by calcitonin and sodium phosphate. In some patients in whom exploration is unsuccessful or who refuse surgery, long-term phosphate administration may lead to improvement in osteitis fibrosa.[101] This is paradoxical, since the normal response to phosphate administration is a fall in plasma calcium and an increase in parathyroid hormone secretion.

In parathyroid carcinoma, complete surgical cure is usually not achieved. The subsequent course may be complicated by

fractures due to metastases as well as to severe osteitis fibrosa.[312] Intractable hypercalcemia may sometimes respond temporarily to mithramycin but stilbestrol diphosphate, from which stilbestrol is liberated in tissues rich in phosphatase, may be more effective.[356]

A DIAGNOSTIC APPROACH TO VERTEBRAL RAREFACTION AND COLLAPSE

Since osteoporosis is so much more common than either osteomalacia or osteitis fibrosa, and since these diseases are frequently easily recognized by their own positive features, a commonly recurring practical problem is to decide to what lengths one should go, first, in ruling out the occult forms of osteomalacia or osteitis fibrosa (which are treatable) in a patient who seems to have the essentially untreatable condition of osteoporosis, and second, in ruling out occult and possibly treatable causes of osteoporosis, rather than accepting the diagnosis of involutional osteoporosis. We have broken the diagnostic process into eight steps which are illustrated in Figure 13–59 as a flow chart. This is designed as a

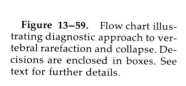

Figure 13–59. Flow chart illustrating diagnostic approach to vertebral rarefaction and collapse. Decisions are enclosed in boxes. See text for further details.

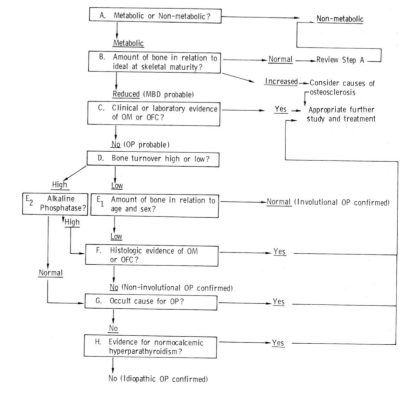

convenient framework to illustrate the underlying logical relationships of the various decisions, not as a rigid and invariant program. In practice, several steps shown as sequential may be taken together and some may be omitted, depending on individual circumstances.

Step A. Is This Metabolic or Nonmetabolic Disease of the Spine?

Very often the presence of some non-metabolic disease will be obvious on the initial clinical and radiographic assessment. If a patient has backache and completely normal x-rays, then metabolic bone disease is unlikely. Occasionally, osteoporosis may cause pain in the back in the absence of changes in vertebral shape, but only in the presence of an unambiguous increase in radiolucency. Pain which is absolutely unremitting always suggests metastatic bone disease of the spine, even if the x-rays show osteoporosis. Sometimes osteomalacia will develop acutely (the special usage of "acute" and "chronic" in the context of bone disease was explained earlier) and cause symptoms and signs before significant radiographic abnormality has developed. Such patients almost always have pain and tenderness in other bones also. As a rule, therefore, pain felt only in the back by a patient with radiographically normal bones is not due to metabolic bone disease. Most problems arise in patients who have some degree of vertebral wedging or compression and some degree of osteoporosis. One important consideration is the number of vertebrae involved. If only one, and the rest of the spine is normal, metabolic bone disease is most unlikely. Isolated vertebral collapse should lead to a careful inquiry for previous trauma. A special form of trauma is that due to a convulsive seizure, either spontaneous (epilepsy) or iatrogenic. This is especially likely to cause mid and upper thoracic vertebral collapse in the presence of an otherwise normal spine.

Other causes of vertebral wedging which may be overlooked are the various causes of so-called epiphysitis, such as irradiation in childhood (Fig. 13–60) and the effects of delayed epiphyseal closure. In a young adult male, a stiff painful back is likely to be due to ankylosing spondylitis. The x-rays may be normal or may be reported to show osteoporosis. Gaucher's disease may cause a gener-

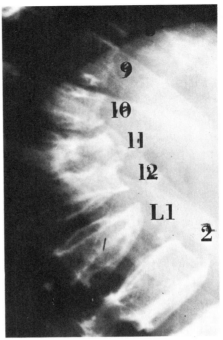

Figure 13–60. Spine of woman aged 22 who had irradiation for a Wilms' tumor in childhood. Some of the vertebrae resemble those of severe idiopathic osteoporosis (see Fig. 13–51).

alized reduction in vertebral density, with multiple wedging and collapse closely resembling osteoporosis, but changes in other bones are more characteristic.[171]

Erythroid hyperplasia, most commonly secondary to hemolytic anemia, may cause endosteal resorption and loss of both trabecular and cortical bone. The distribution of this varies with age; it is commonly in the hands and feet in infancy, the skull in older children, and the ribs, spine and pelvis in adults.[233] In older patients, metastatic bone disease is the most worrying condition to exclude before concluding that vertebral rarefaction is metabolic; it can cause symptoms for many months before specific radiographic signs are apparent. Spinal metastases usually arise from breast, bronchus, thyroid, kidney, prostate or stomach. Lymphoma and allied conditions may produce a similar clinical and radiographic picture. Apart from careful physical examination, two procedures may be especially helpful in this context. In the absence of recent vertebral fracture, a positive bone scan strongly suggests metastatic rather than metabolic bone disease, but the scan will not distinguish between metastatic and non-metastatic causes of fracture. A positive scan may also be found in Paget's disease, but this diagnosis should be obvious on x-ray. Secondly, in metastatic disease, electromyography may show evidence of posterior nerve root involvement with normal anterior roots, because the pedicles are so often involved.[243]

Myelomatosis requires special consideration because this sometimes exactly mimics the radiographic features of involutional osteoporosis, owing to diffuse proliferation of plasma cells throughout the spine, rather than to the more usual focal proliferation. Work-up to exclude myelomatosis should include testing of urine for Bence Jones protein, complete blood count and sedimentation rate, and serum protein electrophoresis. If suspicion of myeloma is sufficiently great, electrophoresis of urinary proteins after concentration, estimation of plasma immunoglobulin, and aspiration of bone marrow may be needed.

If metabolic bone disease is a possibility, x-ray of the hands, plasma calcium, inorganic phosphate and alkaline phosphatase should be ordered, with the precautions mentioned earlier. If any of these are abnormal, one may omit Step B and proceed immediately to Step C. If the plasma calcium is elevated in a patient presenting with a vertebral lesion, consider the conditions given in Table 13–14. If the plasma calcium is not raised, then either a low calcium, low phosphorus, or raised alkaline phosphatase suggests the possibility of osteomalacia. Occasionally, a raised alkaline phosphatase is the only clue to hyperparathyroidism,[134] but unrecognized Paget's disease is a more likely explanation.

Step B. Is the Amount of Bone Reduced in Relation to Normal Values at Skeletal Maturity for the Patient's Sex and Race?

The difficulties in determining the mineral content of bone from standard x-rays have already been mentioned, and some objective assessment is always desirable. Radiographic photodensitometry of the spine is clearly the most appropriate for vertebral disease, but the semiquantitative assessment of femoral trabeculae is an acceptable alternative and photonabsorptiometry of the forearm is accurate and convenient. Lacking facilities for these, radiographic morphometry of the hands is a valuable substitute, needing no special equipment other than a pair of calipers. The relatively low correlation between cortical bone in the extremities and trabecular bone in the spine must be remembered. Since we are interested in the amount of bone *lost* as well as in the amount of bone *present,* the most desirable comparison to make is with the amount of bone present in the same individual at the time of skeletal maturity. In practice, we have to make use of normal values at skeletal maturity established in a group of individuals of the same sex and background, interpreted in light of the patient's height and of the various nutritional, endocrine and other factors which affect the accumulation of bone during growth. With the result of assessment of amount of bone by whatever means, the patient can be categorized into one of three groups: 1) Amount of bone increased; the various metabolic and non-metabolic diseases associated with osteosclerosis must be reviewed (see page 702); 2) Amount of bone normal; if the assessment was made by radiographic photodensitometry or photonabsorptiometry, the possibility of an aberrant result due to superimposition of zones of increased and reduced density must be considered; this is especially likely in renal osteodystrophy and some cases of osteomalacia. If this possibility is excluded, the initial decision to classify the patient as metabolic rather than nonmetabolic must be reviewed. If this decision is supported by abnormalities of serum calcium, phosphorus and alkaline phosphatase, it may be correct to proceed to Step C despite a normal value. However, if the calcium, phosphorus and alkaline phosphatase are all normal, one should return to Step A and reconsider alternative diagnoses. At this juncture a vertebral biopsy may be needed to resolve the diagnostic problem.[197] 3) Amount of bone reduced; proceed to Step C.

Step C. Is There Radiographic or Laboratory Evidence of Osteomalacia or Osteitis Fibrosa?

At this stage, a full metabolic bone survey should be ordered. Other evidence of hyperparathyroidism, primary or secondary, may be sought by obtaining a 24-hour urine calcium, phosphorus and creatinine, interpreted as explained earlier, and a plasma parathyroid hormone assay if possible. Further evidence of osteomalacia might come from a dietary history, a low plasma 25-hydroxy D_3, and evidence of the most likely causes of osteomalacia; namely, malabsorption and chronic renal failure. If any of these studies are abnormal, the possibility of osteomalacia may be sufficient to proceed directly to Step F and order a bone biopsy.

The clinical findings should be reviewed for evidence of hyperthyroidism, Cushing's syndrome, and other known causes of osteoporosis. If urinary calcium is raised, one should consider neoplastic osteolysis, acute idiopathic osteoporosis, high turnover osteoporosis of any cause, normocalcemic hyperparathyroidism, and some rare forms of osteomalacia. If all these tests are normal, then osteoporosis is the most likely diagnosis and the next step is to consider the possibility of high or low bone turnover.

Step D. Is Bone Turnover High or Low?

The best simple test is to examine the hands by magnification radioscopy. Urinary total hydroxyproline may also be helpful, as are radiokinetic studies of calcium accretion and pool size if available. If bone turnover is low or normal, as judged by these tests, then proceed to Step E. If bone turnover is high and the alkaline phosphatase is raised, proceed to Step F. If bone turnover is high and the alkaline phosphatase is normal or only slightly raised, proceed to Step G.

Step E. Is the Amount of Bone Normal for the Patient's Age and Sex?

The studies performed in Step B must now be reviewed, using as a comparison normal controls matched for age as well as sex and race. If the values, although reduced in comparison with those of skeletal maturity, are normal for the patient's age, then involutional osteoporosis (postmenopausal or senile) is accepted as the diagnosis and a decision is made on treatment, in light of the severity of the disease and the presence or absence of symptoms. If the patient is asymptomatic and the vertebral abnormality was found by accident, probably no treatment is needed.

If the amount of bone is significantly reduced in relation to the patient's age, then either the patient has some noninvolutional

cause of osteoporosis or has some atypical form of osteomalacia or osteitis fibrosa with normal chemistry.

Step F. Is There Histologic Evidence of Osteomalacia or Osteitis Fibrosa?

A bone biopsy is the most certain way to resolve the diagnosis at this juncture. The diagnostic value is greatly improved when quantitative assessment of mineralization and resorption is made as described earlier. If osteomalacia or osteitis fibrosa is found, then further study and treatment (as described elsewhere) are undertaken. If the biopsy is normal, then we have arrived by exclusion at the diagnosis of noninvolutional osteoporosis.

Step G. Is There Evidence for any Occult Causes of Osteoporosis?

We assume that overt evidence of hyperthyroidism, Cushing's syndrome, hypogonadism and malabsorption have already been detected at the initial clinical evaluation. It is easy to overlook excess ethanol consumption. The extent to which one should go to rule out a treatable cause depends mainly on the severity of the bone disease and on the patient's age. The simplest routine screening test for hyperthyroidism is a column T_4 and for Cushing's syndrome a morning and evening plasma cortisol. The most accurate screening test for intestinal malabsorption as a cause of bone disease is a quantitative estimation of fecal fat excretion; further evaluation and treatment of any abnormality found are beyond the scope of this text. If these studies are all negative, and there are no family history and no evidence of osteogenesis imperfecta tarda (or tardissima), the diagnosis of idiopathic osteoporosis is established, except for a possible final consideration of normocalcemic primary hyperparathyroidism.

Step H. Is There Evidence of Normocalcemic Hyperparathyroidism?

The previous studies, especially bone biopsy, tests for high turnover osteoporosis, and parathyroid hormone assay should have effectively ruled out hyperparathyroidism. If these studies are equivocal or for any reason cannot be undertaken, further exploration of this possibility may be indicated by means of calcium infusion, EDTA infusion or phosphate loading before finally accepting the diagnosis of idiopathic osteoporosis.

RENAL OSTEODYSTROPHY[301]

The varied osseous manifestations of chronic renal failure are collectively referred to as renal osteodystrophy. This is primarily the result of varying combinations of two major pathologic processes—defective mineralization leading to rickets or osteomalacia, and secondary hyperparathyroidism leading to osteitis fibrosa. Osteosclerosis is common but usually asymptomatic, and osteoporosis is rare in the normal course of chronic renal failure but may be the principal lesion in some patients on maintenance hemodialysis.

Natural History of Renal Osteodystrophy prior to Maintenance Hemodialysis

Although parathyroid hormone secretion begins to rise very early in the course of chronic renal failure it does not initially have a major effect on the bones. Probably all patients who ultimately develop significant osteodystrophy go through a phase during which defective mineralization is the main osseous abnormality and, depending on sociologic and geographic differences in vitamin D nutrition, this phase may be clinically overt, as in Great Britain and other European countries, or asymptomatic, as in the United States and Australia.

As renal function deteriorates, the parathyroid glands continue to enlarge, and parathyroid hormone blood levels rise to a point at which they exert a significant deleterious effect on the bones, osteitis fibrosa develops and worsens, plasma calcium and phosphate levels rise, the mineralization defect may improve to a variable extent, osteosclerosis develops, and soft tissue calcification may appear. Thus, several different clinical courses are possible, even though the underlying sequence of events is the same. The patient may present with rickets or osteomalacia which may continue as the dominant lesion until the patient's death. Alternatively, osteitis fibrosa may supervene, the rickets and osteomalacia healing spontaneously or persisting in a less severe form. In children, severe rickets and osteitis fibrosa may develop more or less together and finally the patient may present with dominant osteitis fibrosa, with no preceding episode of clinically overt rickets or osteomalacia.

Pathogenesis of Renal Osteodystrophy

Since the kidney is the site of the second step in the intermediary metabolism of vitamin D, namely the addition of a hydroxy group in position 1 (p. 615), it is to be expected that progressive loss of functioning renal tissue would be associated with an inability to synthesize 1,25-DHCC. This expectation has been confirmed in both experimental renal failure and human subjects.

Except for the presence of normal amounts of 25-HCC, the effects of nephron destruction and uremia would thus resemble the effects of vitamin D depletion, and impaired calcium released from bone, impaired calcium absorption, hypocalcemia, secondary hyperparathyroidism and impaired mineralization would all be expected.

The mineralization defect of chronic renal failure may also be due in part to the presence of a circulating inhibitor of mineralization.

This has been advanced as an explanation for the lesser incidence of osteomalacia in patients treated with peritoneal dialysis than with hemodialysis. Plasma pyrophosphate levels are raised in uremic patients, but the importance of this remains to be established. In the osteomalacia of renal osteodystrophy, in contrast to other kinds, there seems to be a correlation between the mineralization defect and the degree of hypocalcemia.[279] Other changes in the composition of the plasma, such as metabolic acidosis and deficiency of trivalent phosphate,[82] are probably of lesser importance.

The hypocalcemia of chronic renal failure is due mainly to the impairment of calcium absorption, together with impaired action of parathyroid hormone on the osteocyte-mediated release of calcium, which appears to be defective in the presence of vitamin D deficiency. The increased frequency and severity of hypocalcemia in chronic renal failure, compared with nutritional vitamin D depletion, is probably a function of the increased plasma phosphorus concentration. The subnormal hypercalcemic response to exogenous parathyroid hormone which is characteristic

of chronic renal failure probably results from a
depression of the activity of the individual osteoclast and associated reduction in the linear
resorption rate.[401]

As renal failure advances and the glomerular filtration rate falls, the amount of
phosphate reabsorbed by the tubules falls progressively, so that phosphate excretion per
nephron increases. This homeostatic adjustment enables phosphate excretion to be maintained without significant hyperphosphatemia,
and is mediated by increased parathyroid hormone secretion. This increase can be prevented by dietary phosphate restriction, which
allows a normal plasma phosphate to be maintained without a change in tubular phosphate
reabsorption. Later, when deficiency of 1,25-
DHCC is added, the resultant hypocalcemia
is an additional stimulus to parathyroid hormone hypersecretion and parathyroid gland
hyperplasia.

Secondary hyperparathyroidism thus
serves to maintain normophosphatemia in the
face of a progressive fall in glomerular filtration rate, and to maintain normocalcemia in
the face of progressive depletion of vitamin D
metabolites, and so is truly compensatory. In
some patients with advanced renal failure
parathyroid hormone secretion outstrips these
compensatory demands because normal control mechanisms have been disrupted, leading
to hypercalcemia, a situation sometimes referred to as autonomous hyperparathyroidism
or tertiary hyperparathyroidism.

When the glomerular filtration rate falls to
about 25 per cent of normal, tubular reabsorption of phosphate becomes maximally suppressed, and as the glomerular filtration rate
falls further plasma phosphate must inevitably
rise. From this point, further increases of
parathyroid hormone secretion are no longer
able to alter phosphate reabsorption but continue to increase the removal of calcium and
phosphate from bone. Consequently, a rise in
parathyroid hormone secretion leads to a rise
in plasma phosphate instead of the fall that
occurs in the presence of normal renal function.

Although calcium transfer by the osteocyte shows increased resistance to parathyroid hormone, osteoclasts respond to hormone in much the same way as in primary
hyperparathyroidism. This is the explanation
for the apparent paradoxical association of
hypocalcemia and enhanced osteoclastic resorption. Although plasma parathyroid hor-

mone levels rise very early in the course of
chronic renal failure, radiographically detectable osteitis fibrosa is a relatively late event
because the parathyroid hormone level
required for this is much higher than that
which produces suppression of tubular reabsorption of phosphate.

The main reason for the development of
osteosclerosis is that excess osteoid accumulated during the osteomalasic phase becomes
progressively mineralized as uremic hyperparathyroidism advances. This process may
be facilitated by the replacement of lamellar
bone by woven bone characteristic of severe
osteitis fibrosa.

Clinical Features of Renal Osteodystrophy

Orthopedists may be consulted about
treatment in patients already found to have
renal osteodystrophy, but not infrequently
they may be faced with the patient's initial
complaint and so have to recognize the disorder among patients with a variety of skeletal
symptoms.

In children, significant spinal manifestations are uncommon. The clinical features
resemble those of rickets of late onset, with
the addition of severe impairment of longitudinal growth. The commonest skeletal deformity is genu valgum, but slipped femoral
capital epiphysis is also frequent in adolescents. When severe, these abnormalities result
primarily from the metaphyseal erosion of osteitis fibrosa.

In adults, the effects of renal osteodystrophy on the spine are what one would expect
from a mixture of osteomalacia and osteitis
fibrosa. There may be backache and spinal
tenderness associated with increasing kyphosis and loss of height. In the extremities
there may be diffuse bone pain and tenderness
or localized bone pain related to an osteoclastoma or cyst. This may fracture, especially if
the patient gets a convulsive seizure from
uremia or hypocalcemia. Fractures of other
kinds are no more common in uremic patients
than in the population at large.

Radiographic Features of Renal Osteodystrophy

The severe vertebral changes of renal osteodystrophy are often indistinguishable from

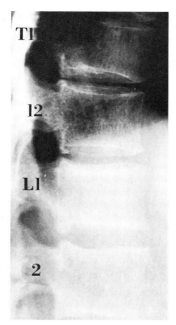

Figure 13–61. Vertebrae of a patient with renal osteodystrophy (both osteomalacia and osteitis fibrosa). Coarse trabeculation resembles pure osteomalacia (compare Fig. 13–23), but with greater end-plate sclerosis in L1 and L2.

those that occur in osteomalacia or severe osteitis fibrosa, but there may be a greater degree of osteosclerosis (Fig. 13–61). In its most severe form, a wide band of sclerosis adjacent to each end plate produces alternating bands of different density, the so called rugger-jersey spine (Fig. 13–27). In other bones, the hands will usually show phalangeal subperiosteal erosion due to secondary hyperparathyroidism. The increased sensitivity of this radiographic sign is important to remember, since the dominant lesion in the bones may be osteomalacia, even when only phalangeal subperiosteal erosion is seen on the x-rays. Lack of awareness of this fact, combined with unwillingness to carry out bone biopsy, has undoubtedly led some workers to underestimate the incidence of uremic osteomalacia in the United States. In children, severe metaphyseal erosion may produce apparent irregularity of the end of the metaphyses, especially if the x-ray beam is slightly misdirected. This may lead to the opposite mistake of attributing radiographic findings of osteitis fibrosa to rickets. This mistake can be avoided by attending to the thickness of the growth plate, which is normal unless rickets is also present,

and to the fact that rickets is most severe in the lower femoral and upper tibial epiphyseal plates, whereas osteitis fibrosa is most severe in the upper femoral and lower tibial.

Diagnosis of Renal Osteodystrophy

This comprises two separate problems; the recognition that chronic renal failure is the underlying cause in patients presenting with osseous manifestations, and the identification of the presence and nature of bone disease in patients known to have chronic renal failure.

RECOGNITION OF CHRONIC RENAL FAILURE. There is a widespread misconception that renal osteodystrophy becomes manifest clinically only in the preterminal phase of uremia, except in the patient whose life is artificially prolonged. In fact, at the onset of osseous symptoms the manifestations of renal disease may be slight and several years of worthwhile life may still be possible. The simplest way to identify chronic renal failure as the cause of orthopedic symptoms is to test the urine for protein in all patients with appropriate clinical manifestations. In addition, the BUN and creatinine should be estimated in all patients with suspected metabolic bone disease.

RECOGNITION OF THE PRESENCE AND TYPE OF BONE DISEASE. The clinical and radiographic basis for the diagnosis have already been mentioned. The only constant biochemical findings, apart from those due directly to renal failure, are a raised alkaline phosphatase level and an increase in urinary total hydroxyproline excretion. In general, both the total calcium and the inorganic phosphate levels are lower in patients with mainly osteomalacia than in those with mainly osteitis fibrosa, but this is of little value in predicting the bone pathology in an individual patient.

Photon-beam absorptiometry is being used increasingly in the recognition of metabolic bone disease. Its usefulness in renal osteodystrophy is limited by the frequent coexistence of osteosclerosis with other lesions, so the above-normal values may be found even in patients with obvious osteitis fibrosa or osteomalacia. Bone biopsy should be done in all patients before vitamin D therapy is considered unless Looser's zones or life-threatening hypocalcemia are present.

In patients with widespread osteitis fibrosa, the differentiation between primary, secondary and tertiary hyperparathyroidism may be difficult. If there is persistent hypercalcemia, by definition the patient does not have secondary hyperparathyroidism. The distinction between the primary and tertiary forms depends mainly on the history and clinical course. If the plasma calcium, or more accurately the ionized calcium, is normal and the serum phosphate is raised, the effect of lowering the serum phosphate by diet plus aluminum-containing antacids should be assessed, since the development of persistent hypercalcemia would then indicate autonomous hyperparathyroidism. Giant cell tumors and cysts and nephrocalcinosis are more common in primary hyperparathyroidism, and associated osteomalacia, osteosclerosis and soft tissue calcification elsewhere are more common in secondary hyperparathyroidism, but these pointers may be unreliable in an individual patient.

The Effect of Maintenance Hemodialysis

Unless appropriate precautions are taken, all patients on maintenance hemodialysis will ultimately develop renal osteodystrophy, but with few exceptions osteomalacia and osteitis fibrosa are preventable. Some patients develop an osseous abnormality which differs from that seen in undialyzed patients. This is characterized by a progressive reduction in bone mass, owing to a profound depression of new bone formation. Affected patients develop painful stress fractures, especially of the metatarsals, ribs, femoral necks and, less frequently, the vertebrae.[302] These fractures heal slowly but with abundant callus formation, as in the osteoporosis of Cushing's syndrome. Histologically, varying degrees of osteomalacia and osteitis fibrosa are often present, but neither vitamin D nor parathyroidectomy is of therapeutic benefit for the osteoporosis.

Treatment of Renal Osteodystrophy

Prophylaxis in the Undialyzed Patient. Graded dietary phosphate restriction, such that the dietary phosphate is progressively reduced in proportion to the falling glomerular filtration rate, will prevent the early increase in parathyroid hormone which otherwise would occur. It is important to monitor this therapy carefully to avoid the induction of phosphate depletion. It would seem logical to administer moderate doses of vitamin D at an early stage, but there is no information on the value or danger of such a policy. The ultimate hope will be that serial measurements of 1,25-DHCC will be possible in all patients and that replacement therapy with 1,25-DHCC will be undertaken when a deficiency is discovered.[61]

Prophylaxis During Maintenance Hemodialysis. In most patients, osteomalacia and osteitis fibrosa can be prevented by maintaining the dialysate calcium concentration at a sufficiently high level and by keeping the predialysis plasma levels of calcium and phosphate within normal limits. No way is yet known of preventing dialysis osteopenia except by abandoning maintenance hemodialysis and proceeding to transplantation.

Treatment of Established Renal Osteodystrophy. Although the dihydroxy metabolites of vitamin D will become the agents of choice, these are unlikely to be widely available for several years. Meanwhile, it is possible to achieve complete healing of rickets and osteomalacia with minimal risk in all patients by using calciferol, provided the appropriate precautions are taken and the correct dosage for individual patients is established. This therapeutic effect is probably dependent not on 1,25-DHCC but on 25-HCC acting directly on gut and bone. As renal failure and secondary hyperparathyroidism progress, a point is reached at which the risks of vitamin D therapy outweigh the benefits.

If the main objective of treatment is to control hypocalcemia and suppress parathyroid hormone secretion, a large calcium supplement, alone or combined with dihydrotachysterol, is the treatment of choice. In a very small number of patients, surgical parathyroidectomy may be required. Some deformities arising from renal osteodystrophy may require orthopedic intervention, but for spinal involvement this is not feasible.

PAGET'S DISEASE OF BONE[29]

Paget's disease of bone (or osteitis deformans) is a localized chronic disturbance which slowly increases the size and frequently changes the shape of the involved bones. It is not strictly a metabolic bone disease, but similar principles underlie its understanding, investigation and treatment. The basic process of the disease is a creeping replacement of normal bone by new bone of abnormal architecture. The newly formed bone is woven bone, which is gradually replaced by lamellar bone, but the same disordered structure is preserved. The etiology is unknown.

Prevalence*

Sir James Paget's original description in 1877, which has been recently reprinted,[298] and often quoted,[115, 415] was written twenty years before x-rays were used in clinical medicine. Such advanced and clinically overt disease is still rare, but Paget's disease may be found by x-rays in 3 to 4 per cent of the population, either at autopsy or by review of radiographs taken in patients over 45 years of age. The great majority of such patients are asymptomatic. In one autopsy series, only one third of the patients had been diagnosed before death and only 5 per cent had required admission to hospital.[84]

The disease rarely begins before age 40. In a collective review of experience in Australia, the youngest patient was 25, 0.7 per cent were under 30, and 3 per cent between 30 and 40 years.[29] The incidence and prevalence increase progressively with age. There is a slight preponderance of females, and the disease occasionally runs in families.

Investigations of prevalence from different countries are rarely comparable in scope or methods, but the available data suggest that the disease is most common in England, Australia, France and Germany, less common in the United States, quite rare in Scandinavian and Mediterranean countries, very rare in Africa, and almost unknown in India and the Far East.

Histogenesis

The disease begins with a zone of increased osteoclastic and osteocytic resorption which slowly spreads out from its origin, extending along and across the bone, always

---

*Prevalence (the fraction of a population who have a disease at one moment in time) is a more appropriate statistic for a nonterminating disease than incidence (the fraction of a population who newly develop a disease in one year). All figures in the literature which purport to be estimates of incidence, are in reality estimates of prevalence.

maintaining a clear demarcation between adjacent, as yet uninvolved and apparently normal, bone and the advancing edge of resorption. This demarcation can be shown by radiographic and histologic examination.[6, 219] However, there is also a phase of pre-Paget bone, so that ahead of the advancing resorption front, the bone shows increased osteocyte death and periosteocytic osteolysis, and altered staining properties suggesting premature aging.[219]

Behind the advancing resorption front, separated in time and space to a varying degree, new woven bone of completely irregular structure is laid down. New woven bone is also formed under the periosteum, which enlarges by cellular proliferation to accommodate the expanding outer margin of the bone.[219] The newly formed bone is immature and structurally weak and is subject to very rapid turnover, with chaotic and randomly dispersed resorption and formation, either of which may predominate. There are numerous osteoid seams, but the appositional rate is normal.[247] Eventually, the characteristic mosaic pattern of irregular cement lines is produced.

Finally, after many years of activity, the disease may become quiescent in a particular part of the bone, usually well behind the advancing front, and the remaining abnormal bone is then gradually subjected to normal remodeling and replacement by normal lamellar bone. This does not alter the spatial disposition or size of the structurally abnormal trabeculae, so that there may be no change in the radiographic appearance. This quiescence may be purely local, the disease continuing to advance at the edge, or, alternatively, the entire disease process may cease. In principle, unless death supervenes, it is then possible for all of the diseased bone to be eventually converted to normal lamellar bone, but preserving the abnormal architecture.

These three phases are sometimes referred to as osteolytic, mixed, and sclerotic, on the basis of the radiographic appearances, but the occurrence of sclerosis in Paget's disease is determined by the cumulative effect of the relative balance between formation and resorption in the second phase of the disease, and transition between the second and third phases cannot be detected radiographically. Also, it must be remembered that, except in the very early and very late stages of the disease, all three phases are going on at the same time but in different places.

Clinical Features

Although virtually any bone in the body can be affected, and involvement can vary from a single bone to almost the entire skeleton, certain patterns are discernible. The most commonly affected sites are the spine, pelvis, skull, femora and tibia.

As already indicated, most patients are asymptomatic; in those who are not, pain due to the stress of weight bearing or muscle action on the involved bone is the dominant complaint as is evident from Paget's original description: "In its earlier periods, and sometimes through all its course, the disease is attended with pain in the affected bones, pains widely variant in severity and variously described as rheumatic, gouty or neuralgic, but not especially nocturnal or periodical."[298] These pains are commonest in the back, hips and lower extremities. It may be difficult to separate pain caused by Paget's disease from pain caused by associated osteoarthritis in the hips or spine. Although Paget's disease does not itself involve joints, joint remodeling may be increased and osteoarthritis is very commonly associated.[115, 219]

There is some involvement of the spine in almost all patients with the disease: "The spine, whether by yielding to the weight of the overgrown skull, or by changes in its own structure, may sink and seem shorter with greatly increased dorsal and lumbar curves."[298] The dorsal kyphosis and enlarged skull, together with lateral and anterior bowing of both femora and both tibiae, comprise the classical appearance of advanced Paget's disease. In one of the earliest accounts of Paget's disease in the United States, four of six cases conformed exactly to this description.[194] Today, this clinical picture is rare; possibly it is not really less common but simply diluted by the much larger number of patients who previously escaped detection.

The complications of Paget's disease will be described very briefly. Deafness is a common symptom due either to eighth nerve compression or, occasionally, to Paget's disease of the ossicles. It has often been claimed that urinary tract stones are common in Paget's disease, but convincing evidence for this is lacking.[29] The skin over involved bone in the extremities is usually warm, and both bone and skin show greatly increased blood flow, occasionally leading to high output cardiac failure. Fractures through involved bone are quite common but usually heal normally. Very rarely, immobilization for fracture or for other reasons may lead to serious hypercalcemia.[6] The most serious complication is osteogenic sarcoma, which is about 30 times more common than in the general population. Nevertheless, it only occurs in 1 to 5 per cent of cases.[29, 115] A rapid increase in swelling and intractable pain are the usual symptoms. The risk of sarcoma is high in the humerus, which is rarely affected by Paget's disease, and low in the spine, which is commonly affected. The spine is the site of only about 3 per cent of Paget's sarcomas.[29]

Neurologic Effects of Paget's Disease

Occasionally, Paget's disease produces serious neurologic disability. This is most commonly caused by compression, either by the enlarged or collapsed vertebral bodies or by encroachment on intervertebral foramina. The role of ischemia of the spinal cord is still uncertain. Patients with spinal cord compression caused by Paget's disease usually have no significant involvement outside the spine and have rarely sought medical advice before the onset of neurologic symptoms.[8] Frequently, multiple adjacent vertebrae are involved and they may be fused, owing to ossification of the intervertebral disc by Pagetic bone, and often also by bony union of adjacent vertebral appendages. The risk of neurologic involvement is inversely related to the frequency with which the vertebrae are involved, being greatest in the cervical spine, where Paget's disease is least common, and least in the lumbar spine, where the disease is most common, the thoracic spine being intermediate in both respects.

The clinical effects naturally depend on the level of the disease. Paget's disease of the occiput may lead to basilar invagination[63, 420] with posterior fossa compression and distortion of the foramen magnum, cerebellar dysfunction, lower cranial nerve lesions, and mild upper cervical cord compression. In the cervical spine, cord compression has occurred in 11 of 40 reported cases; an especially serious situation arises from involvement of the axis,[322] which may produce spastic quadriplegia, usually fatal.[124] Cord compression is most commonly due to Paget's disease of the upper thoracic spine, where the diameter of the spinal canal is relatively smaller than elsewhere. Usually, weakness and numbness develop gradually in both legs at the same time, and there is no sharp sensory level, since compression is spread out over several vertebrae. As well as low back pain, these patients may have aching in the legs, and girdle pains possibly from narrowing of intervertebral foramina.[8] In about three fourths of the cases there has been a good response to laminectomy.[334]

Less commonly, cord compression develops suddenly as a result of collapse of a single vertebra.[350] The increased risk of cord compression caused by vertebral collapse in Paget's disease contrasts with the absence of this complication in the vertebral collapse of osteoporosis. The involved vertebra may be structurally weak even though it contains a greater than normal amount of bone, and when it collapses, the softened bone is squeezed out circumferentially. Nevertheless, vertebral fracture in Paget's disease most commonly does not produce any spinal cord involvement. True compression fractures are less common than mild vertebral wedging associated with osteophytosis.[107]

Paget's disease of the lumbar spine occasionally may cause compression of the cauda equina, a complication which has been reported in five cases.[179, 238] Even less commonly, root compression may arise from foraminal encroachment.[179] Finally, the sciatic nerve may be compressed between an enlarged ischium and lesser trochanter of the femur in external rotation or between the ilium and the piriformis muscle in internal rotation.[179] It must be emphasized that all these neurologic complications are rare and that if Paget's disease is unexpectedly discovered by x-rays done for backache or sciatic pain, it is most likely not the cause of the patient's symptoms.

Radiographic Appearances

These vary with the stage of the disease. A clearly defined osteolytic phase is best seen in the skull (osteoporosis circumscripta) and in the tibia or femur, where a **V**-shaped line may clearly divide normal bone from the advancing resorption front.

An osteolytic phase is only rarely seen in the spine but has been detected in the cervical vertebrae, where it may easily be confused with metastatic disease.

Once woven bone replacement has begun, the x-rays show replacement of cortical bone by striated cancellous type bone with greatly thickened but more widely spaced trabeculae, and irregularly distributed zones of increased and reduced density. There is always expansion of the outline of the bone. A frequent finding in the femora and tibiae are horizontal fissure fractures, often multiple, which extend inwards at right angles to the cortex, especially on the convexity of the involved bone (Fig. 13–62). The fractures bear a superficial resemblance to Looser zones,[10] and heal slowly with little callus formation.

In the vertebrae the cortex is thickened and more dense, especially on the inferior and superior aspects. The appearance may be likened to a picture frame which is filled with coarse and irregular vertical striations (Fig. 13–63). Depending on the balance of formation and resorption, varying degrees of sclerosis may be seen, the most extreme resulting in a so-called ivory vertebra, often an isolated abnormality. Differentiation of Paget's disease

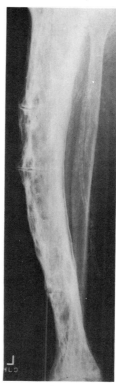

Figure 13–62. Tibia from a man aged 71 with Paget's disease. Note irregular structure, bowing, fissure fractures at right angles of long axis, and vascular calcification.

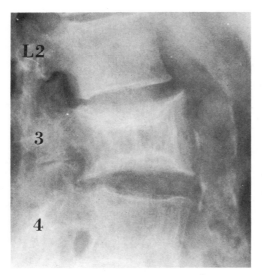

Figure 13–63. Vertebrae from a woman aged 55 with Paget's disease. Note enlargement of L3 with picture-frame appearance. Aortic calcification is also present.

from osteoblastic metastases from prostatic carcinoma may be difficult, but in the latter condition the external size of the vertebra is usually not increased and the vertebral appendages are less often involved.

Laboratory Findings

The most characteristic abnormality is elevation of the serum alkaline phosphatase, which roughly reflects the extent of woven bone osteoblastic activity. Change in alkaline phosphatase is only occasionally of value in detecting the onset of osteogenic sarcoma.[414] Occasionally, the acid phosphatase is also raised, but less so than in prostatic carcinoma with osseous metastases. The urinary total hydroxyproline is also raised, both dialyzable and nondialyzable fractions. Except with immobilization, the plasma calcium is usually normal; a rise is likely to be due to associated primary hyperparathyroidism.

Both alkaline phosphatase and urinary total hydroxyproline correlate fairly well with radiokinetic estimations of bone turnover and provide a convenient method of estimating the activity of the disease process. This is especially useful in following the response to treatment, and in the third phase of the disease, in which activity may subside and even cease altogether, with persistence of gross radiographic changes.

Differential Diagnosis

The diagnosis of Paget's disease is usually obvious. However, the skull findings in osteitis fibrosa and Paget's disease may be indistinguishable. The histologic resemblances and differences between these diseases were discussed on pp. 624 to 626, and it is wise to rule out hyperparathyroidism in all doubtful cases. The spinal changes may be difficult to differentiate from osteosclerotic metastases from carcinoma of the prostate or breast, which should be ruled out at least by physical examination in all cases. Single or multiple sclerotic vertebrae may be produced by a variety of other diseases which are considered in a subsequent section.

Medical Treatment[173, 415]

Until recently, there was no effective treatment for Paget's disease, but there now is a multiplicity of agents which are at least temporarily effective. All are still classified by the FDA as investigational drugs, either completely or specifically for use in the treatment of Paget's disease. The long-term beneficial effects are still unknown, and previous experience with corticosteroids, in which the adverse effects on normal bone greatly outweighed the beneficial effects on the disease, suggests a cautious approach to these newer agents. Although suppression of disease activity and symptomatic relief are readily achieved, evidence that structural improvement occurs in the bone is limited. Some published radiographs which purport to demonstrate improvement, to us merely indicate the natural progress of the disease with increasing sclerosis; however, in a few patients convincing improvement has been obtained. The available histologic evidence for improvement is suspect, since an iliac crest biopsy produces a marked and prolonged disturbance in remodeling of the adjacent bone, irrespective of the effects of any treatment. There is no indication at present for prophylactic therapy in asymptomatic patients, so that most patients with Paget's disease need no treatment. Nevertheless, there are undoubtedly many patients who get sufficient short-term improvement in their symptoms to make treatment worthwhile. Of the available agents, calcitonin appears to us to be the safest and most suitable for general use, but we will also describe briefly the possible alternatives.

AVAILABLE MEDICATIONS

Phosphate. Supplemental phosphate, one to two grams daily, has produced a fall in kinetically determined bone turnover and a reduction in cardiac output in Paget's disease. However, in our view, the unpredictability of the response, the possibility of soft tissue calcification (to which patients with Paget's disease are already prone (Fig. 13–62), and the unpalatability of most available preparations preclude its long-term use in this disease.

Fluoride. Although suppression of disease activity and symptoms is well documented, the response is slow and may not be maximal for at least one year, and does not occur in all patients. Since fluoride may produce exostoses and ligamentous calcification, it should not be used in patients with involvement of the spine or the occiput. In view of the availability of other agents which appear to be more effective, there is now little place for fluoride in the treatment of Paget's disease, except possibly in patients who become refractory to calcitonin.

Mithramycin. This is a cytotoxic agent which appears to be selectively active against osteoclast precursors. It is highly effective in suppressing the activity of the disease, is rapid in onset, and has produced remission of symptoms for up to several years. Nevertheless, the potential seriousness of the side effects, which include thrombocytopenia, elevation of liver enzymes, and uremia, make it unsuitable in our view for general use, even though these effects may be reversible and with very close monitoring permanent toxicity has apparently so far been avoided in the treatment of Paget's disease.

Diphosphonates. These are synthetic analogues of pyrophosphate which are resistant to hydrolysis by pyrophosphatase. They are thought to act by stabilizing the bone crystals and making them less subject to resorption, but their action is probably much more complex. Although the initial biochemical and clinical responses in a few patients have been impressive, too little is yet known of the long-term effects of these agents on normal bone and on mineral physiology generally to recommend their widespread use.

Calcitonin. This agent acts by inhibiting the proliferation of osteoclast precursors and also, at least acutely, by suppressing the resorptive activity of existing osteoclasts. Its main disadvantage is the need for parenteral administration, usually by daily intramuscular injection, although possibly thrice-weekly or even weekly injections would be just as effective. Although transient hypocalcemia may follow each injection, this usually does not lead to parathyroid hyperplasia, at least as judged by the parathyroid secretory response to induced hypocalcemia. Porcine, salmon and human calcitonin have all been successfully used, but the first two may be complicated by the development of antibodies and so become ineffective. Apart from an increase in urinary sediment which could have resulted from the diluent, no significant toxic effects have been encountered. This is not unexpected, since calcitonin is normally present in the body and the enormously high levels found in medullary carcinoma of the thyroid appear to have no harmful effects.

INDICATIONS FOR TREATMENT

Bone Pain. This may be adequately relieved by aspirin or phenylbutazone, but if not, treatment with calcitonin may be tried if the pain is disabling. If, as commonly occurs, it is difficult to decide whether the pain is due to Paget's disease or to associated osteoarthritis, the patient should be warned that no benefit may occur, and if no relief has been obtained within three months, it is unlikely that further treatment will be helpful.

Immobilization. If a patient with Paget's disease requires surgical treatment for fracture or correction of deformity, hypercalciuria and hypercalcemia may develop and lead to nephrolithiasis and renal insufficiency. In this situation, the short-term use of calcitonin has been recommended; probably, phosphate supplements would be equally effective.

Neurologic Symptoms. If the integrity of the spinal cord or cauda equina is threatened and surgical intervention is for any reason impractical, medical treatment should be instituted. Although mithramycin might seem to be the drug of choice in this situation because of its rapid onset of action, surprisingly rapid improvement, especially in sensory deficit, has occurred with calcitonin. Significant improvement in auditory acuity has also been documented. The mechanism of action of this response is unclear; it seems unlikely to be due to a reduction in size of the involved bone within a few weeks or months, and may reflect reduction in vascularity and edema of adjacent soft tissues.

Cardiac Failure. Calcitonin may produce a significant reduction in skin temperature over the affected bones and fall in cardiac output, which would be beneficial if heart failure had supervened.

Deformity. There is no evidence that existing deformity can be affected by treatment, or even that development of deformity in the future may be forestalled. There is a limited amount of evidence that long-term suppression of the disease activity by calcitonin may be followed by the laying down of normal lamellar bone in place of woven bone,[415] which gives some hope that long-term treatment with calcitonin may significantly modify the course of the disease.

DISEASE CHARACTERIZED BY OSTEOSCLEROSIS

Although a reduction in bone mineral content and increased radiolucency is the usual finding in metabolic bone disease, occasionally the opposite situation is found. This is referred to as osteosclerosis, although dense bones are not always physically harder or stronger than normal.

Osteosclerosis arises in two principal ways. During growth, the normal processes of resorption which occur during modeling may be so retarded that they fail to keep pace with the rate of growth. Histologically there may be immature bone persisting beyond its normal life span, and radiographically there may be characteristic changes in the external shape of the bones. The alkaline phosphatase is usually normal for the patient's age. Such a defect may be generalized, or may occur only in certain bones; there is no good evidence that excess calcitonin is involved. Second, there may be abnormal formation and accumulation of woven bone, which for obvious reasons can only take place in the marrow cavity. During the active phase of this process the alkaline phosphatase is usually raised, as normally happens with increased woven bone osteoblastic activity. Although hypermineralization of periosteocytic bone and plugging of haversian canals may lead to locally increased density which can be detected by microradiography, the increase is too small to produce radiographically detectable osteosclerosis.

Many causes of osteosclerosis do not properly fall within the scope of metabolic bone disease. Nevertheless, even in situations such as metastatic malignancy there is probably some biochemical stimulus to abnormal bone cell behavior. The same general principle operates as with osteolytic metastases—the response of the bone is directly mediated by normal bone cells, not by the invading cells.

Osteopetrosis

This is characterized by a generalized increase in bone density which begins during growth. Genetically there are at least two different forms, which probably have a different pathogenesis. The classical form is characterized by autosomal recessive inheritance, early onset, anemia, cranial nerve compression, and poor prognosis. The more recently recognized tarda form is characterized by autosomal dominant inheritance, late onset, little disability, and normal life expectancy. Both types show considerable variability in severity, which had led some workers to propose still further subdivision.[221]

CLASSICAL OSTEOPETROSIS (ALBERS-SCHOENBERG DISEASE). There is a generalized defect of bone resorption, owing to a marked depression of the linear resorption rate. This leads to persistence of the primary spongiosa in the marrow cavity, defective transverse tubulation of the long bones, owing to failure of endosteal resorptive remodeling, defective longitudinal tubulation with trumpeting of the metaphyses, owing to failure of periosteal resorptive modeling, and failure of cranial foramina to enlarge at a normal rate. Within the cortex there is normal formation of circumferential lamellae and primary and secondary haversian systems made of normal lamellar bone, but there is diminished turnover, with reduction in the appositional rate as well as in the linear resorption rate, and fewer resorption spaces.[143, 333]

Radiographic Findings in the Spine. There are increased density and marked widening of the end plate, visible at an early age (Fig. 13–64). In older children there may be exaggerated waisting of the vertebral bodies, the so-called spool-shaped vertebrae, but otherwise little abnormality in shape, since the normal changes depend on continued periosteal apposition rather than periosteal resorptive modeling. Consequently, there are usually no clinical findings directly related to the spine. In later life, the centra may be less dense, producing horizontal stripes resembling those of renal osteodystrophy (Fig. 13–65), but in more severe cases the vertebral bodies may be uniformly dense.

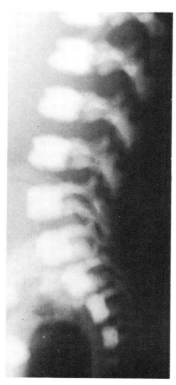

Figure 13–64. Spine from a patient aged six months with osteopetrosis. Note generalized increase in density with widening of the end plates.

to proptosis, mental retardation and convulsive seizures.

The hematologic manifestations result from encroachment on the marrow space leading to a leukoerythroblastic anemia with extramedullary hematopoiesis, with enlargement of the spleen, liver and, sometimes, lymph nodes. In many cases there is a significant or even dominant hemolytic component to the anemia, which may benefit from corticosteroid therapy or splenectomy.

The prognosis is poor; most patients die before the age of 20 from anemia, infection or raised intracranial pressure, but long survival is possible—patients still alive at 38 years and 57 years are on record.[95, 143]

Laboratory Findings. Apart from findings related to the anemia, laboratory findings are usually normal. Inevitably, there is an abnormally positive balance for calcium, owing to a marked reduction of both urinary and fecal calcium excretion. Attempts to induce calcium depletion by diet and cellulose phosphate, a divalent cation binding agent, have produced suggestive evidence of improvement in the radiographic appearances, but no long-term benefit has yet been documented. The occurrence of tetany on such a regimen is con-

Radiographic Findings in Other Bones. There is a generalized increase in density. In severe cases, this is uniform, with no distinction between cortex and lamellae, but in mild cases, some areas of lesser density may be discerned. There is failure of metaphyseal flaring, leading to progressive widening of the shaft, the Erlenmeyer flask deformity, or trumpeting. Occasionally, rachitic changes are seen at the growth plate. In some cases, alternating zones of lucent and dense bone suggest cyclical changes in the severity of the disease.[123]

Clinical Features. Positive clinical findings fall into three groups; orthopedic, neurologic, and hematologic. In the extremities there may be genu valgum, pectus deformities, increased liability to fracture, and sometimes the epiphyseal signs of rickets. The skull may show frontal bossing, and osteomyelitis of the mandible is common.

The neurologic manifestations result from failure of foramina to enlarge and, consequently, nerve compression leading to optic atrophy and blindness, deafness and facial palsy. Failure of the skull to enlarge may lead

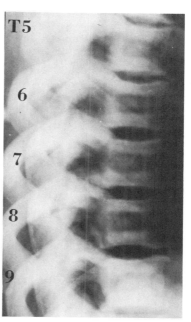

Figure 13–65. Spine from patient aged 37 with osteopetrosis showing end plate sclerosis and appearance resembling rugger-jersey spine of renal osteodystrophy.

sistent with failure of the bone cells to respond normally to parathyroid hormone,[97] but the renal tubular response to parathyroid hormone is normal.[339]

Diagnosis. In infancy there is essentially no differential diagnosis, but in survivors to adult life there may be a close resemblance to myelofibrosis, which can be most easily resolved by studying the family.

OSTEOPETROSIS TARDA.[221] This is usually discovered in late childhood or early adult life. In half of the cases there are no symptoms, and diagnosis is made accidentally or as a result of a family survey. In the remainder, there may be increased liability to fracture, occasionally resulting in deformity,[180] bone pain, osteomyelitis, and cranial nerve palsy. The radiographic findings are in general similar to the classic form, but are frequently less severe. The spine is more likely to show horizontal banding, and trumpeting of the metaphyses is less prominent because of the later age of onset. Mild cases may show longitudinal striation at the metaphyses resembling osteopathia striata.[199] In the pelvis and the extremities, and sometimes in the vertebrae, there may be a double cortical contour, the bone within a bone appearance. These findings are all symmetrical, a useful point in differential diagnosis. The laboratory findings pertaining to the bone are normal, with the exception of a raised acid phosphatase;[221] there is no anemia.

Histologic study shows persistence of the primary spongiosa, but the static evidence of remodeling seems normal. The bone may also be qualitatively abnormal, the osteons separating freely at the cement lines.

Response to exogenous parathyroid hormone is normal; whether this reflects a fundamental difference in pathogenesis from the infantile form or whether remodeling osteoclasts (predominant in the adult) respond differently from modeling osteoclasts (predominant in the child) in this disease is unclear.

Pyknodysostosis

This disease has only recently been delineated, but was diagnosed retrospectively in the painter Toulouse-Lautrec.[258] It combines some of the features of osteopetrosis and of cleidocranial dysostosis. In the spine there may be kyphoscoliosis, anomalous segmentation of the posterior elements of the vertebrae, end-plate thickening and sclerosis, and exaggerated anterior notching as in osteopetrosis.[116] The stature is short, primarily because of short extremities. There is increased liability to fracture, and most of the bones are dense. There is also separation of the cranial sutures, persistence of fontanelles, obtuseness of the mandibular angle and hypoplasia of the terminal phalanges. The basic defect is similar to that of osteopetrosis, but affects only modeling on the endosteal surface. There is failure of transverse tubulation, but normal longitudinal tubulation with no persistence of the primary spongiosa. There is no encroachment on the bone marrow. Haversian remodeling is virtually normal, except for a moderate depression of the radial resorption rate, but marked depression of both appositional rate and resorption rate are found on the cortical endosteal surface.[346]

Hyperostosis Corticalis Generalisata (Van Buchem's Disease)

This is characterized by late onset of increased density and increased size of affected bones due to irregular thickening and sclerosis of the cortex. In the spine, the appearance resembles osteopetrosis, but the spinous processes are more dense than the bodies of the vertebra, whereas the reverse is the case in osteopetrosis.[397]

The main bones affected are the skull, mandible, clavicles, ribs, and the diaphyses of the long bones. The earliest clinical manifestation is thickening and enlargement of the chin in early adolescence. Symptoms are usually few, but perceptive deafness, optic atrophy and facial palsy appear in some patients. The bone marrow is not involved and life expectancy is normal. Alkaline phosphatase is raised, and urinary total hydroxyproline is normal or slightly increased. Elevation of plasma calcitonin has been found in two cases.[398]

Osteofluorosis

This is a crippling disease resulting from prolonged ingestion of excess fluoride. It is endemic in certain areas of the world where there is a combination of a high content of fluoride in the natural water supply (4 ppm) and an increased consumption of water because of a hot and dry climate. Fluoride intake in tea and other foods grown in high fluoride soil is probably also important.[23, 359] The first reports of fluorosis in man referred to industrial exposure,[278] but this is now rare. Osteofluorosis is rare in the United States, but may occur in patients with abnormally high water intake due to diabetes insipidus or chronic renal failure.[228] Osteofluorosis may also complicate the osteodystrophy occurring during maintenance hemodialysis.

CLINICAL AND RADIOGRAPHIC FEATURES. Although there is generalized osteosclerosis, especially in the spine, the clinical effects result primarily from exostosis and ligamentous calcification. Usually it takes at least 20 years to develop significant clinical effects, but with extremely severe exposure the disease may begin in children. Spinal manifestations are then of progressive stiffness of the neck and back without pain; increasing kyphosis, progressing to generalized flexion and eventually complete fixation of the spine. This fixation is caused by ossification or calcification of the interspinous and longitudinal ligaments and the capsules of the apophyseal joints, and exostoses especially at sites of muscle and tendon attachment.[358] Radiographic evidence of secondary hyperparathyroidism may be seen at any age but especially in children.[388]

In adults the symptoms are similar, with stiffness of the back and neck, but the orthopedic manifestations are generally less severe, although kyphosis, increasing hip and knee flexions and fixation of the thoracic cage are common. Severe crippling occurs in about one fifth of the cases, and in about one case in 10 the clinical findings are dominated by a progressive radiculomyelopathy,[357] with weakness of the legs and spasticity due to spinal cord and root compression by osteophytes, exostoses and calcified ligaments. The anteroposterior diameter of the spine may be reduced in places to as little as 3 mm. The general appearance and effects are similar to those described for adults with familial hypophosphatemic vitamin D refractory rickets (p. 680), but are much more severe. The same diseases must be considered in the differential diagnosis (p. 679).

In epidemiological surveys, useful signs are the presence of dental fluorosis and ossification of the interosseous membrane in the forearm.[222]

LABORATORY FINDINGS. There are reduced urinary calcium and increased alkaline phosphatase and positive calcium balance.[376] There may be biochemical evidence of secondary hyperparathyroidism.

The histological features are complex, and the most complete description is based on iatrogenic osteofluorosis in patients with osteoporosis.[34] The bones are harder and more resistant to cutting and may show a yellow-brown discoloration due to a lipogenic pigment. Metaplastic woven bone is found in the medullary cavity, within the haversian canals, and also in tendons. Osteoid seams of moderate thickness (up to 20μ) are much more frequent on periosteal, haversian and endosteal surfaces.[118] The accumulation of seams is due partly to a reduction in the appositional rate and partly to the increased duration of the remodeling cycle. The extent of resorption is decreased on the periosteal surface and increased in Haversian systems.[118] Many small resorption spaces switch over to formation before they are fully completed.

The bone is of poor physical quality, with wider cement lines, more degenerating osteocytes and empty lacunae, increased areas of hypermineralization and more microfractures: paradoxically there also may be areas of increased periosteocytic low density bone, possibly due to secondary hyperparathyroidism. In contrast to osteopetrosis there is no increased liability to overt fracture, possibly because the patients are so disabled that they do not encounter the normal trauma of daily life.

Miscellaneous Causes of Osteosclerosis

Osteosclerosis occurring in renal osteodystrophy, primary hyperparathyroidism and Paget's disease has already been mentioned. These conditions should give rise to no diagnostic problems but should always be ruled out when vertebral osteosclerosis is discovered accidentally during some unrelated radiographic procedure.

Other conditions which need to be considered in the differential diagnosis are myelosclerosis,[249] mastocytosis,[183] lymphoma, myeloma, metastatic malignancy and heavy-metal poisoning. There are also many other known causes of osteosclerosis which have been omitted because they do not affect the vertebrae. In myelosclerosis, massive splenomegaly is usual, with other signs of extramedullary hematopoiesis, and there is no family history. In the neoplastic conditions there may be spinal cord compression. This may also occur in Paget's disease, fluorosis, fibrous dysplasia, osteoclastoma, and in adults with familial hypophosphatemia, but not in osteopetrosis or in osteosclerosis complicating other metabolic bone disease. In myelomatosis, either diffuse or localized osteosclerosis may occur in contrast to the usual finding of primarily osteolytic lesions.[80] Even with osteosclerosis the alkaline phosphatase is usually normal in myelomatosis; this is virtually the only situation in which increased woven bone formation is accompanied by a normal instead of a raised alkaline phosphatase.

MISCELLANEOUS METABOLIC OR PARAMETABOLIC CONDITIONS

Here we consider a heterogeneous collection of disorders in which there is some metabolic abnormality or which may need to be considered in the differential diagnosis of metabolic bone disease proper.

Fibrous Dysplasia

In this condition there is localized proliferation of primitive mesenchymal cells within the medullary canal, leading to osteoclastic destruction and replacement of bone by fibrous tissue. Fibrous dysplasia was first differentiated from osteitis fibrosa cystica by Hunter and Turnbull in 1932,[204] and termed osteitis fibrosa disseminata by Albright.

The histological findings resemble the brown tumors of osteitis fibrosa cystica, but there may be islands of cartilage within the lesions. Both monostotic and polyostotic forms are described, but there is probably no fundamental difference between them since both forms may occur in the same family.[126]

The symptoms are local pain, deformity due to expansion of the lesion outside the boundary of the bone and pathologic fractures. The lesions enlarge rapidly during childhood and usually stop growing at skeletal maturity. In one series only 5 of 24 patients showed any progression after followup of as long as 30 years.

The spine is only rarely involved, but large cystic lesions in the lumbar spine[174] and sclerotic lesions in the cervical spine[77] have

been described, and sometimes spinal cord compression may result.[387] In one extraordinary case there was extensive spinal involvement with severe kyphoscoliosis.[59] The most common other sites are the ends of the long bones (Shepherd's-crook deformity of the upper femora), occiput, facial bones and pelvis. Multiple lesions may increase the bone circulation sufficiently to produce high output cardiac failure as in Paget's disease. About one case in 20 of polyostotic fibrous dysplasia shows the special features of Albright's syndrome, in which the lesions are unilateral, accompanied by a characteristic irregularly shaped (coast of Maine) pigmentation on the same side as the lesions, and precocious puberty leading to premature epiphyseal fusion and short stature.[6] More commonly, a variety of other endocrinopathies may be associated, for which a hypothalamic origin has been suggested. These include hyperthyroidism, acromegaly or gigantism, diabetes, and primary hyperparathyroidism. This last, occurring in 6 of 80 cases in three large series,[117] is of particular interest. The lesions of fibrous dysplasia are apparently unaffected by parathyroid hormone, neither progressing more rapidly than normal nor regressing after successful parathyroid surgery.

Except for associated hyperparathyroidism, the plasma calcium and phosphorus are normal. The alkaline phosphatase may be raised and urinary total and peptide-bound hydroxyproline may be increased with extensive disease.[42]

Usually no treatment is feasible, but curettage of a cyst and filling with bone chips may be needed if a pathological fracture occurs. Irradiation is ineffective.[126]

Fibrogenesis Imperfecta Ossium

This condition is due to an acquired abnormality of bone collagen leading to replacement of normal bone by abnormal bone which fails to mineralize properly, producing severe disability. The disease was first identified in autopsy material,[24] and was subsequently diagnosed retrospectively in a patient first encountered in 1931; the details of this case have recently been published.[166] The disease was not recognized during life until much later,[25] and so far only six patients have been so diagnosed, five of them males. The onset is usually in the fifth decade, with increasingly severe pain and tenderness in the hips and back, aggravated by movement and weight-bearing, with increased liability to fracture, loss of height due to vertebral compression, and kyphosis. The pain eventually becomes so severe that the patient becomes bedridden and develops severe weakness and muscle wasting.

Skeletal radiographs show a generalized abnormality of trabecular bone, which is mottled, striated and coarse, with alternating areas of increased and decreased density and extreme thinning of the cortex (Figs. 13–66 and 13–67). There is a superficial resemblance to Paget's disease,[136] but every bone in the body is affected, and there is no expansion of the outline of the bone. Very similar radiographic appearances, but with normal bone collagen, have been observed in association with macroglobulinemia.[378] Laboratory findings include raised sedimentation rate, normal plasma calcium and phosphorus, raised alkaline phosphatase, and raised urinary total hydroxyproline.

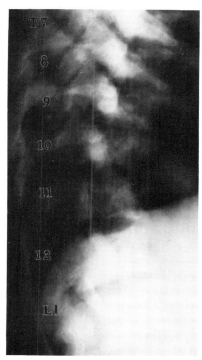

Figure 13–67. Spine from a patient aged 56 with fibrogenesis imperfecta ossium. Note coarse and irregular structure, somewhat resembling Paget's disease or osteitis fibrosa, but affecting every bone.

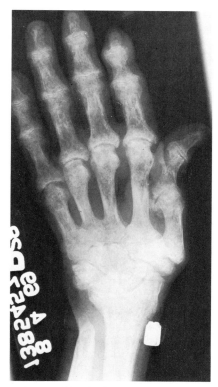

Figure 13–66. Hands from a patient aged 56 with fibrogenesis imperfecta ossium. Note extremely abnormal trabecular structure, cortical thinning and involvement of every bone.

Bone histology shows accumulation of unmineralized bone which, by ordinary microscopy without special stains, may be indistinguishable from normal osteoid, but in which the collagen in the matrix is abnormal in amount, quality and arrangement. Examination under polarized light shows an almost complete lack of normal birefringence; this is the cardinal finding required to establish the diagnosis, and does not occur in any other disease.[25] There is a marked reduction in the amount of collagen in the matrix; the collagen present is very immature and lacks normal crosslinking and is consequently abnormally soluble.[188] Finally, the collagen fibrils are randomly arranged, as in woven bone. Depending on the duration of the disease, islands of normal birefringent lamellar bone may persist, but they are surrounded by the abnormal material, with apparently sudden transition between the two. Although most of the abnormal bone is unmineralized, a feature which has suggested that the disease should be classified as a form of osteomalacia, mineralization is still possible, although it proceeds extremely slowly, and in some areas the abnormal bone may, in fact, be hypermineralized. This is made possible by the reduction in the amount of collagen, so leaving more room for mineral deposition.[25] The appositional rate in one case was reduced only to about 50 per cent of normal, and osteoid seams were greatly thickened, indicating a much greater uncoupling of mineralization and matrix synthesis rates than is normal in osteomalacia.[136] Many Haversian systems show seams extending right from the cement lines.

In some cases there may be a partial therapeutic response to vitamin D, with symptomatic improvement, increased mobility, increased thickening of the cortices and a fall in urinary total hydroxyproline to normal.[25, 136]

Axial Osteomalacia

This condition is characterized by a coarsening and spongelike appearance of trabecular bone in the axial skeleton, that is in the spine, pelvis and ribs.[142] Generally, the cervical spine is involved most severely and there is generalized flattening and wedging of the vertebrae. Again there may be a superficial resemblance to Paget's disease. Clinically, there may be slight ache in the neck, but symptoms are minimal and may be completely absent, and there is no progression even after many years.[85] Bone biopsy reveals wide osteoid seams up to 100μ thick, which are normally birefringent.[85] Remodeling dynamics show a three- to fivefold increase in the number of seams, with a proportionate increase in the number of resorption spaces, and an approximately 50 per cent reduction in appositional rate.[142] The findings are more suggestive of increased activation and turnover than of osteomalacia, so that the name may be somewhat inappropriate, but no alternative has been proposed. The laboratory findings are all normal. Five of six published cases have come from one institution, which suggests that awareness of this condition is not widespread.

Hereditary Hyperphosphatasia[122, 392]

This is a progressive, severe osteopathy beginning in early infancy, in which there are marked thickening of the bones, enlargement of the skull, symmetrical bowing of the tibiae, flaring of the ribs, shortness of stature, difficulty in walking, and high tone deafness. The spine may show kyphoscoliosis and shortening of the neck and exaggerated lumbar lordosis. The radiographic appearances are somewhat similar to Paget's disease, with enlargement, striation and coarsening of trabeculae. The vertebrae are radiolucent, and show increased biconcavity. Bone histology reveals extremely rapid turnover, with complete replacement of lamellar bone by woven bone in the cortex, but preservation of normal lamellar bone in the trabeculae.[217] The appositional rate may be increased twofold.[392] The high turnover is confirmed by laboratory findings of gross increases in urinary total hydroxyproline excretion of up to 100 mg per kg of body weight or almost 200 times the normal adult rate, and about 20 to 30 times the normal rate for growing children. This is accompanied by a disproportionate increase in the excretion of glycyl proline. The alkaline phosphatase is very high, and accretion as determined by strontium kinetics is also accelerated. Hyperuricemia and hyperuricosuria may also be found, probably due to the liberation of nucleic acids from the extremely high bone turnover, which is higher in this disease than in any other.

This disease has been described under many different names, such as familial osteoectasia, familial hyperostosis, hyperostosis corticalis juvenalis, and juvenile Paget's disease. Although there is a clinical radiographic and biochemical resemblance to Paget's disease, the involvement of every bone in the body and the envelope specific abnormality indicate that it must have a different pathogenesis. In one case, an excellent therapeutic response to human calcitonin was found.[417]

Hydroxylysine Deficient Collagen Disease

Although only two cases of this disease have been described, it is of great potential interest because it is the first time that a clear-cut biochemical abnormality has been identified in kyphoscoliosis. The disease in two siblings is characterized by severe kyphoscoliosis, joint dislocation and hyperextensibility of the skin, thin scars, a high arched palate and pectus excavatum, but without ectopia lentis or cardiovascular abnormalities.[240, 311] Clinically, the disease represents a combination of some features of the Ehlers-Danlos syndrome, and some of the Marfan syndrome. Both patients have a severe gibbus from T11 to L2.

The collagen in both skin and bone is deficient in hydroxylysine. Normally, lysine is incorporated into protocollagen and is then hydroxylated within the protocollagen molecule. In this disease, the enzyme which accomplishes this hydroxylation, namely lysyl protocollagen hydroxylase, is deficient. The abnormal collagen shows impaired crosslinking, and somewhat resembles that found in experimental lathyrism, in which scoliosis may also develop.

Kyphoscoliosis is a feature of both osteogenesis imperfecta and homocystinuria,[267] (described in relation to osteoporosis), Marfans syndrome and the Ehlers-Danlos syndrome,[37] but in all these conditions the bone deformity has been thought to result from ligamentous laxity and postural realignment, rather than from some abnormality of the bone itself.

The identification of a biochemical abnormality in collagen in a closely similar disease will undoubtedly prompt more detailed investigation of all these heritable disorders of connective tissue. Also, further biochemical study of idiopathic scoliosis might be profitable, since in this disease there appears to be a significant increase in total hydroxyproline excretion in both sexes between the ages of 11 and 18, and a still further increase produced by spinal traction or spinal fusion.[423]

Hypophosphatasia

This is a rare, genetically determined disease of which the principal features are impaired mineralization of bone and diminished alkaline phosphatase activity in the blood and tissues. The diagnosis is confirmed by demonstrating increased urinary excretion of phosphoethanolamine and pyrophosphate. Three clinical varieties have been described, classified according to the age of onset.[139, 257]

INFANTILE. The abnormality is present at birth or develops within six months, with failure to thrive, respiratory distress due to flail chest, poor growth, short extremities, rachitic deformities such as costochondral beading, and increased liability to fracture. Usually, the spine is not involved. Hypercalcemia, the cause of which is unexplained, is often present. Death usually occurs before one year of age. Differentiation from other, even rarer, causes of fatal, short-lived dwarfism, several of which have characteristic spi-

nal manifestations, may be important for genetic counseling.[203]

LATER CHILDHOOD. The disease is less severe, presenting with genu valgum and moderate growth impairment. Kyphosis may be noted in some cases. There may be premature loss of deciduous teeth and cranial synostosis. Spontaneous improvement in the severity of the disease may occur with the passage of time.

ADULT ONSET. The patient may present with stiffness and weakness of the back and pain in the back and extremities. There may be a history of repeated fractures and of mild rickets in childhood, possibly with residual stigmata of rachitic deformities. The spine may be abnormally straight, with loss of the thoracic curvature and prominence of the sternum.[43] In other cases, the thoracic curvature may be exaggerated and scoliosis may also be found. Paravertebral ligamentous calcification has been present in half the reported adult cases.[213] Various abnormalities in the shape of the vertebrae have been described. Some show relative vertical elongation and others relative anteroposterior elongation. In other bones there may be appearances resembling Looser zones, especially in the femur. Anterior femoral bowing is present in the majority of patients. The serum calcium is normal.

In some cases, the clinical and radiographic findings in the spine have resembled those of idiopathic osteoporosis, with wedging and compression and generalized reduction in density and increasing biconcavity of the porotic rather than the malacic type.[310] Bone remodeling dynamics show a normal appositional rate and turnover reduced by about 25 per cent.[310] Osteoid seams may be increased in number and thickness.[213]

In patients with a history of childhood rickets, Looser zones and paravertebral calcification, the clinical picture may closely resemble that of adults with familial hypophosphatemic vitamin D refractory rickets (q.v.).

ADDENDUM

Since this manuscript was completed a number of important advances have taken place.

1. A patient with vitamin D dependency was found to respond very well to an exceedingly small dose of 1,25 dihydroxy D_3, having needed much larger amounts of the parent

vitamin and of the 25 hydroxy derivatives.[139a] This finding strongly suggests that, at least in this patient, the disease was due to a defect in 1 hydroxylation of 25 hydroxy D_3 in the kidney, thus bringing the condition into line with other examples of specific enzyme deficiency.

2. The beneficial effect of estrogens in slowing down the development of postmenopausal osteoporosis has now been documented in an adequately controlled study.[1a] The effects were greatest when begun soon after the menopause, and if treatment was delayed for more than ten years no benefit could be demonstrated. In some patients an actual increase in bone mineral content was claimed.

3. Convincing evidence has been given of radiographic improvement of Paget's disease treated with human calcitonin.[112a] The external diameter of affected bones may diminish and the bone structure rendered more normal. Of special interest is that an increase in net resorption on the periosteal envelope could be produced by an agent whose major effect is usually thought to be suppression of bone resorption. One possible explanation is that there are two populations of mesenchymal precursor cells. Proliferation of the abnormal cells is suppressed by calcitonin, thus allowing the normal cells and their derivatives to produce normal remodeling of the abnormal bone.

Collections*

A. Calcium Metabolism and Metabolic Bone Disease. I. Macintyre (ed.), Clinics in Endocrinology and Metabolism, *1*(1)1–328, 1972.

B. Clinical Aspects of Metabolic Bone Disease. B. Frame, A. M. Parfitt and H. Duncan (eds.). Amsterdam, Excerpta Medica, 1973, ICS #270.

C. Drug Treatment of Bone. S. Wallach (ed.). Seminars in Drug Treatment. *2*(1)1–146, 1972.

D. Osteoporosis. U. S. Barzel, (ed.). New York, Grune and Stratton, 1970.

E. Symposium on Metabolic Bone Disease. J. C. Hohl (ed.). Ortho. Clin. N. Amer. *3*(3)501–792, 1972.

F. The Biochemistry and Physiology of Bone. 2nd Edition, G. H. Bourne (ed.). New York, Academic Press, 1972.

---

* Throughout the numbered references in this chapter these publications will be referred to by letter; e.g., 14. Arnaud, C. D. . . . *B*, 281–290.

References

1. Adams, P., Davies, G. T., and Sweetnam, P.: Osteoporosis and the effects of aging on bone mass in elderly men and women. Quart. J. Med. *39*:601–615, 1970.

1a. Aitken, J. M., Hart, O. M., and Lindsay, R.: Oestrogen replacement therapy for prevention of osteoporosis after oophorectomy. Brit. Med. J. *3*:515–518, 1973.

2. Aitken, R. E., Kerr, J. L., and Lloyd, H. M.: Primary hyperparathyroidism with osteosclerosis and calcification in articular cartilage. Amer. J. Med. *37*:813–820, 1964.

3. Albright, F., Aub, J. C. and Bauer, W.: Hyperparathyroidism: A common and polymorphic condition as illustrated by 17 proved cases from one clinic. J.A.M.A. *102*:1276–1287, 1934.

4. Albright, F., Smith, P. H. and Fraser, R.: A syndrome characterized by primary ovarian insufficiency and decreased stature. Amer. J. Med. Sci. *204*:625–648, 1942.

5. Albright, F.: A page out of the history of hyperparathyroidism. J. Clin. Endocr. *8*:637–657, 1948.

6. Albright, F., and Reifenstein, E. G.: The Parathyroid glands and Metabolic Bone Disease. Selected Studies. Baltimore, Williams & Wilkins Co., 1948.

7. Albright, J. A., and Grant, J. D.: Studies of patients with osteogenesis imperfecta. J. Bone Joint Surg. *53A*:1415–1425, 1971.

8. Aldren-Turner, J. W.: The spinal complication of Paget's disease. Brain *63*:321–349, 1940.

9. Ali, S. Y., Sajdera, S. W., and Anderson, H. C.: Isolation and characterization of calcifying matrix vesicles from epiphyseal cartilage. Proc. Nat. Acad. Sci. *67*:1513–1520, 1970.

10. Allen, M. L., and John, R. L.: Osteitis deformans (Paget's disease). Fissure fractures—their etiology and clinical significance. Radiology *38*:109–115, 1937.

11. Ardran, G. M.: Bone loss not demonstrable by radiography. Brit. J. Radiol. *4*:107–109, 1951.

12. Armstutz, H. C., and Sissons, H. A.: The structure of the vertebral spongiosa. J. Bone Joint Surg. *51B*:540–550, 1969.

13. Arnaud, C., Maijer, R., Reade, T., Scriver, C. D., and Whelan, D. T.: Vitamin D dependency: an inherited postnatal syndrome with secondary hyperparathyroidism. Pediatrics *46*:871–879, 1970.

14. Arnaud, C. D., Goldsmith, R. S., Sizemore, G. W., Oldham, J. W., Bischoff, J., Larsen, J. A., and Bordier, P.: Studies in characterizations of human parathyroid hormone and hyperparathyroid serum—practical considerations. *B*, 281–290.

15. Arnold, J. S., Frost, H. M., and Buss, R. O.: The osteocyte as a bone pump. Clin. Orthop. *78*:47–55, 1971.

16. Arnold, J. S., Bartley, M. H., Tont, S. A., and Jenkins, D. P.: Skeletal changes in aging and disease. Clin. Orthop. *49*:17–38, 1966.

17. Arnstein, A. R.: Regional osteoporosis. *E*, 585–600.

18. Arnstein, A. R., Frame, B., and Frost, H. M.: Recent progress in osteomalacia and rickets. Ann. Int. Med. *67*:1296–1330, 1967.

19. Atkinson, P. J., Weatherell, J. A., and Weidman, S. M.: Changes in density of the human femoral cor-

tex with age. J. Bone Joint Surg. *44B*:496–502, 1962.

20. Avioli, L. V., McDonald, J. E., and Lee, S. W.: The influence of age on the intestinal absorption of [47]Ca in women and its relation to [47]Ca absorption in postmenopausal osteoporosis. J. Clin. Invest. 44:1960–1967, 1965.

21. Avioli, L., and Haddad, J. G.: Vitamin D: Current Concepts. Metabolism 22:507–531, 1973.

22. Avioli, L. V.: Intestinal absorption of calcium. J.A.M.A. *219*:345–355, 1972.

23. Azar, H. A., Wucho, C. K., Bayyuk, S. I., and Bayyuk, W. B.: Skeletal sclerosis due to chronic fluoride intoxication. Cases from an endemic area of fluorosis in the region of the Persian Gulf. Ann. Int. Med. *55*:193–200, 1964.

24. Baker, S. L.: Fibrogenesis imperfecta ossium. J. Bone Joint Surg. *38B*:378–417, 1956.

25. Baker, S. L., Dent, C. E., Friedman, M., and Watson, L.: Fibrogenesis imperfecta ossium. J. Bone Joint Surg. *48B*:804–825, 1966.

26. Ballin, M.: Parathyroidism in reference to orthopaedic surgery. J. Bone Joint Surg. *15*:120, 1933.

27. Balsan, S., Guivarch, J., Dartois, A. M., and Royer, P.: Rachitisme Vitamino-resistant associe a une Neurofibromatose probable chez un Enfant. Arch. Franc. Pediat. *24*:609–632, 1967.

28. Barnett, E., and Nordin, B. E. C.: The radiologic diagnosis of osteoporosis. A new approach. Clin. Radiol. *11*:166–174, 1962.

29. Barry, H. C.: Paget's Disease of Bone. London, Livingstone, 1969.

30. Bartter, F. C.: Bone as a target organ: toward a better definition of osteoporosis. Perspect. Biol. Med. *16*:215–231, 1973.

31. Barzel, U. S.: The skeleton, the parathyroid hormone and acid base metabolism. *B*, 346–353.

32. Baud, C. A.: Submicroscopic structure and functional aspects of the osteocyte. Clin. Orthop. *56*:227–236, 1968.

33. Bauer, W.: Hyperparathyroidism: A distinct disease entity. J. Bone Joint Surg. *15A*:135–141, 1933.

34. Baylink, D. J., and Bernstein, D. S.: Effects of fluoride therapy in metabolic bone disease—a histologic study. Clin Orthop. *55*:51–85, 1967.

35. Baylink, D. J., and Wergedal, J. E.: Bone formation by osteocytes. Amer. J. Phys. *221*:669–678, 1971.

36. Baylink, D., Stauffer, M., Wergedal, J., and Rich, C.: Formation, mineralization and resorption of bone in vitamin D deficient rats. J. Clin. Invest. *49*:1122–1134, 1970.

37. Beighton, P., and Moran, H.: Orthopaedic aspects of the Ehlers-Danlos syndrome. J. Bone Joint Surg. *51B*:444–453, 1969.

38. Belanger, L. F.: Osteocytic osteolysis. Calc. Tiss. Res. *4*:1–12, 1969.

39. Bell, G. H., Dunbar, O., and Beck, J. S.: Variations in strength of vertebrae with age and their relation to osteoporosis. Calc. Tiss. Res. *1*:75–86, 1967.

40. Bergofsky, F. H., Turner, G. M., and Fishman, A. P.: Cardiorespiratory failure in kyphoscoliosis. Medicine *38*:263–317, 1959.

41. Bernstein, D. S., Sadowsky, N., Hegsted, D. M., Gari, C. D., and Stone, F. D.: Prevalence of osteoporosis in high- and low-fluoride areas in North Dakota. J.A.M.A. *198*:499–504, 1966.

42. Berry, H. K., Silverman, F. N., and Marnell, R. T.: Polyostotic fibrous dysplasia associated with collagen peptiduria. *B*, 478–483.

43. Bethune, J. E., and Dent, C. E.: Hypophosphatasia in the adult. Amer. J. Med. *28*:615–621, 1960.

44. Bhandarkar, S. D., and Nordin, B. E. C.: Effect of low-calcium diet on urinary calcium in osteoporosis. Brit. Med. J. *5272*:145–147, 1962.

45. Bick, E. M., and Copel, J. W.: Fractures of vertebrae in the aged. Geriatrics *5*:74–81, 1950.

46. Bijvoet, O. L. M., and Van der Sluys Veer, J.: The interpretation of laboratory tests in bone disease. *A*, 217–238.

47. Biltz, R. M. and Pellegrino, E. D.: The chemical anatomy of bone. J. Bone Joint Surg. *51A*:456–466, 1969.

48. Birge, S. J., Keutmann, H. T., Cuatnercasos, P., and Whedon, G. D.: Osteoporosis, intestinal lactase deficiency and low dietary calcium intake. New Eng. J. Med. *276*:445–448, 1967.

49. Birtwell, W. M., Magsanen, B. F., Fenn, P. A., Torg, J. S., Tourtellotte, C. D., and Martin, J. H.: An unusual hereditary osteomalacic disease—pseudo-vitamin D deficiency. J. Bone Joint Surg. *52A*:1222–1228, 1970.

50. Black, J. R., Ghormley, R. K., and Camp, J. D.: Senile osteoporosis of the spinal column. J.A.M.A. *117*:2144–2150, 1941.

51. Blumcke, S., and Niedorf, H. R.: Histochemical and fine structural studies on the cornea with osteogenesis imperfecta congenita. Virchows Arch. Abt. B Zellpath. *11*:124–132, 1972.

52. Bollet, A. J.: Epidemiology of osteoporosis. Arch. Intern. Med. *116*:191, 1965.

53. Bonucci, E., Denis-Matrajt, H., Tun Chot, S., and Hioco, D. M.: Bone structure in osteomalacia with special reference to ultrastructure. J. Bone Joint Surg. *51B*:511–528, 1969.

54. Bonucci, E.: The locus of initial calcification. Clin. Orthop. *78*:108, 1971.

55. Bordier, P. J., and Tun Chot, S.: Quantitative histology of metabolic bone disease. *A*, 197–216.

56. Bostrom, H., Edgren, B., Nilsonne, U., and Wester, P. O.: Metabolic and orthopedic treatment of a case of adult nonfamilial hypophosphatemia with severe osteomalacia. Acta Orthop. Scand. *39*:238–260, 1968.

57. Boukhris, R. and Becker, K. L.: Calcification of the aorta and osteoporosis. J.A.M.A. *219*:1307–1311, 1972.

58. Boyde, A.: Scanning electron microscope studies of bone. *F*, Vol. I:259–310.

59. Bradfield, E. W. C.: A case of generalized fibrocystic disease of the bones. Brit. J. Surg. *19*:192–202, 1930.

60. Brandner, M. W.: Normal values of the vertebral body and intervertebral disc index in adults. Amer. J. Roent. *114*:411–415, 1972.

61. Brickman, A. S., Coburn, J. W., and Norman, A. W.: Action of 1,25-dihydroxycholecalciferol, a potent kidney-produced metabolite of vitamin D_3, in uremic man. New Eng. J. Med. *287*:891–895, 1972.

62. Bromley, R. G., Dockstern, N. L., Arnold, J. S., and Lee, W. S. S.: Quantitative histological study of human lumbar vertebrae. J. Geriat. *21*:537–543, 1966.

63. Bull, J. W. D., Nixon, W. L. B., Pratt, R. T. C., and Robinson, P. K.: Paget's disease of the skull and

secondary basilar impression. Brain *32*:10–22, 1959.

64. Bullamore, J. R., Wilkinson, R., Gallagher, J. C., and Nordin, B. E. C.: Effect of age on calcium absorption. Lancet, 2:535–537, 1970.

65. Burkholder, P. K., DuBoff, E. A. and Felmanowicz, E. V.: Nontropical sprue with secondary hyperparathyroidism. Amer. J. Dig. Dis. *10*:75–83, 1965.

66. Burrows, H. J., and Graham, G.: Spinal osteoporosis of unknown origin. Quart. J. Med. *14*:147–1945.

67. Bywaters, E. G. L., Dixon, A. St. J., and Scott, J. T.: Joint lesions of hyperparathyroidism. Ann. Rheum. Dis. *22*:171–187, 1963.

68. Caffey, J.: Pediatric X-ray diagnosis. Fifth Edition, Chicago, Year Book Medical Publishers, 1967.

69. Caldwell, R. A.: Observation in the incidence, etiology and pathology of senile osteoporosis. J. Clin. Path. *15*:421–431, 1962.

70. Cameron, D. A.: The ultrastructure of bone. *F*, Vol. 1: 191–236.

71. Camp, J. D.: Osseous changes in hyperparathyroidism. J.A.M.A. *99*:1913–1917, 1932.

72. Caniggia, A., Gennari, G., Bornello, G., Bencini, M., Cesari, L., Poggi, C., and Escabar, S.: Intestinal absorption of calcium-47 after treatment with oral oestrogen-gestogens in senile osteoporosis. Brit. Med. J. *4*:30–31, 1970.

73. Caniggia, A., Gennari, G., Piantelli, F., and Vattimo, A.: Initial increase of plasma radioactive calcium after intravenous injection of calcitonin in man. Clin. Sci. *43*:17–180, 1972.

74. Carstairs, L. S.: Radiology *In* Nassim. R., and Burrows, H-J.: Modern trends in disease of the vertebral column. pp. 210–244, London, Butterworth, 1959.

75. Casuccio, C.: Concerning osteoporosis. J. Bone Joint Surg. *44B*:453–463, 1962.

76. Chalmers, J.: Osteomalacia. J. Roy. Coll. Surg. Edinb. *13*:255–275, 1968.

77. Charlton, W. S., and Cramer, E.: An unusual case of fibrous dysplasia of the skull and upper cervical part of the spine. Med. J. Aust. *50*(1):503–504, 1963.

78. Chesnut, C. M., Nelp, W. B., Denney, J. D., and Sherrard, D. J.: Measurement of total body calcium (bone mass) by neutron activation analysis: applicability to bone wasting disease. *B*, 50–54.

79. Chrisman, O. D., Snook, G. A., and Walker, H. R.: Paget's disease as a differential diagnosis in sciatica. Clin. Orthop. *37*:154–159, 1964.

80. Clarisse, P. D. and Staple, T. W.: Diffuse bone sclerosis in multiple myeloma. Radiology *99*:327–328, 1971.

81. Cloutier, M. D., Hayles, A. B., Riggs, B. L., Jowsey, J., and Bickel, W. H.: Juvenile osteoporosis: Report of a case including a description of some metabolic and microradiographic studies. Pediatrics *40*:649–655, 1967.

82. Cochran, M., and Nordin, B. E. C.: Role of acidosis in renal osteomalacia. Brit. Med. J. *2*:276–279, 1969.

83. Cohen, J., and Harris, W. H.: The three-dimensional anatomy of haversian systems. J. Bone Joint Surg. *40A*:419–434, 1958.

84. Collins, D. H.: Paget's disease of bone. Incidence and subclinical forms. Lancet *2*:51, 1956.

85. Condon, J. R., and Nassim, J. R.: Axial osteomalacia. Postgrad. Med. J. *47*:817–820, 1971.

86. Cooke, A. M.: Osteoporosis. Lancet *1*:877–936, 1955.

87. Cooper, R. R., Milgrim, J. W., and Robinson, R. A.: Morphology of the osteon. J. Bone Joint Surg. *48A*:1239, 1966.

88. Cotmore, J. M., Nichols, G., and Wuthier, R. E.: Phospholipid-calcium phosphate complex: Enhanced calcium migration in the presence of phosphate. Science *172*:1339–1341, 1971.

89. Cox, R. W., and Grand, R. A.: The structure of the collagen fibril. Clin. Orthop. *67*:172–187, 1969.

90. Cropp, G. J. A.: Hypermetabolism in osteogenesis imperfecta. *B*, 308–313.

91. Cuervo, L. A., Pita, J. C., and Howell, D. S.: Ultramicroanalysis of pH, P_{CO2} and carbonic anhydrase activity at calcifying sites in cartilage. Calc. Tiss. Res. *7*:220–231, 1971.

92. Curtiss, P. H., Clark, W. S., and Herndon, C. H.: Vertebral fractures resulting from prolonged cortisone and corticotropin therapy. J.A.M.A. *156*:467–469, 1954.

93. Davis, M. D., Lanzl, L. H., and Cox, A. B.: The detection, prevention and retardation of menopausal osteoporosis. *D*, 140–149.

94. Dawson, J. W. and Struthers, J. W.: Generalized osteitis fibrosa with parathyroid tumors and metastatic calcification. Edin. Med. J. *30*:421–564, 1923.

95. Denison, E. K., Peters, R. L., and Reynolds, T. B.: Portal hypertension in a patient with osteopetrosis. Arch. Intern. Med. *128*:279–283, 1971.

96. Dent, C. E., Engelbrecht, H. E., and Godfrey, R. C.: Osteoporosis of lumbar vertebrae and calcification of abdominal aorta in women living in Durban. Brit. Med. J. *4*:76–80, 1968.

97. Dent, C. E., Smellie, J. M., and Watson, L.: Studies in osteopetrosis. Arch. Dis. Child. *40*:7–15, 1965.

98. Dent, C. E., and Hodson, C. J.: Radiological changes associated with certain metabolic bone diseases. Symposium, Generalized Softening of Bone Due to Metabolic Causes. Brit. J. Radiol. *27*:605–618, 1954.

99. Dent, C. E.: Rickets (and osteomalacia), nutritional and metabolic (1919–69). Proc. Roy. Soc. Med. *63*:401–408, 1970.

100. Dent, C. E., and Watson, L.: Osteoporosis. Postgrad. Med. J. *42* (suppl): 582–608, 1966.

101. Dent, C. E.: Some problems of hyperparathyroidism. Brit. Med. J., 2:1419–1425; 1495–1500, 1962.

102. Dent, C. E., and Stamp, T. C. B.: Hypophosphatemic osteomalacia presenting in adults. Quart. J. Med. *40*:303–329, 1971.

103. Dent, C. E., and Friedman, M.: Idiopathic juvenile osteoporosis. Quart. J. Med. New Ser. *34*:177–210, 1965.

104. Dent, C. E., Round, J. M., and Stamp, T. C. B.: Treatment of sex linked hypophosphataemic rickets (SLHP). *B*, 427–432.

105. Dequeker, J.: Bone loss in normal and pathological conditions. Leuven, Leuven University Press, 1972.

106. DeSeze, S., Lichtwitz, A., Bordier, P., Hioco, D., and Mazatraud, M.: Le syndrome de Looser-Milkman. Etude de 60 cas. Sem. Hop. Paris *34*:2005, 1962.

107. Dickson, D. D., Camp, J. D. and Ghormley, R. K.: Osteitis deformans: Paget's disease of the bone. Radiology 44:449–470, 1945.

108. Doty, S. B., and Schofield, B. H.: Electron microscopic localization of hydrolytic enzymes in osteoclasts. Histochem. J. 4:245–258, 1972.

109. Doyle, F. H., Gutteridge, D. H., Joplin, F. G. and Fraser, R.: An assessment of radiologic criteria used in the study of spinal osteoporosis. Brit. J. Radiol. 40:241–250, 1967.

110. Doyle, F. H., Brown, J., and Kaibanne, C.: Relation between bone mass and muscle weight. Lancet, 1:391–393, 1970.

111. Doyle, F. H.: Involutional osteoporosis. A, 143–168.

112. Doyle, F. H.: Radiological assessment of endocrine effects in bone. Radiol. Clin. N. Amer. 5:289, 1967.

112a. Doyle, F. H., Pennock, J., Greenberg, P. B., Joplin, G. F., and MacIntyre, I.: Radiological evidence of a dose-related response to long term treatment of Paget's disease with human calcitonin. Brit. J. Radiol. 47:1–8, 1974.

113. Drogula, K. H., and Dettmer, N.: The effect of anabolic hormones as shown in bone obtained by biopsy from patients with generalized osteopathies. Arzneimittelforschung 14:1212–1218, 1964.

114. Duncan, H.: Osteoporosis in rheumatoid arthritis and corticosteroid induced osteoporosis. E, 571–584.

115. Duncan, H.: Paget's disease of bone (osteitis deformans). In Tice's Practice of Medicine, Vol. 5, New York, Hoeber, 1969, Chapter 54.

116. Dusenberry, J. F., and Kane, J. J.: Pyknodysostosis. Report of three new cases. Amer. J. Roent. 94:717–723, 1967.

117. Ehrig, U., and Wilson, D. R.: Fibrous dysplasia of bone and primary hyperparathyroidism. Ann. Int. Med. 77:234–238, 1972.

118. Epker, B. N.: A quantitative microscopic study of bone remodeling and balance in a human with skeletal fluorosis. Clin. Orthop. 55:87–95, 1967.

119. Epker, B. N., and Frost, H. M.: The nature of bone resorption and formation in normalcy and disease. Henry Ford Hosp. Med. J. 16:29–39, Spring 1968.

120. Epstein, F. H.: Calcium and the kidney. Amer. J. Med. 45:700–714, 1968.

121. Eugenidis, N., Olah, A. J., and Haas, H. G.: Osteosclerosis in hyperparathyroidism. Radiology 105:265–275, 1972.

122. Eyring, E. J., and Eisenberg, E.: Congenital hyperphosphatasia. J. Bone Joint Surg. 50A:1099–1117, 1968.

123. Fairbank, H. A.: Osteopetrosis. J. Bone Joint Surg. 30B:339–356, 1968.

124. Feldman, F., and Seaman, W. B.: The neurologic complications of Paget's disease in the cervical spine. Amer. J. Roent. 105:375–382, 1969.

125. Finby, N., and Archibald, R. M.: Skeletal abnormalities associated with gonadal dysgenesis. Amer. J. Roent. 89:1222, 1963.

126. Firat, D. and Stutzman, L.: Fibrous dysplasia of the bone. Review of twenty four cases. Amer. J. Med. 44:421–429, 1968.

127. Follis, R. H.: Skeletal changes associated with hyperthyroidism. Bull. Johns Hopkins Hosp. 92:405–422, 1953.

128. Ford, J. A., Calhoun, E. M., Mikutosh, W. B., and Dunnigan, M. G.: Biochemical response of late rickets and osteomalacia to a chupatty-free diet. Brit. Med. J. 3:446–447, 1972.

129. Forland, M., Strandjord, N. M., Paloyan, E., and Cox, A.: Bone density studies in primary hyperparathyroidism. Arch. Intern. Med. 122:236–240, 1968.

130. Foss, M. V. L., and Byers, P. D.: Bone density, osteoarthrosis of the hip and fracture of the upper end of the femur. Ann. Rheum. Dis. 31:259–264, 1972.

131. Foster, G. V., Byfield, P. G., and Gudmundsson, T. V.: Calcitonin. A, 93–124.

132. Foster, G. V., Doyle, F. H., Bordier, P., and Matrajt, H.: Effect of thyrocalcitonin on bone. Lancet, 2:1428–1432, 1966.

133. Fourman, P., and Royer, P.: Calcium Metabolism and the Bone. Oxford, Blackwell Scientific Publications, 1968.

134. Frame, B., Foroozanfar, F., and Patton, R. G.: Normocalcemic primary hyperparathyroidism with osteitis fibrosa. Ann. Intern. Med., 73:253–257, 1970.

135. Frame, B., Guiang, H. L., Frost, H. M., and Reynolds, W. A.: Osteomalacia induced by laxative (phenolphthalein) ingestion. Arch. Intern. Med. 128:794–796, 1971.

136. Frame, B., Frost, H. M., Pak, C. Y. C., Reynolds, W., and Argen, R. S.: Fibrogenesis imperfecta ossium. New Eng. J. Med. 285:769–772, 1971.

137. Frame, B.: Metabolic bone disease as a cause of neck ache and back ache. Proceedings of Conference in Neckache and Backache in association with Neurologic Surgery. Springfield, C. C Thomas, 1970.

138. Frame, B., and Nixon, R. K.: Bone marrow factors in osteoporosis. D, 238–250.

139. Fraser, D.: Hypophosphatasia. Amer. J. Med. 22:430–446, 1957.

139a. Fraser, D., Kooh, S. W., Kind, H. P., Holick, M. F., Tanaka, Y., and DeLuca, H. F.: Pathogenesis of hereditary vitamin D dependent rickets. An inborn error of vitamin D metabolism involving defective conversion of 25 hydroxy vitamin D to 1 α 25 dihydroxy vitamin D. New Eng. J. Med. 289:817–822, 1973.

140. Fraser, S. A., Smith, D. A., Anderson, J. B., and Wilson, G. M.: Osteoporosis and fractures following thyrotoxicosis. Lancet, 1:981–983, 1971.

141. Frost, H. M.: Postmenopausal osteoporosis: the evolution of our concepts of its cause. Henry Ford Hosp. Med. J. 20:83–90, 1972.

142. Frost, H. M., Frame, B., Armand, R. S., and Hunter, R. B.: Atypical axial osteomalacia. Clin. Orthop. 23:283–295, 1962.

143. Frost, H. M., Villanueva, A. R., Teth, J., and Eyring, E.: Tetracycline-based analysis of bone remodeling in osteopetrosis. Clin. Orthop. 65:203–217, 1969.

144. Frost, H. M.: The origin and nature of transients in human bone remodeling dynamics. B, 124–137.

145. Frost, H. M.: The Physiology of Cartilaginous, Fibrous and Bony Tissue. Springfield, C. C Thomas, 1972.

146. Frost, H. M.: Bone Remodelling and Its Relationship to Metabolic Bone Disease. Springfield, C. C Thomas, 1973.

147. Frost, H. M.: Managing the skeletal pain and disability of osteoporosis. E, 561–570.

148. Frost, H. M.: Presence of microscopic cracks in

vivo in bone. Henry Ford Hosp. Med. Bull., 8(1):25–35, 1960.

149. Frost, H. M.: Osteocyte death *in vivo*. J. Bone Joint Surg. 42(1):138–143, 1960.

150. Frost, H. M.: Micropetrosis. J. Bone Joint Surg. 42A(1):144–150, 1960.

151. Frost, H. M., Villanueva, A. R., and Roth, H.: Halo volume. Henry Ford Hosp. Med. Bull. 8(2):228–238, 1960.

152. Frost, H. M.: The osteoporoses: A definition of term and concepts. Henry Ford Hosp. Med. Bull. 10(2):315–337, 1963.

153. Frost, H. M.: Tetracycline-based histological analysis of bone remodelling. Calc. Tiss. Res. 3(3):211–217, 1969.

154. Frost, H. M.: Musculoskeletal pain. *In* Facial Pain, C. C. Alling (ed.). Philadelphia, Lea and Febiger, 1968, pp. 9–22.

155. Fujita, T., Orimo, H., Okano, K., and Yoshikawa, M.: Clinical application of parathyroid hormone radioimmunoassay. *B*, 281–290.

156. Funsten, R. V.: Certain arthritic disturbances associated with parathyroidism. J. Bone Joint Surg. 15:112–119, 1933.

157. Gallagher, J. C., Bulusu, L., and Nordin, B. E. C.: Oestrogenic hormones and bone resorption. *B*, 266–273.

158. Garn, S. M.: The Earlier Gain and the Later Loss of Cortical Bone. Springfield, C. C Thomas, 1970.

159. Garn, S. M.: The course of bone gain and the phases of bone loss. *E*, 503–520.

160. Garn, S. M., Poznanski, A. K., and Nagy, J. M.: Bone measurement in the differential diagnosis of osteopenia and osteoporosis. Radiology 100:409–518, 1971.

161. Garnett, E. S.: An absolute measurement of in vivo bone density. *B*, 44–47.

162. Gersh, I. and Catchpole, H. R.: The nature of ground substance of connective tissue. Persp. Biol. Med. 3:282–312, 1960.

163. Gershon-Cohen, J.: Asymptomatic fractures in osteoporotic spines of the aged. J.A.M.A. 153:625–627, 1953.

164. Ghormley, R. K., Sutherland, C. G., and Pollock, G. A.: Pathological fractures. J.A.M.A. 107:2112, 1937.

165. Glorieux, F. H., Scriver, C. R., Reade, T. M., Goldman, H., and Roseborough, A.: Use of phosphate and vitamin D to prevent dwarfism and rickets in x-linked hypophosphatemia. New Eng. J. Med. 287:481–487, 1972.

166. Golding, F. C.: Fibrogenesis imperfecta. J. Bone Joint Surg. 50B:619–622, 1968.

167. Goldsmith, N. F., Johnston, J. O., Ury, H., Vose, G., and Colbert, C.: Bone-mineral estimation in normal and osteoporotic women. J. Bone Joint Surg. 53A:83–100, 1971.

168. Goldsmith, R. S.: Laboratory aids in the diagnosis of metabolic bone disease. *E*, 545–560.

169. Gong, J. K., Arnold, J. S., and Cohn, S. H.: Composition of trabecular and cortical bone. Anat. Rec. 149:325–332, 1964.

170. Gooding, C. A., and Ball, J. H.: Idiopathic juvenile osteoporosis. Radiology 93:1349–1350, 1969.

171. Greenfield, G. B.: Bone changes in chronic adult Gaucher's disease. Amer. J. Roent. 110:800–807, 1970.

172. Griffith, G. C., Nichols, G., Asher, J. D., and Flan-

agan, B.: Heparin osteoporosis. J.A.M.A. 193:91, 1965.

173. Haddad, J. G.: Paget's disease of bone: problems and management. *E*, 775–786.

174. Hall, P.: Albright's syndrome in an adult male. Brit. Med. J., 2:1159–1162, 1962.

175. Hancox, N. M.: The Biology of Bone. Cambridge, Cambridge University Press, 1972.

176. Harris, W. H., and Heaney, R. P.: Skeletal renewal and metabolic bone disease. N. Eng. J. Med. 28:193–202, 253–259, 303–311, 1969.

177. Harris, W. H., Heaney, R. P., Jowsey, J., Cockin, J., Akins, C., Graham, J., and Weinberg, E. H.: Growth hormone: the effect on skeletal renewal in the adult dog. Calc. Tiss. Res. 10:1–13, 1972.

178. Hart, F. D.: The stiff aching back. The differential diagnosis of ankylosing spondylitis. Lancet 1:740–742, 1968.

179. Hartman, J. T. and John, D. F.: Paget's disease of the spine with cord and nerve root compression. J. Bone Joint Surg. 48A:1079–1084, 1966.

180. Hasenhuttl, K.: Osteopetrosis. J. Bone Joint Surg. 44A:359–370, 1962.

181. Hattner, R., and Frost, H. M.: Mean skeletal age: its calculations and theoretical effects on skeletal tracer physiology and on the physical characteristics of bone. Henry Ford Hosp. Med. Bull. 11(2):201–216, 1963.

182. Hattner, R., Epker, B. N., and Frost, H. M.: Suggested sequential mode of control of changes in cell behavior in adult bone remodelling. Nature 206(4983):489–490, 1965.

183. Havard, C. W. H., and Scott, R. B.: Urticaria pigmentosa with visceral and skeletal lesions. Quart. J. Med. 28:459–472, 1959.

184. Haymowitz, A., and Horwitz, M.: The miscible calcium pool in metabolic bone disease, in particular acromegaly. J. Clin. Endocr. 24:4–14, 1964.

185. Heaney, R. P.: A unified concept of osteoporosis: A second look. *D*, 257–265.

186. Heaney, R. P.: Measurement of skeletal remodelling by means of bone seeking isotopes. *B*, 154–164.

187. Heaton, K. W., Lever, J. V., and Barnard, D.: Osteomalacia associated with cholestyramine therapy for postileectomy diarrhea. Gastroenterology 62:642–646, 1972.

188. Henneman, D. H., Pak, C. Y. C., and Bartter, F. C.: Collagen composition, solubility and biosynthesis in fibrogenesis imperfecta ossium. *B*, 469–472.

189. Henneman, D. H., Pak, C. Y. C., Bartter, F. C., Lifschitz, M. D., and Sanzenbacher, L.: The solubility and synthetic rate of bone collagen in idiopathic osteoporosis. Clin. Orthop., 88:275–282, 1972.

190. Henneman, P. H., and Wallach, S.: A review of the prolonged use of estrogen and androgens in postmenopausal and senile osteoporosis. Arch. Intern. Med. 100:715, 1957.

191. Henneman, P. H.: Treatment of postmenopausal osteoporosis with gonadal steroids. *C*, 15–20.

192. Hernberg, C. A.: Treatment of postmenopausal osteoporosis with estrogens and androgens. Acta Endocr. 34:51–57, 1960.

193. Herring, G. M.: The organic matrix of bone. *F*, Vol. I:128–190.

194. Herwitz, S. H.: Osteitis deformans, Paget's disease. Bull. John Hopkins Hosp. 24:263–274, 1913.

195. Hess, A. F.: Rickets Including Osteomalacia and Tetany. Philadelphia, Lea and Febiger, 1929.

196. Highman, J. H., Sanderson, P. H., and Sutcliffe, M. M. L.: Vitamin D resistant osteomalacia as a cause of cord compression. Quart. J. Med. 39:529–537, 1970.

197. Higinbotham, N. L.: An assessment of spinal biopsy. In Nassim, R. and Burrows, H.-J.: Modern Trends in Disease of the Spinal Column. London, Butterworth, 1959, pp. 287–292.

198. Hill, L. F.: Phytic acid and serum calcium. Lancet, 2:769, 1972.

199. Hinkle, C. L. and Beiler, D. D.: Osteopetrosis in adults. Amer. J. Roent. 74:46, 1955.

200. Holtrop, M. E., and Weinger, J. M.: Ultrastructural evidence for a transport system in bone. In Calcium, Parathyroid Hormone and the Calcitonins, R. V. Talmage, and P. L. Munson (eds.), Amsterdam, Excerpta Medica, 1972.

201. Holtrop, M. E.: The ultrastructure of the epiphyseal plate. II. The hypertrophic chondrocyte. Calc. Tiss. Res. 9:140–151, 1972.

202. Hossain, M., Smith, D. A. and Nordin, B. E. C.: Parathyroid activity and postmenopausal osteoporosis. Lancet, 1:809–811, 1970.

203. Houston, C. S.: Fatal neonatal dwarfism. J. Can. Assoc. Radiol. 23:45–61, 1972.

204. Hunter, D., and Turnbull, H. M.: Hyperparathyroidism: generalized osteitis fibrosa with observations upon the bones, the parathyroid tumour and normal parathyroid glands. Brit. J. Surg. 12:202–284, 1930.

205. Hurwitz, L. J., and Banerji, N. V.: Basilar impression of the skull in patients with adult coeliac disease and after gastric surgery. J. Neurol. Neurosurg. Psychiat. 35:92–96, 1972.

206. Hurwitz, L. J. and Shepherd, W. H. J.: Basilar impression and disordered metabolism of bone. Brain 59:223–234, 1966.

207. Hurxthal, L. M.: Measurement of anterior vertebral compressions and biconcave vertebrae. Amer. J. Roent. 53:635–644, 1968.

208. Hurxthal, L. M., and Vose, G. P.: The relationship of dietary calcium intake to radiographic bone density in normal and osteoporotic persons. Calc. Tiss. Res. 4:245–256, 1969.

209. Hurxthal, L. M., Vose, G. P., and Dotter, W. E.: Densitometric and visual observations of spinal radiographs. Geriatrics 24:93–106, 1969.

210. Jackson, C. E., and Frame, B.: Diagnosis and management of parathyroid disorders. E, 691–712.

211. Jackson, H. C.: Nerve endings in the human lumbar spinal column and related structures. J. Bone Joint Surg. 48A:1272, 1966.

212. Jackson, W. P. U.: Osteoporosis of unknown cause in younger people. J. Bone Joint Surg. 40B:420–441, 1958.

213. Jardon, O. M., Burney, D. W., and Fink, R. L.: Hypophosphatasia in an adult. J. Bone Joint Surg. 52A:1477–1484, 1970.

214. Jaworski, Z. F., Meunier, P., and Frost, H. M.: Observations on two types of resorption cavities in human lamellar cortical bone. Clin. Orthop. 83:279–285, 1972.

215. Jaworski, Z. F., and Lok, E.: The rate of osteoclastic bone erosion in Haversian remodelling sites of adult dog's rib. Calc. Tiss. Res. 10:103–112, 1972.

216. Jaworski, Z. F.: Pathophysiology, diagnosis and treatment of osteomalacia. E, 623–652.

217. Jett, S., and Frost, H. M.: Tetracycline-based measurements of the bone dynamics in the rib of a girl with hyperphosphatasia. Henry Ford Hosp. Med. J. 16:325–338, 1968.

218. Joffe, N.: Some radiological aspects of scurvy in the adult. Brit. J. Radiol. 34:429–434, 1961.

219. Johnson, L. C.: Morphologic analysis in pathology: The kinetics of disease and general biology of bone. In Bone Biodynamics, H. M. Frost (ed.) Boston, Little, Brown and Co., 1964, pp. 543–654.

220. Johnston, C. C., Smith, D. M., Nance, W. E., and Bevan, J.: Evaluation of radial bone mass by the photon absorption technique. B, 28–36.

221. Johnston, C. C., Lavy, N., Lord, T., Vellios, F., Merritt, A. D., and Deiss, W. P.: Osteopetrosis. A clinical, genetic, metabolic and morphologic study of the dominantly inherited benign form. Medicine 47:149–167, 1968.

222. Jolly, S. S., Singh, B. M., Mathers, D. C., and Malhotra, K. C.: Epidemiological, clinical and biochemical study of endemic dental and skeletal fluorosis in Punjab. Brit. Med. J. 2:427–429, 1968.

223. Jones, G.: Radiological appearances of disuse osteoporosis. Clin. Radiol. 20:345–353, 1969.

224. Jowsey, J.: Age changes in human bone. Clin. Orthop. 16:210–217, 1960.

225. Jowsey, J.: Microradiography. A morphological approach to quantitating bone turnover. B, 114–123.

226. Jowsey, J. and Gordan, G.: Bone turnover and osteoporosis. F, Vol. III:202–239.

227. Julkunen, H., Hernonen, O. P., and Pyorala, K.: Hyperostosis of the spine in an adult population. Ann. Rheum. Dis. 30:605–612, 1971.

228. Juncos, L. I., and Donadio, J. V.: Renal failure and fluorosis. J.A.M.A. 222:783–785, 1972.

229. Juster, M., Oligo, N., Laval-Jeantet, M.: Lisére préosseux et tissu ostéoide. In L'osteomalacie Hioco, D. (ed). Paris, Masson et cie, 1967.

230. Kalayjian, D. B., and Cooper, R. R.: Osteogenesis of the epiphysis. Clin. Orthop. 85:242–256, 1972.

231. Kalu, D. N., Pennock, J., Doyle, F. H., and Foster, G.: Parathyroid hormone and experimental osteosclerosis. Lancet, 1:1363–1366, 1970.

232. Keele, D. K., and Vose, G. P.: Bone density in nonambulatory children. Follow up after termination of treatment with sodium fluoride, inorganic phosphates and oxymethalone. Amer. J. Dis. Child. 121:204–206, 1971.

233. Kellerhouse, L. E., and Linarzie, L. R.: Bone manifestations of hematologic disorders. Med. Clin. N. Amer. 49:203–228, 1965.

234. Kellett, C. E.: Glissonian rickets. Arch. Dis. Childh. 9:233–246, 1934.

235. Kellgren, J. H.: On the distribution of pain arising from deep somatic structures with charts of segmental pain areas. Clin. Sci. 4:35–46, 1939.

236. Kempinsky, W. H.: Osteoporotic kyphosis with paraplegia. Neurology 8:181, 1958.

237. Keynes, W. M., and Caird, F. I.: Hypocalcemic primary hyperparathyroidism. Brit. Med. J. 1:208–211, 1970.

238. Klenerman, L.: Cauda equina and spinal cord compression in Paget's disease. J. Bone Joint Surg. 48B:365–370, 1966.

239. Kooh, S. W., Cumming, W. A., Fraser, D., and Fornasier, L.: Transient childhood osteoporosis of unknown cause. *B*, 329–332.

240. Krane, S. M., Pinnell, S. R., Erbe, R. W., and Glimcher, M. J.: A disorder of connective tissue resulting from lysyl protocollagen hydroxylase deficiency. *B*, 473–477.

241. Krane, S. M., Munoz, A. J., and Harris, E. D.: Urinary polypeptides related to collagen synthesis. J. Clin. Invest. *49*:716, 1970.

242. Kranendonk, D. H., Jurist, J. M. and Lee, H. G.: Femoral trabecular patterns and bone mineral content. J. Bone Joint Surg. *54A*:1472–1478, 1972.

243. LaBan, M. M., Dworkin, H. J., and Shevitz, H. A.: Metastatic disease of the spine: electromyography and bone scan in early detection. Arch. Phys. Med. and Rehab. *53*:232–235, 1972.

244. Lacroix, P.: The internal remodelling of bones. *F*, Vol. III:119–144.

245. Lafferty, F. W., Spencer, G. E., and Pearson, O. H.: Effects of androgens, estrogens and high calcium intakes on bone formation and resorption in osteoporosis. Amer. J. Med. *36*:514–528, 1964.

246. Lapatsanis, P., Deliyanni, V., and Doxiadis, S.: Vitamin D deficiency rickets in Greece. J. Pediat. *73*:195, 1968.

247. Lee, W. R.: Bone formation in Paget's disease. A quantitative microscopic study using tetracycline markers. J. Bone Joint Surg. *49B*:146–153, 1967.

248. Lehninger, A. L.: Mitochondria and calcium ion transport. Biochem. J. *119*:129–138, 1970.

249. Leonard, B. J., Israels, M. C. G., and Wilkinson, J. F.: Myelosclerosis. A clinicopathologic study. Quart. J. Med. *26*:131–148, 1957.

250. Lievre, J. A., Lievre, Mme. J. A., and Camus, J. P.: Etude de l'action du phenylpropionate de 19-nor androstenolone sur le tissu osseux humain au cours de l'osteoporose. IV Conference Des Maladies Rhumatismales — Aix-x Les-Bains. 1964.

251. Lindenfelser, R., Hasselkus, W., Haubert, P., and Kronert, W.: Zur osteogenesis imperfecta congenita. Virchows Arch. Abt. B. Zellpath. *11*:80–89, 1972.

252. Little, K., Kelly, M., and Court, A.: Studies on bone matrix in normal and osteoporotic bone. J. Bone Joint Surg. *44B*:503–519, 1962.

253. Loomis, W. F.: Rickets. Sci. Amer. *223*:77–91, 1970.

254. Lovett, R. W.: The roentgenographic appearances in rickets. J.A.M.A. *65*:2062–2067, 1915.

255. Lumb, G. A., Mawer, E. B., and Stanbury, S. W.: The apparent vitamin D resistance of chronic renal failure. A study of the physiology of vitamin D in man. Amer. J. Med. *50*:421, 1971.

256. Lutwak, L.: Nutritional aspects of calcium metabolism in man. Corn. Vet. *58*(suppl):136–148, 1968.

257. MacPherson, R. I., Kroeker, M., and Houston, C. J.: Hypophosphatasia. J. Can. Assoc. Radiol. *23*:16–26, 1972.

258. Maroteaux, P., and Lamy, M.: The malady of Toulouse-Lautrec. J.A.M.A. *191*:715–717, 1965.

259. Mather, H. G.: Hyperparathyroidism with normal serum calcium. Brit. Med. J. *2*:424–425, 1953.

260. Matthews, J. L., and Martin, J. H.: Intracellular transport of calcium and its relationship to homeostasis and mineralization. Amer. J. Med. *50*:589–597, 1971.

261. Mawer, E. B. and Holmes, E. B.: Rickets in Glasgow Pakistanis. Brit. Med. J. *3*:177–178, 1972.

262. Maxwell, J. P.: Further studies in adult rickets (osteomalacia) and foetal rickets. Proc. Roy. Soc. Med. *28*:265–300, 1935.

263. Mazess, R. B. and Cameron, J. R.: Growth of bone in school children: comparison of radiographic morphometry and photon absorptiometry. Growth *36*:77–92, 1972.

264. Mazess, R. B., Judy, P. R., Wilson, C. R., and Cameron, J. R.: Progress in clinical use of photon absorptiometry. *B*, 37–43.

265. McConkey, B., Fraser, G. M., Bligh, A. S., and Whiteley, H.: Transparent skin and osteoporosis. Lancet *1*:693–695, 1963.

266. McGeown, M. G.: Severe hyperparathyroid bone disease without apparent involvement of the kidneys. Lancet *2*:799–802, 1962.

267. McKusick, V. A.: Heritable disorders of connective tissue. St. Louis, C. V. Mosby, 1966.

268. Meema, H. E.: The interrelationship between cortical bone thickness, mineral mass and mineral density in human radius: A roentgenologic-densitometric study. *In* Progress in Bone Mineral Measurement, U.S. Dept. of H.E.W., Bethesda, Maryland, 1968, 139–157.

269. Meema, H. E., Harris, C. K., and Powell, R. E.: A method for determination of bone-salt content of cortical bone. Radiol. *82*:986–997, 1966.

270. Meema, H. E. and Reid, D. B. W.: The relationship between skin and cortical bone thickness in old age with special reference to osteoporosis and diabetes mellitus: a roentgenographic study. J. Geront. *24*:28–32, 1969.

271. Meema, H. E., and Meema, S.: Comparison of microradioscopic and morphometric findings in the hand bones with densitometric findings in the proximal radius in thyrotoxicosis and in renal osteodystrophy. Invest. Radiol. *7*:88–96, 1972.

272. Meema, H. E., and Meema, S.: Prevention of postmenopausal osteoporosis by hormone treatment of the menopause. Can. Med. Assoc. J. *99*:248–251, 1968.

273. Mellors, R. C.: Electron microprobe analysis of human trabecular bone. Clin. Orthop. *45*:157–167, 1966.

274. Melvin, K. E. W., Tashjian, A. H. and Bordier, P.: The metabolic significance of calcitonin secreting thyroid carcinoma. *B*, 193–201.

275. Merz, W. A., and Schenk, R. K.: Quantitative structural analysis of human cancellous bone. Acta. Anat. *75*:54–66, 1970.

276. Meunier, P. J., Branchi, G. G. S., Edouard, C. M., Gerieve, J. C., Courpron, P., and Vignon, G. E.: Bony manifestations of thyrotoxicosis. *E*, 745–774.

277. Meunier, P., Aaron, J., Edouard, C., and Vignon, G.: Osteoporosis and the replacement of cell populations of the marrow by adipose tissue. Clin. Orthop. *80*:147–154, 1971.

278. Moller, P. V., and Gudjonnssen, S. V.: Massive fluorosis of bones and ligaments. Acta Radiol. Scand. *13*:269, 1932.

279. Morgan, D. B.: Osteomalacia, renal osteodystrophy and osteoporosis. Springfield, C. C Thomas, 1973.

280. Morgan, D. B.: Calcium and phosphorus transport

across the intestine. *In* Malabsorption, Girdwood, R. H. and Smith, A. W. (eds.). University of Edinburgh Pfizer Medical Monographs 4. Baltimore, Williams and Wilkins, 1969.

281. Moss, A. J., Waterhouse, C., and Terry, R.: Gluten-sensitive enteropathy with osteomalacia but without steatorrhea. N. Eng. J. Med. *272*:825–830, 1965.

282. Munck, O.: Osteoporosis due to malabsorption of calcium responding favorably to large doses of vitamin D. Quart. J. Med. *33*:209–221, 1964.

283. Murphy, E. A.: A scientific viewpoint on normality. Perspect. Biol. Med. *9*:333, 1966.

284. Nathanson, L., and Levitan, A.: Deformities and fractures of the vertebrae as a result of senile and presenile osteoporosis. Amer. J. Roent. *46*:197, 1941.

285. Neuman, W. F., and Neuman, M. W.: The chemical dynamics of bone mineral. Chicago, Univ. of Chicago Press, 1958.

286. Newton-John, H. F., and Morgan, D. B.: The loss of bone with age, osteoporosis and fractures. Clin. Orthop. *71*:229–252, 1970.

287. Nilsson, B. E.: Parity and osteoporosis. Surg. Gynec. Obstet. *129*:27–28, 1969.

288. Nordin, B. E. C.: International patterns of osteoporosis. Clin. Orthop. *45*:17–30, 1966.

289. Nordin, B. E. C., and Peacock, M.: Role of kidney in regulation of plasma calcium. Lancet, *3*:1280–1283, 1969.

290. Nordin, B. E. C.: Clinical significance and pathogenesis of osteoporosis. Brit. Med. J. *1*:571–576, 1971.

291. Nordin, B. E. C., Young, M. M., Denilly, B., Ormandroyd, P., and Sykes, J.: Lumbar spine densitometry methodology and results in relation to the menopause. Clin. Radiol. *19*:459–464, 1968.

292. Nordin, B. E. C., Hodgkinson, A., and Peacock, M.: The measurement and the meaning of urinary calcium. Clin. Orthop. *52*:293–322, 1967.

293. Nordin, B. E. C.: Osteomalacia, osteoporosis and calcium deficiency. Clin. Orthop. *17*:235, 1960.

294. Nordin, B. E. C., and Roper, A.: Post pregnancy osteoporosis. A syndrome? Lancet *1*:431, 1955.

295. Nordin, B. E. C., and Smith, D. A.: Pathogenesis and treatment of osteomalacia. *In* L'Osteomalacie, Hioco, D. (ed). Paris, Masson et cie, 1967, p. 48.

296. Oppenheimer, A.: Rickets of the spinal column. International Radiol. Rev. *8*:332–339, 1939.

297. Owen, M.: The origin of bone cells. Internat. Rev. Cytol. *28*:213–238, 1970.

298. Paget, J.: On a form of chronic inflammation of bone (osteitis deformans). Reprinted in Clin. Orthop. *49*:3–16, 1966.

299. Pak, C. Y. C., and Bartter, F. C.: Treatment of osteoporosis with calcium infusion. *C*, 39–46.

300. Parfitt, A. M., and Frame, B.: Treatment of rickets and osteomalacia. *C*, 83–116.

301. Parfitt, A. M.: Renal osteodystrophy. Ortho. Clin. N. Amer. *3*:681–698, 1972.

302. Parfitt, A. M., Massry, S. G., Winfield, A. C., DePalma, J., and Gordon, A.: Osteopenia and fractures occurring during maintenance hemodialysis. A new form of renal osteodystrophy. Clin. Orthop. *87*:287–302, 1972.

303. Parfitt, A. M.: Hypophosphatemic vitamin D refractory rickets and osteomalacia. Ortho. Clin. N. Amer. *3*:653–680, 1972.

304. Parfitt, A. M.: The quantitative approach to bone morphology. A critique of current methods and their interpretation. *B*, 86–94.

305. Park, E. A.: Some aspects of rickets. The Blackader Lecture. Can. Med. Assn. J. *26*:3–15, 1932.

306. Parsons, J. A., and Potts, J. T.: Physiology and chemistry of parathyroid hormone. *A*., 33–78.

307. Pellegrino, E. D., and Biltz, R. M.: The composition of human bone in uremia. Medicine *44*:397–418, 1965.

308. Pentecost, R. L., Murray, R. A., and Bradley, H. H.: Fatigue, insufficiency and pathologic features. J.A.M.A. *187*:1001–1004, 1964.

309. Phang, J. M., Berman, M., Finerman, G. A., Neer, R. M., Rosenberg, L. E., and Hahn, T. J.: Dietary perturbation of calcium metabolism in normal man: Compartmental analysis. J. Clin. Invest. *48*: 67–77, 1969.

310. Pimstone, B., Eisenberg, E., and Silverman, J.: Hypophosphatasia: genetic and dental studies. Ann. Intern. Med. *65*:722–729, 1966.

311. Pinnell, S. R., Krane, S. M., Kenzova, J. E., and Glimcher, M. J.: A heritable disorder of connective tissue, hydroxylysine-deficient collagen disease. New Eng. J. Med. *286*:1013–1020, 1972.

312. Pisar, D. E.: Parathyroid carcinoma with endocrine function—report of a case. *B*, 229–231.

313. Pita, J. C., Cuervo, L. A., Madruga, J. E., Muller, F. J., and Howell, D. S.: Evidence for a role of proteinpolysaccharides in regulation of mineral phase separation in calcifying cartilage. J. Clin. Invest. *49*:2188–2197, 1970.

314. Posen, S., Kleerekoper, M., and Cornish, C.: Serum alkaline phosphatase in the diagnosis of metabolic bone disorders. *B*, 74–79.

315. Potts, J. T., Habener, J. F., Segre, G. V., Niall, H. D., Tregear, G. W., Leutmann, H. T., and Powell, D. A.: Parathyroid hormone: chemical and immunochemical studies in relation to biosynthesis, secretion and metabolism of the hormone. *B*, 208–214.

316. Powell, R. C., and Deiss, W. P.: Symptomatic osteomalacia secondary to clinically occult causes. Ann. Intern. Med. *54*:1280–1289, 1961.

317. Prineas, J. W., Mason, A. S., and Henson, R. A.: Myopathy in metabolic bone disease. Brit. Med. J. *1*:1034, 1036, 1965.

318. Pritchard, J. J.: General histology of bone. *F*, Vol. I, 1–20.

319. Pritchard, J. J.: The osteoblast. *F*, Vol. I, 21–44.

320. Pyrah, L. N., Hodgkinson, A., and Anderson, C. K.: Primary hyperparathyroidism. Brit. J. Surg. *53*:234–316, 1966.

321. Ragab, A. H., Frech, R. S., and Ketti, T. J.: Osteoporotic fractures secondary to methotrexate therapy of acute leukemia in remission. Cancer *25*:580–585, 1970.

322. Ramanurthi, B., and Visvanathan, G. S.: Paget's disease of the axis causing quadriplegia. J. Neurosurg. *14*:580–583, 1957.

323. Ramser, J. R., Frost, H. M., and Smith, R.: Tetracycline-based measurement of the tissue and cell dynamics in the rib of a 25-year-old man with active acromegaly. Clin. Orthop. *49*:169–172, 1966.

324. Ramser, J. R., Villanueva, A., and Frost, H. M.: Cortical bone dynamics in osteomalacia, measured by tetracycline bone-labeling. Clin. Orthop. *49*:89–102, 1966.

325. Rich, C., Bernstein, D. S., Gates, S., Heaney, R. P., Johnston, C. C., Rosenberg, C. A., Schnaper, H. W., Tewksbury, R. B., and Williams, G. A.: Factors involved in an objective study of the efficacy of treatment of osteoporosis. Clin. Orthop. 46:63–66, 1956.

326. Richelle, L. J., and Onkelinx, C.: Recent advances in the physical biology of bone and other hard tissues. In Mineral Metabolism; an advanced treatise, Vol. III. Comar, C. L., and Bronner, F. (eds). New York, Academic Press, 1969.

327. Riggs, B. L., Kelly, R. J., Kinney, V. R., Scholz, D. A., and Bianc, A. J.: Calcium deficiency and osteoporosis. J. Bone Joint Surg., 49A:915–924, 1967.

328. Riggs, B. L., Randall, R. V., Wahner, H. W., Jowsey, J., Kelly, P. J., and Singh, M.: The nature of the metabolic bone disorder in acromegaly. J. Clin. Endocr. 34:911–918, 1972.

329. Riggs, B. L., Jowsey, J., and Kelly, P. J.: Quantitative microradiographic study of bone remodeling in Cushing's syndrome. Metab. 9:773–780, 1966.

330. Riggs, B. L., Jowsey, J., Goldsmith, R. S., Kelly, P. J., Hoffman, D. L., and Arnaud, C. D.: Short- and long-term effects of estrogen and synthetic anabolic hormone in postmenopausal osteoporosis. J. Clin. Invest. 51:1659–1663, 1972.

331. Riggs, B. L., and Jowsey, J.: Treatment of osteoporosis with fluoride. C, 27–34.

332. Riggs, B. L., Jowsey, J., Kelly, P. J., and Hoffman, D. L.: Treatment for postmenopausal and senile osteoporosis. Med. Clin. N. Amer. 56:989–997, 1972.

333. Robichon, J., Wiley, J. J., and Germain, J. P.: Osteopetrosis. Can. J. Surg. 11:424–430, 1968.

334. Robinson, R. G.: Paraplegia due to Paget's disease (osteitis deformans). Brit. Med. J. 2:542–544, 1953.

335. Rockoff, S. D., Zeitner, A., and Albright, J.: Radiographic trabecular quantitation of human lumbar vertebrae in situ. II. Relation to bone quantity, strength and mineral content (preliminary results). Invest. Radiol. 2:339–352, 1967.

336. Rockoff, S. D., Sweet, E., and Bleustein, J.: The relative contribution of trabecular and cortical bone to the strength of human lumbar vertebrae. Calc. Tiss. Res. 3:163–175, 1969.

337. Rose, G. A., Lumb, F. H., and Dent, C. E.: Discussion on generalized aches and pain from metabolic bone diseases. Proc. Roy. Soc. Med. 50:371–380, 1957.

338. Rose, G. A.: Some thoughts on osteoporosis and osteomalacia. Sci. Bas. Med. Ann. Rev. 252–275, 1967.

339. Rosen, J. F. and Haymovitz, A.: Liver lysosomes in congenital osteopetrosis. J. Pediat. 81:518–527, 1972.

340. Rosen, J. F., and Finberg, L.: Vitamin D dependent rickets: actions of parathyroid hormone and 25-hydroxy cholecalciferol. B, 388–393.

341. Rowland, R. E., Marshall, J. H., and Jowsey, J.: Radium in human bone: the microradiographic appearance. J. Radiat. Res. 10:323–336, 1959.

342. Rubin, P.: Dynamic classification of bone dysplasia. Chicago, Year Book Medical Publishers, 1964.

343. Russell, G. G., and Fleisch, H.: Inorganic pyrophosphate and pyrophosphatases in calcification and calcium homeostasis. Clin. Orthop. 69:101–117, 1970.

344. Rutishauser, E., and Mayno, G.: Physiopathology of bone tissue: the osteocytes and fundamental substance. Bull. Hosp. Joint Dis. 12:468–490, 1951.

345. Samachson, J.: Basic requirements for calcification. Nature 221:1247–1248, 1969.

346. Sarnsethsiri, P., Hitt, O. C., Eyring, E. J., and Frost, H. M.: A tetracycline-based study of bone dynamics in pycnodysostosis. Clin. Orthop. 74:301–312, 1971.

347. Saville, P. D.: Osteoporosis: An overview. B, 293–392.

348. Schenk, R. K., Olah, A. J., and Merz, W. A.: Bone cell counts. B, 103–113.

349. Scherft, J. P.: The lamina limitans of the organic matrix of calcified cartilage and bone. J. Ultrastruct. Res. 38:318–331, 1972.

350. Schreiber, M. H., and Richardson, L. A.: Paget's disease confined to one lumbar vertebra. Amer. J. Roent. 90:1271–1276, 1963.

351. Seftel, H. C., Malkin, C., Schmaman, A., Abrahams, C., Lynch, S. R., Charlton, R. W., and Bothwell, T. H.: Osteoporosis, scurvy and siderosis in Johannesburg Bantu. Brit. Med. J. 1:642–646, 1966.

352. Seliger, W. G.: Tissue fluid movement in compact bone. Anat. Rec. 166:247–255, 1970.

353. Shaw, M. T., and Davies, M.: Primary hyperparathyroidism presenting as spinal cord compression. Brit. Med. J. 4:230–231, 1968.

354. Sherman, M.: The nerves of bone. J. Bone Joint Surg. 45A:522, 1963.

355. Shifrin, L. Z.: Correlation of serum alkaline phosphatase with bone formation rates. Clin. Orthop. 70:212–215, 1970.

356. Sigurdsson, G., Woodhouse, W. J. Y., Taylor, S., and Joplin, G. F.: Stilboestrol diphosphate in hypercalcaemia due to parathyroid carcinoma. Brit. Med. J. 1:27–28, 1973.

357. Singh, A. and Jolly, S. S.: Endemic fluorosis with particular reference to fluorotic radiculomyelopathy. Quart. J. Med. 30:357–372, 1961.

358. Singh, A., Das, R., Hayret, S. S., and Jolly, S. S.: Skeletal changes in endemic fluorosis. J. Bone Joint Surg. 44B:806–815, 1962.

359. Singh, A., Jolly, S. S., Bansal, B. C., and Mathur, C. C.: Endemic fluorosis. Medicine 42:229–246, 1963.

360. Singh, M., Nagrath, A. R., and Maini, P. S.: Changes in trabecular pattern of the upper end of the femur as an index of osteoporosis. J. Bone Joint Surg. 52A:457–467, 1970.

361. Singh, M., Riggs, B., Beabout, J. W., and Jowsey, J.: Femoral trabecular pattern index for evaluation of spinal osteoporosis. Ann. Intern. Med. 77:63–67, 1972.

362. Skeels, R. T.: The reversibility of osteoporosis in Cushing's disease. A case report. J. Clin. Endocr. 18:61–64, 1958.

363. Smith, D. A., Anderson, J. B., Shimmins, J., Speurs, C. F., and Barnett, E.: Changes in metacarpal mineral content and density in normal male and female subjects with age. Clin. Radiol. 20:23–31, 1969.

364. Smith, J. F.: Parathyroid adenomas associated with malabsorption syndrome and chronic renal disease. J. Clin. Path. 23:362–369, 1970.

365. Smith, R., and Stern, G.: Myopathy, osteomalacia and hyperparathyroidism. Brain 90:593, 1967.

366. Smith, R.: The pathophysiology and management of rickets. *E*, 601–622.

367. Smith, R. W., Rizek, J., and Frame, B. with Mansour, J.: Determinants of serum antirachitic activity. Amer. J. Clin. Nutr. *14*:98–108, 1964.

368. Smith, R. W., and Taft, P. M.: Relationship of vertebral size to fracture in osteoporotic spines. Henry Ford Hosp. Med. J. *15*:101–106, 1967.

369. Smith, R. W., and Rizek, J.: Epidemiologic studies of osteoporosis in women of Puerto Rico and Southeastern Michigan with special reference to age, race, national origin and to other related or associated findings. Clin. Orthop. *45*:31–48, 1966.

370. Smith, R. W., Eyler, W. R., and Mellinger, R. W.: On the incidence of senile osteoporosis. Ann. Intern. Med. *52*:773–781, 1960.

371. Smith, R. W., and Frame, B.: Concurrent axial and appendicular osteoporosis: Its relation to calcium consumption. N. Eng. J. Med. *273*:73–78, 1965.

372. Smith, R. W., and Walker, R. R.: Femoral expansion in aging woman: implications for osteoporosis and fractures. Science *145*:156–157, 1964.

373. Solomon, G. F., Dickerson, W. T., and Eisenberg, E.: Psychologic and osteometabolic responses to sex hormones in elderly osteoporotic women. Geriatrics *15*:46–60, 1960.

374. Sotaniemi, E. A., Hakkarainen, H. K., Puranen, J. A., and Lahle, R. O.: Radiologic bone changes and hypocalcemia with anticonvulsant therapy in epilepsy. Ann. Intern. Med. *77*:389–394, 1972.

375. Spencer, H., Menczel, J., Lewin, I., and Samachson, J. D.: Absorption of calcium in osteoporosis. Amer. J. Med. *37*:223–234, 1964.

376. Srikantia, S. G., and Siddiqui, A. H.: Metabolic studies in skeletal fluorosis. Clin. Sci. *28*:477–485, 1965.

377. Stamp, T. C. B., Round, J. M., Rowe, D. J. F., and Haddad, J. G.: Plasma levels and therapeutic effect of 25-hydroxycholecalciferol in epileptic patients taking anticonvulsant drugs. Brit. Med. J. *4*:9–12, 1972.

378. Stanley, P., Baker, S. L., and Byers, P. D.: Unusual bone trabeculation in a patient with macroglobulinaemia simulating fibrogenesis imperfecta ossium. Brit. J. Radiol. *44*:305–315, 1971.

379. Stanbury, S. W.: Osteomalacia. *A*, 239–266.

380. Steinbach, H. L., Feldman, R., and Goldberg, M. B.: Acromegaly. Radiology *72*:535–549, 1959.

381. Steinbach, H. L.: Roentgenology of the skeleton in the aged. Radiol. Clin. N. Amer. *3*:277–292, 1965.

382. Steinbach, H. L., Kolb, F. O., and Gilfielan, R.: A mechanism of the production of pseudofractures in osteomalacia (Milkman's syndrome). Radiology *62*:388–395, 1954.

383. Stevens, J. Freeman, P. A., Nordin, B. E. C., and Barnett, E.: The incidence of osteoporosis in patients with femoral neck fracture. J. Bone Joint Surg. *44B*:520–523, 1962.

384. Stevenson, C. J., Bottoms, E., and Shuster, S.: Skin collagen in osteogenesis imperfecta. Lancet, *1*:860–861, 1970.

385. Talmage, R. V.: Calcium homeostasis-calcium transport-parathyroid action. Clin. Orthop. *67*:210–224, 1969.

386. Taylor, S.: Hyperparathyroidism. *A*, 79–92.

387. Teng, P., Gross, G. W., and Hewman, C. M.: Compression of spinal cord by osteitis deformans (Paget's disease) giant cell tumor, and polyostotic fibrous dysplasia (Albright's syndrome) of vertebrae. J. Neurosurg. *8*:482–493, 1951.

388. Teotia, M., Teotia, S. P. S., and Kurwa, K. D.: Endemic skeletal fluorosis. Arch. Dis. Child. *46*:686–691, 1971.

389. Teotia, S. P. S.: Nutritional osteomalacia in Northern India. Abstract submitted to International Symposium on Clinical Aspects of Metabolic Bone Disease, Detroit, 1972.

390. Termine, J. D.: Mineral chemistry and skeletal biology. Clin. Orthop. *85*:207–241, 1972.

391. Thalassinos, N. C., Wicht, S. and Joplin, G. F.: Secondary hyperparathyroidism in osteomalacia. Brit. Med. J. *1*:76–79, 1970.

392. Thompson, R. C., Gaull, G. E., Horwitz, S. J., and Schenk, R. K.: Hereditary hyperphosphatasia. Amer. J. Med. *47*:209–219, 1969.

393. Tseng, T. C., Daeschner, C. W., Singleton, E. B., Rosenberg, H. S., Cole, V. W., Hill, L. L., and Brennan, J. C.: Liver diseases and osteoporosis in children. J. Pediat. *59*:684–709, 1961.

394. Urist, M. R., Gurvey, M. S. and Fareed, D. O.: Long-term observations on aged women with pathologic osteoporosis. *D*, 3–37.

395. Vaishnava, H., and Rizvi, S. N. A.: Nutritional osteomalacia in immigrants in an urban community. Lancet *2*:1147, 1971.

396. Vaishnava, H. and Rizvi, S. N. A.: Primary hyperparathyroidism associated with nutritional osteomalacia. Amer. J. Med. *46*:640–645, 1969.

397. Van Buchem, F. S. P., Hadders, H. N., Hansen, J. F., and Woldring, M. L.: Hyperostosis corticalis generalisata. Report of seven cases. Amer. J. Med. *33*:387–397, 1962.

398. Van Buchem, F. S. P.: The pathogenesis of hyperostosis corticalis generalisata and calcitonin. Konink. Nederl. Akad. van Wetenschappen Proc. Series C. *73*:243–253, 1970.

399. Vaughan, J. M.: The Physiology of Bone. Oxford, Oxford Univ. Press, 1970.

400. Villanueva, A. R., Ilnicki, L., Duncan, H., and Frost, H. M.: Bone and cell dynamics in the osteoporoses: A review of measurements by tetracycline bone labeling. Clin. Orthop. *49*:135–150, 1966.

401. Villanueva, A. R., Jaworski, Z. F., Hitt, O., Sarnsethsiri, P., and Frost, H. M.: Cellular level bone resorption in chronic renal failure and primary hyperparathyroidism. Calc. Tiss. Res. *5(4)*:289–304, 1970.

402. Villanueva, A. R., and Frost, H. M.: Bone formation in human osteogenesis imperfecta, measured by tetracycline bone labeling. Acta Orthop. Scand. *41*:531–538, 1970.

403. Virtama, P., Gästrin, G., and Teokka, A.: Biconcavity of the vertebrae as an estimate of their bone density. Clin. Radiol. *13*:128–131, 1962.

404. Wachman, A., and Bernstein, D. S.: Diet and osteoporosis. Lancet *1*:958–959, 1968.

405. Waine, H., Bennett, G. A., and Bauer, W.: Joint disease associated with acromegaly. Amer. J. Med. Sci. *209*:672–687, 1945.

406. Wakamatsu, E. and Sissons, H. A.: The cancellous bone of the iliac crest. Calc. Tiss. Res. *4*:147–161, 1969.

407. Walker, A. R. P.: The human requirement of calcium: should low intakes be supplemented? Amer. J. Clin. Nutr. 25:518–520, 1972.

408. Wallach, S., Aloia, J., and Cohn, S.: Treatment of osteoporosis with calcitonin. C, 21–26.

409. Weick, M. T.: A history of rickets in the United States. Amer. J. Clin. Nutr. 20:1234–1241, 1967.

410. Wells, I. C., and Gambal, D. A.: Vitamin D-dependent serum factor promoting calcium uptake by bone. Proc. Soc. Exp. Biol. Med. 127:1006, 1968.

411. Whitehouse, W. J., Dyson, E. D., and Jackson, C. K.: The scanning electron microscope in studies of trabecular bone from a human vertebral body. J. Anat. 108:481, 1971.

412. Whitson, S. W.: Tight junction formation in the osteon. Clin. Orthop., 86:206–213, 1972.

413. Wills, M. R., Richardson, R. E., and Paul, R. G.: Osteosclerotic bone changes in primary hyperparathyroidism with renal failure. Brit. Med. J. 1:252–255, 1961.

414. Woodard, H. Q.: Long term studies of the blood chemistry in Paget's disease of bone. Cancer 12:1226–1237, 1959.

415. Woodhouse, N. J. Y.: Paget's disease of bone. A, 125–142.

416. Woodhouse, N. J. Y., Doyle, F. H., and Joplin, G. F.: Vitamin D deficiency and primary hyperparathyroidism. Lancet 2:283–286, 1971.

417. Woodhouse, N. J. Y., Fisher, M. T., Sigurdsson, G., Joplin, G. F., and MacIntyre, I.: Paget's disease in a 5-year-old: Acute response to calcitonin. Brit. Med. J. 4:267–269, 1972.

418. Wu, K., and Frost, H. M.: Bone formation in osteoporosis. Arch. Pathol. 88:508–510, 1969.

419. Wu, K., Jett, S., and Frost, H. M.: Bone resorption rates in rib in physiological, senile and postmenopausal osteoporoses. J. Lab. Clin. Med. 69:810–818, 1967.

420. Wycis, H. T.: Basilar impression. A case secondary to advanced Paget's disease with severe neurologic manifestations. Successful surgical result. J. Neurosurg. 1:299–305, 1944.

421. Young, R. W.: The control of cell specialization in bone. Clin. Orthop. 45:153–156, 1966.

422. Yu, J. S., Walker-Smith, J. A., and Burnard, E. D.: Rickets: A common complication of neonatal hepatitis. Med. J. Austr. 1:790, 1971.

423. Zorab, P. A., Clark, J., Cotrel, Y., and Harrison, A.: Bone collagen turnover in idiopathic scoliosis estimated from total hydroxyproline excretion. Arch. Dis. Child. 46:828–832.

CHAPTER 14

Arthritis of the Spine

ARTHRITIC DISORDERS OF THE SPINE
NATHAN SMUKLER, M.D.

Thomas Jefferson University

ANKYLOSING SPONDYLITIS

Introduction

Ankylosing spondylitis is a chronic inflammatory disease which characteristically involves the sacroiliac and spinal joints, but also other musculoskeletal structures, the eyes and, rarely, the heart. Prior to 1960 this disease was usually referred to as rheumatoid spondylitis in the American literature, as it was considered a spinal variant of rheumatoid arthritis. However, as ankylosing spondylitis patients were more critically studied, it became clear they could be differentiated from those with rheumatoid arthritis on the basis of numerous findings; these included the characteristic spinal involvement, predilection for young men, absence of rheumatoid factor and subcutaneous nodules, and failure to respond to certain drugs which are valuable in the management of rheumatoid arthritis patients. The eponyms von Bechterew arthritis and Marie-Strumpell's disease also have been applied to this disease on the basis of the clinical and clinicopathologic studies published by these physicians during the last decade of the nineteenth century. Further confusion has been added by the use of numerous synonyms, including pelvospondylitis ossificans and spondylitis ankylopoietica. However, from this plethora of synonyms and eponyms, ankylosing spondylitis has emerged as the generally accepted name for this disease.

The incidence of ankylosing spondylitis in the general population has been variously estimated at 1 to 3 per 1000, with young men composing the segment of population at greatest risk.[1-3] In numerous series the ratio of men to women ranges from 4 to 1 to 15 to 1.[4-6] The incidence of ankylosing spondylitis *vis-a-vis* rheumatoid arthritis varies from 1 in 13 to 1 in 19, as noted in Boland's summary, garnered from several arthritis centers in the United States.[7] Ankylosing spondylitis patients, however, are more likely to be encountered in military than civilian practice as a corollary of the predilection for young men.[7] Baum and Ziff found ankylosing spondylitis to be less common among American blacks than whites (ratio of 1:4) and noted that it is extremely rare in African blacks.[8] On the basis of these observations, they have theorized that, since there is a genetic predisposition to this disease, the incidence among black Americans is a reflection of an admixture of genes.

The onset of ankylosing spondylitis is usually in the third decade; but it may appear during the second decade, and there are rare reports of its appearance during the first.[9] However, the onset is not always in the early decades; Wilkinson and Bywaters reported the apparent onset after the age of 39 in 11 per cent of their series of 222 patients.[10]

There is little known concerning the pathogenesis or etiology of ankylosing spondylitis and this, in all likelihood, is at least partially the result of emphasis on the investigation of the more prevalent and generally more crippling disease, rheumatoid arthritis. Numerous studies have shown that there is a familial predisposition to ankylosing spondylitis and perhaps the most impressive investigations have been those carried out in families of ankylosing spondylitis patients belonging to North American Indian tribes.[2, 11, 12, 12a] However, these studies have failed to identify a usual pattern of inheritance for a single mendelian gene defect and raise the possibility of a polygeneic defect or an additional etiologic factor or factors. Evidence for one genetic factor in this disease has been recently defined by HL-A antigen typing.

HL-A antigens are genetically determined and can be identified by a typing procedure based on a toxic reaction of lymphocytes after exposure to an incompatible serum antibody. Schlosstein et al. found HL-A antigen of the W-27 type in 88 per cent of 40 ankylosing spondylitis patients and 8 per cent of controls.[12b] Similarly, Brewerton et al. noted this antigen in 95 per cent of 75 ankylosing spondylitis patients and 4 per cent of controls.[12c] An observation pertinent to these findings is that approximately 5 per cent of the Caucasian population has HL-A antigen of the W-27 type, but that less than 1 per cent of this population develops ankylosing spondylitis. It appears then that individuals with W-27 antigen are at increased risk to develop ankylosing spondylitis, but multiple etiologic factors are operative, as most individuals positive for W-27 antigen do not develop ankylosing spondylitis. The W-27 antigen appears to have great promise as a marker to identify those with genetic susceptibility to develop ankylosing spondylitis, but it is not currently known how the antigen contributes to the pathogenesis of the disease. It has been suggested that individuals with this antigen have an unusual susceptibility to react immunologically to the etiologic factor. Another hypothesis implicates a similarity in molecular structure of the W-27 antigen and the etiologic factor predisposing to an immunological cross-over reaction.[12b]

Histocompatibility antigen W-27 frequency has also been found to be significantly increased in patients with spondylitis associated with ulcerative colitis or regional enteritis, psoriasis and Reiter's syndrome.[12d, e, f, g] Thus a hereditary factor may underlie the similar spinal involvement found in many patients with these apparently diverse entities.

There have been numerous investigations attempting to prove that a microbiologic agent harbored in the genitourinary tract and disseminated to the sacroiliac joints through the pelvic lymphatics is the cause of ankylosing spondylitis. Interest in this concept was undoubtedly stimulated by reports of instances in which ankylosing spondylitis appeared to follow an episode of non-specific urethritis.[13] Although such patients may have had Reiter's syndrome, there are, nevertheless, definite similarities between the spondylitis associated with Reiter's triad and ankylosing spondylitis (see page 752), and the relationship between these spinal disorders remains unknown. Studies to determine a link between genitourinary tract infection and ankylosing spondylitis, to date, have not produced any convincing evidence to support this hypothesis.[14, 15] It is conceivable that a still unidentified infectious agent, such as a virus which is causally related to or disseminated as a result of the urethritis, is the etiologic factor in this disease. Such a virus could be pathogenetic as a result of its long survival in tissue, or by inducing an autoimmune reaction.

Pathology

Knowledge of the pathology of the spinal joints in ankylosing spondylitis has been limited by their inaccessibility for biopsy and the infrequency with which they are examined postmortem. In particular, there has been little opportunity to study the sequence of histological changes during the early and active phases of this disease. Blumberg and Ragan could not find evidence of a single study of this disease among over 10,000 autopsies, and only one biopsy among a total of 16,000 performed at the Columbia-Presbyterian Hospital in New York during the period from 1906 to 1956.[4] Cruickshank has approached this problem by studying biopsies of radiographically identified arthritis localized to the manubriosternal joint and postmortem specimens from the symphysis pubis and spines of ankylosing spondylitis patients.[16] The manubriosternal joint and the symphysis pubis are classified as synchondroses or fibrocartilaginous joints without a capsule, and thus they are analogous to the disc joints of the spine. There is, however, evidence of a rudimentary capsule at the symphysis pubis, and this joint may represent a transitional state between a synchondrosis and a diarthrodial joint. The sacroiliac joint is generally classified as a diarthrodial joint, but its capsule is rudimentary and perhaps it too falls in the transitional category.

Cruickshank, on the basis of his findings in the manubriosternal joint and the symphysis pubis, has evolved the following concept of the pathology of the synchondroses in ankylosing spondylitis.[16] Initially, there is an osteitis localized to the joint margins characterized by chronic inflammatory cells and vascular fibrous (granulation) tissue. At this stage, bone surrounding the early lesion shows osteoclastic resorption, and radiographs of the specimens show osteoporosis. Next, there is extensive replacement of subchondral bone and fibrocartilage by fibrous tissue which manifests little evidence of inflammation. Erosions of the joint surfaces are found on some of the radiographs of these lesions. The final or healing stage is ossification and obliteration of the joint and the radiographs show sclerosis and ankylosis (Fig. 14–1).

In postmortem studies of the disc joints of the spine, Cruickshank found ossification to be the most prevalent change.[16] In joints showing limited change, the ossification was confined to a strip at the anterior or posterior surface of the discs, although in some in-

stances both of these surfaces were involved. These bony strips originated close to a vertebral border and extended for varying distances over the height of the disc, and in some instances spanned the disc. Osseous changes of this type give rise to the radiographic finding of syndesmophytes, and involvement of the lateral aspects of several contiguous discs in the dorsolumbar area will yield a "bamboo spine." Ossification of the vertebral body also may occur, and is usually localized to the anterior surface adjacent to the disc. In a few specimens, fibrous tissue had replaced much of the disc and adjacent parts of the vertebral bodies, and presumably less extensive changes of this type preceded the disc ossification. It is, therefore, likely that the same sequence of events takes place in these spinal joints as had been noted in the manubriosternal joints and symphysis pubis. However, the predominance of the osseous phase in the disc joints may reflect a greater duration of disease in these specimens, which were all obtained at autopsy (Fig. 14–2).

The studies of Ball have suggested that certain anatomical factors account for the particular localization of the lesions in ankylosing spondylitis.[17] Biopsies of tender areas localized to the iliac crest, greater trochanter and patella in ankylosing spondylitis patients have revealed inflammatory lesions localized to the site of a bone-ligament junction or enthesis. The normal enthesis is characterized by a

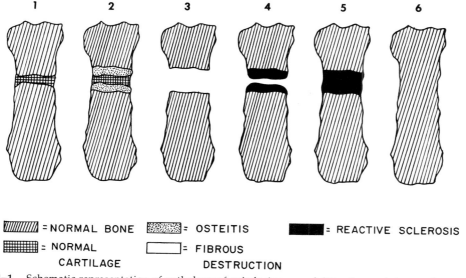

Figure 14–1. Schematic representation of pathology of ankylosing spondylitis at manubriosternal joint. *1,* Normal joint; *2,* osteitis at subchondral margins; *3,* fibrous destruction; *4,* early reactive sclerosis (reossification); *5,* late reactive sclerosis (reossification) and ankylosis; *6,* resorption of sclerosis and ankylosis.

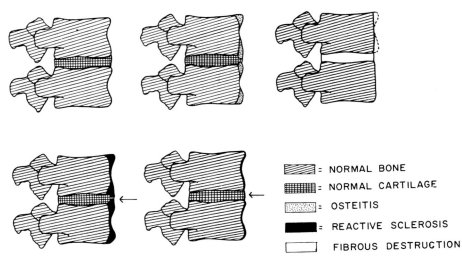

= NORMAL BONE

= NORMAL CARTILAGE

= OSTEITIS

= REACTIVE SCLEROSIS

= FIBROUS DESTRUCTION

Figure 14–2. Schematic representation of pathology of ankylosing spondylitis at lumbar vertebra. *Upper left,* normal; *upper center,* osteitis; *upper right,* fibrous destruction and squaring; *lower left,* reactive sclerosis (reossification) restoring normal contour and syndesmophyte formation (arrow); *lower right,* partial resorption of reactive sclerosis and syndesmophyte (arrow).

transition from densely fibrous ligament to cartilage, calcified cartilage and bone. Capillary vessels pass through the enthesis to reach bone, and both anatomical and physiological studies indicate that this is a site with considerable capacity for blood flow and metabolic activity.[17-20] Only the very outer layers of the fibrocartilaginous discs have a blood supply, and the juncture of this vascularized fibrocartilage with the vertebra, in a sense, forms an enthesis. In diarthrodial joints, the junction of the joint capsule and bone also simulates an enthesis. It has been hypothesized that the lesions of ankylosing spondylitis tend to localize at these junctions of fibrous and bone tissue.

Ball's contentions have been supported by postmortem studies of 13 patients.[17] In the spine, inflammatory and erosive lesions analogous to those described by Cruickshank[16] were noted in the outer portion of the annulus at or near the junction of the annulus and the vertebra. These lesions appeared to heal with deposition of new bone in the outer layers of the annulus, thus forming syndesmophytes and conforming to Cruickshank's osseous phase. Findings also suggested that these syndesmophytes enlarge as a result of activation of an inflammatory process at their tip. These studies do not support the possibility that syndesmophytes are the sequelae of an inflammatory reaction which originates in the anterior

longitudinal ligament and then spreads to the contiguous vertebral flanges and discs. However, syndesmophyte formation is most marked on the anterior surface of the vertebral bodies, and the connective tissue lining the anterior longitudinal ligament may be a factor in this localization. Ossification of the capsules of apophyseal joints was also observed. In one of these joints, the ossification was localized to the capsule-bone junction, presumably reflecting prior inflammation at this site, and thus was analogous to other enthesis lesions. In these specimens synovitis was minimal or absent, although proliferative synovitis similar to that of rheumatoid arthritis has been found in both peripheral and spinal joints of ankylosing patients. The cartilage in the apophyseal joints showing capsular ossification was either intact or replaced to some degree by enchondral ossification.

The pathologic changes which precede osseous ankylosis of the sacroiliac joints are obscure due to the rarity of study of these joints during the early phase of involvement. Ball, on the basis of one of his postmortem studies and by analogy to his findings in the apophyseal and disc joints, has suggested the following.[17] There is initially inflammation followed by ossification of the joint capsule, and then endochondral ossification of the articular cartilage which ultimately leads to ankylosis.

Support for this concept was found in the postmortem study of a 22-year-old man known to have ankylosing spondylitis for four years. One portion of his sacroiliac joint was enclosed in a 1 mm thick shell of bone and there was evidence of endochondral calcification of the adjacent cartilage. This concept of sacroiliac pathology will require further support before it can be accepted, as it is possible that proliferative synovitis may also be an antecedent of sacroiliac destruction in this disease.

The peripheral joints in ankylosing spondylitis show changes indistinguishable from those of rheumatoid arthritis, including proliferative synovitis, pannus formation and, ultimately, fibrous and bony ankylosis.[16, 17, 21]

CLINICAL FEATURES

Onset

Pain localized to the sacrum, buttocks and thighs is the usual initial manifestation of ankylosing spondylitis in adult patients. The buttock and thigh pain may be unilateral or bilateral, or it may alternate from side to side; however, typical sciatica with radiation of pain into the calf and foot rarely, if ever, occurs. In most patients (60 to 75 per cent in several series) the onset is insidious, and is characterized by a mild to moderate, dull ache; alternatively, there may be a sudden attack of severe pain.[5, 6, 10] Occasionally, patients may relate the onset of backache to a strain or trauma; however, careful review will usually disclose prior symptoms, and such incidents may serve to aggravate preexisting disease. The initial course may be marked by one or more remissions of the pain lasting for weeks or months, and in some instances severe exacerbations of up to two weeks may be superimposed on mild symptoms. Also, the severity of pain tends to vary during the course of a single day, being most severe for the first few hours after arising and recurring in the late afternoon and evening. If this early pain reflects the lumbar spine, in addition to the sacroiliac joints, it will be aggravated by motion but rest will not afford complete relief. Perhaps the most helpful early clue to the diagnosis of ankylosing spondylitis is classical "rheumatic" or "fibrositic" stiffness. Such stiffness, initially localized to the low back, is most severe during the early morning hours, then relieved for a period of time only to re-

turn with the approach of evening. Periods of rest provoke this symptom, and these patients may awaken at night with stiffness of such severity that it necessitates getting out of bed and limbering up before returning to sleep.

Other areas of the spine, peripheral joints, sites of tendon attachment and occasionally the eyes, may also be the initial sites of symptoms. Pain and stiffness reflecting involvement of the dorsal spine, rib cage joints, or cervical spine may be the first complaint. In these patients there is almost always radiographic evidence of disease of the sacroiliac joints which, however, are asymptomatic possibly as a result of mild involvement or a high pain threshold. In a series reported by Sigler et al., initial symptoms were localized to the dorsal spine in 5 per cent and to the cervical spine in 13 per cent; in 15 per cent the onset was marked by diffuse spinal symptoms.[5]

In approximately 20 per cent of patients the first symptoms are localized to the root (hip and shoulder) or peripheral joints. However, in children there is an even greater tendency for the initial manifestations to localize to limb joints. Schaller et al., for example, noted the onset of ankylosing spondylitis in joints peripheral to the shoulders and hips in four of seven children aged seven to 12.[9] Pain localized to the plantar surface of the heel is not an uncommon presenting symptom and in 2 per cent of patients uveitis antedates musculoskeletal symptoms.[5]

Rarely, systemic symptoms such as asthenia, low grade fever and weight loss may be associated with the onset of ankylosing spondylitis.

SACROILIAC JOINTS

Detection of disease of the sacroiliac joints by clinical evaluation is difficult and this undoubtedly contributes to the frequent delay in diagnosis of ankylosing spondylitis. The sacroiliac joints have a broad sensory supply which includes branches from L4 through S2 roots, and pain may be referred throughout the distribution of these nerves. Low back, buttock and thigh pain originating in the sacroiliac joints may easily be attributed to lumbar spine or hip disease. Also, the sacroiliac joints are difficult to evaluate by physical diagnostic procedures because of their deep set position and limited motion. Newton has described three brief, simple tests which he feels are reasonably reliable in detecting active inflammation of the sacroiliac joints.[22] He has found them to be positive in a high proportion of patients tested during the first four or five years of disease and negative in those with radiographic evidence of ankylosis or long standing and, likely, quiescent disease. Newton also suggests that tenderness is an unreliable and inconstant sign of sacroiliac disease, and that many of the tests designed to evaluate these joints also stress the lumbar spine or hip.[22] For the first two tests the patient is lying in a supine position. In the first test, the examiner places his palms over the anterior aspect of each ilium, and applies pressure in a posterior direction. In the second test, the examiner's palms are placed on the lateral aspects of the ilia, and pressure is directed toward the midline of the body. These tests are positive when there is pain localized to the lumbosacral or sacroiliac region, buttock or thigh. However, pain localized to areas where the hands compress the pelvis or the midline posteriorly at the site where the sacrum contacts the table are of no consequence. It is emphasized that these tests should be performed on a firm surface to prevent posterior displacement of the sacrum, which stresses the lumbosacral joint. Also, if there is a marked lumbar lordosis, this area should be supported with a pillow or folded blanket to eliminate stress upon this portion of the spine. The third test is performed with the patient in the prone position. The hands, one superimposed on the other, are applied to the mid-portion of the sacrum, and firm pressure is exerted in an anterior direction. Criteria for a positive test are similar to those for the first two tests. If two of these three tests are positive, it is very likely that there is disease of the sacroiliac joints.

LUMBAR SPINE

Involvement of the lumbar spine is manifested by local pain and stiffness, referred pain to the buttocks and thighs and, usually, the earliest dependable physical signs of spinal disease. Tenderness of the paraspinal muscles and spinous processes, pain on motion, and limited motion are early findings, and later there may be straightening of the lumbar lordosis, almost complete or complete loss of spinal motion, and atrophy of the paraspinal muscles.

The Schober test as modified by Macrae and Wright is probably the best approach to quantitating the loss of lumbar motion.[23] In the modified Schober test the lumbosacral junc-

tion is identified and points 10 cm above and 5 cm below are marked on the skin while the patient is standing erect. The patient then maximally flexes his lumbar spine, and the distance between the marks is remeasured. In the original test, skin marks were made at the lumbosacral junction and 10 cm cephalad to this point; however, the modified test provides the following advantages: 1) the skin 5 cm caudad to the lumbosacral junction is tightly tethered, and the marker at this point is not likely to ride up with forward flexion of the spine; 2) the use of markers above and below the lumbosacral junction minimizes error due to faulty identification of this site. Macrae and Wright, utilizing this technique, observed a mean distraction of 6.27 cm among a group of 342 subjects including patients with ulcerative colitis and their relatives and spouses; however, they emphasized that allowances must be made for variations due to age, sex and weight.[23] In the group of patients studied by these workers, there were six with classical x-ray findings of ankylosing spondylitis and all had limited spinal motion as defined by this test. Twelve patients with spinal x-ray findings only of sacroiliitis had normal lumbar spinal motion by this criterion; however, they were classified as false negatives. There were also five patients (1.5 per cent) with false positive tests.

DORSAL SPINE AND RIB CAGE

In this area disease may involve the costovertebral, costotransverse, and manubriosternal joints in addition to the spine. Pain originating in the spine or posterior rib joints may be localized to the spine or be referred to the chest or abdomen, the referred component generally spreading in a circumferential manner rather than penetrating directly anteriorly. Also, the pain arising from the manubriosternal joint and localized referred pain to the chest or abdomen may be attributed to intrathoracic or intraabdominal disease. Additional symptoms may include a feeling of chest tightness and stiffness and difficulty in taking a deep breath.

Limitation of chest expansion due to disease of the costovertebral joints is the most reliable indication of thoracic spine involvement. This may be an early finding, antedating symptoms or radiological evidence of thoracic involvement. Chest expansion measured at the nipple line should be at least 5 cm in normal young men; however, this cannot be utilized as a standard for all patients, as Moll and Wright have shown that chest expansion decreases with aging and in the presence of obesity and pulmonary disease.[24] Tenderness of paraspinal muscles and spinous processes, and pain on rotation of this portion of the spine are additional early signs. Atrophy of the dorsal paraspinal muscles in association with similar change in the lumbar area will yield an "ironed out" appearance of the back, and with progressive long-standing disease the dorsal spine may develop a kyphotic configuration (Fig. 14–4).

Patients with a destructive lesion localized to one or perhaps two of the lumbar or dorsal vertebrae as a manifestation of ankylosing spondylitis, will have a different clinical presentation.[25-27] It may be stated at this point that the origin of these lesions has not been clarified. They are generally considered to be caused by an extensive destructive fibrous tis-

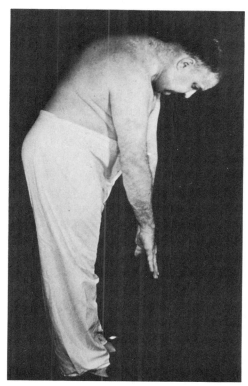

Figure 14–4. Patient with long-standing ankylosing spondylitis showing maximum forward bending attainable by flexion of the lumbar and dorsal spine. There is a marked cervicodorsal kyphosis.

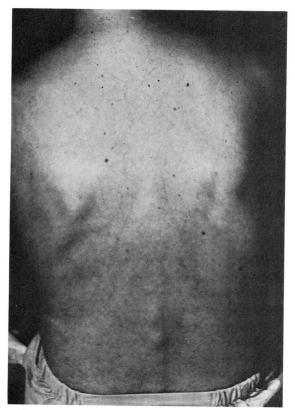

Figure 14–3. Paraspinal muscle atrophy yielding "ironed out" appearance in patient with ankylosing spondylitis involving the lumbar and dorsal spine.

sue reaction; however, some believe them to be secondary to excessive stress in an unankylosed portion of a severely involved spine.[26, 27] In these patients, generally with clinical and radiological evidence of long-standing disease, there is acute onset of localized lumbar or dorsal spine pain, or well-localized referred abdominal or chest pain. The referred pain may be interpreted as arising in the abdomen or chest, but a history of aggravation by spine motion, deep breathing, or walking or standing will point to the spinal origin. On examination, there is likely to be tenderness localized to one or two spinous processes and pain on forced extension of the spine. These lesions may be associated with spinal cord compression, and neurological examination is mandatory.

CERVICAL SPINE

Pain, stiffness and limitation of motion are the usual manifestations with involvement of the cervical spine. The pain may be local or at the usual sites of referred pain for the cervical spine, including the occiput, epaulet, interscapular and upper chest areas. Spinous process tenderness and pain on motion are the earliest physical findings; however, limitation of motion which may progress to ankylosis, eventually develops. An occasional ankylosing spondylitis patient will first seek medical advice when severe cervical restriction becomes a problem at work or while driving. Flexion deformity may be prominent and the entire cervical dorsal spine may be aligned in a single kyphotic curve (Fig. 14–4). Patients with a significant curve of this type develop compensatory flexion at the hips and knees in order to maintain their peripheral vision.

Dislocation of the atlantoaxial joint may occur in ankylosing spondylitis, with clinical manifestations that are generally similar to those found in association with rheumatoid disease of this articulation (see page 765). However, Sharp and Purser have noted that ankylosing spondylitis patients are likely to show more striking cervical and occipital clinical findings, including: 1) forward flexion of the head; 2) forward displacement of the head, with loss of usual contour in the occipital region; and 3) rotation and lateral tilting of the head.[28] These authors also report that patients with this flexion deformity may experience a sensation of the head "falling forward."

Trauma

These spines are extremely vulnerable to trauma, and seemingly insignificant strains and falls may lead to fracture at any level. Following trauma these patients should be observed carefully for signs of spinal cord compression.[29]

Neurological Involvement

It is appealing to explain the diffuse pain frequently encountered in ankylosing spondylitis patients on the basis of nerve root or spinal cord involvement, for conceivably the spine inflammation could spread to or distort these structures. However, the usual absence of motor or sensory nerve impairment suggests that nerve involvement is not an important pain mechanism. Paraplegia in these patients is usually secondary to fracture of the brittle spine. Lorber et al., however, have

described a patient with a history of ankylosing spondylitis for 20 years who developed paraplegia in association with a destructive fibrous tissue reaction involving two midthoracic vertebrae.[25] The fibrous tissue, which was negative for acid-fast organisms and fungi on culture, was considered to be an aspect of ankylosing spondylitis.

Matthews, in a recent report, described two patients of his own, and an additional six gleaned from the literature, who had a cauda equina syndrome in association with ankylosing spondylitis.[30] These patients showed evidence of motor and sensory impairment of the sacral and coccygeal roots, particularly manifested as sphincter disturbances. However, subsequent survey of a large group of patients failed to reveal additional examples of this type of involvement. Postmortem study of one of the cauda equina syndrome patients revealed prominent arachnoid cysts which eroded the lower lumbar vertebrae and the roof of the sacrum, and some of the nerve roots showed evidence of fibrosis and demyelinization. There also was suggestive evidence of similar arachnoid cysts on myelograms from a few other patients with cauda equina involvement. The author believes that an inflammatory reaction, presumably an aspect of the basic disease, involves the meninges and is the forerunner of the nerve damage and the arachnoid cysts. It is clear, however, that if meningeal involvement does occur in ankylosing spondylitis, it is generally not associated with clinically detectable nerve damage.

Extra-Spinal Musculoskeletal Disease

Involvement of extra-spinal joints, including the root joints (hips and shoulders) and peripheral joints, is common in ankylosing spondylitis. The percentage of patients with extra-spinal joint disease varies in reports from several clinics, and this in all likelihood is related to differences in criteria for joint involvement. It is a reasonable generalization that extra-spinal arthritis marks the onset of ankylosing spondylitis in 20 per cent and is present at some time during the course of disease in 50 per cent of patients. In children and teenagers, there is even greater involvement of these joints, particularly at the outset, but also during the course of disease. Typically, the arthritis is asymmetrical, transient, lasts weeks to months, involves a few weight-bearing joints, and does not progress to deformity or loss of joint function. Although the extra-spinal joint disease is generally benign, recent studies by McEwen et al.,[31] Riley et al.,[32] and Glick[33] have shown that radiological evidence of joint disease is not uncommon. In Riley's study, among 54 patients with onset of disease under age 21, there was radiographic evidence of involvement of root joints in 35 per cent and of peripheral joints in 37 per cent; however, in patients with onset after age 21, radiological findings were less frequent.

The extra-spinal arthritis was found most frequently in the metatarsophalangeal joints. Glick's retrospective radiological study of the hip joints of 240 patients revealed abnormalities in one third, and although the changes were generally mild, 12 per cent showed ankylosis.[33] The hip joints are an exception to the generalization that extra-spinal joint disease is mild in ankylosing spondylitis.

Extra-articular bone lesions in the locale of tendon or ligament attachments may develop at numerous sites including the calcanei, greater trochanters, ischial tuberosities and ribs. Pain at the posterior or plantar surface of the heel, and marked discomfort on sitting secondary to tenderness at the ischial tuberosity are manifestations of this type of lesion.

Extra-Musculoskeletal Disease

Recurrent iritis, cardiovascular disease characterized by aortitis and carditis and, rarely, pulmonary disease are the significant forms of extra-musculoskeletal disease in ankylosing spondylitis. Recurrent iritis is noted in 25 per cent of patients and in perhaps two per cent it is the initial manifestation, antedating other symptoms by months or years.[6, 10] The attacks are generally unilateral, but recurrent episodes may affect either eye, although serious visual impairment is uncommon. Palpitation, tachycardia, ECG evidence of conduction defects, and pericarditis may be early signs of cardiovascular involvement and precede the murmur of aortic regurgitation, which is the most characteristic finding of "spondylitic" heart disease. Clinical, laboratory and pathologic studies of these patients indicate that they have a unique form of cardiac involvement which is neither a sequela of rheumatic fever nor related to other recognized forms of heart disease. Postmortem examination of such patients has disclosed

aortic ring dilatation and an inflammatory and destructive lesion in the media of the proximal aorta reminiscent of syphilitic medial necrosis. In Graham and Smythe's series of 519 patients, the overall prevalence of aortic regurgitation was four per cent; however, among patients with disease of 30 years' duration, it increased to 10 per cent.[34] This cardiac disorder was often a source of disability in those in whom 15 years had elapsed since the detection of heart disease, and in some instances it was the cause of death.

Although limited mobility of the rib cage and thoracic spine does not tend to compromise pulmonary function in ankylosing spondylitis (AS) patients, nevertheless the respiratory system may not be spared, for fibrotic lung disease may occur in these patients. This pulmonary lesion appears to be a rare finding in AS patients who have had spinal involvement for many years. The radiographic findings are generally limited to the upper lung fields, and although bilateral involvement is usual the disease may be unilateral at the outset. Early, there are fine nodules and areas of fibrosis but the lesions are characteristically progressive and areas of consolidation and cavitation usually develop. On histologic examination the earliest change appears to be interstitial fibrosis, but later there are areas of dense fibrosis with distortion of lung parenchyma and cavitation.[34-37]

The pulmonary fibrosis in these patients appears to be a manifestation of ankylosing spondylitis. Although it is attractive to suspect that the limited thoracic excursions found in this disease might be a predisposition to infection, there is no evidence that a microbiologic agent is responsible for this fibrotic reaction. The cavitary lesions are frequently colonized by aspergilli, but these fungi are almost certainly secondary invaders. Also, there is no evidence that this is a tuberculous lesion, and it is likely that prior reports of increased pulmonary tuberculosis among AS patients have included some with this entity.[37] Finally, this did not appear to be a post-irradiation fibrosis, as only a small percentage of these patients have received x-ray therapy for their spinal disease.[37]

There is no effective treatment for this pulmonary fibrosis; however, the generally poor prognosis for these patients may be modified if antifungal agents such as 5-fluorocytosine amphotericin-B prove effective in eradicating aspergilli from these lesions.

Clinical Laboratory Studies

Clinical laboratory studies, with exception of the erythrocyte sedimentation rate (ESR), are not helpful in the diagnostic work-up or ankylosing spondylitis. The ESR is elevated in approximately 80 per cent of patients during the first few years of illness and also at other times when there is active disease; however, during the overall course of the disease, there are likely to be periods when this test is normal.[6] Wilkinson and Bywaters,[10] in a follow up study of 138 patients, found normal values in 52 per cent. In this same study, it was noted that the Westergren ESR is practically always elevated, and frequently quite highly in those with extraspinal articular disease; however, it was rarely over 40 mm per hour in those with disease limited to the spine. Rheumatoid factor, as determined by the latex flocculation test and other techniques, is invariably negative in ankylosing spondylitis patients and thus is a helpful test in distinguishing between ankylosing spondylitis and rheumatoid arthritis. Synovial fluid obtained from peripheral joints is of the Class II type (poor viscosity, poor mucin clot and increased WBC's) and is similar to that found in rheumatoid arthritis and many other inflammatory joint diseases.

It is unlikely that the spinal fluid would be studied during the diagnostic workup of an ankylosing spondylitis patient; however, it should be noted that spinal fluid protein may be elevated in this disease.[38,39]

Radiology

The diagnosis of ankylosing spondylitis is ultimately based on radiographic findings in the absence of clinical findings or laboratory tests which are pathognomonic for this disease. A rote approach to the varied and complex radiographic findings in this disease may be avoided if the basic pathology of ankylosing spondylitis is kept in mind. The pathology of this disease has been presented in a previous section; however, certain aspects may be recalled at this point. Cruickshank has described a sequence of three pathologic findings in the synchondroses: 1) osteitis manifest radiographically as osteoporosis; 2) fibrous tissue replacement of bone and cartilage which appears as osteolysis on x-rays; 3) ossification giving rise to the radiographic finding of bony sclerosis or joint ankylosis.[16] The

studies of Ball indicate that these reactions tend to localize at enthesis (bone-ligament junctions) or their equivalent, including the junction of the vascular outer fibers of the annulus of the intervertebral disc with vertebral body and the bone-capsule junction of diarthrodial joints.[17] This author finds that the diarthrodial joints, including the apophyseal joints of the spine, may be involved by two different pathologic reactions. In some instances there is a reaction similar to that of rheumatoid arthritis, a proliferative synovitis marked by pannus formation and erosions of cartilage and bone. However, in other instances an inflammatory reaction appears to begin at the bone-capsule junction and progresses to ossification of the capsule, while the articular cartilage is replaced by endochondral bone formation.

It is not clear which of the aforementioned processes account for the destruction of sacroiliac joints in ankylosing spondylitis, but the radiographic findings reflect the sequence of inflammation, bone destruction and ossification. The earlist findings in the sacroiliac joints may include patchy osteoporosis, irregular loss of subchondral cortex on the iliac side of the joint, widening of the joint space and erosions (Fig. 14–4). These early changes can be explained as the expression of an active inflammatory and destructive process which does not involve the joint in a uniform manner. Clearly the radiograph catches only one phase of this process and this accounts for the patchy and irregular distribution of the findings as well as the absence of one or more of these findings on a particular film. Berens also includes patchy subchondral sclerosis, usually localized to the iliac side of the joint, among the early radiographic findings (Fig. 14–5).[40] This sclerosis reflects the earliest phase of the ossification reaction. The late involvement is marked by increasing sclerosis of the joint margins, irregular bridging of the joint and, in many instances, complete obliteration of the joint space (Fig. 14–6).

There is discrepancy in the literature concerning the relationship of the clinical onset of ankylosing spondylitis to the earliest detection of radiographic findings in the sacroiliac joints. It has been suggested by some workers that the first radiographic signs of sacroiliac disease might not appear until many months or years after the onset of back pain.[7] However, Berens and Romanus and Yden believe on the basis of clinical and radiographic studies

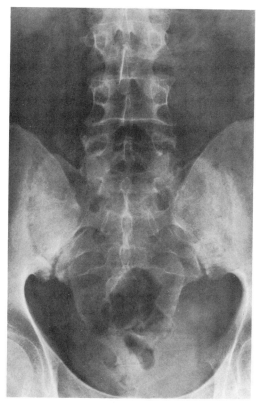

that careful radiographic evaluation of these joints will reveal changes concomitant with or shortly after the onset of back pain.[40, 41] If the initial films are negative, they should be repeated after six months, as they will almost certainly show changes in the presence of ankylosing spondylitis. Ankylosing spondylitis without sacroiliac joint involvement apparently does occur but is extremely rare. Polley and Slocumb[42] noted this in nine of 1035 patients and Romanus and Yden[41] in one of 117 patients; however, for practical purposes this diagnosis can be excluded if radiographs of the sacroiliac joints are normal. The sacroiliac joint involvement is characteristically bilateral; however, in some patients the changes may be more advanced on one side. In such instances of unequal or even unilateral involvement, followup studies will eventually disclose bilateral disease.

Sacroiliac findings in the young may be misinterpreted if changes related to growth are not considered. Carter and Loewi, in a study of x-rays from normal children, have shown that there is narrowing of the joint space and change in appearance of the joint margins with aging.[43] These joints are widest in children up to nine years of age, and in the 10-to-14-year-old age group there is some narrowing and the joint margins become less distinct. In those aged 14 to 20, the joint margins are likely to be obscured by the lateral sacral epiphyses.

Figure 14–5. Moderately early changes in the sacroiliac joints in ankylosing spondylitis. Widening and irregularity of the joint spaces and sclerosis are present.

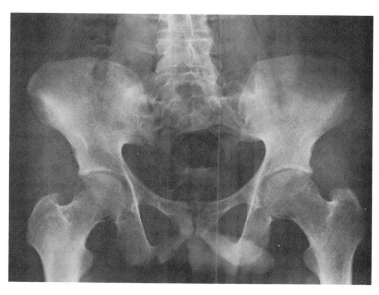

Figure 14–6. Fusion of the sacroiliac joint spaces in the late stage of sacroiliitis of ankylosing spondylitis. Note that the sclerosis has resorbed. There is slight narrowing of the left hip joint.

It is beyond this reviewer's competence to discuss radiographic techniques but it is necessary to emphasize that Berens and Grainger have indicated that routine AP studies of the lumbosacral spine and views obtained during intravenous pyelograms, barium enemas, and other specialized studies are often inadequate for evaluation of the sacroiliac joints.[40, 44] Grainger has emphasized the value of the prone (PA) study, for in this position the x-rays tend to pass through the plane of the joint, whereas in the supine (AP) view they tend to cross it.[44]

The value of angling the x-ray toward the head or feet to fully visualize this elongated joint has been stressed by Berens.[40] He has recommended two techniques: 1) a supine position with the x-ray angled 30 degrees toward the head; and 2) a prone study with x-rays angled 20 degrees in the direction of the feet.

Radiographic manifestations of the sequential changes of inflammation, destruction and repair by ossification at the junction of the outer portion of the annulus of the disc and the vertebral body may be seen on lateral films of the spine. Rarely, it is possible to see evidence of erosion and sclerosis localized to the upper or lower anterior corner of the vertebra, but the prominent finding is the square appearance of the anterior surface of the vertebra due to loss of the vertebral flanges (Fig. 14-7). Eventually the reparative process takes over, with evidence of sclerosis, restoration of the bony flange, and syndesmophyte formation (Fig. 14-8). Romanus and Yden have referred to these changes as anterior spondylitis;[41] however, a similar process may involve the lateral and posterior aspects of the vertebra, giving rise to syndesmophytes and in some instances a "bamboo" appearance. On the lateral aspects of the spine the destructive process is apparently less severe and squaring is not noted on frontal x-rays.

Squaring and syndesmophytes rank just behind the sacroiliac joint changes in diagnostic importance, and certain details of these findings deserve emphasis. Squaring may be missed if the patient is studied after repair has begun. Squaring and syndesmophytes are usually first noted at the lumbosacral and lumbodorsal junctions but their overall appearance is in a cephalad progression, and at times the cervical spine may be involved. Frontal, lateral and oblique views of the first lumbar

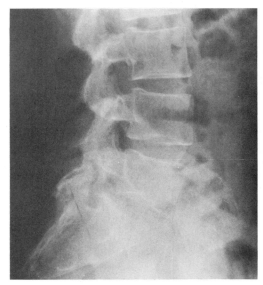

Figure 14-7. Squaring of the anterior surface of the fourth and fifth lumbar vertebrae in ankylosing spondylitis. The square appearance reflects an osteitis and fibrous reaction which has destroyed the bony flange at the upper and lower anterior surfaces of the involved vertebrae.

and lower dorsal vertebrae are valuable in detecting small syndesmophytes (Figs. 14-9, 14-10 and 14-11).[40] Romanus and Yden found that the time required for syndesmophytes to completely bridge the intervertebral disc varies greatly; those growing most rapidly required a minimum of a year and others appeared to grow intermittently and required several years.[41] Finally, it is necessary to appreciate that the vertically oriented syndesmophytes and the horizontally disposed osteophytes, which develop in relation to disc degeneration and protrusion have an entirely different pathogenesis and significance (Figs. 14-12 and 14-13). Occasionally, they may be difficult to distinguish on the radiographs but the overall findings in the spine should indicate their pathogenesis.

The inflammatory, destructive, and reparative phases of ankylosing spondylitis may lead to many additional radiographic findings but they are generally less characteristic and prevalent than the sacroiliac and disc joint changes. Among these findings are ossification localized to the transverse and spinous processes of the vertebra and iliolumbar and interspinous ligaments, generalized osteoporosis, narrowing of the intervertebral discs, and, rarely, an extensive destructive process involving one more vertebrae and adjacent discs. Extensive ossification of the interspinous ligaments accompanied by ossification of numerous apophyseal joints and connective tissue strands between these joints may lead to elongated parallel strips or tracks on frontal views of the spine (Fig. 14–14). Apophyseal joint involvement may be manifested by erosions, narrowing of the joint space and ankylosis, but these changes are difficult to delineate radiographically.

Radiographic evidence of dislocation of the atlantoaxial joint may be noted, but Sharp and Purser have found this lesion to be less prevalent in ankylosing spondylitis than in rheumatoid arthritis.[28] The radiographic criteria are considered on page 766.

Radiographic findings related to extraspinal musculoskeletal disease will be consid-

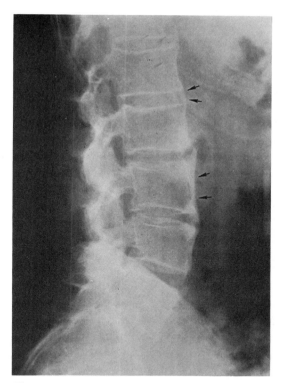

Figure 14–9. Lumbar spondylitis in ankylosing spondylitis. There is calcification of the prevertebral space (lower arrows) and a syndesmophyte (upper arrow).

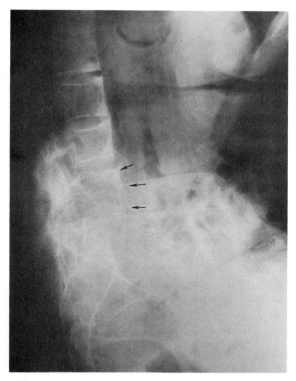

Figure 14–8. Sclerotic changes localized to the anterior surface of the vertebrae in ankylosing spondylitis. These changes reflect fibrous destruction and reactive sclerosis. The usual concavity of the anterior surface is lost and convexity is present due to resorption (arrows). Eventual restoration of the normal contour of the vertebrae may occur.

ered only briefly. Disease of the extraspinal joints is marked by changes similar to those of rheumatoid arthritis, with the exception of the hip joints, Forestier et al. noted an unusual, possibly specific, form of hip disease limited to patients under 40 years of age which is manifested by osteoporosis and eventually ankylosis with only minimal narrowing of the joint space.[45] These authors also described hip joint disease characterized by cartilage space narrowing and destructive changes in the femoral head and acetabulum in patients over 40 years of age (Fig. 14–15). The calcaneus is the most frequent site of extraspinal bone–tendon junction lesions in this disease. Radiographic signs of calcaneal disease may include: 1) erosions localized to the attachment site of the achilles tendon or plantar fascia; 2) generalized osteoporosis; 3) calcification and later spur formation at the plantar fascia attachment site; and 4) a rim of new bone formation at the posterior surface of the calcaneus (Fig. 14–16). Also bone–soft tissue attachment lesions at the pelvic brim or ischial tuberosity may be mani-

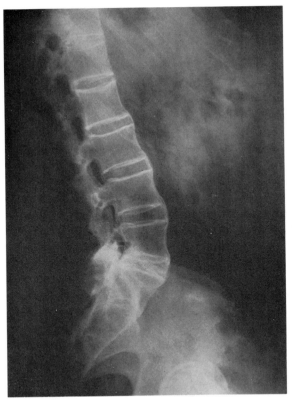

Figure 14–10. Lumbar spondylitis in ankylosing spondylitis. The anterior surfaces of the discs are bridged by syndesmophytes and there is modest osteoporosis of the vertebral bodies.

fested by irregular fuzzy new bone formation or "whiskering" (Fig. 14–17).

In summary, the diagnosis of ankylosing spondylitis is dependent upon detection of the radiographic changes indicative of bilateral sacroiliitis. Additionally, it is almost always possible to detect radiographic evidence of involvement of the vertebral bodies and discs as straightening of the anterior surface of the vertebrae and syndesmophytes.

Course of Disease

The course of ankylosing spondylitis in the pelvis and spine is characterized by initial involvement of the sacroiliac joints and progressive upward extension in the spine. The upward spread is not necessarily stepwise, for there is radiographic evidence that the vertebrae at the lumbodorsal junction are affected before the more caudal section of the lumbar

spine. The disease is rarely, if ever, confined to the sacroiliac joints and generally extends to involve the cervical spine; however, this may occur over a period of from five to 30 years.

Variations in disease activity, progressive spinal deformity and extraspinal joint disease, which is generally short lived and non-destructive, also characterize the course of ankylosing spondylitis. The overall course of disease is intermittent, with active phases, as defined by symptoms and radiographic findings, being interspersed with periods of inactivity of months' or even years' duration. There is also progressive spinal deformity with passage of years, and it is not clear whether this can be modified or prevented by present day treatment programs. The extraspinal joint disease is for the most part short lived and benign; however, hip involvement may progress to destruction or ankylosis with its attendant crippling.

The majority of ankylosing spondylitis patients can lead a reasonably normal life as

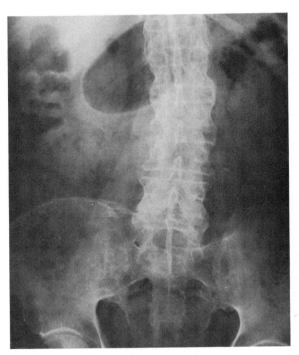

Figure 14–11. Syndesmophytes in ankylosing spondylitis. There are numerous syndesmophytes in various stages of development at the lateral aspects of the discs. Progression of this involvement will yield a "bamboo" spine. Fusion of the sacroiliac joints is present.

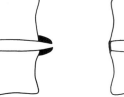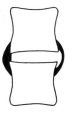

Figure 14–12. Osteophytes compared to marginal and non-marginal syndesmophytes.

OSTEOPHYTES

MARGINAL SYNDESMOPHYTES

NON-MARGINAL SYNDESMOPHYTES

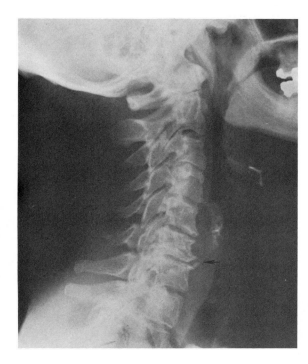

Figure 14–13. Horizontally disposed osteophytes (arrow) in spondylosis of the cervical spine.

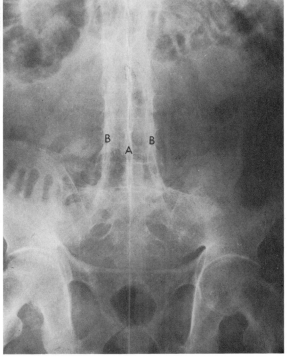

Figure 14–14. "Trolley track" configuration in ankylosing spondylitis. The parallel vertical white lines reflect ossification of the interspinous ligaments (A) and capsules of the apophyseal joints, as well as strands of connective tissue extending between these joints (B). The sacroiliac joints are fused.

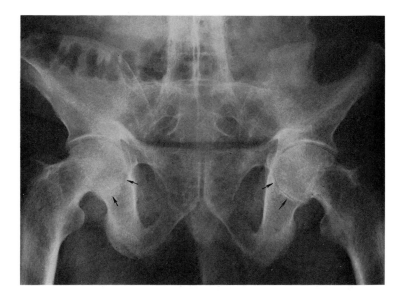

Figure 14–15. Hip joint involvement in a 48-year-old man who had ankylosing spondylitis for 30 years. There is narrowing of the cartilage space at the medial and inferior aspect of each joint (arrows). The sacroiliac joints are fused.

indicated by their ability to engage in sedentary occupations; in addition, this disease does not appear to shorten the life span. Blumberg and Ragan's study of 121 ankylosing spondylitis patients followed for from two to 35 years showed that 92 (76 per cent) were able to support themselves and their families.[4] However, spinal involvement was not the limiting factor in the remaining 24 patients, who were not gainfully employed; 12 had severe disease of the hips and the remainder were limited by a variety of non-rheumatic problems including psychiatric disease. It is clear from this study, and also from the one by Wilkinson and Bywaters,[10] that the prognosis for reasonable functional capacity in ankylosing spondylitis is quite good if the hip joints are spared. The disease does not appear to shorten life expec-

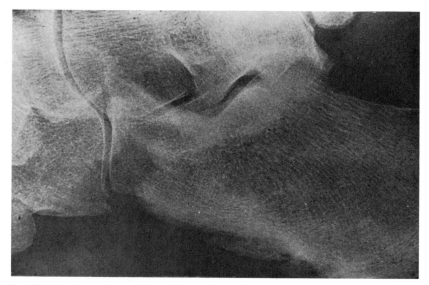

Figure 14–16.   Calcification and spur formation at plantar fascia attachment site in ankylosing spondylitis.

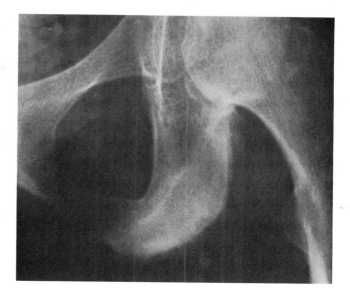

Figure 14–17. Fuzzy new bone formation or "whiskering" localized to the left ischial tuberosity in ankylosing spondylitis.

tancy or cause death except in patients with aortic, myocardial or lung involvement.

Diagnosis

The diagnosis of ankylosing spondylitis is suggested by the symptoms and clinical findings, which have been reviewed; but, in essence, the combination of low back, buttock and thigh pain along with protracted stiffness ("fibrositic" or "rheumatic") points to this disease. However, the diagnosis is ultimately dependent upon the demonstration of radiological findings which are highly indicative if not pathognomonic for this disease. The diagnosis can usually be clarified reasonably early in the course of disease, as radiographic evidence of bilateral sacroiliitis is usually present within six months of the onset of low back pain. It is not clear how long a lag period may exist between the onset of disease and radiographic evidence of sacroiliitis, when the initial involvement is in the extraspinal joints. The clinical laboratory is of little help in diagnosis, and it may be reiterated that although the ESR is often elevated, it may be normal during many periods throughout the course of this disease.

Differential Diagnosis

The differential diagnosis of ankylosing spondylitis widely encompasses those dis-

eases marked by stiffness and aching of the back or polyarthritis; however, in this section we will emphasize entities which by virtue of their clinical manifestations or radiographic findings or both would be most likely to be confused with ankylosing spondylitis. In addition, other entities which might be confused with ankylosing spondylitis but which have not been considered in other portions of this review will be cited in this section. Also, the reader will be referred to the appropriate section for diseases which although characterized by back pain are less likely to be confused with ankylosing spondylitis. Ankylosing spondylitis must be considered in the differential diagnosis of polyarthritis, particularly in children and young men, and appropriate spine x-rays must be obtained if this disease is to be identified; however, a review of the various diseases characterized by polyarthritis is beyond the scope of this review.

TRAUMATIC, DEGENERATIVE AND DEVELOPMENTAL DISORDERS. Patients with ankylosing spondylitis can generally be rather easily delineated from those with the commoner traumatic degenerative and developmental disorders of the spine. In young men, the presence of low back, buttock and thigh pain as manifestations of ankylosing spondylitis will raise the possibility of lumbosacral strain, herniated disc, or structural abnormalities such as spondylolisthesis; whereas patients in the fourth or, rarely, the fifth decade will have to be differentiated primarily from those with spondylosis. It has been previously noted that spondylitics may relate the onset of their pain to a traumatic incident, but on detailed questioning will recall prior stiffness and pain; however, such an anamnesis is unlikely in young men with post-traumatic conditions. Stiffness and muscle spasm may occur in all of these disorders, but protracted morning stiffness which can be "worked out" during the day only to return at evening or during the night is characteristic of ankylosing spondylitis.

Historical details serve as helpful clues but ultimately the differential diagnosis of these disorders is dependent upon examination of the spine and the nervous system, and on radiological studies. It may be reemphasized at this point that ankylosing spondylosis patients do not manifest signs of nerve root compression, and within six to 12 months of onset of their disease they are likely to show radiographic evidence of sacroiliitis. A possible source of confusion in older individuals is obliteration of the sacroiliac joints on a nonspecific, probably degenerative, basis; however, these subjects will not have additional radiographic evidence of spondylitis.

SACROILIAC DISEASE IN PARAPLEGIA. Paraplegics may develop sacroiliac changes presumably as a result of degeneration associated with chronic mechanical stress. Wright, Catterall and Cook, in a radiologic study of 38 paraplegic men, noted sacroiliac joint abnormalities, primarily joint space narrowing but without erosions or ankylosis, in 12.[46] The authors attributed these changes to the effect of chronic mechanical stress mediated during lying, sitting and crutch walking upon a pelvis devoid of muscular support and osteoporotic. Also, there did not appear to be any correlation between the sacroiliac changes and urinary tract infection which these patients are so prone to develop.

ADULT RHEUMATOID ARTHRITIS (see also page 757). Ankylosing spondylitis patients may manifest peripheral arthritis without obvious spinal involvement at the outset of their disease, and in these instances diagnosis will depend upon or even have to await the characteristic radiographic findings in the spine. Such patients would be likely to have an asymmetrical arthritis involving a few large joints and a negative test for rheumatoid factor. Therefore, it is important to list ankylosing spondylitis among the various diseases which must be considered in the differential

TABLE 14–1. POLYARTHRITIS— DIFFERENTIAL DIAGNOSIS

Primary osteoarthritis
Rheumatoid arthritis and other general connective tissue disorders
Psoriatic arthropathy
Ankylosing spondylitis
Reiter's syndrome
Rheumatic fever
Crystal induced arthritis (urate, pyrophosphate)
Colitic arthritis
Arthritis with vasculitis (serum sickness, hepatitis, Schonlein-Henoch purpura, etc.)
Arthritis with neoplasia
Gonococcal arthritis (rarely other microbiologic agents)
Polymyalgia rheumatica
Endocrine arthropathy (Hypothyroid, acromegaly)
Others, including sarcoidosis, multiple myeloma, lipoid dermatoarthritis, familial Mediterranean fever and Behçet's syndrome.

diagnosis of polyarthritis (see Table 14–1). The presence of low back pain and stiffness in these patients would point to ankylosing spondylitis, but these symptoms may be absent, evanescent or obscured by the peripheral joint involvement. Ultimately, the delineation of ankylosing spondylitis from the various diseases listed in Table 14–1 must be based on periodic clinical and radiological evaluation to define involvement of the sacroiliac joints and lumbodorsal spine. Limitation of lumbar spine motion and thoracic excursions are early findings which point to ankylosing spondylitis. Radiologic evidence of bilateral sacroiliitis is strong evidence for ankylosing spondylitis. This finding is usually present within six months or a year of the onset of ankylosing spondylitis, although this interval conceivably may be longer when peripheral arthritis is the initial manifestation. Rheumatoid arthritis patients may also exhibit radiographic evidence of sacroiliitis, at times bilateral and similar to that found in ankylosing spondylitis, but this is not usually manifested until five or more years after onset of disease.[47] The diagnosis of ankylosing spondylitis is clinched by radiographic findings of spondylitis in the lumbodorsal spine, as this portion of the spine is spared in rheumatoid arthritis patients. Particularly helpful early signs of ankylosing spondylitis in this area are straightening of the anterior surface of the vertebrae and syndesmophytes.

JUVENILE RHEUMATOID ARTHRITIS (see also page 769). The onset of ankylosing spondylitis in adolescents and children is not infrequently marked by peripheral arthritis, and in these instances differentiation from juvenile rheumatoid arthritis may be impossible until the characteristic clinical and radiographic spinal findings of ankylosing spondylitis are manifested. Ansell has described children considered to have juvenile rheumatoid arthritis for many years who ultimately developed ankylosing spondylitis.[48] Ankylosing spondylitis is not likely to develop in children of less than five years of age, and this may be a helpful differential point, as juvenile rheumatoid arthritis has its peak incidence of onset at from one to three years of age. At the outset of disease acute neck pain and stiffness would suggest juvenile rheumatoid arthritis, whereas symptoms and signs related to the sacroiliac joints and lumbodorsal spine would point to ankylosing spondylitis. Also, high fever, rash, and involvement of the wrist or finger joints would point to juvenile rheumatoid arthritis.[49]

Although the characteristic radiographic findings of ankylosing spondylitis will ultimately distinguish between these diseases, the following factors may be emphasized: 1) The likely interval between onset of ankylosing spondylitis in children and radiologically detectable sacroiliitis has not been clarified, and repeated examinations may be required; 2) radiological evaluation of the sacroiliac joints in children and adolescents is hampered by developmental changes; 3) radiological evidence of bilateral sacroiliitis has been de-

scribed in juvenile rheumatoid arthritis; and 4) the lumbodorsal spine is not involved in juvenile rheumatoid arthritis, and this is a crucial differential point. Radiographic findings in the cervical spine in these two diseases also differ somewhat; there is a greater tendency for apophyseal joint ankylosis in juvenile rheumatoid arthritis patients (see page 770).

COLITIC, PSORIATIC AND REITER'S SPONDYLITIS (see also pages 746, 749, and 752). Spondylitis identical to that of ankylosing spondylitis may occur in patients with ulcerative colitis and regional enteritis, and also, but with perhaps minor radiologic differences, in those with psoriasis and Reiter's syndrome. These forms of spondylitis can be identified only if there is past or present evidence of the associated disease, and it is clear that in some instances spondylitis may precede the appearance of psoriasis or colitis.

OSTEITIS CONDENSANS ILII. Osteitis condensans ilii is a lesion localized to the area of the sacroiliac joints which is identifiable only on the basis of its roentgen features; it may be confused with the sacroiliitis of ankylosing spondylitis. The characteristic x-ray finding is a bilateral or, rarely, unilateral triangle-shaped area of sclerosis in the medial portion of the ilium; the base of the triangle is in juxtaposition to the sacroiliac joint and the apex extends laterally into the auricular portion of the ilium (Fig. 14–18). These lesions vary in size from a small area localized to the medial inferior aspect of the ilium to those

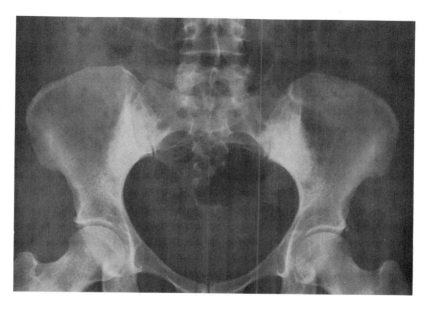

Figure 14–18. Osteitis condensans ilii in a 46-year-old woman. There is extensive sclerosis of the medial aspect of each ilium: however, the sacroiliac joints and the sacrum do not appear to be involved. The symphysis pubis is sclerotic and widened.

which involve the entire juxta-articular area of the ilium and extend to the region of the pubic ramus.[50] Clearly, these large areas of sclerosis are not likely to be confused with lesions of ankylosing spondylitis. It appears that in a small proportion of patients the sacrum is affected, but it is generally held that the sacroiliac joint is not involved.[50] Thompson (see below) believes that if there is involvement of the sacroiliac joints as clearly defined by widening, erosions or osteoporosis, then a diagnosis of osteitis condensans ilii is not tenable and ankylosing spondylitis is likely.[51]

A definitive survey study for the prevalence of osteitis condensans ilii is lacking, but in a review of 3260 x-rays of Japanese patients, including a large proportion who had been exposed to atomic radiation, this entity was found in 1.6 per cent.[50]

The etiology of osteitis condensans ilii is unknown and there is only scant knowledge of the pathology of this lesion. It has been theorized that osteitis condensans ilii is secondary to mechanical stress upon the soft tissues and circulation of the sacroiliac joint during pregnancy, as the vast majority of these lesions are found in women; there is also a concept that these lesions are most likely to be symptomatic during pregnancy. However, the occasional detection of osteitis condensans ilii in nulliparous women and in men is inconsistent with this theory. Urinary tract infection has also been implicated, but this has not been supported by studies in a large series of patients.[51,52] Thompson in a clinical and radiological followup of 20 women with a diagnosis of osteitis condensans ilii eventually classified seven as having ankylosing spondylitis.[53] All seven of these patients showed radiological evidence of sacroiliitis, and in four there was intermittent elevation of the sedimentation rate, while two showed progressive stiffness of the spine. It is postulated that these women have a limited or abortive form of ankylosing spondylitis which may be delineated from osteitis condensans ilii. Jolkunen and Rokkanen have biopsied the ilium adjacent to the sacroiliac joint in three patients with ankylosing spondylitis and three with osteitis condensans ilii and observed the same pathology in both of these lesions.[54] This limited study suggests that the bone reacts similarly in these two diseases, but these authors emphasize this must not be construed that the diseases are the same or that they reflect a single etiology.

It is not clear that osteitis condensans ilii is a source of back pain. For example, this lesion may be apparent on x-rays obtained during the course of barium enemas, intravenous pyelograms and other specialized studies that are not part of an evaluation for backache.[50] It has been stressed that patients with backache and osteitis condensans ilii may have a more likely source for their pain which is detectable on x-rays or by clinical examination.[55] However, many observers believe osteitis condensans ilii is a source of low back pain. This issue is unresolved and it is prudent to exclude other causes of backache in patients with radiologic evidence of this lesion.

INFECTION AND NEOPLASIA. There are two aspects of ankylosing spondylitis which may simulate a localized infection. The first of these occurs early in the course of disease when there may be asymmetrical radiological evidence of sacroiliitis, with one joint clearly involved and absent or equivocal findings in the other. In such instances, the apparent unilateral sacroiliac disease raises the possibility of a pyogenic or tuberculous infection, for the early radiologic findings in all of these conditions are similar except for bilateral involvement.[44] The situation can usually be clarified by followup radiographs at six-month, or even shorter, intervals to ascertain if there is involvement of the other sacroiliac joint or additional evidence of ankylosing spondylitis. A more intensive approach is indicated, however, in the presence of findings highly suggestive of pyogenic infection such as severe pain localized to or radiating from one sacroiliac joint or persistent fever or leukocytosis. It may be emphasized at this point that localized pyogenic infection of the musculoskeletal system may develop in the absence of chills, fever and leukocytosis, particularly in the very young or old. In instances when pyogenic infection of the sacroiliac joint is suspected, x-rays should be repeated at brief intervals for evidence of a rapidly destructive process, and blood cultures should be obtained. A therapeutic trial with an appropriate antibiotic and an open biopsy for histological and bacteriological studies may also be warranted. Persistent unilateral sacroiliac joint disease and a positive tuberculin test, of course, point to a tuberculous etiology and in such instances a biopsy is indicated.

Destructive lesions involving one or more lumbar or dorsal vertebrae and their adjacent discs are the second manifestation of ankylosing spondylitis which may have to be differentiated from injection or neoplasia. These lesions develop in patients with advanced clinical and radiological evidence of ankylosing spondylitis, and a destructive lesion of vertebra(e) and disc(s) in this setting is likely to be a manifestation of the underlying disease; however, the clinical and radiological findings will not serve to distinguish such lesions from those due to neoplasia or infection. In these situations, it is not possible to make a blanket statement as to whether to proceed with biopsy for histological and bacteriological studies; the decision must be based on careful clinical, laboratory and radiological evaluation of each patient.

DISEASES WITH AN "OSSIFYING" DIATHESIS. There are a group of entities, for the most part very rare, with a proclivity for ossification of the spine and perispinal ligaments, and with clinical and radiological findings that are in some respects similar to those of ankylosing spondylitis. Forestier and Lagier have referred to an "ossifying diathesis" in these disorders, but there is no evidence of a common etiologic or pathogenetic factor among them.[56] Included in this category are ankylosing hyperostosis, fluorosis, hypoparathyroidism, congenital hypophosphatemia and a rare familial disorder described by Sharp.[62]

Ankylosing Hyperostosis. See page 785.

Fluorosis. Patients absorbing unusual amounts of fluoride may develop progressive stiffness, limitation of motion and forward flexion of the spine resembling ankylosing spondylitis. Exposure to industrial or other fluoride, or a high fluoride content in the drinking water, a situation that occurs particularly in areas of India and Africa, are usual factors in increased fluoride absorption.[57] Osteosclerosis and formation of exostoses, usually initially apparent in flat bones, as in the pelvis and jaw, and in the vertebrae, are the major manifestations of excessive fluoride deposition in bones. The spine eventually becomes rigid, with evidence of fusion of the vertebral bodies and calcification of the paraspinal ligaments. The radiographic changes in the spine and pelvis include extensive sclerosis which may obliterate the sacroiliac joints, osteophytosis and ligament calcification. The extensive uniform osteosclerosis, which eventually involves extremity bones, and the absence of erosions in the sacroiliac joints are helpful points in distinguishing fluorosis from ankylosing spondylitis.[57]

Hypoparathyroidism. Pain, stiffness and limited motion of the spine, hips and shoulders suggestive of ankylosing spondylitis have been reported rarely in patients with idiopathic or secondary hypoparathyroidism and pseudohypoparathyroidism. For example, a patient reported by Jimenea et al. showed clinical findings of spinal ankylosis and kyphosis and limited chest expansion, although there was no radiographic evidence of sacroiliitis.[58] Skeletal radiographic studies of these patients have shown calcification of soft tissues, particularly spinal ligaments, and osteosclerosis with varying involvement of the spine, hip and shoulder girdles and limbs. The sacroiliac joints were partially obliterated in some instances. Absence of classical radiographic findings of sacroiliitis and clinical and laboratory evidence of hypoparathyroidism were helpful in delineating these patients.

The mechanism of the calcification and ossification in these patients is unknown. Todd et al. have theorized that there may be a predisposition to calcification and ossification in a group of genetic, possibly related disorders including idiopathic and pseudo forms of hypoparathyroidism, myositis ossificans progressiva, hereditary multiple exostoses, multiple epiphyseal dysplasias and familial calcification of the basal ganglia.[59]

Treatment with vitamin D and calcium may result in symptomatic improvement of the spine pain and stiffness.

Hypophosphatemic Rickets. Persons with the x-linked dominant type of hypophosphatemic rickets on reaching middle age may manifest pain in the low back and hip area, with severe restriction of motion of all segments of the spine and multiple peripheral joints.[60] This finding, which may be attributed to ankylosing spondylitis, reflects hyperostotic osteomalacia associated with the persistent underlying defect. X-rays show sclerosis and a coarsened trabecular pattern of bone, particularly obvious in the pelvis, lumbar vertebrae and phalanges of the hand, and ossification of perispinal and periarticular soft tissues. In addition, the sacroiliac and apophyseal joints may be obliterated. The peculiar stature of these individuals and the chemical abnormality point to the correct diagnosis.

Myositis Ossificans Progressiva. Children with this rare hereditary disorder may show marked limitation of spinal motion as a result of bone deposition in paravertebral muscles. In addition, fusion of the vertebral bodies and apophyseal joints of the cervical spine, in one instance associated with fusion of the sacroiliac joints, has been reported in these children.[61] X-rays indicating diffuse ectopic bone formation in the muscles is diagnostic of this disease.

Heredofamilial Vascular and Articular Calcification. The progeny of a consanguineous marriage with a propensity for calcification and ossification of spinal and peripheral joints and their surrounding soft tissues, and with clinical and x-ray findings somewhat reminiscent of ankylosing spondylitis, have been reported.[62] Calcification of medium-sized arteries was also prominent in these patients. Spinal x-rays showed extensive vertebral bridging, but the classical pattern of sacroiliitis and spondylitis associated with ankylosing spondylitis was not present.

PAGET'S DISEASE. Paget's disease, although it may be marked by low back pain and x-ray findings of deossification and sclerosis of the bony pelvis, is easily differentiated from ankylosing spondylitis. The clinical and laboratory findings of Paget's disease, including onset in middle age, absence of protracted stiffness of the spine, normal chest expansion and elevated alkaline phosphatase during the active phase of the disease, are not likely to be confused with those of ankylosing spondylitis. Furthermore, the radiographic findings in the pelvis serve to clearly distinguish between these diseases. The radiographic findings of Paget's disease in the pelvis feature combina-

tions of diffuse, patchy or linear sclerosis, coarsened trabeculae and rarefaction. Although these findings may be noted in the area of the sacroiliac joints, they do not suggest sacroiliitis for they are uniformly part of a more extensive reaction in the bony pelvis (Fig. 14–19). In addition, obliteration of the sacroiliac joints, syndesmophyte formation and squaring of the anterior surfaces of vertebrae are not features of Paget's disease.

ACRO-OSTEOLYSIS. Erosion and sclerosis of the sacroiliac joints has been described in workers who develop acro-osteolysis and Raynaud's phenomenon while engaged in the processing of polyvinyl chloride resins.[63] This toxic reaction has been noted in only a small proportion of the individuals who handle these resins, suggesting a genetic factor in the development of this toxicity. The toxic reaction in these workers is characterized by the radiographic finding of lytic lesions at the tips of the distal phalanges in the hands, Raynaud's phenomenon and thickening of the skin of the hands. Synovial thickening at the wrist and erosive lesions at the ulnar styloid, calcaneus and patella have also been reported. Dodson et al. carefully evaluated four patients with this toxic reaction and noted erosion and sclerosis of the sacroiliac joints in each of them; however, the overall incidence of sacroiliac involvement in this entity is not known.[63] It is unlikely that sacroiliac disease found in association with this toxic reaction will be attributed to ankylosing spondylitis if the history

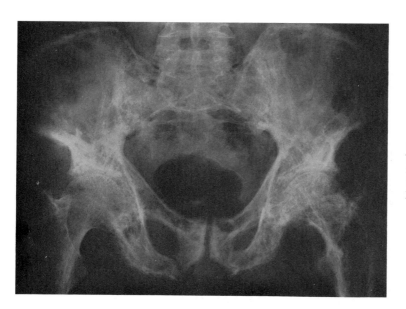

Figure 14–19. Paget's disease of the pelvis and left hip and femur. There is diffuse sclerosis and areas of rarefaction. Note the linear configuration of the sclerosis. The sacroiliac joints are not obliterated.

of Raynaud's phenomenon is elicited, the hands are x-rayed and the occupational background is reviewed.

SARCOIDOSIS. Low or mid-back pain as a manifestation of vertebral sarcoidosis has rarely been reported.[64, 65] These patients have had evidence of pulmonary sarcoidosis on chest x-ray except in one instance in which the spinal lesion preceded radiographic findings of sarcoidosis. The usual radiographic finding is a lytic lesion with sclerotic margins in one or more vertebral bodies; however, vertebral collapse, disc narrowing, destruction of pedicles and a paraspinal soft tissue mass have also been noted. Sarcoid involvement of the sacroiliac joint has not been reported. It is not likely that sarcoidosis of the vertebrae will be confused with ankylosing spondylitis, and this rare lesion of the spine is included only for the sake of completeness.

WHIPPLE'S DISEASE. See page 784.

OCHRONOSIS. See page 787.

FAMILIAL MEDITERRANEAN FEVER. See page 789.

BEHCET'S SYNDROME. See page 789.

SCHEUERMANN'S DISEASE. See page 361.

Treatment

INTRODUCTION. In the absence of a therapeutic agent which completely suppresses the inflammatory process of ankylosing spondylitis, treatment is based on agents which ameliorate pain and stiffness and on a program of rest and exercise to maintain motion and prevent deformity. Despite the lack of a curative drug, the prognosis is generally favorable, as: 1) the overall natural course of the disease is benign and the majority of patients may be gainfully employed, particularly if the hips and knees are spared; and 2) therapeutic agents which are reasonably safe and effective are available. Treatment will be considered under the heading of rest-exercise program, therapeutic exercise and anti-rheumatic drug therapy.

REST-EXERCISE PROGRAM. In developing a therapeutic program, one must attempt to establish a proper balance of rest and exercise, as both modalities contribute to the wellbeing of these patients. Avoidance of fatigue and tension related to excessively long working hours or emotional stress is appropriate to the management of all chronic rheumatic diseases, and to some degree adequate rest may

be insured by eight to nine hours of sleep each night. It is clear that strenuous occupations that might entail lifting, carrying and straining are contraindicated, as are vigorous contact sports. Hart, however, has pointed out that immobilization of the spine, accomplished by plaster of paris jackets, braces or even prolonged bed rest, leads to early and unusually severe loss of spinal motion.[66] Similarly, absolutely sedentary occupations that require long hours of sitting at a desk or bench also seem to accelerate loss of spinal motion. Patients engaged in such sedentary occupations should have the opportunity to be up and about for mild exercise several times during the course of the day. An ideal occupation would permit non-strenuous activities, such as walking, bending and twisting. Calabro et al. indicate that swimming is an ideal activity, and in some instances tennis and badminton are permissible.[67] This approach must be modified if the hips or knees are involved, as frequent weight-bearing activities are deleterious for these joints.

THERAPEUTIC EXERCISE. Therapeutic exercise is another approach to maintenance of spinal motion and prevention or correction of deformity. Hart has indicated that perhaps the best approach to these objectives is exercise that is included in the patient's daily occupational or recreational activities, but exercise is a valuable alternative or supplement.[66] The basic objectives of the exercise program are to maintain a straight spine and maximum respiratory excursions. Various exercises which strengthen the extensor muscles of the spine are valuable in the first instance, and there are several exercises to stress the accessory respiratory muscles. Patients should be taught these exercises by a physical therapist who is well versed in the "spondylitis routine." This may be accomplished during a period of hospitalization or by regular outpatient visits to a department of physical therapy, and supervision should be continued until the entire exercise program is "down pat." The attending physician should follow his patient carefully during the instruction period and caution the therapist if too vigorous a program has resulted in increased pain. The patient must be encouraged to arrange his daily schedule so that there are two or three periods of time set aside for exercises; they should not be fitted into free moments. It is also helpful if the therapist is revisited at four-to-six-month intervals for reinforcement and perhaps modification of the program. Knee and hip exercises should also be stressed if these joints are involved.

ANTI-RHEUMATIC AGENTS. *Aspirin.* Aspirin should be utilized initially, as it may be effective in controlling pain and stiffness and is relatively non-toxic and inexpensive. The optimum dosage is just below that which produces symptoms of mild toxicity. Adults and teenagers may begin treatment with three tablets (0.9 gm) QID and then the total dosage—not each dose—may be increased by one or two tablets every few days until tinnitus or mild hearing loss is noted. At this point, treatment is discontinued for 24 hours and restarted at a total dosage of one or two tablets less than that which produced toxicity. If morning stiffness is a particular problem, the total dosage should be divided into five portions, including one at 3 or 4 A.M. Aspirin is an irritant to the upper gastrointestinal mucosa, and the following precautionary measures should be utilized: 1) each dose of aspirin should be taken after a meal or with 8 ounces of milk or skim milk; 2) an antacid should be prescribed one hour after meals and at bedtime. An occasional patient may develop indigestion secondary to upper gastrointestinal irritation with even small doses of aspirin, and in these patients a trial with enteric coated aspirin is indicated. This program is not applicable to young children, who may ignore tinnitus and other early signs of aspirin toxicity. Children may be treated with 40 mg of aspirin per pound per day in divided doses which usually affords an adequate blood level of 25 to 30 mg per 100 ml. Salicylate toxicity is unlikely with this dosage regimen.

Phenylbutazone (Butazolidin). Phenylbutazone is probably the most effective agent available for the treatment of ankylosing spondylitis; however, rarely it may induce a serious toxic reaction, and thus its use is justified only after a trial of aspirin, and only at the lowest possible effective maintenance dosage. Initially, treatment with 100 mg TID or QID for one or two weeks will control pain and stiffness and then a maintenance dosage of 200 mg or preferably 100 mg per day may be utilized.

Toxic effects of phenylbutazone include irritation and ulceration of the upper gastrointestinal tract, edema secondary to salt and water retention and a pruritic maculopapular rash; however, bone marrow depression leading to agranulocytosis is the most serious complication. Patients taking 300 to 400 mg daily should have weekly complete blood counts; however, for those on a maintenance dosage of 100 mg per day, CBC's may be obtained at three or four week intervals. A sharp drop in the number of granulocytes, the appearance of immature forms, or any other abnormality is an indication for cessation of treatment and review of the hematological picture. Phenylbutazone should be taken with meals or milk and be accompanied by antacid therapy as outlined for aspirin. This drug may react synergistically with the coumarin-like drugs to antagonize coagulation factors and, thus, extreme caution must be exercised if these drugs are used simultaneously.

There is little experience with the use of phenylbutazone in children, and it is probably preferable to use aspirin for these patients.

Indomethacin (Indocin). Indomethacin appears to be an effective agent for the management of ankylosing spondylitis. It is probably somewhat less potent but also less toxic than phenylbutazone. Some workers prefer a trial with indomethacin before resorting to phenylbutazone, and we have noted an occasional patient to respond more favorably to indomethacin.

During the early phases of indomethacin treatment, some patients experience nausea or headache; however, with continued use these symptoms tend to clear. These early symptoms may frequently be bypassed by initiating treatment with a 25 mg capsule at bedtime and then adding 25 mg each week, to be spaced throughout the day, until a total dosage of 100 to 150 mg is attained. Control of pain and stiffness can usually be attained with 100 to 150 mg daily, and 50 to 100 mg per day is the usual maintenance range. Indomethacin, like aspirin and phenylbutazone, irritates the upper gastrointestinal tract, and precautions as outlined for those drugs should be utilized. There is some evidence that long-term usage of indomethacin may be associated with the development of corneal deposits and retinal disturbances, and patients receiving such therapy should have an examination by an ophthalmologist every six to 12 months.

Corticosteroids, Corticotropin and Radiation Therapy. Corticosteroids and adrenocorticotropin have a very limited role, and x-ray therapy has been generally abandoned in the treatment of ankylosing spondylitis. Although the hormones will control pain and stiffness in this disease, side effects are inevitable; whereas the other agents are effective and side effects are rare. Uveitis, however, occasionally requires the systemic use of steroids or corticotropin. The use of x-ray radiation, although effective, has been abandoned, as it is associated with a significant incidence of leukemia.

For surgical considerations of treatment see pages 790 to 809.

References

Introduction

1. West, H. F.: Etiology of ankylosing spondylitis, Ann. Rheum. Dis. 8:143–148, 1949.
2. Hersh, A. H., Stecher, R. M., Solomon, W. M., Wolpaw, R., and Hauser, H.: Heredity in ankylosing spondylitis. A study of fifty families. Am. J. Hum. Gen. 2:391–408, 1950.
3. Lawrence, J. S.: The prevalence of arthritis. Brit. J. Clin. Pract. 17:699–705, 1963.
4. Blumberg, B., and Ragan, C.: The natural history of rheumatoid spondylitis. Medicine 35:1–31, 1956.
5. Sigler, J. W., Bluhm, G. B., Duncan, H., and Ensign, D. C.: Clinical features of ankylosing spondylitis. Clin. Ortho. Rel. Res. 74:14–19, 1971.
6. Ogryzlo, M. A., and Rosen, P. S.: Ankylosing (Marie-Strumpell) spondylitis. Postgrad. Med. J. 45:182–188, 1969.
7. Boland, E. W.: Ankylosing spondylitis. In Arthritis and Allied Conditions. 7th edition, Hollander, J. L. (ed.), Philadelphia, Lea and Febiger, 1966, pp. 633–655.
8. Baum, J., and Ziff, M.: The rarity of ankylosing spondylitis in the black race. Arth. Rheum. 14:12–18, 1971.
9. Schaller, J., Bitnum, S., and Wedgewood, R. J.: Ankylosing spondylitis with childhood onset. J. Pediat. 74:505–516, 1969.
10. Wilkinson, M., and Bywaters, E. G. L.: Clinical features and course of ankylosing spondylitis. Ann. Rheum. Dis. 17:209–228, 1958.
11. DeBlecourt, J. J., Polman, A., and DeBlecourt-Meindersma, T.: Hereditary factors in rheumatoid arthritis and ankylosing spondylitis. Ann. Rheum. Dis. 20:215–223, 1961.
12. Emery, A. E. H., and Lawrence, J. S.: Genetics of ankylosing spondylitis. J. Med. Genet. 4:239–244, 1967.
12a. Gofton, J. P., Robinson, H. S., and Trueman, G. E.: Ankylosing spondylitis in a Canadian Indian population. Ann. Rheum. Dis. 25:525–527, 1966.
12b. Schlosstein, L., Terasaki, P. I., Bluestone, R., and Pearson, C. M.: High association of an HL-A antigen, W-27, with ankylosing spondylitis. New Eng. J. Med. 228:704–706, 1973.
12c. Brewerton, D. A., Hart, F. D., Nicholls, A. et al.: Ankylosing spondylitis and HL-A 27. Lancet 1:904–907, 1973.
12d. Morris, R. I., Metzger, A. L., Bluestone, R., and Terasaki, P. I.: HL-A-W-27—a useful discriminator in the arthropathies of inflammatory bowel disease. New Eng. J. Med. 290:1117–1119, 1974.
12e. Brewerton, D. A., Nicholls, A., Caffrey, M., et al.: HL-A 27 and arthropathies associated with ulcerative colitis and psoriasis. Lancet 1:956–958, 1974.

12f. Brewerton, D. A., Nicholls, A., Oates, J. K., et al.: Reiter's disease and HL-A 27. Lancet 2:996–998, 1973.
12g. Woodrow, J. C.: HL-A and Reiter's syndrome. Lancet 2:671–672, 1973.
13. Ford, D. K.: The natural history of arthritis following venereal urethritis. Ann. Rheum. Dis. 12:177–197, 1953.
14. Mason, R. M., Murray, R. S., Oates, J. K., and Young, A. C.: Prostatitis and ankylosing spondylitis. Brit. Med. J. 1:748–751, 1958.
15. Grimble, A. and Lessoj, M. H.: Anti-prostate antibodies in arthritis. Brit. Med. J. 2:263–264, 1965.

Pathology

16. Cruickshank, B.: Pathology of ankylosing spondylitis. Clin. Ortho. Rel. Res. 74:43–58, 1971.
17. Ball, J.: Enthesopathy of rheumatoid and ankylosing spondylitis. Ann. Rheum. Dis. 30:213–222, 1971.
18. Peacock, E. E., Jr.: A study of the circulation in normal tendons and healing grafts. Ann. Surg. 149:415–428, 1959.
19. Rathbun, J. B., and McNab, I.: The microvascular pattern of the rotator cuff. J. Bone Joint Surg. 52B:540–553, 1970.
20. Davies, D. V., and Young, L.: The distribution of radioactive sulphur (S35) in the fibrous tissues, cartilages and bones of the rat following its administration in the form of inorganic sulphate. J. Anat. (Lond.) 88:174–183, 1954.
21. Wagner, T.: The microscopic appearance of synovial membranes in peripheral joints in ankylosing spondylitis. Rheumatologia 8:209–215, 1970.

Clinical Features

22. Newton, D. R. L.: Discussion on the clinical and radiological aspects of sacro-iliac disease. Proc. Roy. Soc. Med. 50:850–853, 1957.
23. Macrae, I. F., and Wright, V.: Measurement of back movement. Ann. Rheum. Dis. 28:584–589, 1969.
24. Moll, J. M. H., and Wright, V.: An objective clinical study of chest expansion. Ann. Rheum. Dis. 31:1–8, 1972.
25. Lorber, A., Pearson, C. M., and Rene, R. M.: Osteolytic vertebral lesions as a manifestation of rheumatoid arthritis and related disorders. Arth. Rheum. 4:514–532, 1961.
26. Cawley, M. I. D., Chalmers, T. M., and Ball, J.: Destructive lesions of vertebral bodies. Ann. Rheum. Dis. 30:539–540, 1971.
27. Kanefield, D. G., Mullins, B. P., Freehafer, A. A., Furey, J. G., Herenstein, S., and Chamberlin, W. B.: Destructive lesions of the spine in rheumatoid ankylosing spondylitis. J. Bone Joint Surg. 51:1369–1375, 1969.
28. Sharp, J., and Purser, D. W.: Spontaneous atlanto-axial dislocation in ankylosing spondylitis and rheumatoid arthritis. Ann. Rheum. Dis. 20:47–77, 1961.
29. Woodruff, F. P., and Dewing, S. B.: Fracture of the cervical spine in patients with ankylosing spondylitis. Radiology 80:17–21, 1963.
30. Matthews, W. B.: Neurological complications of ankylosing spondylitis. J. Neurol. Sci. 6:561–573, 1968.
31. McEwen, C., DiTata, D., Lingg, C., Porini, A., Good, A., and Rankin, T.: Ankylosing spondylitis and spondylitis accompanying ulcerative colitis, regional enteritis, psoriasis and Reiter's disease: A

comparative study. Arthr. Rheum. 14:291–318, 1971.

32. Riley, M. J., Ansell, B. M., and Bywaters, E. G. L.: Radiological manifestations of ankylosing spondylitis according to age at onset. Ann. Rheum. Dis. 30:138–148, 1971.

33. Glick, E. N.: A radiological comparison of the hip joint in rheumatoid arthritis and ankylosing spondylitis. Proc. Roy. Soc. Med. 59:1229–1231.

34. Graham, D. C., and Smythe, H. A.: The carditis and aortitis of ankylosing spondylitis. Bull. Rheum. Dis. 9:171–174, 1958.

35. Campbell, A. H., and MacDonald, C. B.: Upper lobe fibrosis associated with ankylosing spondylitis. Brit. J. Dis. Chest 59:90–101, 1965.

36. Jessamine, A. G.: Upper lobe fibrosis in ankylosing spondylitis. Canad. Med. Assn. J. 98:25–29, 1968.

37. Davies, D.: Ankylosing spondylitis and lung fibrosis. Quart. Jour. Med. 41:395–417, 1972.

Laboratory Radiology

38. Boland, E. W., Headley, N. E., and Hench, P. S.: The cerebro-spinal fluid in rheumatoid spondylitis. Ann. Rheum. Dis. 7:195–199, 1948.

39. Ludwig, A. O., Short, C. L., and Bauer, W.: Rheumatoid arthritis as a cause of increased cerebro-spinal fluid protein. New. Eng. J. Med. 228:306–310, 1943.

40. Berens, D. L.: Roentgen features of ankylosing spondylitis. Clin. Orth. Rel. Res. 74:20–33, 1971.

41. Romanus, R., and Yden, S.: Pelvo-spondylitis Ossificans. Chicago, Year Book Medical Publishers, 1955.

42. Polley, H. F., and Slocumb, C. H.: Rheumatoid spondylitis, a study of 1035 cases. Ann. Intern. Med. 26:240–249, 1947.

43. Carter, M. E., and Loewi, G.: Anatomical changes in normal sacro-iliac joints during childhood and comparison with the changes in Still's disease. Ann. Rheum. Dis. 21:121–134, 1962.

44. Grainger, R. G.: Discussion on the clinical and radiological aspects of sacro-iliac disease. Proc. Roy. Soc. Med. 50:854–858, 1957.

45. Forestier, J., Jacqueline, F., and Rotes Querol, J. (Translated by DesJardins, A. U.): Ankylosing Spondylitis. Springfield, Ill., Charles C Thomas, 1956.

Differential Diagnosis

46. Wright, V., Catterall, R. D., and Cook, J. B.: Bone and joint changes in paraplegic men. Ann. Rheum. Dis. 24:419–431, 1965.

47. Dilsen, N., McEwen, C., Poppel, M., Gersh, W. J., DiTata, D., and Carmel, P.: A comparative roentgenologic study of rheumatoid arthritis and rheumatoid (ankylosing) spondylitis. Arth. Rheum. 5:341–368, 1962.

48. Ansell, B. M.: Still's disease followed in adult life. Proc. Roy. Soc. Med. 62:912–913, 1969.

49. Ladd, J. R., Cassidy, J. T., and Martel, W.: Juvenile ankylosing spondylitis. Arth. Rheum. 14:579–590, 1971.

50. Numaguchi, Y.: Osteitis condensans ilii, including its resolution. Radiology 98:1–8, 1971.

51. Szabados, M. D.: Osteitis condensans ilii, report of 3 cases associated with urinary tract infection. J. Florida Med. Assn. 34:95–99, 1947.

52. Wells, J.: Osteitis condensans ilii. Amer. J. Roentgen. 76:1141–1143, 1956.

53. Thompson, M.: Osteitis condensans ilii and its differentiation from ankylosing spondylitis. Ann. Rheum. Dis. 13:147–156, 1954.

54. Julkunen, H., and Rokkanen, P.: Ankylosing spondylitis and osteitis condensans ilii. Acta. Rheum. Scand. 15:224–231, 1965.

55. Gillespie, H. W., and Lloyd-Roberts, G.: Osteitis condensans. Brit. J. Radiol., 26:16–21, 1953.

56. Forestier, J., and Lagier, R.: Ankylosing hyperostosis of the spine. Clin. Orth. Rel. Res. 74:65–83, 1971.

57. Steinberg, C. L., Gardner, D. E., Smith, F. A., and Hodge, H. C.: Comparison of rheumatoid (ankylosing) spondylitis and crippling fluorosis. Ann. Rheum. Dis. 14:378–384, 1955.

58. Jimenea, C., Frame, B., Chaykin, L. B., and Siglor, J. W.: Spondylitis of hypoparathyroidism. Clin. Orth. Rel. Res. 74:84–89, 1971.

59. Todd, J. N., III, Hill, S. R., Jr., Nickerson, J. F., and Fingley, J. O.: Hereditary multiple exostoses, pseudo-hypoparathyroidism and other genetic defects of bone calcium and phosphorus metabolism. Amer. J. Med. 30:289–298, 1961.

60. Kellgren, J. H., Stanbury, W., and Hall, L. quoted by Hart, F. D.: The stiff aching back. The differential diagnosis of ankylosing spondylitis. Lancet, 1:740–742, 1968.

61. Hamilton, E. B. D., quoted by Hart, F. D.: The stiff aching back. The differential diagnosis of ankylosing spondylitis. Lancet, 1:740–742, 1968.

62. Sharp, J.: Heredo-familial vascular and articular calcification, Ann. Rheum. Dis. 13:15–27, 1954.

63. Dodson, V. N., Dinman, B. D., Whitehouse, W. M., Nasr, A. N. M., and Magnuson, H. J.: Occupational acroosteolysis, III. A clinical study. Arch. Envir. Health 22:83–91, 1971.

64. Zener, J. C., Alpert, M., and Klainer, L. M.: Vertebral sarcoidosis. Arch. Intern. Med. 111:696–702, 1963.

65. Berk, R. N., and Brower, T. D.: Vertebral sarcoidosis. Radiology 82:660–663, 1964.

66. Hart, F. D.: The treatment of ankylosing spondylitis. Proc. Roy. Soc. Med. 48:207–210, 1955.

67. Calabro, J. J., Maltz, B. A., and Sussman, P.: Ankylosing spondylitis. Am. Fam. Phys./GP 2:80–89, 1970.

COLITIC ARTHRITIS

Introduction

Approximately 20 per cent of ulcerative colitis patients and 5 per cent of those with regional enteritis have evidence of arthritis involving either the peripheral joints or the spine.[1] In this discussion peripheral arthritis will refer to involvement of extraspinal joints including the hips and shoulders, and spondylitis will refer to the sacroiliac and spinal joints. The terms colitic arthritis, colitic peripheral arthritis and colitic spondylitis will refer to joint disease associated with ulcerative colitis or regional enteritis. The etiology and pathogenesis of the peripheral arthritis associated with these intestinal disorders is unknown, but the tendency of the joint and bowel disease to flare up almost simultaneously suggests they are related and not the chance association of two diseases. Erythema nodosum is noted in approximately 5 per cent of patients with these bowel disorders, but it is five times more likely to occur in those who manifest peripheral arthritis.[1] The association of erythema nodosum and arthritis in these patients suggests the possibility of a hypersensitivity reaction in the pathogenesis of the joint disease. Such a hypersensitivity reaction could be an underlying factor of the entire disease process, including the bowel involvement, or a factor only in the joint disease. The etiology of colitic spondylitis will be considered in a subsequent portion of this discussion. These bowel disorders and the associated arthritis are likely to develop in young adults; however, the onset may occur in the middle aged, aged or in children. Wright and Watkinson and McEwen et al. have found that colitic peripheral arthritis occurs with equal frequency in men and women, but McEwen and his co-workers noted that colitic spondylitis is more frequent in men.[2, 3]

Peripheral Arthritis

The peripheral arthritis characteristically is marked by an acute onset, involves a few weight-bearing joints, most frequently the ankles and knees, follows a migratory pattern and subsides in less than a month. There are numerous variations from this prototype: numerous joints may be involved, the small joints of the hands and feet may be affected, the duration may be up to a year, and in some instances the involvement is limited to arthralgia. In many instances, but particularly with transient involvement, there is no permanent damage to the joints. Bywaters and Ansell and McEwen et al. noted that 25 to 50 per cent of these patients develop radiographic or clinical evidence of permanent joint damage, but the latter workers have emphasized that the damage is often minimal and not incapacitating.[4, 5]

Pyoderma gangrenosum and ocular involvement, in the form of conjunctivitis or uveitis, are additional extra-gastrointestinal findings in these bowel disorders. Pyoderma gangrenosum is noted in 5 per cent of these patients, and the incidence does not increase in those with peripheral joint disease. The incidence of ocular involvement is about 5 per cent in the overall population of these patients

but, according to McEwen, it increases to 15 per cent in those with peripheral arthritis.[1]

The peripheral arthritis is related to several aspects of the bowel disease. The onset of arthritis is generally concomitant with or follows closely after the onset of bowel disease, although in some instances it may not develop until a year or more after the onset of intestinal involvement.[6] Approximately 10 per cent of patients will develop arthritis as the initial manifestation of their disease; however, in such instances subsequent bouts of arthritis are likely to be associated with intestinal flare ups.[1] The tendency of joint and bowel disease to flare up together is a striking aspect of colitic peripheral arthritis, and has been noted in the majority of patients. Wright and Watkinson noted that peripheral arthritis is four times more frequent in those with chronic symptoms of ulcerative colitis than in those in whom the course was featured by acute fulminating attacks.[7] These authors also found an increase in the frequency of peripheral arthritis in patients in whom the bowel disease was complicated by perianal disease or pseudopolyps. Finally, McEwen has noted that the average number of attacks of peripheral arthritis was highest during the first year after onset (1.4 per year) and then tended to diminish during subsequent years.[1]

The diagnosis of colitic peripheral arthritis is dependent upon appreciating and recognizing the relationship between joint and bowel disease. In instances in which joint disease occurs initially, the diagnosis will remain in abeyance until bowel disease is evident. If migratory joint disease presents prior to the onset of bowel disease, it is likely to be confused with rheumatic fever. The latex flocculation test and other tests for rheumatoid factor are negative in colitic arthritis and a positive test raises the possibility of the rare association of rheumatoid arthritis and one of these bowel diseases. Joint fluid is of the Class II or inflammatory type.

COLITIC SPONDYLITIS

Introduction

Clinical and radiographic evidence of spondylitis has been noted in patients with ulcerative colitis and regional enteritis in a greater frequency than would be expected by chance alone. Wright and Watkinson studied 234 patients with ulcerative colitis and found evidence of sacroiliitis in 17.9 per cent, while

4.7 per cent of a control series showed these changes.[8, 9] Among these patients, there were also 3.8 per cent with findings typical of ankylosing spondylitis and no examples of this in the control group. Study of ankylosing spondylitis patients for evidence of ulcerative colitis reveals an incidence of up to 3.9 per cent; however, in one study of such patients there was radiographic evidence of ulcerative colitis in 18 per cent, although only a third of this group had symptoms compatible with this disease.[10, 11] McEwen et al., in a study of 38 patients with colitic spondylitis (34 ulcerative colitis and four regional enteritis), found that 61 per cent had clinical or radiological evidence of permanent damage to at least one peripheral joint, indicating that spondylitis in these patients is likely to be associated with extraspinal joint disease.[5] The incidence of spondylitis among regional enteritis patients has been studied less intensively; Ansell and Wigley noted this association in 5 per cent of 91 patients.[12] It is not clear whether patients with spondylitis and bowel disease have the association of two diseases or a form of spondylitis specific for these intestinal disorders. Similarity of the clinical and radiographic findings to those of ankylosing spondylitis in these patients, and the fairly frequent onset of spine disease prior to bowel involvement, suggest the possibility of two diseases. This concept is also supported both by the greater proportion of men with spondylitis and bowel disease and by failure of the spondylitis to remit after bowel resection. McEwen, however, believes that the tendency of the spondylitis to flare up in association with exacerbation of the bowel in 25 per cent of his patients and the overall incidence of spondylitis in these intestinal disorders suggest a specific form of spondylitis.[1]

Although it is an attractive theory, there has been no solid evidence to support the contention that there is dissemination of an infectious agent from the genitourinary tract or bowel through the pelvic lymphatics to involve the sacroiliac joints and spine in Reiter's syndrome, ankylosing spondylitis and these bowel diseases.

Recent studies have indicated that patients manifesting chronic inflammatory bowel disease and spondylitis have an increased incidence of the HL-A antigen W-27 found so prevalently (approximately 90 per cent) in patients with ankylosing spondylitis. Brewerton found this antigen in 13 of 18 patients with ulcerative colitis and clinical and radiographic evidence of spondylitis, whereas patients with ulcerative colitis with or without peripheral arthritis had an incidence comparable to a control population ($p < .00003$).[3a] Morris in a somewhat similar study utilizing patients with either ulcerative colitis or regional enteritis found the W-27 antigen in six of eight patients with spondylitis but not in those with only bowel disease or colitic peripheral arthritis ($p < .003$).[3b] Studies to date strongly suggest that 0.6 per cent of the male Caucasian population at large with the W-27 antigen will develop ankylosing spondylitis. However, these investigations of patients with ulcerative colitis and regional enteritis strongly suggest there will be a several-fold increase over the predicted 0.6 per cent incidence of spondylitis in individuals with W-27 antigen who develop inflammatory bowel disease.

The clinical and radiographic findings in colitic spondylitis are similar to those described for ankylosing spondylitis (see page 721). McEwen et al., in a clinical and radiographic study, have observed marked similarity in the findings in ankylosing spondylitis and colitic spondylitis, and they have pointed out certain features which may distinguish these two types of spondylitis from that in Reiter's syndrome and psoriasis (see pages 749–752).[5] It was also noted in this study that 40 per cent of 38 patients considered to have colitic spondylitis developed spinal involvement prior to the onset of bowel disease by an average interval of 8 years. Colitic spondylitis is generally progressive and unrelated to the vagaries of the bowel disease; however, as has been noted in 25 per cent of patients, the spine and bowel manifestations flared simultaneously.

Treatment

Peripheral arthritis and ulcerative colitis or ileitis are likely to flare concomitantly, and appropriate treatment of the bowel disease will generally control both facets of the exacerbation. The peripheral arthritis is generally short lived and benign, and is not an indication for bowel resection. However, persistent or destructive arthritis would be a point in favor of colectomy in a patient with severe chronic debilitating bowel disease.

Colitic spondylitis tends to be progressive irrespective of the state of the bowel disease, and treatment measures outlined for ankylosing spondylitis may generally be employed (see page 743). If corticosteroids are required in the management of the bowel disease, they will also relieve spinal symptoms; however, they are not indicated for control of back pain or stiffness. Progressive spondylitis is not ameliorated by colectomy and is not an indication for such surgery.

PSORIATIC ARTHRITIS

Introduction

Patients with psoriasis may develop inflammatory joint disease, generally designated as psoriatic arthritis, which appears to be specific for those with this skin disease. The earliest reference to psoriatic arthritis appeared in the French literature during the latter part of the nineteenth century. Numerous contemporary studies have also indicated an unusual incidence of arthritis in association with psoriasis.[13] For example, Leczinsky noted that among a population of psoriatic patients, the prevalence of inflammatory arthritis was 6.8 per cent.[14] The interpretation of these studies was difficult, however, as it was not clear what proportion of these patients represented the chance association of psoriasis and rheumatoid arthritis or other specific types of polyarthritis. As pointed out by Wright and Moll, rheumatoid factor has been helpful in delineating psoriatic arthritis as a specific entity.[13] The absence of this factor in the majority of patients with psoriasis and inflammatory arthritis is inconsistent with the thesis that these patients represent chance association of psoriasis and rheumatoid arthritis. The age of onset of this disease is generally in the second or third decade, with a sex ratio slightly in favor of women.

The etiology and pathogenesis of psoriatic arthritis have not been clarified. There is a genetic predisposition to psoriatic dermatitis, and the pattern of inheritance indicates that polygenic factors are involved. There are also numerous reports suggesting a hereditary predisposition to psoriatic arthritis. For example, the prevalence of psoriatic arthritis among first degree relatives of patients with this entity has been found to be almost fifty times greater than the estimated prevalence in the general population.[13] HL-A antigen typing has yielded further support for the presence of genetic factors in both psoriasis and the rheumatic disorders associated with this entity. Patients with psoriasis appear to have an increased incidence of the A-13 and W-17 antigens but not of the W-27 type found in

over 90 per cent of patients with ankylosing spondylitis. However, a study of patients with psoriatic arthritis revealed the presence of the W-27 antigen in 10 of 41 patients with peripheral arthritis, 4 of 10 with sacroiliitis and 9 of 10 with spondylitis. Thus, it appears that in patients with psoriasis and possessing the W-27 antigen there is strong likelihood of developing arthritis, particularly spondylitis.[3a]

There are many theories of the pathogenesis of psoriatic arthritis, but none has been clearly demonstrated to be operative in this disease. Psoriatic skin lesions tend to develop at sites of trauma or irritation, an example of the Koebner effect. Buckley and Raleigh have suggested that joints, since they are subjected to mechanical stress, may also be the site of a Koebner effect, and that conceivably the interaction of local stress and a systemic factor results in joint inflammation.[15] In support of this thesis, they cite a patient who developed acro-osteolysis following trauma to a finger.

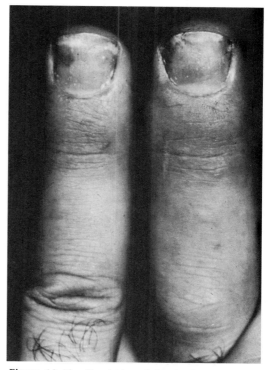

Figure 14–20. Psoriatic arthritis in the finger joints. The joints on the left are normal; however, on the right both the proximal and terminal interphalangeal joints are swollen. Swelling of both interphalangeal joints of a finger may yield a "sausage digit." Note the psoriatic pitting of the finger nails.

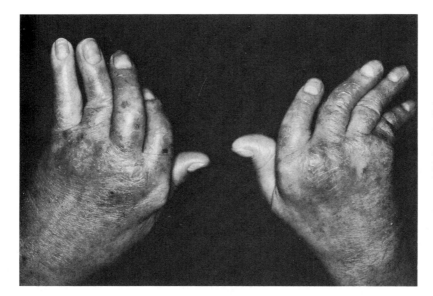

Figure 14–21. Far advanced psoriatic arthritis in the hands. The fingers are somewhat shortened and there is ulnar deviation at the metacarpal phalangeal and proximal interphalangeal joints. Each thumb shows a hyperextension deformity at the interphalangeal joint. Psoriatic involvement of the skin and nails is present.

Clinical Manifestations of Peripheral Arthritis

Wright and Moll, at the University of Leeds, who have carefully followed a large group of patients with this disease, classify them in the following groups:[13]

1. Patients with a predominantly distal interphalangeal arthritis.
2. Patients with classical arthritis mutilans often complicated by digital "telescoping" and involvement of the sacroiliac joints.
3. Patients with a pattern of arthritis indistinguishable from rheumatoid arthritis (Figs. 14–20 and 14–21).

The onset of psoriatic arthritis may be sudden and severe, resembling gout, but the site of this intense involvement is usually the distal interphalangeal joints. Wright and Moll have noted that joint involvement in this disease, particularly at the distal interphalangeal joints, is often limited to a few joints in an asymmetric distribution. Patients with psoriasis and polyarthritis who also have positive tests for rheumatoid factor and possibly rheumatoid nodules are probably best classified as having both psoriasis and rheumatoid arthritis.

The relationship of the onset of arthritis to the presence of skin involvement varies. In the past, it was generally believed that the arthritis either followed or occurred simultaneously with the onset of skin lesions, but it is now recognized that arthritis may be the initial manifestation. Patients presenting with arthritis may pose a difficult diagnostic problem until the skin lesions appear. Clearly, certain patients classified as having seronegative rheumatoid arthritis (absence of rheumatoid factor) ultimately prove to have psoriatic arthritis. Psoriatic arthritis is not necessarily associated with severe skin disease, and in some instances the key to diagnosis may be a single, tiny patch of dermatitis localized to a site of predilection at the elbow, knee or umbilicus.

The diagnosis of psoriatic arthritis is ultimately dependent upon recognition of the association of skin and joint involvement; however, the laboratory findings must also be considered. The value of the rheumatoid factor test in delineating those patients with the association of psoriatic dermatitis and rheumatoid arthritis has been previously cited. Ten to 20 per cent of these patients may have an elevated uric acid, presumably reflecting the proliferation and destruction of skin cells, and this finding may be particularly confusing in those with an acute onset of arthritis.[16] Examination of joint fluid for urate crystals and a therapeutic trial with colchicine may be helpful in resolving this differential diagnosis, but it may be stated that association of arthritis (particularly if interphalangeal joints of the hands are involved) in association with psoriasis points to psoriatic arthritis even in the presence of hyperuricemia.

The radiologic findings in the peripheral joints of patients with psoriatic arthritis are generally similar to those of rheumatoid arthritis; however, there may be changes which are strongly suggestive of psoriatic involvement.

Asymmetry and the tendency to involve distal interphalangeal joints are suggestive of psoriasis (Fig. 14–22). Radiographic findings considered to be strongly indicative of psoriatic arthritis tend to be uncommon; they include: whittling of the terminal phalanges, pencil-in-cup appearance of the finger or toe joints, arthritis mutilans with extensive destruction of articular bone, and extensive destruction of metatarsal, phalangeal and proximal interphalangeal joints of the toes in absence of change in these joints in the fingers.[17]

Spondylitis

Several clinical and radiographic studies have demonstrated that approximately 20 per cent of patients with psoriatic arthritis have radiographic evidence of sacroiliitis or spondylitis, and these findings may rarely be present in patients who manifest only skin involvement. Wright noted that 19 per cent of 103 patients with psoriatic arthritis had evidence of sacroiliitis.[18] McEwen et al., in a study of 39 individuals who ultimately developed spondylitis in association with psoriasis, found that the onset of spondylitis in one third of the patients preceded the appearance of psoriasis by an average time of eight years.[5] It is not clear whether these patients reflect an association of psoriasis and ankylosing spondylitis or spondylitis which is an aspect of the psoriatic involvement. McEwen et al., in their clinical and radiographic study of spondylitis, concluded that spondylitis in patients with psoriasis and Reiter's syndrome had some features which differentiated it from that noted in ankylosing spondylitis and colitic spondylitis (pages 721 and 746).[5] However, this work requires confirmation, and it is clear, at least in some instances, that the spondylitis associated with psoriasis is similar to that of ankylosing spondylitis. Another interesting relationship is that not only are clinical and radiographic features of spondylitis in psoriasis and Reiter's syndrome similar but also the skin lesions of Reiter's syndrome, keratoderma blennorrhagicum, may at times be impossible to differentiate either clinically or histologically from pustular psoriasis.[19]

The sacroiliac and spine disease associated with psoriasis may range from clinically inapparent to highly expressed, resembling ankylosing spondylitis. At times, psoriatic spondylitis may be attended by remarkably lit-

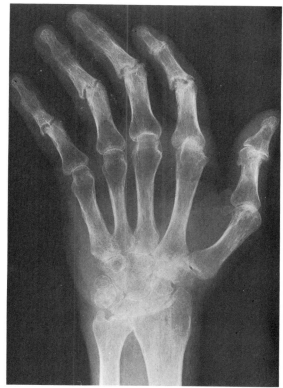

Figure 14–22. Advanced psoriatic arthritis in the hand. There is ankylosis of the third, fourth and fifth terminal interphalangeal joints and destructive arthritis of the proximal interphalangeal joints. The metacarpophalangeal, intercarpal and radiocarpal joints are also affected.

tle in the way of symptoms or clinical signs and, in these instances, there may be a marked discrepancy between clinical and radiographic findings. McEwen et al., found that psoriatic spondylitis, like Reiter's spondylitis, is often mildly expressed with absent or minimal straightening of the lumbar spine and less restriction of chest expansion than is noted with ankylosing spondylitis.[5] Those patients with highly expressed spondylitis have symptoms and clinical and radiographic findings similar to those of advanced ankylosing spondylitis.

Treatment of Psoriatic Arthritis and Spondylitis

Anti-rheumatic drugs of value in the management of psoriatic peripheral arthritis include aspirin, indomethacin, gold, and intra-articular injections of corticosteroids; aspirin and indomethacin, as well as butazolidin will also be of value if there is an associated spondylitis. For peripheral arthritis, aspirin and indomethacin are used in the dosages and with the same precautions as outlined in the treatment of rheumatoid arthritis (page 761) or ankylosing spondylitis (page 743). The treatment for symptomatic spondylitis is similar to that outlined for ankylosing spondylitis (page 743). Patients with peripheral arthritis failing to respond to aspirin or to a maintenance dosage of indomethacin, up to 150 mg. daily, may be considered for gold therapy. Gold, an agent of undoubted value in the management of rheumatoid arthritis is also often effective in controlling the peripheral arthritis associated with psoriasis, but it is not clear as to whether it has any effect on the spinal involvement. It must be emphasized that gold should be utilized only in patients with severe peripheral arthritis, as there are, occasionally, severe toxic reactions associated with the use of this drug. Gold has been reported to exacerbate the psoriatic rash, but we have encountered this on only one occasion and in general have found gold to be very helpful in this disease. The dosages, contraindications, side effects and precautions pertinent to gold therapy should be carefully reviewed before utilizing this agent. Systemic corticosteroids should not be utilized because of their side effects and, in addition, withdrawal or reduction of dosage of these agents leads to severe and at times incapacitating flare up of the skin lesions. Intra-articular injections of hydrocortisone or its analogues are often helpful in management of the peripheral joints, but we believe there should be only three or four such injections into a particular weight-bearing joint during the course of a year.

Methotrexate, a folic acid antagonist, and azathioprine, an immunosuppressive agent, are of possible value in the management of psoriatic arthritis but they should be utilized only in carefully controlled clinical research trials in view of their potential toxicity.[20, 21] Even in the management of psoriatic dermatitis, where it is unquestionably of value, methotrexate is reserved for very resistant patients. The use of methotrexate may be associated with insidious and progressive hepatic fibrosis which is not readily monitored by the usual tests for liver toxicity.

Rest and physical therapy are additional treatment modalities, and in instances of spinal involvement a program of rest and physical therapy as outlined for ankylosing spondylitis may be utilized.

REITER'S SYNDROME

Introduction

Reiter's syndrome comprises the triad of urethritis, conjunctivitis and arthritis, and there may be associated lesions of the skin and mucous membranes. Recurrent episodes, not necessarily manifesting the full triad, are characteristic, and in some instances there may be recurrent uveitis and chronic arthritis or spondylitis. Although the onset is most common between the ages of 20 and 40, the first episode may occur in those over 40, and it has also been described in children. Men appear to be more prone to the disease but difficulty in recognizing the genitourinary manifestations in women may contribute to this discrepancy.

The etiology of Reiter's syndrome is unknown, but there are epidemiological and laboratory findings which suggest that it may be caused by an infectious agent. The syndrome may follow outbreaks of bacillary dysentery; there is, however, no evidence of dissemination of the bacilli, although conceivably they may initiate a hypersensitivity reaction or the inflamed bowel may allow for the dissemination of an unknown pathogen. Clearly relating Reiter's syndrome to bacillary dysentery are the report of Paronen, describing 344 such patients after an epidemic in Finland, and Noer's description of nine patients following an epidemic which affected 602 crew members of a U.S. Navy cruiser.[22, 23] Many patients appear to develop Reiter's syndrome after a genitourinary infection which in all likelihood is venereally transmitted. Clearly, dissemination of gonococci is not a factor, for Reiter's syndrome may develop following adequately treated gonococcal urethritis. In these instances there may be an additional infectious agent or the gonococcal infection may permit dissemination of a non-invasive pathogen. It may be emphasized that urethritis occurs with both the postdysenteric and the venereal forms of this disease. Finally, adding to the epidemiological muddle is evidence that Reiter's syndrome may develop in the absence of previous dysentery or sexual exposure.

There are laboratory findings which relate two groups of microbiological agents to Reiter's syndrome, but in neither instance has it been clearly established that they cause this disorder. Members of the Mycoplasma genus have been isolated from the urethra and rarely from the joints of these patients; however, these organisms may also be found in the genitourinary tract in other diseases and in normal persons.[24] In 1966 Schacter et al. isolated an apparently new strain of Bedsonia from the synovial membrane, synovial fluid, urethra or conjunctiva of five of eight patients with Reiter's syndrome.[25] One of these isolates repeatedly produced arthritis when injected into the knee of a monkey. However, efforts to confirm these promising studies have not been fruitful. Also militating against the likelihood that these chlamydiae are the etiologic agents in this disease is the failure of patients to respond to tetracycline, an antibiotic which is rapidly effective against this group of organisms. In summation, the etiology of Reiter's syndrome remains to be clarified, but it is likely that an infectious agent, possibly several, may cause this disorder.

HL-A typing of affected individuals suggests there may be a hereditary factor in the etiology of Reiter's syndrome.[25a, b] Brewerton, having noted a 95 per cent incidence of HL-A antigen of the W-27 type in ankylosing spondylitis patients and stimulated by similar clinical findings in ankylosing spondylitis and Reiter's syndrome, as arthritis, sacro-iliitis, spondylitis, uveitis, and aortitis, investigated the HL-A typing of Reiter's syndrome patients. The W-27 antigen was found in 76 per cent of 33 patients, and among a similar number of controls and patients with nonspecific urethritis the incidence was 9 per cent and 6 per cent, respectively.[25a] Thus, in this study there was a highly significant association of W-27 antigen and Reiter's syndrome. Also, the Reiter's patients were a heterogeneous group including those with early disease, chronic peripheral arthritis, sacro-iliitis, and spondylitis and there appeared to be an increased incidence of the W-27 antigen in all categories.

We have previously cited evidence that Reiter's syndrome may be caused by an infectious agent, and now there is evidence of genetic similarity among patients with this entity. On the basis of these observations, it may be theorized that certain individuals have a genetic propensity to develop the various facets of this syndrome after exposure to a particular microbiological agent or even to a variety of agents. There is perhaps some support for this theory in the finding of only a 9 per cent incidence of W-27 antigen in patients with uncomplicated, non-specific urethritis, an entity which in all likelihood is due to a microbiological agent. It is possible that HL-A positive patients who have non-specific urethritis develop Reiter's syndrome as a sequela to this presumably infectious entity.

The diagnosis of Reiter's syndrome is dependent upon recognition of the triad of genitourinary, ocular and rheumatic manifestations; however, some will accept two of the triad in association with typical skin or mucous membrane lesions. This syndrome is likely to be missed if any of the manifestations are evanescent or separated from the others by an unusually long interval. Onset of Reiter's syndrome may follow within 11 to 30 days after an episode of dysentery, and following sexual exposure there is an average two-week delay before the appearance of urethritis and another two weeks before the onset of joint disease.[22, 26] Any one of the triad may be the presenting manifestation, although urethritis is the most common initial feature; in some instances all may appear almost simultaneously. The three components usually develop within a period of four weeks, although at times a longer period is encompassed.

The arthritis of Reiter's syndrome is marked by an acute onset and by the generally asymmetrical involvement of a few joints; the large joints, the joints of the mid-foot, the metatarsophalangeals and the interphalangeals of the toes are those most frequently affected (Fig. 14–23). The hip joints are usually spared. Extraarticular involvement localized to the attachment of the achilles tendon or the plantar fascia, to periarticular tendons, or seemingly to a portion of or an entire joint capsule are common and may be the presenting complaint.[27] Low back pain may occur and heralds the onset of sacroiliitis; however, the sacroiliitis may be asymptomatic or perhaps overshadowed by the other joint manifestations (see below). The rheumatic manifestations may last for only a few weeks or, in rare cases, up to a year, but three months is the average duration. Repeated episodes are quite common, may or may not be preceded by sexual exposure and often are unaccompanied by other features of the syndrome. Joint damage may follow the initial or subsequent attacks and this is most likely to be clinically apparent in feet manifested by chronic swelling and deformity, including pes planus and cock-up toes. In some instances there appears to be a chronic active arthritis, again frequently in the feet, and it is not clear whether this represents a chronic active process, superimposition of subacute episodes or residual joint damage.[27]

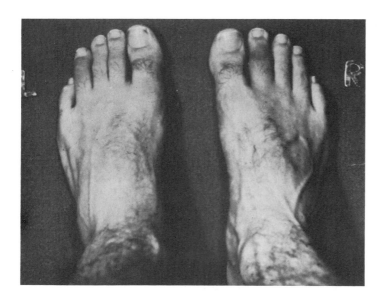

Figure 14–23. Acute arthritis of Reiter's syndrome. The terminal interphalangeal joint of the left fourth toe and the proximal interphalangeal joint of the right second toe are swollen and dusky. Involvement of the interphalangeal joints of the toes is unusual in rheumatoid arthritis.

Diagnosis of this arthritis is likely to be a problem only if the other manifestations of the syndrome are obscure or absent. Recurrent episodes, limited to arthritis, pose a difficult problem if the entity was not recognized during the initial or earlier episodes. The tendency to involve the achilles tendon attachment site or the undersurface of the heel is helpful but these sites may also be involved in ankylosing spondylitis, rheumatoid and psoriatic arthritis, and gout. Absence of rheumatoid factor will help in differentiating from rheumatoid arthritis. Synovial fluid is typically Class II (inflammatory); however, the absence of urate and pyrophosphate crystals rules out crystal synovitis, a diagnosis which may be suspect, in view of the acute onset. Differentiation from psoriatic arthropathy may be impossible, as the keratotic lesions of Reiter's disease may evolve into lesions which cannot be differentiated from psoriasis.[19]

The genitourinary, ocular, skin and mucous membrane lesions of Reiter's syndrome will be considered only briefly. The urethritis and conjunctivitis may range from asymptomatic and inapparent to severe and purulent, with all intervening gradations. Cystitis and prostatitis are additional manifestations in men, while women may develop cystitis and pelvic inflammatory disease. Recurrent uveitis is not uncommon and frequently is associated with recurrent arthritis or spondylitis. The classic skin lesion keratoderma blennorrhagicum most frequently is localized to the plantar surface of the feet but

may also involve the extensor surfaces of the feet, legs, hands and fingers. These lesions which develop in approximately 10 per cent of patients initially consist of small macules which then enlarge to keratotic plaques (Fig. 14–24).[27] Lesions of the glans penis in the area of the meatus occur in approximately 25 per cent of patients.[28] Typical keratoderma occurs in circumcized patients; however, the uncircumcized may manifest balanitis circinata, round shallow ulcers with raised borders. These skin lesions in association with arthritis are strongly suggestive of Reiter's syndrome. The mucous membrane lesions of the oral cavity are marked by erythema and erosions and are quite non-specific; however, they may be helpful from a diagnostic standpoint in the absence of one of the characteristic findings.

Reiter's Spondylitis

A high percentage of patients with Reiter's syndrome show radiographic evidence of sacroiliitis, at times asymmetrical or even unilateral, but it is clear that a smaller proportion develop spondylitis (Fig. 14–25). In this discussion sacroiliitis and spondylitis will not be used interchangeably; spondylitis will be used in an inclusive sense to indicate sacroiliac and vertebral joint disease. Studies by Marche, Ford, Murray, Oates and Young, and Reynolds and Csonka have shown radiographic evidence of sacroiliitis which ranged from 20 to 80 per cent among patients with

Reiter's syndrome.[29-32] Oates and Young, in a study of 78 patients, found definite evidence of sacroiliitis in 45 per cent, doubtful changes in 11 per cent and normal joints in 44 per cent.[33] This study also suggested that the incidence of sacroiliitis increased in relation to the time span after the initial episode of the syndrome. Thus, the average elapsed time after onset of disease in patients with sacroiliitis was 13.4 years and only 4.8 years in those with normal sacroiliac joints. It has also been shown that the prevalence of sacroiliitis associated with Reiter's syndrome is greater in patients with a history of recurrent epidoses of peripheral arthritis than among those with but a single attack of arthritis.

Finally, Ford and many others have shown that radiographic study of the spine in Reiter's syndrome patients will yield a greater prevalence of sacroiliitis than spondylitis.[30]

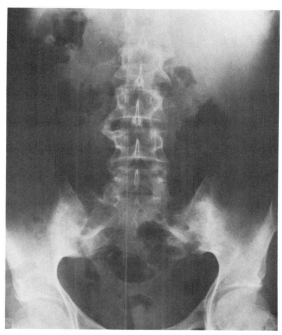

Figure 14–25. Spondylitis associated with Reiter's syndrome. The sacroiliac joints are sclerotic and almost fused, and there is unilateral osseous bridging between L-3 and L-4. Asymmetric osseous bridging is characteristically found in both Reiter's syndrome and psoriatic spondylitis, and probably represents atypical syndesmophyte formation. Smaller syndesmophytes are noted in the upper lumbar area.

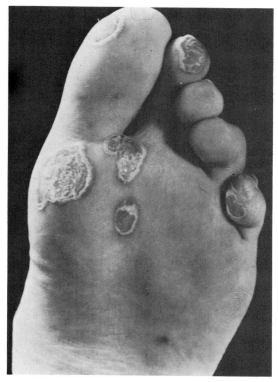

Figure 14–24. Keratodermia blenorrhagicum in Reiter's syndrome. There are keratotic plaques in the metatarsal area and also at the tips of the first, second and fifth toes. (Courtesy of Dr. Chitranjan Ranowat, and The Arthritis Foundation.)

In some patients with Reiter's syndrome, sacroiliitis and spondylitis are asymptomatic, while others present symptoms indistinguishable from those of advanced ankylosing spondylitis. We have previously noted that low back pain in association with an episode of Reiter's syndrome is strongly suggestive of sacroiliitis; but in the series reported by Oates and Young less than 50 per cent of those with definite radiographic evidence of sacroiliitis complained of back pain.[33] Overall, the symptoms, signs and radiographic findings are similar to those noted in ankylosing spondylitis (see page 721 and following); however, in patients with Reiter's syndrome the disease appears to be less severe and extensive.

In a recent clinical and radiographic study McEwen et al. reviewed and compared 29 patients with ankylosing spondylitis, 38 with colitic spondylitis, 34 with Reiter's syndrome and 39 with spondylitis associated with psoriasis.[5] On the basis of this study, patients fell into two distinct groups. The ankylosing spondylitis and colitis patients formed one group and those with Reiter's and psoriasis the second. In brief summation, the ankylosing spondylitis and colitis patients had a more severe form of spondylitis, with early radiological evidence of bilateral sacroiliac disease, and also a greater tendency to syndesmophyte formation and squaring of vertebrae. This same group also had more obvious clinical signs, including a greater tendency to lumbar spine straightening and kyphosis, and a greater decrease in chest expansion. They also noted a variation in the types of syndesmophytes in these two groups. The ankylosing spondylitis and colitis patients almost exclusively showed marginal syndesmophytes while the Reiter's and psoriasis patients had both marginal and non-marginal syndesmophytes (Fig. 14–12).

Finally, the spinal involvement in ankylosing spondylitis and colitis is ascending and progressive, whereas it is patchy in Reiter's and psoriasis (Fig. 14–25). The presence of sacroiliitis in association with one or a few asymmetrical, large, non-marginal osteophytes suggests the possibility of the spondylitis associated with Reiter's syndrome.

In a young man who develops progressive spondylitis after an episode of non-specific urethritis, it is difficult to distinguish between post-Reiter's spondylitis and ankylosing spondylitis. King and Mason suggest that it is usually possible to differentiate these diseases if details concerning the course of illness are available.[27] Points suggestive of Reiter's syndrome are recurrent episodes of peripheral arthritis and mild spinal symptoms and findings. Also, the spine involvement in Reiter's, as noted above, is likely to be patchy, whereas in ankylosing spondylitis it is generally ascending and progressive. Conjunctivitis, oral lesions and keratoderma do not occur in ankylosing spondylitis, but both diseases may be marked by recurrent bouts of uveitis. The radiographic studies of McEwen et al. suggest an additional approach to this differentiation but a larger series of patients will have to be studied in order to validate this categorization.[5]

TREATMENT

Aspirin and other non-steroidal anti-inflammatory drugs are utilized in the management of the rheumatic manifestations of Reiter's syndrome. Aspirin, indomethacin, and butazolidin, are utilized in the same dosages and with the same precautions outlined for the treatment of rheumatoid arthritis (page 761) or ankylosing spondylitis (page 743). For symptomatic spondylitis the treatment program is similar to that outlined for ankylosing spondylitis. There is evidence that immunosuppressive agents including azathioprine, cyclophosphamide, and methotrexate suppress the dermatitis and peripheral arthritis of Reiter's syndrome. However, it is clear that these drugs must be reserved for extremely severe and protracted disease which has failed to respond to full trials of conservative treatment agents. The various toxic and potentially lethal side effects of the immunosuppressive drugs must be considered in relation to a disease that is almost always self limited. Also to be kept in mind is the cidal effect of cyclophosphamide upon reproductive cells, as Reiter's syndrome is primarily a disease of the young.

References

1. McEwen, C.: Arthritis accompanying ulcerative colitis. Clin. Orthop. 57:9–17, 1968.
2. Wright, V., and Watkinson, G.: Articular complications of ulcerative colitis. Am. J. Proct. 17:107–115, 1966.
3. McEwen, C., Lingg, C., Kirsner, J. B., and Spencer, J. A.: Arthritis accompanying ulcerative colitis. Am. J. Med. 6:923–941, 1962.
3a. Brewerton, D. A., Nichols, A., Caffrey, M., et al: HL-A 27 and arthropathies associated with ulcerative colitis and psoriasis. Lancet 1:956–958, 1974.
3b. Morris, R. I., Metzger, A. L., Bluestone, R. and Terasaki, P. I.: HL-A-W-27—a useful discriminator in the arthropies of inflammatory bowel disease. New Eng. J. Med. 290:1117–1119, 1974.
4. Bywaters, E. G. L., and Ansell, B. M.: Arthritis associated with ulcerative colitis. Ann. Rheum. Dis. 17:169–183, 1958.
5. McEwen, C., DiTata, D., Lingg, C., Porini, A., Good, A., and Rankin, T.: Ankylosing spondylitis and spondylitis accompanying ulcerative colitis, regional enteritis, psoriasis and Reiter's disease. Arthritis Rheum. 14:291–318, 1971.
6. Wilske, K. R., and Decker, J. L.: The articular manifestations of intestinal disease. Bull. Rheum. Dis. 15:362–365, 1965.
7. Wright, V., and Watkinson, G.: The arthritis of ulcerative colitis. Medicine 38:243–259, 1959.
8. Wright, V., and Watkinson, G.: The arthritis of ulcerative colitis. Brit. Med. J. 2:670–675, 1965.
9. Wright, V., and Watkinson, G.: Sacro-iliitis and ulcerative colitis. Brit. Med. J. 2:675–680, 1965.
10. Hart, F. D.: The ankylosing spondylopathies. Clin. Orthop. 74:7–13, 1971.
11. Jayson, M. I. V., and Bouchier, I. A. D.: Ulcerative colitis with ankylosing spondylitis. Ann. Rheum. Dis. 27:219–224, 1968.
12. Ansell, B. M., and Wigley, R. A. D.: Arthritic mani-

festations in regional enteritis. Ann. Rheum. Dis. 23:64–72, 1964.
13. Wright, V., and Moll, J. M. H.: Psoriatic arthritis. Bull. Rheum. Dis. 21:627–632, 1971.
14. Leczinsky, C. G.: The incidence of arthropathy in a ten-year series of psoriasis cases. Acta Derm. Venereol. (Stockh.) 28:483–487, 1948.
15. Buckley, W. R., and Raleigh, R. L.: Psoriasis with acroosteolysis. New Eng. J. Med. 261:539–541, 1959.
16. Baker, H., Golding, D. N., and Thompson, M.: Psoriasis and arthritis. Ann. Intern. Med. 58:909–925, 1963.
17. Avila, R., Pugh, D. G., Slocumb, C. H., and Winkelman, R. K.: Psoriatic arthritis: a roentgenologic study. Radiology 75:691–701, 1960.
18. Wright, V.: Psoriatic arthritis: a comparative study of rheumatoid arthritis and arthritis associated with psoriasis. Ann. Rheum. Dis. 20:123–131, 1961.
19. Wright, V., and Reed, W. B.: The link between Reiter's syndrome and psoriatic arthritis. Ann. Rheum. Dis. 23:12–21, 1964.
20. O'Brien, W. M., Van Scott, E. J., Black, R. L., Eisen, A. Z., and Bunim, J. J.: Clinical trial of Amethopterin (methotrexate) in psoriatic and rheumatoid arthritis (preliminary report). Arthritis Rheum. 5:312, 1962. (Abstr.).
21. Levy, J., Paulus, H. E., Barnett, E. V., Sokoloff, M., Bangert, R., and Pearson, C. M.: A double-blind controlled evaluation of azathioprine treatment in rheumatoid arthritis and psoriatic arthritis. Arthritis Rheum. 15:116–117, 1972, (Abstr.).
22. Paronen, I.: Reiter's disease—A study of 344 cases observed in Finland. Acta. Med. Scand. 133(suppl. 212):1–114, 1948.
23. Noer, H. R.: An "experimental" epidemic of Reiter's syndrome J.A.M.A. 197:693–698, 1966.
24. Engleman, E. P., and Weber, H. M.: Reiter's syndrome. Clin. Orthop. 57:19–29, 1968.
25. Schacter, J., et al: Isolation of Bedsoniae from the joints of patients with Reiter's syndrome. Proc. Soc. Exp. Biol. Med. 122:283–285, 1966.
25a. Brewerton, D. A., Nichols, A., Oates, J. K., et al: Reiter's Disease and HL-A 27. Lancet, 2:996–998, 1973.
25b. Woodrow, J. C.: HL-A and Reiter's Syndrome. Lancet, 2:671–672, 1973.
26. Csonka, G. W.: The course of Reiter's syndrome. Brit. Med. J. 1:1088–1090, 1958.
27. King, A. J., and Mason, R. M.: Reiter's disease. In Textbook of the Rheumatic Diseases. Copeman, W. S. C. (ed.), Baltimore, Williams & Wilkins, 1969, pp. 366–384.
28. Hancock, J. A. H., and Mason, R. M.: Reiter's disease. In Progress in Clinical Rheumatology. Dixon, A. St. J. (ed.), Boston, Little, Brown and Co., 1965, pp. 201–219.
29. Marche, J.: L'atteinte des articulations sacro-iliaques dans le syndrome "dit" de Reiter. Rev. Rhum. 17:449–451, 1950.
30. Ford, D. K.: Arthritis and venereal urethritis. Brit. J. Vener. Dis. 29:123–133, 1953.
31. Murray, R. S., Oates, J. K., and Young, A. C.: Radiological changes in Reiter's syndrome and arthritis associated with urethritis. J. Fac. Radiol. (Lond.) 9:37–43, 1958.
32. Reynolds, D. F., and Csonka, G. W.: Radiological aspects of Reiter's syndrome (venereal arthritis). J. Fac. Radiol. (Lond.) 9:44–49, 1959.
33. Oates, J. K., and Young, A. C.: Sacro-iliitis in Reiter's disease. Brit. Med. J. 1:1013–1015, 1959.

RHEUMATOID ARTHRITIS

As an introduction to rheumatoid arthritis, we will consider present concepts of the pathogenesis of rheumatoid synovitis. Intensive investigations during the past three decades have yielded histological, immunopathological and immunochemical findings which strongly implicate the immune system in the pathogenesis of rheumatoid arthritis. Histologically, one of the characteristic features of rheumatoid synovitis is infiltration by lymphocytes and plasma cells—cell types associated with immune reactions. In some instances the lymphocytes are aggregated into follicle-like structures, thus resembling lymphoid tissues reacting to an antigenic stimulus. By fluorescent antibody tracing techniques, it has been shown that plasma cells of rheumatoid synovitis synthesize IgG and IgM immunoglobulins and that some of the IgM immunoglobulins have rheumatoid factor activity.[1] Thus, there is evidence of antibody production in the rheumatoid joint. Next, we may consider studies which point to formation of complexes of antibody, antigen and complement in these joints. IgG, IgM and complement have been detected in the synovial membrane and synovial fluid leukocytes evidently as immune complexes.[2,3,4] Further evidence of intra-articular immune complexes is based on the immunochemical analysis of protein aggregates that have been found in rheumatoid synovial fluids.[5] The major component of the aggregated protein appears to be IgG, but cold precipitable fractions of the fluid have revealed aggregates containing IgG, IgM, DNA, and complement.[6,7] Also, consistent with presence of intra-articular immune complexes which bind complement are studies which have shown that the ratio of synovial complement to serum complement in RA is lower than in other arthritides.[8]

These findings all point to an intra-articular immune reaction and are the background for the following hypothetical schema of the pathogenesis of rheumatoid arthritis: An unknown antigen localizing at the synovial surface stimulates formation of antibodies directed against it. The subsequent formation of complexes of antigen and antibody binds complement and attracts polymorphonuclear leukocytes into the joint space. The leukocytes ingest the complexes but for unexplained reasons disintegrate and release their lysosomal enzymes into the joint. It has been postulated that these enzymes are responsible for at least some of the inflammatory, proliferative, and destructive changes which characterize rheumatoid joint disease.

While the proposed schema is an attractive one, it does not account for many aspects of rheumatoid inflammation. A key point of this hypothesis is the postulation of an inciting antigen, likely a microbiologic agent; however, such an antigen has not been detected despite intensive investigation. Also, the schema does not account for the chronicity of rheumatoid inflammation. Persistence of the inciting antigen is possible but seems unlikely, for it is difficult to believe that such a chronically entrenched factor would consistently evade detection. It has been proposed that after the inciting antigen has been destroyed or carried away a substance associated with the inflammatory process may serve as a continuing source of antigenic stimulation. Possible sources of a chronic antigenic stimulus include: 1) molecules such as gamma globulin or fibrin which tend to accumulate at inflammatory lesions and may conceivably undergo slight structural alteration at such sites; 2) DNA or other molecules released from disintegrating leukocytes; 3) complexes consisting of a newly synthesized or accumulated molecule (possibly gamma globulin, fibrin, or DNA) and IgG antibody. In support of the possibility that DNA may be a chronic antigenic stimulus are the facts that it can be found in cold precipitable aggregates from rheumatoid arthritis synovial fluid, and that antibody to nuclear material including DNA has been found in the serum of rheumatoid arthritis patients.[6,7]

It is particularly intriguing to consider a specific accumulation of IgG or an immune complex containing IgG as the antigenic substance as it allows for incorporation of rheumatoid factor of either Ig or IgM variety into the aforementioned schema of rheumatoid inflammation. In this vein, it may be reasoned that rheumatoid factor, which has anti IgG activity, is synthesized in response to the presence of intra-articular IgG and that complexes of rheumatoid factor and IgG are ultimately formed. It is quite possible that such complexes bind complement and thus could activate mechanisms which mediate synovitis and joint destruction. The possibilities that have been cited are consistent with our present understanding of these factors as well as immunochemical and immunopathological studies which suggest that complexes containing RF are present in rheumatoid arthritis joints.

It is furthermore unclear why rheumatoid inflammation tends to localize to synovial lined joints. It has been proposed that this localization reflects certain functional and anatomical features of joints which favor: 1) trapping of antigenic substances; 2) the egress of such materials from the circulation; and 3) the proliferation of immunologically active cells. The phagocytic capability of the majority of the synovial lining cells and similar capability of the endothelial cells of the synovial circulation suggest that the joints are likely sites for the deposition of antigenic substances.[8,9,10] Gaps have been observed between the synovial lining cells and may facilitate the deposition of antigens in the joint space.[9,10] Other possible contributory factors include the absence of a membrane in relation to synovial lining cells and the porous nature of the synovial microcirculation.[11,12] An interesting possibility is that the stress of motion and weight bearing in joints may produce a mild degree of traumatic inflammation which facilitates the egress of various molecules into the synovial interstitium and joint space. Finally, the loose connective tissue just below the synovial lining cells is a favorable site for proliferation of immunologically active cells.

Before leaving this topic, it is pertinent to note that knowledge of the pathogenesis of rheumatoid inflammation provides us with a rational basis for devising treatment modalities. If we can block or modify certain steps in the pathogenesis of the inflammatory process without harming the host, we, in all likelihood, will be able to suppress the disease activity and thereby hopefully prevent the crippling and disability which too frequently ensue.

Peripheral Joints

Rheumatoid arthritis (RA) is a systemic disease characterized by protracted morning stiffness and a symmetrical polyarthritis involving both small and large joints. The onset of the arthritis is usually insidious and, although any combination of joints may be affected, knee, metacarpophalangeal and proximal interphalangeal joints (Figs. 14–26 and

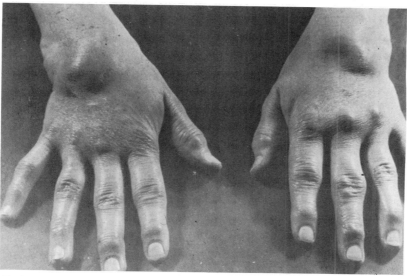

Figure 14–26. Early rheumatoid arthritis involving the metacarpophalangeal and proximal interphalangeal joints of the fingers, the interphalangeal joints of the thumbs, and the extensor tendon sheaths at the wrists. Note that the metacarpophalangeal joint swelling has obliterated the gutters between the metacarpal heads, and the tendon sheath involvement has resulted in swelling over each wrist.

14–27) of the hands and metatarsophalangeal of the feet are the usual sites of early involvement. Almost all patients experience fatigue, but other systemic manifestations, such as weight loss and low grade fever are less common. Rheumatoid nodules localized most frequently to the extensor surface of the forearm or the olecranon bursa are present in from 10 to 20 per cent of patients. The course is generally marked by progressive involve-

ment of the joints, with loss of motion or instability and eventual deformity; however, these changes may evolve over periods of months or many years (Fig. 14–28). Exacerbations and partial remissions are likely to mark the first year or two of illness. There may, however, be marked variation from the typical picture. The onset may be acute or characterized by episodes of joint involvement lasting a day or two (palindromic rheumatism), or longer episodes

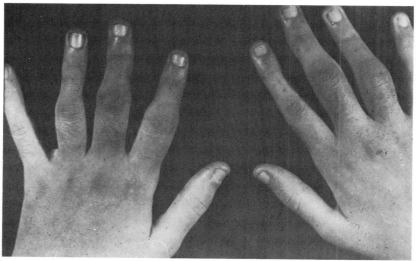

Figure 14–27. Moderately advanced rheumatoid arthritis marked by swelling and flexion of proximal interphalangeal joints.

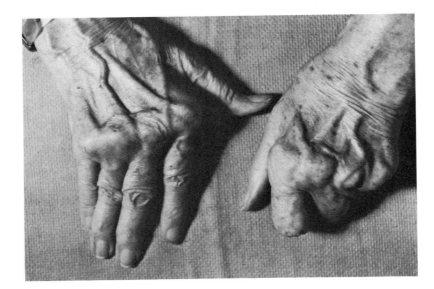

Figure 14-28. Far advanced rheumatoid arthritis. The left hand shows fixed flexion deformities at the proximal interphalangeal joints and swelling of the metacarpophalangeal joints. Ulnar deviation of the fingers and subluxation and swelling of the metacarpophalangeal joints are prominent in the right hand. There is marked muscle atrophy in the dorsum of each hand.

persisting for weeks (episodic RA). Rarely, the arthritis is limited to one or a few joints, and visceral or vascular disease may dominate the clinical course.

The latex flocculation test and other tests to detect rheumatoid factor (RF) are positive in 70 to 80 per cent of patients with definite or classical rheumatoid arthritis as defined by American Rheumatism Association criteria and, therefore, its presence will tend to support a diagnosis of RA in patients with suggestive evidence of this disease.[13] However, these tests do not constitute an absolute criterion for establishing or ruling out the diagnosis of RA. Determining the titer of RF, utilizing a tube dilution technique, may be helpful as high titers are often found in RA patients, whereas the titer is likely to be low when it occurs in other diseases. RA patients with positive tests for this factor will usually have this finding from the outset of their disease, but rarely the test may turn positive a year or two after onset. Rheumatoid factor may also be detectable in patients with generalized connective tissue disorders, and chronic granulomatous and infectious diseases. Among these diseases the percentage of patients with positive tests is usually less than 25 per cent; subacute bacterial endocarditis is an exception with 50 per cent or more of patients having positive reactions.[14] Approximately 25 per cent of RA patients will have positive tests for antinuclear factor and an additional 5 per cent will have a positive LE test.[15]

The synovial fluid is of the Class II or inflammatory type, but there is a wide range of findings, reflecting the intensity of the synovitis. As an example, the WBC averages 10,000 to 20,000 cells, but counts as high as 60,000, as in septic effusions, may be noted. Also, the synovial fluid WBC may be below 10,000 in early or mild disease.[15] Rheumatoid synovial fluid findings are non-specific; the RA cells or inclusion body cells described by Hollander et al. in these effusions may also be detected in other diseases.[16]

Radiographic findings, although not specific, are helpful both diagnostically and in following the course of disease. Deossification, joint space narrowing and erosions are the usual findings, and subchondral deossification and erosions in the hands may be present after three months of joint involvement (Figs. 14-29 to 14-32).

Joint biopsy findings are diagnostic only in very rare instances when a rheumatoid nodule is included in the specimen. The findings of lining cell proliferation, villous formation and aggregates of plasma cells and lymphocytes are strongly suggestive of RA, but not diagnostic, as they may also be found in other diseases. In some instances, specimens from rheumatoid joints lack these findings and the disorder may be interpreted only as nonspecific synovitis.

The diagnosis of rheumatoid arthritis is likely to be difficult in those with atypical joint involvement and in those without rheumatoid

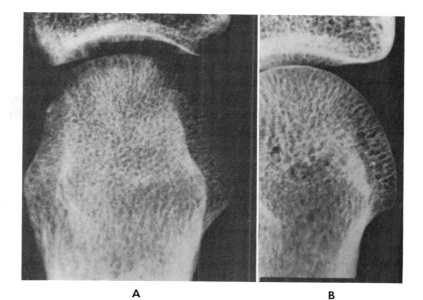

Figure 14–29. Loss of articular cortical bone in rheumatoid arthritis. *A,* The cortical margin at the radial aspect of the metacarpal head has been lost. *B,* The normal appearance of the cortex at the radial aspect of the metacarpal head is shown for comparison. Deossification of this type may be noted three months after onset of joint involvement.

A   B

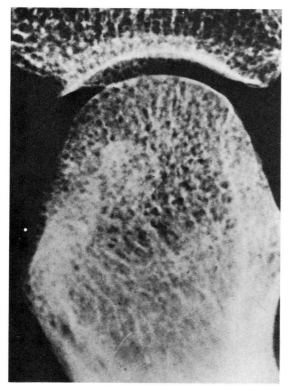

Figure 14–30. Loss of articular bone and early erosion in rheumatoid arthritis. There is deossification of the articular cortex at the radial aspect of the metacarpal. A small erosion has developed on the radial aspect of the phalange just distal to the joint space.

factor. Such patients will have to be considered in relationship to the diagnostic possibilities listed in Table 14–1, and appropriate clinical laboratory and radiographic investigations will be required in order to differentiate between these various disorders. However, patients who ultimately prove to have other diseases, including systemic lupus erythematosus, scleroderma, polymyositis and psoriatic and colitic arthritis, may present with joint involvement similar to that of RA or in the general connective tissue (collagen) diseases with positive tests for RF. In these patients, the correct diagnosis can be established only when the more characteristic aspects of their diseases become apparent.

Treatment

A detailed consideration of the management of rheumatoid arthritis will not be presented: however, the basic treatment program and certain drugs useful in this disease will be outlined. All adult patients presenting with rheumatoid arthritis should have a basic program comprising rest, physical therapy, and a maximally effective dosage of aspirin.

Rest for rheumatoid arthritis patients includes systemic rest, a general supportive measure, and joint rest, a time honored

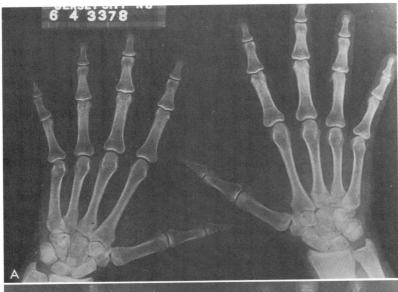

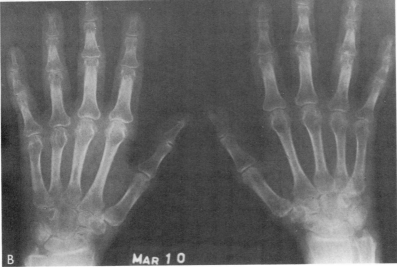

Figure 14–31. Moderately progressive rheumatoid arthritis in the hands. *A,* There is moderate narrowing of the cartilage space of the radiocarpal joints. *B,* Twenty-six months later cartilage space narrowing is present at the radiocarpal, metacarpophalangeal and proximal interphalangeal joints and there is marked juxta-articular deossification.

therapy, more likely to be employed by orthopedic surgeons than medically oriented physicians. Systemic rest for these patients may be accomplished in a variety of ways, but reduction of daily activities and allaying the anxiety, which is often engendered by this disease, are two useful methods. Measures of value in providing progressive restriction of activity include: 1) elimination of activities unessential to the patient's role as a wage earner, homemaker or student; 2) naps; 3) partial reduction of the working day; 4) partial bed rest; and 5) complete bed rest. With respect to relieving the anxiety associated with rheumatoid arthritis, the best approach is probably counseling and support by a physician who is familiar with the

natural course and therapy of rheumatoid arthritis.

The second type of rest, joint rest, may also be accomplished by a variety of techniques, including reduction or elimination of repetitive joint motions during the daily routine, use of splints, braces, canes, crutches, and bed rest. Those patients with minimal evidence of disease activity, as manifested by joint inflammation, morning stiffness, fatigue, and debility, and without evidence of joint destruction require little in the way of rest. Other patients should have a graded program of rest directly related to the degree of disease activity and/or permanent joint destruction. For example, patients with modest disease activity may be managed by restriction of extracurricular activities. Whereas those with intensely active disease will require complete bed rest. The rest program, however, should not be static; it is altered in relation to changes in disease activity and progression of joint destruction. Also, the physician should not be rigid in prescribing rest, particularly restriction of activities, for these patients. Most patients will gratefully accept the increased rest, but some will become depressed and in such instances less stringent restrictions are a reasonable compromise.

The physical therapeutic modality of prime importance in rheumatoid arthritis patients is non-weight-bearing exercise. It is utilized to maintain or increase articular motion and muscle power. Therapeutic exercise, like rest, must be prescribed and altered in relation to disease activity; however, in this instance the relationship is inverse. Patients with marked activity are restricted to passive motion and muscle-setting exercises; with moderate activity, repetitive isometric exercises against gravity are utilized; and with minimal activity, exercises against resistance are permissible. Therapeutic exercise is also indicated for joints which have sustained permanent damage; the intensity of the program is regulated by the severity of concomitant synovitis in these damaged joints.

Aspirin therapy for rheumatoid arthritis patients should provide for: 1) the highest dosage that can be tolerated, 2) frequent administration, and 3) measures to protect the gastrointestinal tract. It is pertinent to briefly consider the background for this program. Rheumatoid arthritis patients almost always experience increasing relief of joint pain and stiffness as aspirin dosage is raised. It is not possible, however, to recommend a maximally effective dosage, as patients vary with respect to both the amount of aspirin necessary to yield a particular serum salicylate concentration and the serum salicylate level at which toxicity develops. Put in another way, two patients receiving the same daily dosage of aspirin may attain quite different serum salicylate levels and only the lower level may be associated with toxicity. Thus, optimum aspirin therapy requires a titration to determine the highest daily dosage that is unassociated with symptoms of toxicity. The requirement of frequent doses relates to studies which have shown that after ingestion of 600 mg. of aspirin there is a maximum serum level at two hours and a steady decline over the next twelve hours.[17] It is clear that rheumatoid arthritis patients who ingest a dose of aspirin on retiring will have a suboptimal blood concentration during the early morning hours, when joint pain and stiffness are at a maximum. Frequent administration, including a dose at 3 or 4 A.M., will serve to maintain salicylate levels, particularly during the important early morning hours. Aspirin is quite often

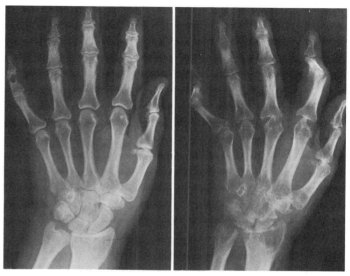

Figure 14–32. Severely progressive rheumatoid arthritis in the hands. *A,* The radiograph of the right hand appears normal except for questionable narrowing of the cartilage space of the radiocarpal joint. *B,* Sixteen months later there is extensive deossification, erosion and cartilage space narrowing at the radiocarpal, intercarpal, metacarpophalangeal and proximal interphalangeal joints of the right hand. The ulnar styloid process has also been eroded.

A   **B**

toxic to the upper gastrointestinal tract, with resultant indigestion, bleeding or peptic ulceration.

It is established that aspirin has a local irritating effect on the upper gastrointestinal mucosa; however, systemic effects of this drug resulting in an altered quality of gastric mucus and decreased platelet adhesiveness may also contribute to these toxic reactions.[18] In any event, it is recommended that aspirin be ingested with food and fluid to reduce its concentration in the stomach and, in addition, antacid therapy should be utilized in an effort to protect the mucosa of the stomach.

The following is a prototype aspirin dosage program for adult rheumatoid arthritis patients that will fulfill these requirements. Treatment should be initiated with 900 mg. of aspirin (600 mg. for those over 60 years of age) five times per day. The doses to be taken immediately after meals and at bedtime and 3 or 4 A.M. with a glass of milk or skim milk. If after a week of treatment there is no evidence of toxicity, such as tinnitus, decreased hearing acuity, dizziness or nausea, the total daily dosage is then raised by a single tablet every two or three days. The increments should, of course, be evenly distributed among the various doses. With the onset of toxicity, aspirin is withdrawn for a period of 24 hours and then restarted at daily dosage totaling two tablets less than the toxic dosage.

Certain aspects of this program of aspirin therapy require qualification. It should not be utilized in children, as the previously cited symptoms are not a reliable guide to toxicity in the young. Also, there is nothing sacrosanct about the aspirin dosage determined by the initial trial, and further adjustment may be necessary. In instances when nausea is the major manifestation of toxicity, a trial of enteric coated aspirin is indicated, as this symptom may reflect gastrointestinal rather than central nervous system toxicity. Tinnitus, which is usually the most reliable guide to toxicity, may be an unreliable sign in the aged and those with decreased hearing acuity. Such patients should be monitored by serum salicylate determinations; concentrations between 15 and 30 mg. per cent are considered to be effective in rheumatoid patients. We have not found that patients object to a 3 or 4 A.M. dose; they usually awaken spontaneously but failing this may resort to an alarm clock. Finally, it is recommended that these pa-

tients utilize an antacid one hour after meals and at bedtime.

If a four to six week trial of the basic program fails to afford marked relief of joint pain and stiffness, treatment with an additional drug is instituted and aspirin is continued, although in a somewhat lower dosage supplemented by an additional drug. It is our routine to first utilize an antimalarial, either chloroquine or hydroxychloroquine. If this agent fails, we turn to gold. Finally, corticosteroids are employed. These drugs are all potentially toxic and the dosages for rheumatoid arthritis patients, contraindications, precautions during treatment, and various side effects must be carefully reviewed before treatment is initiated. Indomethacin (Indocin) appears to benefit some rheumatoid arthritis patients and may be tried if aspirin proves ineffective, either before resorting to the drugs outlined above or as a supplement to them when they prove only moderately effective. The occasional central nervous system toxic effects of indomethacin (headache, psychic reactions, dizziness) can often be avoided if there is an initial dose of 25 mg. at bedtime and then weekly increments of 25 mg. The additional doses are evenly distributed throughout the day and continued until there is relief of symptoms or a maximum dosage of 150 mg. per day is attained. Also, Indomethacin is a gastric irritant and should be ingested with food or a glass of milk and along with antacid therapy.

Azathioprine (Imuran) and cyclophosphamine (Cytoxan) show promise as treatment agents for this disease, but severe toxicity limits their use. Very active disease and failure to respond to the basic program, supplemented by full trials of the drugs noted above and meticulous monitoring for side effects are minimal requirements for their use.

RHEUMATOID SPONDYLITIS

Rheumatoid spondylitis (rheumatoid arthritis of the spine) is usually manifested in the cervical spine or sacroiliac joints, with only rare involvement of other portions of the spine. Symptoms related to the cervical spine or sacroiliac involvement are rarely a presenting or early manifestation, but the cervical spine disease may be a source of pain, disability and even death. In this section the anatomy, pathology, pathophysiology and clinical and radiologic findings pertinent to involvement of various areas of the spine will be presented. The reader is reminded that rheumatoid spondylitis may be differentiated from ankylosing spondylitis on the basis of clinical and radiological findings.

Cervical Spine (Atlantoaxial Joint)

Radiographic study of the cervical spine in several series of patients has disclosed evidence of atlantoaxial subluxations (AAS) in approximately 25 per cent.[19, 21] Although in one series this lesion was noted more frequently, these patients were not a representative sample, as the manifested severe peripheral rheumatoid arthritis.[22] These studies also indicate that AAS is likely to occur in patients with severe disease, but long duration does not appear to be a predisposing factor. Boyle has noted this lesion early in the course of disease; in a prospective study of 122 patients, there were two who developed AAS within two years of onset.[23] It is not clear, however, that corticosteroids are a predisposing factor, as they are used in patients with the severest disease.

Before considering the clinical and radiological manifestations of AAS, it is necessary to briefly review the anatomy of this joint, and its derangement by rheumatoid inflammation. The atlas is an atypical vertebra consisting of a ring of bone without a body. The structure analogous to the body of the atlas lies just behind the anterior portion of this ring; it is a bony protuberance, the odontoid process, which extends from the axis below. This unique arrangement permits the skull and atlas to rotate widely as a unit on the remainder of the cervical spine. A strong transverse ligament suspended in hammock fashion from the lateral masses of the ring of the atlas holds the odontoid in juxtaposition to the anterior portion of this ring. The odontoid process is also fixed in position by the cruciate ligament, extending from the axis to the border of the foramen magnum, and the alar ligaments which extend from the odontoid process to the occipital condyles. Anterior and posterior to the odontoid in its position between the atlas and the transverse ligament are synovial structures variously described as joints or bursae (Fig. 14–33). Rheumatoid inflammation of these synovial structures may lead to erosion or even extensive destruction of the odontoid, or marked weakening and laxity of the transverse ligament, and in patients with long-standing disease there may also be weakening of the lateral attachments of the

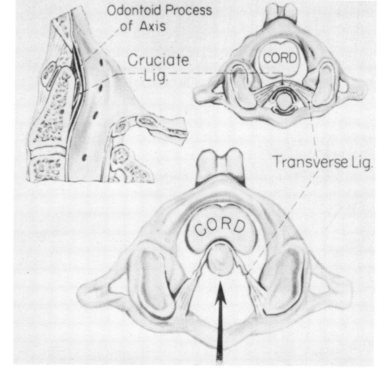

Figure 14–33. *Above,* there is normal anatomy of the atlantoaxial joint, and *below,* subluxation of this joint with compression of the spinal cord.

transverse ligament. The inflammatory changes at the atlantoaxial (AA) joint may lead only to mild instability; however, with progressive involvement there may be a forward slip of the entire bony ring, which in some instances causes compression of the spinal cord (Fig. 14–33). Rarely, severe inflammation in the AA joint area may result in backward slip of the atlas; in this instance the bony ring overrides the odontoid or there is extensive destruction of the odontoid or anterior portion of the ring of the atlas. Also, the odontoid process may rarely herniate upward to the skull and foramen magnum. Forward slippage of the atlas may distort the course of the vertebral arteries, leading to alteration of blood flow or even thrombosis in these vessels, and the subsequent impairment of blood flow in the vertebral arteries may be a factor in the myelopathy associated with AA joint disease. Atlantoaxial subluxation may also result in compression or distortion of the second cervical nerve and an associated occipital neuralgia.

Atlantoaxial subluxation is often symptomatic, and at times is associated with neurological signs of spinal cord disease. Neck pain or occipital headaches are common, and at times the pain may be referred anteriorly to the region of the forehead or eyes. Boyle has found the pain to be continuous, uninfluenced by activity, and not relieved by bed rest.[23] In instances of marked subluxation, sudden movement of the head may cause paresthesias or intense pain. The test described by Sharp and Purser is helpful in evaluating dislocation of the AA joint.[24] The patient is seated, and encouraged to hold his head firmly; the examiner places one hand over the forehead and the index finger of the other hand on the spinous process of the axis; then, firm pressure is applied to the forehead while supporting the neck with the opposite hand. A gliding posterior displacement of the head is indicative of AAS, as the normal cervical spine does not yield with this maneuver.

Quadriplegia is a rare manifestation of AAS, but many patients manifest signs of spinal cord disease. Stevens et al., utilizing increased deep tendon reflexes as criteria, noted that 24 of 36 patients with AAS had myelopathy, but only 10 of these 24 had extensor plantar reflexes.[25] These authors emphasize the difficulty of evaluating muscle strength and tone in patients with peripheral joint disease. However, others, utilizing more stringent criteria for myelopathy, found this complication less frequently in such patients. Conversely, Meikle and Wilkinson found no evidence of spinal cord disease in three patients with severe (12 mm) AAS.[21] Further indication of the perplexing relationship between AAS and spinal cord disease is found in the aforementioned study of Stevens et al.[25] It was noted that there was evidence of myelopathy in 10 of 66 rheumatoid arthritis patients without radiographic evidence of AAS, and in only three of these could the finding be related to subaxial cervical spine disease. These discrepancies suggest that other factors, including normal variations in the width of the spinal canal, vertebral artery distortion and inflammatory swelling of the dura, also influence the development of myelopathy.

Under special circumstances, patients with AAS may develop quadriplegia or even

A

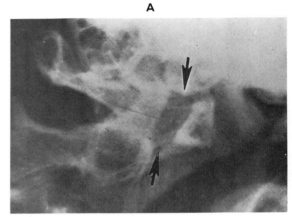

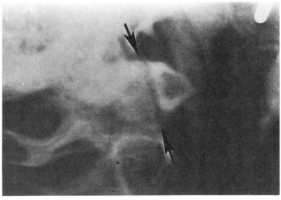

B

Figure 14–34. Subluxation of the atlantoaxial (AA) joint in rheumatoid arthritis. A, with cervical spine in flexion there is a 7 mm subluxation of the AA joint (arrow). B, in the same patient, with the cervical spine extended the AA joint appears to be normal (arrow).

die. These patients are particularly vulnerable to sudden jerks of the neck related to falls or other accidents. Severe distortion of the relaxed neck during unconsciousness due to any cause may have similar dire results, and anesthetists must be wary of this potential in RA patients undergoing surgery.

A distance of 3 mm or greater between the atlas and odontoid is generally considered to be indicative of AAS. The distance is measured from the midpoint of the posterior surface of the anterior ring of the atlas to the nearest point on the odontoid. A distance of less than 3 mm is generally regarded as normal, but Boyle cites a limit of up to 4 mm as being acceptable in patients under 45 (Fig. 14–34).[23]

Treatment of AAS must be individualized and based upon the severity of symptoms and evidence of spinal cord disease. Patients with radiographic findings of AAS, but without symptoms or evidence of spinal disease may be observed. Patients with local or referred pain usually respond to a snug felt collar or a rigid collar; however, severe unrelenting pain calls for a consideration of surgery. Patients similar to those just described but with evidence of cord disease, such as hyperactive reflexes, ankle clonus and absent plantar reflexes, may be treated with a rigid support and a period of bed rest; but these individuals require careful follow up and deserve a neurosurgical consultation. Evidence of progressive myelopathy warrants surgical intervention.

Cervical Spine (Subaxial)

The neurocentral joints, or joints of Luschka, which are lined by synovial tissue, are a feature only of the cervical spine and appear to account for the tendency of rheumatoid inflammation to involve this portion of the spine while the dorsal and lumbar portions are generally spared. For example, Conlon et al. noted that 60 per cent of 845 rheumatoid arthritis patients had signs or symptoms of neck involvement, and radiographic studies have indicated that even if atlantoaxial subluxations are excluded in these patients, there are often findings considered indicative of rheumatoid involvement.[19] Ball's studies indicate that the cervical spine involvement arises from these neurocentral joints which are clefts lined with synovial tissue located in the lateral margin of the disc, just at the point where it contacts the neurocentral lip.[26] Pannus arising from these joints may destroy portions of disc and vertebra, and the resultant weakening of the disc joints predisposes to subluxation.

Involvement of the subaxial portion of the cervical spine may be marked by pain, local signs and findings indicative of nerve root or spinal cord compression. The pain may be experienced in the neck or radiate to the interscapular area, chest, shoulder or arm. Lateral motion of the neck is likely to be painful and somewhat limited, and there may be tenderness of one or more spinous processes. Loss of disc stature and subluxation may be

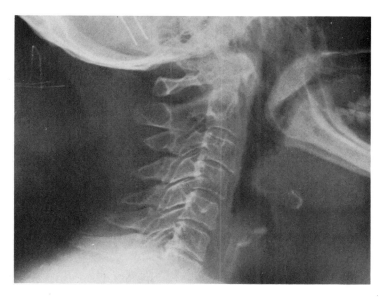

Figure 14–35. Rheumatoid spondylitis in a woman with peripheral rheumatoid arthritis of 21 years' duration. There is narrowing of numerous discs without osteophyte formation.

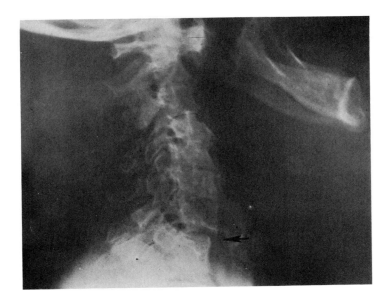

Figure 14–36. Advanced rheumatoid spondylitis with marked narrowing of multiple discs and subluxation of C-7 on T-1.

associated with signs of nerve root or spinal cord disease, but these findings may be difficult to elicit in patients with extensive peripheral joint damage.

Radiographic evidence of rheumatoid spondylitis in the subaxial portion of the cervical spine is marked by dislocations, erosions and disc narrowing (Figs. 14–35 and 14–36). Miekle and Wilkinson, in a study of 118 RA patients, found evidence of subaxial dislocation of greater than 1 mm in 26.3 per cent, end plate erosions in 15.3 per cent and narrowed discs in 72.9 per cent.[21] These authors, however, point out that in a control group of patients with cervical spondylosis, there were similar findings both in kind and percentage, and thus it is not clear that the findings in the RA group are indicative of rheumatoid involvement. It was pointed out that multiple subluxations and particularly subluxations at the C2–C3 level are very suggestive of rheumatoid disease. This study did not confirm the opinion of Conlon et al. and Sharp et al. that disc space narrowing without osteophyte formation is more common in rheumatoid cervical spine disease than in spondylosis.[19, 27] Vertebral body erosions and apophyseal joint changes are difficult to evaluate on routine films of the cervical spine, and are thus of little practical value.

Lumbodorsal Spine

Rheumatoid involvement of the dorsal and lumbar spine is limited to rare instances in which one or more of these vertebrae are involved by a destructive granulomatous lesion. Baggenstoss et al. and Lorber et al. have described rheumatoid arthritis patients with typical subcutaneous nodules who developed vertebral lesions of this type.[28, 29] The lesions appear to originate in the vertebral marrow and may extend to destroy the vertebral end plate. On microscopic examination there is vascular granulation tissue with discrete areas showing typical or atypical rheumatoid nodules.

The clinical manifestations include local and referred pain which is accentuated by motion or straining, pain on forced motion of the spine, and spinous process tenderness. Radiographically these lesions are impossible to differentiate from neoplasms and infections. Lawrence and Sharp described additional radiographic findings but these are probably non-specific.[30]

Sacroiliac Joints

Although rheumatoid arthritis patients sometimes show radiographic evidence of sacroiliac disease this involvement is rarely symptomatic. Martel and Duff noted radiographic evidence of sacroiliac disease in 13 of 40 RA patients, including four in whom the involvement was severe and resembled ankylosing spondylitis.[22] Similarly, Dilsen et al. noted sacroiliac disease in 27 of 97 patients, and in 19 the involvement was bilateral; however, this did not appear to be an early feature and was found in most instances in patients who had had RA for five years.[31] It is not clear why the sacroiliac disease is not clinically apparent; it may be ignored in view of more pressing peripheral joint disease or it may be attributed to hip involvement. The radiographic findings typically consist of unilateral or bilateral erosions without sclerosis; ankylosis is unusual (Fig. 14–37).

Diagnosis

The diagnosis of rheumatoid spondylitis is usually apparent on the basis of accompanying peripheral joint disease and laboratory findings as have been outlined. In instances when rheumatoid spondylitis is associated with atypical or minimal peripheral joint disease, it may be necessary to depend heavily on the presence of rheumatoid factor and the radiographic findings to establish the correct diagnosis.

JUVENILE RHEUMATOID ARTHRITIS

Introduction

Juvenile rheumatoid arthritis (JRA) is probably best defined as chronic polyarthritis of unknown etiology with onset prior to age 16. There is no universally accepted diagnostic criterion or any laboratory test which is highly indicative of this disease, and it is quite possible that diverse diseases are being lumped together under this heading. A familial predisposition to JRA is suggested by the increased finding of seronegative (rheumatoid factor negative) polyarthritis and ankylosing spondylitis among the parents, grandparents and siblings of these patients.[32] JRA is an uncommon disease, less prevalent than its adult counterpart; however, it is one of the commonest causes of crippling among children. The peak incidence of onset is from one to three years, with a range from six months to 16 years; the ratio of girls to boys is approximately 2:1.[33]

Before considering the clinical characteristics of JRA it is pertinent to point out that arthritis in young children and infants is often difficult to detect and evaluate. A reluctance to crawl or walk, a guarded position, and crying whenever limbs are moved are suggestive of arthritis in this age group.

Calabro, in a study of 100 children at the Jersey City Medical Center, has found that at the onset of this disease the clinical features can generally be classified into one of three categories.[33] The acute or Still's type of onset. which made up 20 per cent of the group, was characterized by daily remittent fever, often in the range of 104 to 105° F, adenopathy and splenomegaly, an evanescent macular or slightly papular rash involving the trunk and extremities, and leukocytosis. Joint disease in this group may be absent, mild and inapparent, or florid. Myocarditis or pericarditis may also

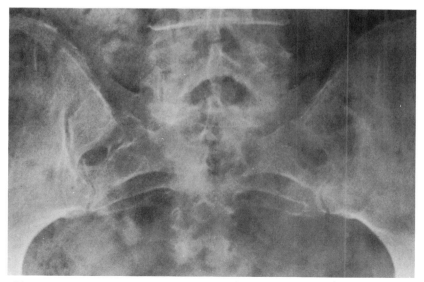

Figure 14–37.   Rheumatoid sacroiliitis. There is marked narrowing and minimal sclerosis of the left sacroiliac joint in a patient with longstanding rheumatoid arthritis. The right sacroiliac joint is normal.

be noted in these children. The second category which made up approximately one half of the group, had a polyarticular onset with involvement of at least four joints. The knees, wrists, ankles and elbows were often affected initially. In some instances there was symmetrical involvement of large and small joints reminiscent of adult rheumatoid arthritis; however, patterns atypical for adult RA, including asymmetric involvement of large joints, involvement of the terminal interphalangeal joints of the hands and migratory arthritis, were also noted. The remaining patients had an onset characterized by monoarticular disease of at least four weeks' duration. Involvement of a large joint, particularly the knee, was usual, but occasionally a single metatarsophalangeal joint or a proximal interphalangeal joint of the hand was affected. These patients, as well as those with polyarticular onset, are less likely to have systemic manifestations, but occasionally there may be low grade fever, a typical rash, or lymphadenopathy and splenomegaly. Calabro has stressed that 15 to 20 per cent of patients with JRA may develop uveitis, usually after the onset of arthritis.[33] It is most common in those with monoarticular disease, and these patients, in particular, should be checked periodically by an ophthalmologist, as the onset of uveitis in these children may not be obvious.

Course

Study of this same group of children has also indicated that the subsequent course of their disease can generally be categorized into one of four types.[33] Remission characterizes the monocyclic course, in which there is a single episode without sequelae, and also the polycyclic, in which there are exacerbations lasting weeks or months. The remaining patients follow either a polyarticular course, not unlike adult RA, or an oligoarthritic course, characterized by persistent involvement of less than four joints. Children, irrespective of their type of onset, may follow any of these courses. However, those with an acute onset are most likely to have a polycyclic or polyarticular course, whereas polyarticular disease at the outset is likely to remain polyarticular, although there is occasionally a monocyclic course, and a monoarticular onset is often associated with an oligoarticular course.

The prognosis for JRA patients with respect to functional impairment and survival is quite good. Ansell found absent or minimal evidence of functional impairment in 70 of 90 girls and 52 of 59 boys evaluated 15 years after onset of their disease.[34] It was also noted that only 17 in an original group of 168 had died prior to the 15 year followup evaluation. Systemic infections and amyloidosis were the most frequent causes of death among these patients.

Growth disturbances reflecting joint inflammation and the systemic effects of the disease are not uncommon in JRA patients. Bone development may be retarded or stimulated, and discrepancies in limb length are often found. The cause of the underslung jaw seen in many of these children is not known but may reflect involvement of the mandibular growth centers.

Radiological Findings

The radiological findings in JRA are nonspecific. Soft tissue swelling and juxtaarticular osteoporosis are usual early findings, and periosteal thickening is more common and erosions less common than in adult RA (Fig. 14-38). Martel et al. have stressed the impor-

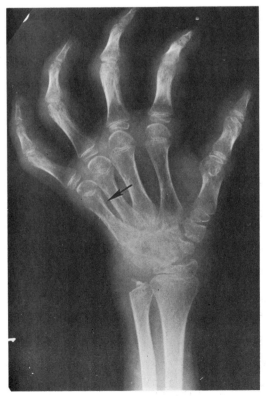

Figure 14–38. Subperiosteal bone apposition in juvenile rheumatoid arthritis (arrow).

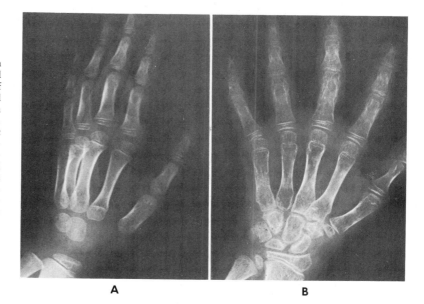

Figure 14–39. Carpal growth retardation in juvenile rheumatoid arthritis (JRA). *A,* Radiograph of six-year-old child shows carpal development consistent with chronological age of two years. *B,* Radiograph of same child at age nine, there is carpal development consistent with the chronological age indicating that normal maturation has ensued. This radiograph, however, shows stigmata of JRA, particularly rectangle-shaped proximal phalanges due to subperiosteal bone apposition.

A   B

tance of evidence of retardation or acceleration of bone development (Fig. 14–39).[35]

Diagnosis

There is no pathognomonic clinical or laboratory criterion indicative of JRA, and the diagnosis must be based upon observation of a compatible clinical picture and exclusion of diseases which may present in a similar manner. The clinical laboratory will afford little help. Rheumatoid factor is present in only a small percentage of JRA patients, probably less than 10 per cent, and it is most commonly found in older children with severe disease. Antinuclear antibody tests may be positive in approximately 10 to 20 per cent of these patients, however, the titer is likely to be low. Synovial fluid is of the Class II or inflammatory type. Patients with an acute or Still's type onset, with fever as the predominant manifestation, are often enigmas, and the gamut of infectious and neoplastic diseases likely in children must be considered. If the acute onset is marked by prominent joint and skin manifestations, the differential diagnosis will encompass systemic lupus erythematosus and various vasculitides, including Henoch-Schonlein purpura and hypersensitivity angiitis. Leukemia will have to be ruled out in those with a high WBC, adenopathy, splenomegaly, and joint pain. Patients with a polyarticular onset will raise such diagnostic considerations as rheumatic fever,

serum sickness and sarcoidosis. Juvenile rheumatoid arthritis at its outset may be particularly difficult to differentiate from rheumatic fever. However, the evolving clinical features of JRA, including remittent fever, evanescent rash and protracted arthritis, contrast with the persistent fever, erythema marginatum, endocarditis and brief migratory arthritis of rheumatic fever and provide the basis for differentiation of these diseases. The antistreptolysin-o titer may be a confusing point in this differentiation if it is not appreciated that elevated titers are not infrequently found in JRA. Those with a polyarticular or monoarticular onset may ultimately prove to have ankylosing spondylitis or the arthritis associated with ulcerative colitis, regional enteritis or psoriasis; however, these diagnoses cannot be established until the basic disease becomes obvious. A monoarticular onset always raises the possibility of septic, tuberculous or fungal arthritis. In these instances, skin testing, appropriate bacteriological studies and, at times, joint biopsy are in order. Villonodular synovitis is a rare cause of monoarticular knee disease in children.

Treatment

The management of JRA patients may be difficult, as it entails treatment of a protracted illness and also dealing with the emotional and financial problems which may stress the families of these patients. Most physicians who have dealt with large groups of these patients have advocated a team approach; the team to be headed by a pediatrician or rheumatologist and to include a physiatrist or orthopedic surgeon, ophthalmologist, physical therapist and social worker. It is clear, however, that patients with mild and limited forms of this disease can be managed successfully by an interested physician, particularly if he has access to appropriate consultants.

Rest integrated with a program of exercises to maintain joint range of motion and muscle strength is a basic part of the treatment program. Splints can be utilized to control pain and prevent or correct deformity. Aspirin therapy is often effective in these patients; it may be initiated at a dosage of 60 mg per pound daily for a few days and then maintained at a level of 40 mg per pound per day. Toxicity is not likely to develop at this maintenance dosage, but small children should be observed for hyperventilation and other signs of salicylism. Patients not responding to aspirin may be treated with gold salts, but corticosteroids are rarely utilized because of their side effects and tendency to retard growth. Antimalarials, indomethacin and phenylbutazone have not been recommended for use in JRA patients. Although these children should be cared for at home so that they may learn to interact with the family, they may require hospitalization for management of severe exacerbations or intensive rehabilitation.

Spondylitis Associated with Juvenile Rheumatoid Arthritis

Cervical spine and sacroiliac disease is common in JRA patients; however, radiographic studies suggest that the cervical spine involvement differs from that found in adult disease. These children, particularly ones with polyarthritis, may develop stiffness and pain on motion of the cervical spine early in the course of their disease, and later there may be severe restriction of motion or ankylosis. Ansell found radiographic evidence of cervical spine involvement in 66 per cent of 147 children with disease of at least 10 years' duration.[36] Studies of Ansell, and Ziff et al. indicate that apophyseal joint changes, particularly fusion, are the most frequent finding; it was also noted that the percentage of fusions at each level increased from caudad to cephalad (Fig. 14–40).[36, 37] Poorly developed cervical vertebrae was the next most common finding and was particularly likely to occur in children who had the onset of their disease while quite young (Fig. 14–41).[35] Posterior subluxations, vertebral body fusions and atlantoaxial subluxations were less commonly encountered. These findings contrast with the frequent atlantoaxial and subaxial anterior subluxations and vertebral body erosions which characterize adult rheumatoid cervical spondylitis.

Radiographic evidence of sacroiliitis is not uncommon in JRA, but it is practically

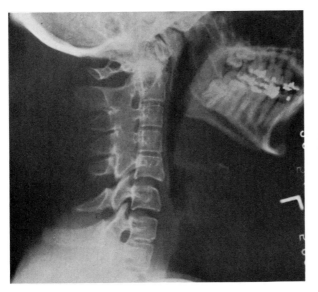

Figure 14–40. Ankylosis of multiple posterior elements of upper cervical spine in spondylitis associated with juvenile rheumatoid arthritis. Note that the bodies and disc spaces of the fused vertebrae are smaller due to underdevelopment.

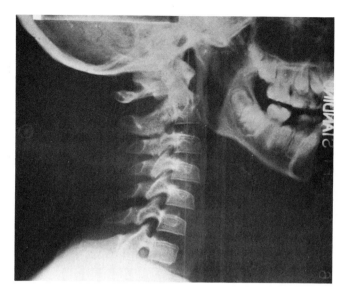

Figure 14–41. Cervical spondylitis in juvenile rheumatoid arthritis marked by poor development of the vertebral bodies.

always asymptomatic. Carter noted changes ranging from marginal irregularity and sclerosis to erosions and finally to ankylosis indicative of probable or definite sacroiliac disease in 23.7 per cent of 202 children with JRA.[38] None of these children had clinical or radiologic findings of ankylosing spondylitis in the lumbar or dorsal spine; however, it is possible that some of them will eventually develop that disease.

The diagnosis of rheumatoid spondylitis in children is based upon recognition of compatible extraspinal joint disease and systemic features in conjunction with the x-ray findings. Early involvement of the cervical spine and absence of changes in the dorsal and lumbar spine are helpful in differentiating this disease from ankylosing spondylitis.

References

Rheumatoid Arthritis

1. Mellors, R. C., Heimer, R., Corcos, J. et al: Cellular origin of rheumatoid factor. J. Exp. Med. *110*:875–886, 1959.
2. Fish, A. J., Michael, A. F., Gewarz, H. and Good, R. A.: Immunopathologic changes in rheumatoid arthritis synovium. Arthritis Rheum. *92*:267–280, 1966.
3. Hollander, J. L., McCarty, D. J., Astorga, G., et al: Studies on the pathogenesis of rheumatoid joint inflammation. Ann. Intern. Med. *62*:271–291, 1965.
4. Vaughan, J. H., Barnett, E. V., Sobel, M. V., and Jacox, R. F.: Intracytoplasmic inclusions of immunoglobulins in rheumatoid arthritis and other diseases. Arthritis Rheum. *11*(2):125–134, 1968.
5. Winchester, R. J., Agnello, V., and Kunkel, H. G.: The joint-fluid γG globulin complexes and their relationship to intra-articular complement diminution. Ann. N.Y. Acad. Sci. *168*:195–203, 1969.
6. Barnett, E. V., Bluestone, R., Cracchiolo, A., et al: Cryoglobulinemia and disease. Ann. Intern. Med. *73*:95–107, 1970.
7. Marcus, R. L., and Townes, A. S.: The occurrence of cryoproteins in synovial fluid; The association of a complement-fixing activity in rheumatoid synovial fluid with cold-precipitable protein. J. Clin. Invest. *50*:282–293, 1971.
8. Ruddy, S. and Austen, K. F.: The complement system in rheumatoid synovitis. I. An analysis of complement component activities in rheumatoid synovial fluids. Arthritis Rheum. *13*:713–723, 1970.
9. Norton, W. L., and Ziff, M.: Electron microscopic observations on the rheumatoid synovial membrane. Arthritis Rheum. *9*:589–610, 1966.
10. Southwick, W. V., and Bensch, K. G.: Phagocytosis of colloidal gold by cells of synovial membrane. J. Bone Joint Surg. *53A*:729–741, 1971.
11. Schumacher, H. R.: The microvasculature of the synovial membrane of the monkey. Arthritis Rheum. *12*:387–404, 1969.
12. Suter, E. J., and Majno, G.: Ultrastructure of the joint capsule in the rat: presence of two kinds of capillaries. Nature (London) *202*:920–921, 1964.
13. Ropes, M. W., et al.: 1958 revision of diagnostic criteria for rheumatoid arthritis. Bull. Rheum. Dis. *9*:175–176, 1958.
14. Messner, R. P., Laxdal, T., Quie, P. G., and Williams, R. C.: Rheumatoid factors in subacute bacterial endocarditis — bacterium, duration of disease or genetic predisposition? Ann. Intern. Med. *68*:746–756, 1968.

15. Cohen, A. S., and Comerford, F. R.: Laboratory studies in the diagnosis of rheumatoid arthritis. Med. Clin. N. Amer. 52:539–548, 1968.
16. Hollander, J. L., McCarty, D. J., and Rawson, A. J.: The "R. A. cell," "ragocyte" or "inclusion body cell." Bull. Rheum. Dis. 16:382–383, 1965.

Rheumatoid Spondylitis

17. Fremont-Smith, K.: Metabolism pharmacology and toxicology of salicylates. In Proceedings of the Conference on Effects of Chronic Salicylate Administration, edited by Lamont-Havers, R. W. and Wagner, B. M. U.S. Dept. Health, Education & Welfare, 1966.
18. Menguy, R.: Gastric mucosa injury by aspirin. Gastroenterology, 51:30–31, 1966.
19. Conlon, P. W., Isdale, I. C., and Rose, B. S.: Rheumatoid arthritis of the cervical spine. Ann. Rheum. Dis. 25:120–126, 1966.
20. Mathews, J. A.: Atlanto-axial subluxation in rheumatoid arthritis. Ann. Rheum. Dis. 28:260–265, 1969.
21. Meikle, J. A. K., and Wilkinson, M.: Rheumatoid involvement of the cervical spine. Ann. Rheum. Dis. 30:154–161, 1971.
22. Martel, W., and Duff, I. F.: Pelvo-spondylitis in rheumatoid arthritis. Radiology 77:744–756, 1961.
23. Boyle, A. C.: The rheumatoid neck. Proc. Roy. Soc. Med. 64:1161–1165, 1971.
24. Sharp, J., and Purser, D. W.: Spontaneous atlanto-axial dislocation in ankylosing spondylitis and rheumatoid arthritis. Ann. Rheum. Dis. 20:47–77, 1961.
25. Stevens, J. C., Cartlidge, N. E. F., Saunders, M., Appleby, A., Hall, M., and Shaw, D. A.: Atlanto-axial subluxation and cervical myelopathy in rheumatoid arthritis. Quart. J. Med. 40:391–408, 1971.
26. Ball, J.: Enthesopathy of rheumatoid and ankylosing spondylitis. Ann. Rheum. Dis. 30:213–222, 1971.
27. Sharp, J., Purser, D. W., and Lawrence, J. S.: Ann. Rheum. Dis. 17:303–313, 1958.
28. Baggenstoss, A. H., Bickel, W. H., and Ward, L. E.: Rheumatoid granulomatous nodules as destructive lesions of vertebrae. J. Bone Joint Surg., 43A:601, 1952.
29. Lorber, A., Pearson, C. M., and Rene, R. M.: Osteolytic vertebral lesions as a manifestation of rheumatoid arthritis and related disorders. Arthritis Rheum. 4:514–532, 1961.
30. Lawrence, J. S., and Sharp, J.: Lumbar spine. In Radiological Aspects of Rheumatoid Arthritis. Carter, M. E. (ed.), Amsterdam, Excerpta Medica Foundation, 1963, pp. 239–250.
31. Dilsen, N., McEwen, C., Poppel, M., Gersh, W. J., DiTata, D., and Carmel, P.: A comparative roentgenologic study of rheumatoid arthritis and rheumatoid (ankylosing) spondylitis. Arthritis Rheum. 5:341–368, 1962.
32. Ansell, B. M., Bywaters, E. G. L., and Lawrence, J. S.: A family study in Still's disease. Ann. Rheum. Dis. 21:243–252, 1962.
33. Calabro, J. J., and Marcheasano, J. M.: The early natural history of juvenile rheumatoid arthritis. Med. Clin. N. Amer. 52:567–591, 1968.
34. Ansell, B. M.: Still's disease followed into adult life. Proc. Roy. Soc. Med. 62:912–913, 1969.
35. Martel, W., Holt, J. F., and Cassidy, J. T.: The roentgenologic manifestations of juvenile rheumatoid arthritis. Amer. J. Roentgenol. 88:400–423, 1962.
36. Ansell, B. M.: The cervical spine in juvenile rheumatoid in post-pubertal patients with rheumatoid arthritis of juvenile onset. Ann. Rheum. Dis. 15:40–45, 1956.
37. Ziff, M., Contreras, V., and McEwan, C.: Spondylitis toid arthritis. In Radiological Aspects of Rheumatoid Arthritis. Carter, M. E. (ed.) Amsterdam, Excerpta Medica Foundation, 1963, pp. 233–234.
38. Carter, M. E.: Sacro-iliitis in Still's disease. Ann. Rheum. Dis. 25:105–120, 1962.

GOUT

Hyperuricemia and precipitation of urates in the tissues or urine are the background of the various clinical manifestations of gout, including acute and chronic arthritis, tophi, renal stones and nephropathy. Patients having an underlying disease or some other discernible factor which accounts for their hyperuricemia are classified as having secondary gout. Rapid cellular turnover in various myeloproliferative disorders, certain drugs, particularly thiazide diuretics, and long-term renal dialysis are likely to be the background of secondary gout encountered in general clinical practice. In the majority of gouty patients the cause of hyperuricemia is inapparent, and these individuals are classified as having primary gout. There is now evidence, however, that patients with primary gout are really a heterogeneous group with diverse mechanisms of overproduction and underexcretion of uric acid to account for their hyperuricemia. For example, a deficiency of the enzyme hypoxanthine-guanine phosphoribosyltransferase (HG-PRT) serves as a marker to identify a subgroup of patients among those with primary gout.[1,2] The enzyme HG-PRT apparently facilitates the reutilization of the purine bases guanine and hypoxanthine during the course of nucleic acid synthesis. This enzyme also appears to limit uric acid production; however, the mechanism of this activity is unknown. One possibility is that the enzyme facilitates the formation of the nucleotides of guanine and hypoxanthine, which in turn inhibit the early stages of purine production. It has also been proposed that the activity of this enzyme pre-empts 5-phosphoribosylpyrophosphate for nucleotide regeneration, thus limiting the availability of this material as a substrate during the early phases of the metabolic pathway leading to uric acid formation.[3] There is an almost complete deficiency of HG-PRT in children with the Lesch-Nyhan syndrome, who characteristically show severe hyperuricemia, mental deficiency, spasticity, choreoathetosis and a tendency for self-mutilation.[4] A less complete deficiency of this enzyme has also been described in 21 adult men with severe gout, thus delineating these individuals from the overall group of primary gout. Characteristically, in Greene's study of patients with a partial deficiency of HG-PRT there was severe articular and renal gout with onset in early adulthood (average age 20 years); however, mental deficiency, seizures or evidence of spinocerebellar disease was also noted in those with more marked partial deficiency of HG-PRT.[5] The findings in these patients also suggest that HG-PRT deficiency is associated with mental and neurological aberrations, but pathogenetic mechanisms interrelating this enzyme deficiency and central nervous system abnormality have not been elucidated.

Although there is evidence of familial predisposition to primary gout, determination of its mode of inheritance will apparently have to await delineation of the various entities which make up this disorder. The partial HG-PRT deficiency elucidated by Greene appears to be present in less than 2 per cent of primary gout patients. Studies of pedigree of patients with the Lesch-Nyhan syndrome indicate that it is an x-linked recessive defect.[6]

The various pathologic lesions of gout all appear to be secondary to deposition of urates in the tissues, and although additional aspects of the pathogenesis of these lesions have been elucidated, there are also many aspects which remain to be clarified. Tophi are foreign body granulomas, varying from a few mm to a few cm in diameter which form about a nidus of urate crystals. Tophus formation appears to have a direct relationship to the level and duration of hyperuricemia, although there are exceptions to this rule. It is not clear why tophi develop preferentially in articular bone, periarticular structures or subcutaneous tissues. Although articular cartilage is resistant to tophus formation, it may be extensively damaged in chronic gouty arthritis. Encrustations of uric acid on the cartilage surface, tophi in subchondral bone and pannus are likely to account for the cartilage destruction in chronic gouty involvement of the joints.

McCarty, Seegmiller and Howell, Weissman, and Nies and Melmon have cited a variety of pathogenetic mechanisms that may be involved in acute gouty synovitis.[7-10] Basic to all concepts of the genesis of acute gouty synovitis, however, is the presence of urate crystals in the synovium or the joint space. This local accumulation of urates may reflect crystallization from interstitial or synovial fluid, or dissolution of tophi or cartilage encrustations. Many of these crystals are noted to be within polymorphonuclear leukocytes and, although it is likely that this occurs as a result of phagocytosis, intracellular crystallization may be an alternative mechanism.[11, 12] Acute synovitis appears to develop when these crystal-containing leukocytes break down, releasing phlogistic factors. Support for this concept is found in studies which show that the acute synovitis which follows intraarticular injection of urates into normal dogs will not develop in dogs depleted of leukocytes.[13] Other researchers have proposed that urate crystals are phlogistic as a result of activating either the kinin system or the complement system in synovial fluid.[14, 15] However, a role for kinins seems unlikely, as Spilberg has shown urate crystal arthritis can be induced in chickens which lack the kinin activator or lack Hageman factor.[15a]

It has also been proposed that acute gouty synovitis is perpetuated as a result of the metabolic activity of the accumulated leukocytes, which lower the local pH and thus facilitate further urate crystallization.[8]

There are some attractive theories as to the circumstances which predispose to an acute episode of gouty arthritis, but much remains to be elucidated. It is possible that acute gout following unusual physical activity is due to breakdown of articular tophi and encrustations of crystals of urate, with their liberation into the joint space. However, strenuous activity does not precede all or even most episodes of acute gout. Acute gout that develops after severe carbohydrate restriction related to alcoholic debauches or stringent dieting may reflect the lactic acidemia which develops in this setting. The renal tubules excrete lactic acid in preference to uric acid, and the retention of uric acid consequent to increased production and excretion of lactic acid may precipitate the acute arthritis.

Peripheral Joints

Although the classical episode of gout marked by the abrupt onset of pain and swelling of the metatarsophalangeal (MTP) joint of the great toe is usually recognized by both patient and physician, other manifestations of gouty arthritis are less obvious. In approximately 50 per cent of patients the initial episode affects one or perhaps two or three joints other than the first MTP; the tarsals, ankle,

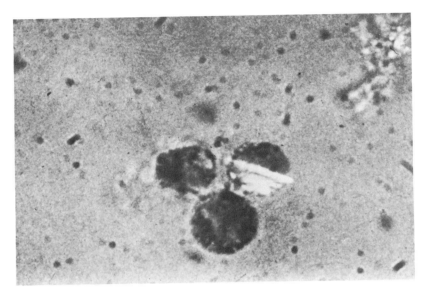

Figure 14–42. Urate crystals in synovial fluid from patient with acute gouty arthritis. Note that the crystals are within a leukocyte: also, the crystals have rounded ends whereas crystals from a tophus have pointed ends. These crystals may be identified by their negative birefringence (yellow color, when parallel to the orienting line of the red plate compensator) when examined by the technique of compensated polarized light microscopy.

knee, wrist and elbow are the usual alternative sites. Onset or exacerbation of gout is less frequently marked by acute generalized polyarthritis and, rarely, at the outset there is an insidious mild polyarthritis or polyarthralgia, and in these instances the diagnosis is likely to be missed. The diagnosis of gouty arthritis may be unequivocally established only by identifying urate crystals in the synovial fluid or joint tissues (Fig. 14–42). Urate crystals cannot be distinguished from calcium pyrophosphate crystals by light microscopy; however, use of a microscope adapted with a red compensator and polarizing lenses permits identification of these crystals on the basis of their optical properties (Figs. 14–43 and 14–44). In many instances, but particularly when the first MTP joint is affected, synovial fluid is not available and other tentatively diagnostic criteria must be utilized. The serum uric acid

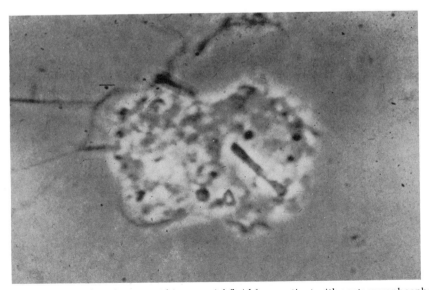

Figure 14–43. Calcium pyrophosphate crystal in synovial fluid from patient with acute pyrophosphate arthropathy. Note that the crystal is within a leukocyte. It is of the needle-shaped or monoclinic type. These crystals may be identified by their positive birefringence (blue color, when parallel to the orienting line of the red plate compensator) when examined by the technique of compensated polarized light microscopy.

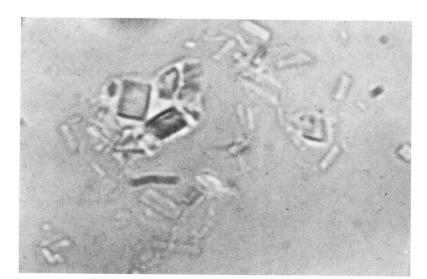

Figure 14–44. Calcium pyrophosphate crystals of the triclinic type in synovial fluid.

is almost always elevated in these patients but this finding does not establish a diagnosis of gout in an individual with joint pain or arthritis. An elevated uric acid may be found in an occasional rheumatoid patient and also in some patients with psoriatic arthritis (see page 749). Diminution of pain in response to colchicine, 1 mg every two hours, until nausea or diarrhea develops or a maximum of 12 mg of the drug has been taken, is suggestive evidence of gout. However, some gouty attacks may not respond to this therapy, particularly in instances when treatment is instituted 24 hours or more after onset of joint pain. Clinical or radiographic evidence of tophi is rarely present at the time of the first acute episode of arthritis. Sharply delimited erosions or punched out areas in the subchondral cortex are suggestive of gout, but these findings are not likely to be present at the outset and they are often difficult to differentiate from the erosions found in RA and the subchondral cysts of osteoarthritis (Fig. 14–45). Although a diagnosis of gout may be based on the clinical findings, the serum uric acid level, response to colchicine, and rarely the radiographic findings, it is always tentative until urate crystals are identified in synovial fluid or tissue.

Chronic gouty arthritis may closely resemble RA or even osteoarthritis (Fig. 14–45). A history of repeated episodes of acute arthritis, although not a constant feature, ele-

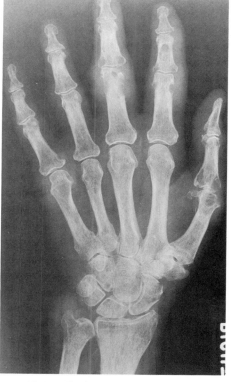

Figure 14–45. Tophaceous gout in the hand. Erosive defects are particularly prominent at the metacarpophalangeal joint and interphalangeal joint of the thumb and at the proximal and middle phalanges of the second and third fingers. These erosions are similar to those in rheumatoid arthritis and osteoarthritis; however, they may be further removed from the joint.

vation of the serum uric acid, and consistent radiographic findings suggest the proper diagnosis. Again, definitive diagnosis depends upon identification of urate crystals in synovial fluid or tissues. If a joint or tophus is biopsied for this purpose, the tissue must be processed in non-aqueous fixatives to preserve the soluble crystals.

Spine

The prevalence of gout of the spine and sacroiliac joints is unknown, reflecting the absence of clearly pathognomonic findings that would distinguish such involvement from other diseases. It is clear that gout does involve these areas; postmortem studies have disclosed urate deposits in the intervertebral discs and vertebrae, and also in the joint space and juxtaarticular bone of the sacroiliac joints.[16] Paraspinal and intraspinal deposits of urates have also been described. One such massive deposit has been noted to disrupt the atlantoaxial articulation and another to compress the spinal cord in the lower dorsal area with resultant paraplegia.[17, 18]

Acute gout involving the spine or sacroiliac joints has rarely been described. A meticulous evaluation of the type described by Malawista et al. may delineate such an episode.[19] In this instance, a 72-year-old woman with tophaceous gout developed severe episodes of pain localized to the area of the left sacroiliac joint, and several examiners noted an area of discrete tenderness at the upper portion of the involved joint. During a two month period, this patient sustained seven such episodes and on each occasion she responded promptly to intravenous colchicine, whereas analgesic compounds did not afford any relief. It would seem likely that acute gout would also localize to the apophyseal joints and neurocentral (Luschka's) joints of the spine, but this is very difficult to prove. A history or findings indicative of acute or chronic gouty arthritis of the limb joints, tophi, hyperuricemia, or response to colchicine would all suggest that acute back pain might be due to gout. There is, however, no combination of these criteria which can be considered pathognomonic of acute gout of the spine or sacroiliac joints and, in final analysis, such a diagnosis must be a clinical judgment based on judicious and meticulous evaluation of the patient's history and findings. It may be emphasized that acute gout does not always respond to colchicine and there is always the possibil-

ity of a spontaneous remission of acute back pain of any etiology in association with colchicine therapy.

The diagnosis of chronic gout of the spine or sacroiliac joints, as in the instance of its acute counterpart, must be based on clinical judgment. Hyperuricemia would be a prerequisite, and tophi in the limb joints, subcutaneous tissues or ears would almost certainly be detectable by clinical examination or on x-rays, as it would be unlikely for a patient to have urate deposits in the spine while sparing all of these structures. The symptoms, clinical findings and radiological findings would be non-specific and likely to resemble spondylosis. However, Malawista et al., in a review of x-rays of patients with limb joint gout, have found sclerosis-rimmed cystic lesions in the juxtaarticular area of the sacroiliac joints which they consider to be characteristic of gout.[17] These findings were noted in seven of 95 patients. The usefulness of colchicine as a diagnostic test in these patients is not clear, for their pain may reflect spinal pathomechanics and traumatic synovitis rather than crystal-induced synovitis.

Any patient who is reasonably suspect for chronic gout of the spine or sacroiliac joints should be treated with uricosuric agents or allopurinol. Treatment of this type could be expected to prevent progression of the spinal involvement or even result in its amelioration.

Treatment

Acute attacks of gouty arthritis will generally respond to short courses of colchicine, phenylbutazone or indomethacin. Colchicine, as has been noted, has some specificity in this disease, but this is no longer an advantage once the diagnosis has been established. Disadvantages of colchicine include frequent ineffectiveness when the acute attack has persisted for 24 hours and the nausea and diarrhea associated with its use, unless the dosage at which gastrointestinal toxicity develops has been established by prior trial. Patients unable to take oral medication, as in the immediate postoperative period, may be treated with a preparation of colchicine developed for intravenous administration (Lilly). The initial dose is usually 2 mg with subsequent injections of 0.5 mg at six-hour intervals as required. The maximum dosage over 24 hours should be less than 4 mg, and injections must be made with caution, as colchicine is very irritating when extruded into the tissues. In most instances acute attacks of gout will respond to phenylbutazone, 200 mg TID for one day and then gradual reduction of dosage and withdrawal over a period of a week. Similarly, indomethacin 50 mg QID for one day, followed by gradual reduction of dosage and withdrawal during the period of a week will often serve to control an acute attack. Details concerning toxic effects and precautions to be taken during treatment should be reviewed before instituting treatment with phenylbutazone or indomethacin (see page 744). Rarely, a patient will not respond to any of these agents, and in such instances three intramuscular injections of 40 units of ACTH, spaced at 8 to 12 hour intervals, will usually be effective. Before withdrawing any of the agents utilized to control the acute attack, it is necessary to institute treatment with small doses of colchicine (0.5 to 1.5 mg daily) to prevent rebound attacks.

The long-term management of hyperuricemia and gout, particularly the indications for uricosuric agents or allopurinol, is beyond the scope of this presentation, and text books of medicine and appropriate articles should be consulted.

References

1. Seegmiller, J. E., Rosenbloom, F. M., and Kelley, W. N.: Enzyme defect associated with a sex-linked human neurological disorder and excessive purine synthesis. Science 155:1682–1684, 1967.
2. Kelley, W. N., Greene, M. L., Rosenbloom, F. M., et al.: Hypoxanthine-guanine phospho-ribosyl-transferase deficiency in gout. Ann. Intern. Med. 70:155–206, 1969.
3. Seegmiller, J. E.: Gout: a biochemical perspective. In Gout A Clinical Comprehensive. Gutman, A. B. (ed.), Medcom. 1971, pp. 26–35.
4. Nyhan, W. L.: Clinical features of the Lesch-Nyhan syndrome. Arch. Intern. Med. 130:186–192, 1972.
5. Greene, M. L.: Clinical features of patients with the "partial" deficiency of the x-linked uricaciduria enzyme. Arch. Intern. Med. 130:193–198, 1972.
6. Nyhan, W. L., Pesek, J., Sweetman, L., et al.: Genetics of an x-linked disorder of uric metabolism and cerebral function. Pediatric Res. 1:5–13, 1967.
7. McCarty, D. J.: The pendulum of progress in gout: from crystals to hyperuricemia and back. Arthritis Rheum. 7:534–541, 1964.
8. Seegmiller, J. E., and Howell, R. R.: The old and new concepts of acute gouty arthritis. Arthritis Rheum. 5:616–623, 1962.
9. Weissman, G.: Molecular basis of acute gout. Hosp. Pract. 6:43–52, 1971.
10. Nies, A. S., and Melmon, K. L.: Kinins and arthritis. Bull. Rheum. Dis. 19:512–517, 1968.
11. McCarty, D. J.: Phagocytosis of urate crystals in gouty synovial fluid. Am. J. Med. Sci. 243:288–295, 1962.
12. Riddle, J. M., Bluhm, G. B., and Barnhart, M. D.: Ultrastructural study of leukocytes and urates in gouty arthritis. Ann. Rheum. Dis. 26:389, 1967.
13. Phelps, P., and McCarty, D. J.: Crystal induced inflammation in canine joints. Part 2, Importance of polymorphonuclear leucocytes. J. Exp. Med. 124:115–125, 1969.
14. Kellermeyer, R. W., and Breckenridge, R. T.: The inflammatory process in acute gouty arthritis: 1 Activation of Hageman factor by sodium urate crystals. J. Lab. Clin. Med. 65:307–315, 1965.
15. Naff, G. B., and Byers, P. H.: Possible implication of complement in acute gout. J. Clin. Invest. 46:1099–1100, 1967 (abstract).
15a. Spilberg, I.: Urate crystal arthritis in animals lacking Hageman Factor. Arthritis Rheum. 17:143–148, 1974.
16. Lichtenstein, L., Scott, H. W., and Leuin, M. H.: Pathologic changes in gout: Survey of 11 necropsied cases. Amer. J. Path. 32:871–896, 1956.
17. Kersley, G. D., Mandel, L., and Jeffrey, M. R.: Gout, an unusual case with softening and subluxation of the first cervical vertebra and splenomegaly. Ann. Rheum. Dis. 9:282–303, 1950.
18. Hall, M. C., and Selin, G.: Spinal involvement in gout. J. Bone Joint Surg. 42A:341–343, 1960.
19. Malawista, S. E., Seegmiller, J. E., Hathaway, B. E., and Sokoloff, L.: J.A.M.A. 194:106–108, 1965.

PYROPHOSPHATE ARTHROPATHY

Introduction

McCarty and Hollander, in 1961, identified calcium pyrophosphate crystals in synovial fluid of patients having attacks of arthritis reminiscent of gout and suggested that this was another example of crystal-induced synovitis which might be appropriately designated as pseudogout.[1] It was soon recognized that pseudogout was similar to the clinical and radiological entity chondrocalcinosis polyarticularis familiaris, described by Zitnan and Sitàj in Czechoslovakia.[2] However, these workers had not detected calcium pyrophosphate crystals in synovial fluid from their patients. Continued study of these patients has indicated that there are two significant clinical phases of this entity: 1) acute episodes of synovitis induced by calcium pyrophosphate crystals and 2) a chronic degenerative arthropathy associated with deposition of these crystals in joint cartilage. The pathogenesis of the acute attacks is in all likelihood quite similar to that of acute gout (see page 774). The mechanism of joint degeneration in this disease is unknown; it has been suggested by some that it is secondary to deposition of calcium pyrophosphate crystals in joint cartilage; but it is also possible that cartilage degeneration is a prerequisite for crystal deposition.[3] In a minority of patients with this entity an associated disease such as hyperparathyroidism, hemochromatosis or gout may be noted; however, these relationships have not been helpful in elucidating the mechanism of pyrophosphate deposition in these patients. This disease does not appear to be inherited, at least on the basis of patients studied in the United States. Zitnan and Sitàj did, however, note a strong familial predisposition in their series from Czechoslovakia.[2] This series included some young patients, whereas generally this disease has been noted in middle-aged or old patients.

There is no general agreement as to the nomenclature of the disease, but the terms acute and chronic pyrophosphate arthropathy seem appropriate, as they indicate both the major manifestations and the chemical composition of the crystalline material which is so important in the pathogenesis of this disease.[4]

The clinical manifestations of acute and chronic pyrophosphate arthropathy are not specific, and diagnosis is based on synovial fluid and radiological findings. The acute arthritis tends to involve one to a few large joints, with a particular propensity for the knees; the first MTP joints, so frequently involved in gout, are generally spared. These acute episodes reach their maximum intensity within 36 hours and generally recede over a period of ten days; longer episodes may reflect superimposition of acute attacks.[3] The manifestations of chronic pyrophosphate arthropathy include swelling, stiffness, aching pain and crepitus on passive motion of the joint, and are indistinguishable from those of osteoarthritis. In many instances, however, patients with the chronic form of this disease have previously sustained attacks of acute pyrophosphate arthropathy.[4] Rarely, this disease may be expressed as a subacute arthritis reminiscent of rheumatoid arthritis.[5]

The diagnosis of acute pyrophosphate arthropathy is dependent upon identification of the characteristic crystals in the synovial fluid. Under light microscopy these crystals appear to be quite similar to urates; however, with compensated polarized light microscopy they exhibit weakly positive birefringence and may thus be distinguished from the negatively birefringent urate crystals (see Figs. 14–42 to 14–44). The remaining synovial fluid findings are non-specific but are of the Class II (inflammatory) type. The majority of patients experiencing attacks of acute pyrophosphate arthropathy will have radiologic evidence of chondrocalcinosis; however, this finding must be interpreted carefully, as chondrocalcinosis

may also occur in association with rheumatoid and gouty arthritis.[6] Radiologic findings indicative of chondrocalcinosis are quite specific and consist of linear punctate or nodular densities localized to cartilage, intraarticular fibrocartilage and capsules of diarthrodial joints and also to the fibrocartilaginous joints (synchondroses). The menisci of the knee and the trapezoid cartilage of the wrist deserve special mention, for they are frequently the site of these opacities. (Figs. 14–46 and 14–47). Chondrocalcinosis may usually be defined by a screening radiographic study which includes an AP view of the pelvis for involvement of the symphysis pubis and lumbar discs and AP views of the knees and wrists.[7, 8]

The diagnosis of chronic pyrophosphate arthropathy is based on clinical findings suggestive of osteoarthritis and radiologic evidence of chondrocalcinosis. In very advanced cases, however, the radiological findings may be obscured by extensive erosion of cartilage. The synovial fluid in chronic pyrophosphate

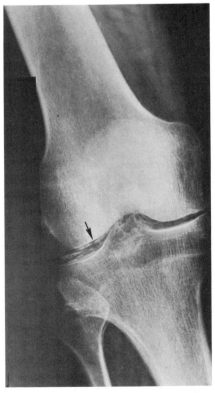

Figure 14–46. Chondrocalcinosis of the knee marked by punctate densities of the menisci and articular cartilage (arrows). Cartilage space narrowing and osteophytes are also present.

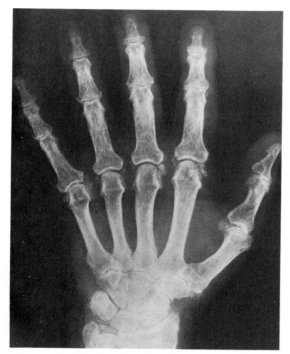

Figure 14–47. Nodular densities in the trapezoid cartilage, first carpometacarpal joint and metacarpophalangeal joints in chondrocalcinosis.

arthropathy is of the Class I (non-inflammatory) type, and only a few pyrophosphate crystals, which are generally extracellular, may be noted. Identification of these crystals is not a prerequisite for the diagnosis of chronic pyrophosphate arthropathy. Patients manifesting acute or chronic pyrophosphate arthropathy or asymptomatic chondrocalcinosis should have appropriate screening tests for hyperparathyroidism, gout and hemochromatosis, as deposition of calcium pyrophosphate in the joints may occur in these diseases.

Acute pyrophosphate arthropathy can generally be controlled by intraarticular injection of hydrocortisone or one of its analogues; however, if such treatment is not practical because of involvement of numerous joints or unfamiliarity with the injection techniques a short course of indomethacin or phenylbutazone may be tried. Phenylbutazone, 100 mg TID or QID, or indomethacin, 25 to 50 mg TID for a period of one week will often be helpful (see precautions outlined on page 744).

The management of chronic pyrophosphate arthropathy is similar to that for osteoarthritis.

The Spine

It is reasonable to suspect that attacks of acute pyrophosphate arthropathy may localize to the synovial tissue-lined joints of the spine, but there are no diagnostic criteria for such episodes. We are not aware of radiological or pathological findings indicative of chondrocalcinosis of the apophyseal or neurocentral (Luschka's) joints which would support the possibility of acute attacks in these areas. However, the absence of such findings may indicate an inability to detect chondrocalcinosis at these sites utilizing standard radiological techniques and a lack of pertinent pathological investigations rather than the absence of pyrophosphate deposition. A likely suspect for acute pyrophosphate arthropathy would be an individual who had repeated episodes of spinal pain and a background of acute attacks in the peripheral joints, or radiological evidence of chondrocalcinosis.

A diagnosis of chronic pyrophosphate arthropathy of the spine is probably indicated in patients with symptoms and signs of spondylosis and chondrocalcinosis of the intervertebral discs (Fig. 14–48). It is apparent, however, that chondrocalcinosis of the spine is not necessarily symptomatic. A clinical and pathologic study of the spines of six patients with idiopathic hemochromatosis, none of whom were known to have had back pain or

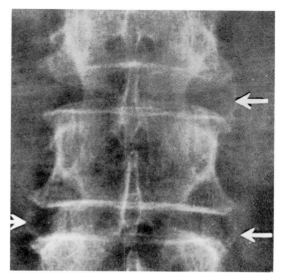

Figure 14–48. Chondrocalcinosis of the spine manifested by densities in the annulus fibrosus (arrows). (From McCarty, D. J., and Haskin, M. E.: Am. J. Roentgenol. Radium Ther. Nuclear Med. *90*:1255, 1963.)

stiffness revealed chondrocalcinosis and associated disc degeneration in four and chondrocalcinosis alone in one.[9] Conversely, progressive stiffness of the spine was a prominent finding among the Czech patients showing a familial predisposition to chondrocalcinosis.[10] Calcification of the lumbar and cervical discs apparent by the third decade was also frequently noted in this group of patients.

References

1. McCarty, D. J., and Hollander, J. L.: Identification of urate crystals in gouty synovial fluid. Ann. Int. Med., 54:452–460, 1961.
2. Zitnan, D., and Sitaj, S.: Chondrocalcinosis articularis Section I. Clinical and radiological study. Ann. Rheum. Dis. 22:142–152, 1963.
3. McCarty, D. J.: Pseudogout, articular chondrocalcinosis, calcium pyrophosphate crystal deposition disease. In Arthritis and Allied Diseases. 7th edition, Hollander, J. H. L. (ed.), Philadelphia, Lea and Febiger, 1966, pp. 947–964.
4. Currey, H. L. F.: Pyrophosphate arthropathy and calcific periarthritis. Clin. Orthop. 71:70–80, 1970.
5. Currey, H. L. F., Key, J. J., Mason, R. M., and Swettenham: Significance of radiological calcification of joint cartilage. Ann. Rheum. Dis. 25:295–306, 1966.
6. Good, A. E., and Rapp, R.: Chondrocalcinosis of the knee with gout and rheumatoid arthritis. New Engl. J. Med. 277:286–290, 1967.
7. McCarty, D. J., and Haskin, M. E.: The roentgenographic aspects of pseudo gout (articular chondrocalcinosis); an analysis of 20 cases. Am. J. Roentgenol. 90:1248–1257, 1963.
8. McCarty, D. J.: Pseudo gout syndrome. Bull. Rheum. Dis. 14:331–334, 1964.
9. Bywaters, E. G. L., Hamilton, E. B. D., and Williams, R.: The spine in idiopathic haemochromatosis. Ann. Rheum. Dis. 30:453–465, 1971.
10. Zitnan, D., and Sitaj, S., quoted by Bywaters, E. G. L., Hamilton, E. B. D., and Williams, R.: The spine in idiopathic haemochromatosis. Ann. Rheum. Dis. 30:453–465, 1971.

LIPOID DERMATOARTHRITIS

Lipoid dermatoarthritis (LDA), or reticulohistiocytoma of the skin and joints, is a destructive arthritis which may involve the peripheral and spinal joints; in all likelihood it reflects a defect in lipid metabolism. The skin lesions and synovial membrane in this disorder are characterized by infiltration of histiocytes and lipid-laden, multinucleated giant cells. Joint destruction presumably reflects invasive and destructive properties of the involved synovium, but this must be clarified by further study. A characteristic serum lipid pattern for these patients has not been defined, although some patients have shown elevations of cholesterol or other lipids or abnormal lipoprotein electrophoresis patterns. Lipoid dermatoarthritis is a rare disease which is likely to develop in patients over 40 years of age; it occurs most frequently in women.

The peripheral arthritis of LDA is polyarticular, involves large and small joints and is likely to be attributed to RA. The destructive nature of the joint disease may be manifested in the hands as "la main en lorgnette" or opera glass deformity, in which the fingers may be distracted and shortened in a manner reminiscent of a telescope. Cutaneous papules or nodules varying in size from 2 mm to 2 cm or xanthelasma are suggestive of this disease, but these findings develop subsequent to the arthritis in two thirds of the patients. In the absence of skin findings, this disease is likely to be attributed to rheumatoid arthritis, but the absence of rheumatoid factor and serum lipid abnormalities are helpful differential points. Ultimately, the diagnosis of lipoid dermatoarthritis must be based on synovial biopsy.

Lipoid dermatoarthritis may involve the spine. Obliteration of the sacroiliac joints and erosions of the apophyseal joints have been noted.[2,3] Also, Martel et al. have described a 47-year-old woman with destruction of the atlas and the odontoid process and body of the second cervical vertebra in association with this disease.[4] These spinal findings may also be noted in ankylosing spondylitis and rheumatoid arthritis; however, the absence of syndesmophytes will help to delineate this disorder from ankylosing spondylitis, and the factors considered in relation to the peripheral joint involvement will aid in distinguishing it from rheumatoid spondylitis.

Although there is no known treatment for lipoid dermatoarthritis, non-weight-bearing exercise and limitation of activity will aid in preserving the joints in this disease.

References

1. Albert, J., Bruce, W., Allen, A. C., and Blank, H.: Lipoid dermato-arthritis. Am. J. Med. 28:661–667, 1960.
2. Johnson, H. M., and Tilden, I. L.: Reticulohistiocytic granulomas of the skin associated with arthritis mutilans. Arch. Dermat. 75:405–417, 1957.
3. Schwartz, E., and Fish, A.: Reticulohistiocytoma: A rare dermatologic disease with roentgen manifestations. Am. J. Roentgenol. 83:692–697, 1960.
4. Martel, W., Abell, M. R., and Duff, I. F.: Cervical spine involvement in lipoid dermato-arthritis. Radiology 77:613–617, 1961.

NEUROPATHIC ARTHROPATHY

Neuropathic arthropathy (Charcot joints) may be regarded as a form of osteoarthritis which develops as a result of impairment of pain or proprioceptive sensation to the joint. It is likely that the joints are traumatized and ultimately destroyed as the result of loss of sensorimotor reflexes which protect the joint from unusual arcs of motion and other abnormal stresses. Tabes dorsalis (neurosyphilis), diabetes, syringomyelia, paraplegia, peripheral neuropathy, congenital insensitivity to pain, and intraarticular corticosteroid therapy are the etiologic factors most frequently associated with neuropathic arthropathy.

The pathology is that of osteoarthritis; however, in advanced disease there may be marked dissolution of the joint, featuring intraarticular fractures, numerous loose bodies, and synovial implants of an osseous or cartilaginous nature.

In patients with neuropathic joint disease, the symptoms, but not the clinical findings, are likely to be camouflaged by the neurological impairment. Pain or instability of the joint is the usual presenting complaint; however, the pain is apt to be mild or moderate and inconsistent with the physical findings. It is likely that this pain arises in periarticular structures which are distorted or stressed as a result of the joint disease. Deformity, effusion, instability, hypermobility and severe crepitus are usual findings, and the range of motion, although abnormal, may be pain free or only minimally painful. The locale of the joint involvement will usually reflect the underlying disorder: the large weight-bearing joints, including the lumbar spine in tabes dorsalis, the foot and ankle in diabetic neuropathy and the wrist in syringomyelia. Diffuse polyarthritis has rarely been reported in association with diabetes or tabes dorsalis.[1, 2] The joint fluid is of the Class I non-inflammatory type; however, at times the fluid may be sanguineous.

The x-ray findings are those of severe osteoarthritis; intraarticular fractures, loose bodies and massive osteophytes are particularly suggestive of neuropathic disease (Fig. 14–49). In the knee, joint crumbling and buckling of a tibial plateau is a clue to this disorder.

Advanced neuropathic joint disease is usually easily recognized on the basis of the clinical and radiographic findings. This diagnosis may be difficult, however, in patients who come to the physician's attention before the characteristic clinical and radiographic findings have evolved and, particularly, if the neurological disease is not apparent. In such patients the diagnosis can be clarified only by careful neurological and rheumatological evaluation.

Spine

Neuropathic arthropathy (Charcot joints) of the spine is likely to be limited to the lumbar

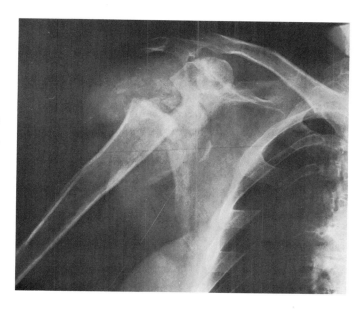

Figure 14–49. Neuropathic arthritis of the shoulder in a patient with syringomyelia. There is disintegration and fragmentation of the humeral head, intra-articular debris and a separation of the acromioclavicular joint. The amputated appearance of the upper end of the humerus is characteristic.

segment and is almost always a sequela of tabes dorsalis; it occurs in approximately 10 to 15 per cent of patients with tabetic arthropathy of peripheral joints, but may also be the only site of involvement.[3] Weakness of the lower extremities and deformity of the spine are early manifestations, but pain localized to the low back, buttocks, and lower extremities is the usual presenting complaint. The weakness and pain reflect compression of nerve root(s), the spinal cord, or cauda equina, but assessment of this involvement is hampered by the underlying tabes dorsalis. Pain in these patients may also reflect spinal instability and stress upon supporting ligaments and muscles. On examination there is likely to be marked deformity and instability of the lumbar spine.[3] Radiographic study of these patients shows advanced spondylosis of the lumbar spine, characterized by compression fractures and extensive sclerosis of the vertebral bodies and large osteophytes (Fig. 14–50).

Diagnosis of neuropathic arthropathy of the lumbar spine is based upon these clinical and radiographic findings in association with clinical and laboratory evidence of tabes dorsalis.

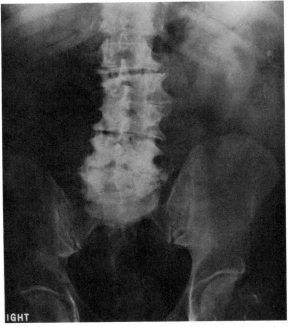

Figure 14–50. Patient with neurosyphilis and neuropathic arthritis (Charcot joint). Advance compression and sclerosis of the vertebral bodies and disc degeneration are present and there is moderate osteophytosis.

Initial treatment is usually a period of bed rest followed by use of a spinal brace; however, intractable pain and evidence of spinal cord compression, particularly if it is progressive, are indications for surgery. Relief of pain and apparent cessation of spinal cord deterioration have been reported after lumbar spine fusion.[3]

References

1. Feldman, M. J., Becker, K. L., Reefe, W. E., and Longo, A.: Multiple neuropathic joints, including the wrist, in a patient with diabetes mellitus. J.A.M.A. *209*:1690–1692, 1969.
2. Beetham, W. P., Kaye, R. L., and Polley, H. F.: A case of extensive polyarticular involvement, and discussion of certain clinical and pathologic features. Ann. Intern. Med., *58*:1002–1012, 1963.
3. Cleveland, M., and Wilson, H. J.: Charcot disease of the spine. J. Bone Joint Surg. *40A*:336–340, 1959.

WHIPPLE'S DISEASE

Whipple's disease (intestinal lipodystrophy) is a rare disease of unknown etiology, although electron microscopic findings and the response of these patients to antibiotic therapy suggest that it is bacterial in origin. Characteristic symptoms include weight loss, diarrhea, arthralgia and abdominal pain, and physical examination is likely to show fever, adenopathy, abdominal distention and skin pigmentation.[1] Approximately two thirds of these patients have rheumatic symptoms and in over a half joint pain antedates the onset of intestinal disease by five or more years. Peripheral joint involvement is marked by an acute onset and monoarticular or polyarticular arthralgia or arthritis. The knees, ankles and fingers are most commonly affected, and in instances of polyarticular disease there is a tendency to bilateral involvement. The joint disease is likely to be episodic and recurrent, with symptoms lasting hours or days but at times longer, and with varying periods between attacks; migratory arthritis has also been described. Residual joint damage is extremely rare. This disease has generally been detected in middle-aged white men.[2, 3]

The diagnosis of Whipple's disease can be established only by demonstrating the macrophages which are characteristic of this disease in the lamina propria of the upper small intestine. Electron microscopic studies indicate that positive PAS staining of these macrophages reflect small bodies, almost certainly bacilli, within and around these phagocytic cells. Peripheral arthritis associated with Whipple's disease appears to be impossible to diagnose until the onset of intestinal disease, as there are no laboratory, radiographic, synovial fluid or synovial histologic findings which serve to identify it. It would seem reasonable to carry out peroral small bowel biopsies—a safe procedure in competent hands—in patients with undiagnosed arthritis, particularly if it is compatible with that described for Whipple's disease.

Spine

There is no evidence that spondylitis of the ankylosing variety is an aspect of Whipple's disease, although radiographic evidence of sacroiliitis has rarely been described in this disease. Kelly and Weisiger, in a review of 64 patients with Whipple's disease and rheumatic manifestations, classified 18 as having spondylitis on the basis of backache (15), x-ray findings (2) or both of these criteria (1).[2] The radiographic findings in two patients, neither of whom had back pain, consisted of bilateral sacroiliac joint fusion, and in the third patient there was unilateral fusion of these joints. It seems clear that further detailed clinical and radiological evaluation of patients with Whipple's disease will be required in order to determine whether sacroiliitis and spondylitis are manifestations of this disease.

References

1. Maizel, H., Ruffin, J. M., and Dobbins, W. O.: Whipple's disease: A review of 19 patients from one hospital and a review of the literature since 1950. Medicine 49:175–205, 1970.
2. Kelly, J. J., and Weisiger, B. B.: The arthritis of Whipple's disease. Arthritis Rheum. 6:615–632, 1963.
3. Wilske, K. R., and Decker, J. L.: The articular manifestations of intestinal disease. Bull. Rheum. Dis. 15:362–365, 1965.

ANKYLOSING HYPEROSTOSIS

Several authors have described the radiologic features of a spinal disorder characterized by intervertebral spurs and bridging without involvement of the discs, apophyseal joints or sacroiliac joints.[1, 3] As might be expected, numerous names have been applied to this entity; however, ankylosing hyperostosis

(AH), suggested by Forestier, is both appropriate and a tribute to the French rheumatologist who has studied this disorder so intensively. In this presentation we have drawn extensively from a recent review by Forestier and his co-worker, Lagier.[3] It is important to delineate AH, a benign, usually asymptomatic or mildly symptomatic disease, from other spinal diseases which have a less favorable prognosis.

The progression of this disease has been defined in Forestier and Lagier's sequential radiographic studies, which indicate that three stages are discernible.[3] Initially, there is slight, barely perceptible, thickening of the anterior surface of the vertebral body and opacities, which may vary from indistinct to well defined, just anterior to the disc space. The second stage is characterized by more obvious prevertebral thickening which extends incompletely over one or both of the adjacent disc spaces, forming a spur. In many instances these spurs have a candle flame configuration. The third and last stage is marked by complete bridging of the disc, initially by extension of a single spur and later by amalgamation of spurs from the adjacent vertebrae. As a by-product of this new bone formation, in portions of the spine the AP diameter may be increased by as much as one fourth to one third. These changes may progress to completion over periods varying from two to 14 years, with the more rapid progression in younger individuals. It has also been noted that a patient may not show the same rate of progression in all affected areas.[3]

The osseous tissue forming the vertebral lamination and the spurs and bridges in this disorder is laid down in paraspinal connective tissue, the peripheral portion of the annulus of the disc, and the deep layers of the anterior spinal ligament. The anterior spinal ligament is not completely ossified and can be identified overlying the involved vertebrae. This bony proliferation is most marked anteriorly but also involves the lateral aspects of the spine; however, the posterior aspects of the vertebrae are rarely affected.[3] Peculiarly, especially in the dorsal area, lateral vertebral involvement is likely to be more extensive on the right than left side. The predominant anterior localization suggests that the anterior longitudinal ligament is a source of connective and vascular tissue which favors the progression of this reaction. Also, it is not clear why the lateral vertebral ossification in the dorsal area is predominantly right sided, although it has been theorized that aortic pulsation may inhibit this process on the left.[3]

The etiology and pathogenesis of AH are unknown but it has been hypothesized that these patients have an "ossifying" diathesis.[3] Butler has cited five instances in which this disease apparently was a sequela to juvenile vertebral epiphysitis (Scheuermann's disease) but it is not clear that this is a common sequence of events.[4] A family with a strong predisposition to this spinal involvement has been described but there is no evidence that this is basically a hereditary disease.[5] A high incidence of AH has been noted among diabetics, but again this observation has not provided any insight into the nature of this disease.[6, 7] Forestier and Lagier, however, have emphasized that, in the absence of evidence of spinal deterioration as disc space narrowing, bony sclerosis and horizontally oriented osteophytes, AH should not be considered a form of osteoarthritis.[3]

It is likely that AH is a relatively common disorder, although prevalence data are not available. It is almost always noted in patients over 50, and when found in younger patients there is likely to be evidence of some predisposing condition such as Scheuermann's disease.

Patients with AH may be asymptomatic or have moderate pain localized to the lumbar and dorsal spine, and stiffness, although it might be anticipated in these patients, is not a prominent complaint. Also, the physical findings are not striking. There may be moderate limitation of spinal motion and increases in the lumbar and dorsal curves; however, these changes may also be consistent with normal attrition of the spine in these aging patients. Sparing of the apophyseal joints and irregular involvement of the spine may account for the paucity of symptoms and findings in this disease.

Radiographic findings of spurs, bridging, and vertebrae thickening, most prominently involving the anterior surface but to a lesser degree the lateral surfaces of the spine, are indicative of this disease (Figs. 14–51 and 14–52). This osseous reaction has a predilection for the lumbar and dorsal vertebrae but the cervical spine may be extensively involved and the curious tendency to spare the left lateral aspect of the dorsal vertebra has been noted. At first these findings may suggest osteoarthritis (spondylosis) or ankylosing spon-

dylitis, and clearly this would be a difficult, if not impossible, differentiation if it were based solely on the configuration of the vertebral lipping. There are prototypes for the osseous projections found in each of these diseases: the thickened spurs and bridges of ankylosing hyperostosis; the horizontally disposed osteophytes of osteoarthritis; and the vertically oriented syndesmophytes of ankylosing spondylitis. But there is also a marked tendency for variation from these basic configurations which in many instances makes it difficult to identify these structures on the basis of morphologic characteristics. Other radiographic findings in the spine, however, should clearly delineate these diseases. Disc space narrowing, sclerosis of the vertebral bodies and narrowing and sclerosis of the apophyseal joints are prominent findings of osteoarthritis but are not features of AH. It is necessary to emphasize that marked hyperostosis suggestive of AH and osteoarthritis of the spine may at times co-exist. Sacroiliitis, straightening of the

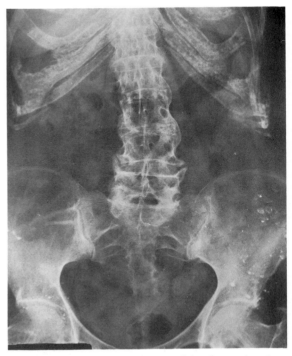

Figure 14–51. The pelvis and lumbar spine in a patient with ankylosing hyperostosis. Osseous spurs are present at the lateral aspects of the discs, and in many instances have formed osseous bridges between adjacent vertebrae. The sacroiliac joints are normal except for moderate sclerosis.

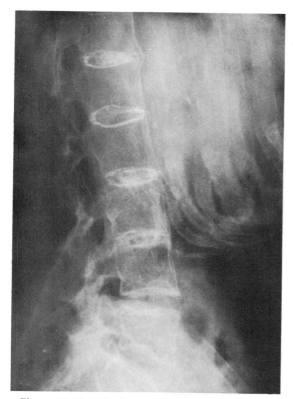

Figure 14–52. The lumbar spine in ankylosing hyperostosis (same patient as in Fig. 14–51). An osseous reaction has formed bridges which span all but the lower two discs.

anterior surface of the vertebra and apophyseal joint narrowing or ankylosis serve to delineate ankylosing spondylitis from ankylosing hyperostosis.

References

1. Bick, E. M.: Vertebral osteophytosis, pathologic basis of its roentgenology. Am. J. Roentgenol. *73*:979–983, 1955.
2. Smith, C. F., Pugh, D. G., and Polley, H. F.: Physiologic vertebral ligamentous calcification: An aging process. Amer. J. Roentgenol. *74*:1049–1058, 1955.
3. Forestier, J., and Lagier, R.: Ankylosing hyperostosis of the spine. Clin. Orthop. *74*:65–83, 1971.
4. Butler, R. W.: Spontaneous anterior fusion of vertebral bodies. J. Bone Joint Surg. *53B*:230–235, 1971.
5. Beardwell, A.: Familial ankylosing hyperostosis with tylosis. Ann. Rheum. Dis. *28*:518–523, 1969.
6. Hajkova, Z., Streda, A., and Skrha, F.: Hyperostotic spondylosis and diabetes mellitus. Ann. Rheum. Dis. *24*:536–543, 1965.
7. Julkunen, H., Karava, R., and Viljanen, V.: Hyperostosis of the spine in diabetes mellitus. Diabetologia *2*:123, 1966.

ALKAPTONURIA AND OCHRONOSIS

Alkaptonuria, the presence of homogentisic acid in urine, and ochronosis, a bluish-black pigmentation of connective tissue, are features of a rare inherited disorder of tyrosine metabolism. Patients manifesting alkaptonuria and ochronosis lack homogentisic acid oxidase, an enzyme vital to tyrosine degradation, and thereby accumulate excessive amounts of homogentisic acid, an intermediate metabolite of tyrosine. Lack of homogentisic acid oxidase is based on a recessive gene defect, and the homozygous state is likely to reflect a consanguineous marriage.[1]

In these patients the connective tissue in various structures, including prominently the joints, skin, blood vessels, and viscera, may be pigmented and distorted as a result of deposition of homogentisic acid or a polymer of this substance. Articular cartilage impregnated with homogentisic acid appears to be quite vulnerable and is likely to fissure and fragment, and eventually be completely eroded from the joint surface. Also, fragments of cartilage may be dispersed throughout the joint and lead to synovial thickening and chondromatosis. Fibrocartilaginous structures, particularly the menisci of the knee and the annulus of the intervertebral disc, may show calcification as well as pigmentation and deterioration.

Clinical Picture

Some patients lacking homogentisic acid oxidase may never have significant symptoms or findings, while others, apparently with greater deficiency of the enzyme, are likely to develop the first evidence of ochronosis when they reach the fourth decade. The disease may be detected in infancy or childhood only if homogentisic acid is identified in the urine (alkaptonuria). Darkly stained diapers, reflecting the black hue which develops in the urine after a period of exposure to oxygen, and positive tests for a reducing substance in the urine in the absence of glucosuria are the usual clues to alkaptonuria. Homogentisic acid may be positively identified in the urine, utilizing a paper chromatographic technique. Slate blue pigmentation of the ears, sclera or skin and discoloration of clothing by axillary sweat are early manifestations of ochronosis. Back pain and stiffness may also be noted early (see below). Peripheral joint disease involving most frequently the knees, at times the shoulders or hips, and usually sparing the joints of the fingers and toes is likely to appear later in the course of this disease. The clinical and radiological findings associated with the peripheral joints are similar to osteoarthritis; however, the meniscus of the knee may be calcified. Locking is a common feature of the knee involvement, reflecting free or tethered cartilaginous or ossified bodies. Cardiac murmurs (15 to 20 per cent) and prostatic calculi are additional manifestations of ochronosis.[1,2]

Spinal Involvement

The musculoskeletal manifestations of ochronosis are likely to be first noted in the spine. Pain, but more prominently stiffness, is noted in the lumbar and eventually the cervical areas of the spine. On examination, there is likely to be marked loss of motion or even rigidity in the lumbar and dorsal spine; however, cervical spine motion is usually retained. The lumbar and cervical lordosis may be reduced, and in some patients there is a generalized kyphosis most marked at the lumbodorsal junction. The rate of progression of this process in the spine varies, but it may involve the entire spine within ten years. In some instances (10 to 15 per cent) the onset of spinal involvement is marked by signs and symptoms of a herniated intervertebral disc, reflecting the weakening of the annulus fibrosus in this disease.[2]

Radiographic evidence of ochronosis in the spine may occur as early as the second or third decade. The characteristic finding is calcification and narrowing of numerous discs, and such involvement in a young patient is practically diagnostic for ochronosis (Fig. 14–53). Osteoporosis of the vertebral bodies is also characteristic and accentuates the radiopaqueness of the calcified discs. In older patients extensive osteophyte formation is likely to develop.

The stiff, deformed spine of ochronotic patients may suggest the diagnosis of ankylosing spondylitis. Furthermore, in some patients with ochronosis there may be involvement of the costovertebral joints, with restriction of thoracic excursions, as in ankylosing spondylitis. However, these two diseases may be easily distinguished on the basis of their charac-

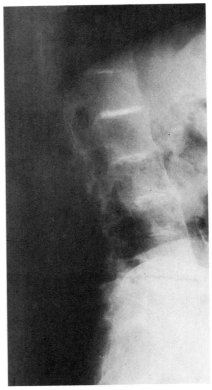

Figure 14–53. Ochronosis of the spine marked by calcification and narrowing of numerous discs.

teristic radiologic findings in the spine. Fusion of the sacroiliac joints, straightening of the anterior surfaces of vertebral bodies and extensive syndesmophyte formation (bamboo spine) are not features of ochronosis.[1,2]

There is no established treatment for ochronosis, but Holdsworth et al. have suggested that a diet low in phenylalanine and tyrosine may ameliorate the rheumatic symptoms.[3]

References

1. Bunim, J. J.: Alkaptonuria, ochronosis and ochronotic arthritis. In Arthritis and Allied Conditions. 6th ed. Hollander, J. L. (ed.), Philadelphia, Lea and Febiger, 1966, pp. 898–906.
2. Laskar, F. H. and Sarginson, K. D.: Ochronotic arthropathy. J. Bone Joint Surg. 52B:653–666, 1970.
3. Holdsworth, D. W., Barry, M. L., and Swyter, J. L.: Treatment of alkaptonuria and ochronotic arthritis with a low phenylalanine-low tyrosine diet. Arthritis Rheum. 10:284, 1967, Abstract.

FAMILIAL MEDITERRANEAN FEVER

Familial Mediterranean fever (FMF) is an inherited disease occurring for the most part in people from eastern Mediterranean countries, including Sephardic Jews, Levantine Arabs, Turks and Armenians. The disease is characterized by acute attacks of peritonitis, pleuritis or synovitis, all accompanied by fever. The abdominal or chest pain associated with serositis is brief, lasting from 12 hours to a few days; however, the arthritis may persist over a much longer period. Episodes of pericarditis and an acute erysipelas-like dermatitis may also be noted. Familial Mediterranean fever patients are undoubtedly included in such categories as benign paroxysmal peritonitis or recurrent polyserositis. Amyloidosis expressed primarily as the nephrotic syndrome may develop in these patients and in some instances is the only manifestation of the underlying disease. Renal amyloidosis associated with familial Mediterranean fever may be fatal in even relatively young patients. The onset of arthritis and other manifestations of this disease is during childhood or adolescence and there is a slightly greater incidence among men.[1]

Peripheral Arthritis

Rheumatic attacks, usually as monoarthritis but rarely as polyarthritis, are noted in 70 per cent of familial Mediterranean fever patients; they may be the only manifestation or interspersed with other facets of the disease. The knee, ankle, hip and shoulder are most frequently affected and in instances of polyarthritis, the distribution is likely to be asymmetric. Para-articular sites, particularly the lower thigh and upper calf may be affected and suggest knee involvement. The joint attacks may last from a few days to a few weeks or, less commonly, for months; there is also marked variability in the periods between attacks, which in some instances may extend for years. Following the attacks, there is generally no residual joint damage, although after prolonged episodes of hip or knee involvement there may be deformity or more likely radiological evidence of deterioration of these joints. Also, muscles of the affected joints may become atrophic during prolonged episodes. Intense pain, exquisite tenderness, swelling and muscle spasm with little tendency for redness and warmth are characteristic of the joint disease.[2]

Clinical laboratory, synovial fluid, and radiographic studies in these patients do not yield specific findings for the arthritis of familial Mediterranean fever, but in some instances a lateral radiograph of the knee shows that the juxtaarticular surface of the femur is marked by linear radiolucency with eggshell-thin borders which may be indicative of this disease. However, the clinical features of the arthritis, the other features of the disease, when present, and the familial and ethnic background of these patients usually serve to clarify the diagnosis.[2]

Spine

There is evidence that the sacroiliac joints and possibly the spine may be involved in familial Mediterranean fever. Heller et al., in a study of the arthritis of familial Mediterranean fever in 24 patients, noted symptoms or signs of sacroiliac disease in four instances and similar evidence of lumbar spine involvement in five patients.[2] Radiographic findings of sacroiliitis and lumbar spondylitis suggestive of ankylosing spondylitis were noted in two patients; a third showed only sacroiliitis. Other studies have shown widening or sclerosis of the sacroiliac joints, irregular calcification of the lumbar paraspinal ligaments and osteitis condensans ilii in familial Mediterranean fever patients.[1, 3, 4] Thus, it is quite likely that young patients may have sacroiliac or spinal disease as a manifestation of familial Mediterranean fever, although the diagnosis in such instances would be dependent upon recognition of more characteristic features of this disease. However, familial Mediterranean fever patients with radiological findings of classical ankylosing spondylitis involving the sacroiliac joints and lumbar spine should probably be classified as having both diseases, at least for the present. Further study will be required to determine whether such radiographic findings may be an aspect of this inherited disease.

References

1. Ehrlich, G. E.: Arthritis of familial Mediterranean fever. In Arthritis and allied conditions. Hollander, J. L., and McCarty, D. J. (eds.), Philadelphia, Lea & Febiger, 1972, pp. 826–831.
2. Heller, H., Gajni, J., Michaeli, D., Shahin, N., Sohar, E., Ehrlich, G., Karten, L., and Sokoloff, L.: The ar-

thritis of familial Mediterranean fever (FMF). Arthritis Rheum. 9:1–17, 1966.

3. Eisinger, J. B., Luccioni, R., Acquaviva, P., Mouland, J. C., and Recondier, A. M.: Maladie périodique et spondylarthrite ankylosante. Marseille Med. *107*:427, 1970.

4. Gajni, J., Sohar, E., and Heller, H.: quoted by Ehrlich, G. E.: Arthritis of familial Mediterranean fever. *In* Arthritis and Allied Conditions. Hollander, J. J. and McCarty, D. J. (eds.), Philadelphia, Lea & Febiger, 1972, pp. 826–831.

BEHCET'S SYNDROME

Behcet's syndrome is a chronic relapsing systemic disease characterized by oral and genital ulcers and iritis. Individuals between the ages of 25 and 40 are most likely to develop this disease but men more frequently than women. It has been found most frequently in the Eastern Mediterranean area, Japan and more recently in the United States. In addition to the basic triad, there may be inflammatory lesions involving the vasculature, including the aorta and vena cava, skin, gastrointestinal tract, nervous system, and articulations. These lesions all appear to reflect an underlying vasculitis. Arteritis, thrombophlebitis, erythema multiforme, erythema nodosum, and enteritis and colitis are among the protean manifestations of this disease. The central nervous system involvement manifested as meningomyelitis, brain stem syndromes, and organic psychosis may be fatal. Laboratory findings include anemia and an increased erythrocyte sedimentation rate, but the diagnosis rests on identification of at least two but preferably three of the diagnostic triad. With respect to treatment, corticosteroids may be tried but are not consistently helpful and immunosuppressives are presently being evaluated.[1, 2]

Arthralgia, myalgia and arthritis are frequent manifestations of Behcet's syndrome and may precede, occur concurrently with, or follow the oral, ocular, and genital findings. Few or many joints may be affected; the large joints, particularly the knees, are involved most frequently but the small joints of the hands and feet may also be involved. The course tends to be subacute or chronic without relapse, and persistence for twenty or more years has been noted. Nonerosive synovitis, effusions, and absence of deformity characterize the joint involvement. The synovial fluid is of the inflammatory (Type II) variety and radiographic findings are nonspecific. Diagnosis depends upon recognition of the characteristic aspects of the syndrome.[1, 3]

Involvement of the sacroiliac joints and spine have been reported in Behcet's syndrome but these findings have not been clearly characterized. Mason and Barnes in a review of their 19 patients with arthritis associated with Behcet's syndrome report one patient with lumbar and three with cervical spine involvement, but the clinical and radiographic manifestations are not defined. In the discussion of this paper there is mention of a series of patients with Behcet's syndrome from Turkey, many of whom had sacroiliac joint involvement. Also, another discussant cited his personal experience of a patient with this disease who had unilateral sacroiliitis.[3]

References

1. O'Duffy, J. D., Carney, J. A., and Deodhar, S.: Behcet's Disease. Ann. Int. Med., *75*:561–570, 1971.
2. Kansu, E., et al.: Behcet's syndrome with obstruction of the venae cavae. A report of seven cases: Quart. Jour. Med. New series XLI, No. 162, 151–168, 1972.
3. Mason, R. M., and Barnes, C. G.: Behcet's syndrome with arthritis. Ann. Rheum. Dis. *28*:95–103, 1969.

SURGICAL CONSIDERATIONS IN ARTHRITIS OF THE CERVICAL SPINE*

ROBERT W. BAILEY, M.D.
University of Michigan

In rheumatoid arthritis and spondylitis rhizomélique, the cervical spine, like other joints, may become involved. Spontaneous dislocations may occur in rheumatoid arthritis and present problems with or without neuro-

logical findings. There are three types of spontaneous dislocations which one may see: a steplike dislocation of the vertebra; atlantoaxial dislocation; and single subluxations between individual vertebrae. Probably atlantoaxial joint dislocations occur more frequently than steplike dislocations. The presence of a steplike dislocation should be sus-

---

*This section has been adapted from R. W. Bailey: The Cervical Spine, published in 1974 by Lea & Febiger; by courtesy of Lea & Febiger.

pected when a bizarre weakness of the hands is found. In such cases, hand weakness may be due to joint involvement, or a portion may be due to involvement of the nerve roots by foraminal encroachment on the roots by the dislocation. Such encroachments may occur at one or more levels. In a study of individuals with rheumatoid arthritis, Martel found a large number of atlantoaxial subluxations.[10] The indication for surgical treatment when atlantoaxial subluxations occur in rheumatoid arthritis is very difficult to define. It must be based on the presence or absence of symptoms. Such symptoms may be pain along the course of the greater occipital nerve with posterior occipital headache, unilateral or bilateral. There may be weakness in the hands and difficulty in walking, reflecting a traction phenomenon on the cord. A number of individuals have been seen in whom a sense of impending doom has been described with certain positions of the head, especially forward flexion of the head on the chest, presumably due to cerebrovascular insufficiency, which is probably due to the disturbance of vertebral arteries.

Abnormal physical findings may or may not be present. There may be weakness in the hands with hyporeflexia in the upper extremities and spasticity in the lower extremities with hyperreflexia and the presence of a pathological reflex such as a Babinski sign. Some symptoms and findings which may be observed in individuals with spontaneous atlantoaxial dislocations with rheumatoid arthritis are illustrated in the following cases: The cause of both steplike dislocations and atlantoaxial dislocations is probably the same. There is inflammation of soft tissue, resulting in their destruction: for example, destruction of the transverse ligament of the odontoid allowing for subluxation of the atlas on the axis. In addition, one may see rather complete resorption of the odontoid, similar to the destructive changes seen in joints elsewhere in rheumatoid arthritis, as for example the small joints of the hands. The decision to carry out atlantoaxial fusion is difficult to make, with atlantoaxial instability in the presence of rheumatoid arthritis. The mere presence of subluxation on flexion and extension films does not in itself warrant a fusion. There must be present symptoms sufficiently significant to warrant subjection of the patient to the hazards of surgery. We have encountered two serious complications in performing atlantoax-

ial fusion for subluxation in rheumatoid arthritis. In one individual, gradual reduction of the atlantoaxial dislocation was achieved after a period of about one month with the patient in skull tong traction on a Stryker frame. The reduction was not complete and at the time of operation, complete reduction was achieved as the wire encircling the neural arch of the atlas was brought around and fixed to the axis. However, as this was being accomplished, spontaneous respirations ceased. The patient remained apneic and required assistance in breathing for better than five minutes, following which spontaneous breathing resumed. The exact mechanism responsible for the apnea appeared to be disturbed medullary function, presumably due to the mechanical factors involved in the reduction. Another serious complication occurred in a 56-year-old woman. She entered the hospital complaining of progressively increasing ataxia and loss of strength in her hands and an unremitting bilateral suboccipital headache. For many years she had been victim of rheumatoid arthritis with multiple joint involvement. On physical examination there was demonstrable weakness in both hands, generalized and disproportionate to the degree of joint involvement. There was hyperreflexia in the lower extremities, and the Babinski sign was present bilaterally. Radiograms revealed dislocation of C-1 on C-2 with forward flexion and a tendency to reduction of the dislocation with extension (Figs. 14–54 and 14–55). She was placed at bed rest, and dramatic improvement occurred within a few weeks. Fusion of C-1 to C-2 was performed using the technique to be described and the operation was performed without any immediate difficulty (Fig. 14–56). For the first 10 postoperative days her course was essentially uneventful. On the eleventh postoperative day, however, she abruptly developed severe headache and began to vomit in an almost projectile manner. Physical examination revealed that cortical blindness had developed, an explanation for which was not clear. This woman had evidence of atherosclerosis elsewhere, and it was thought that she had developed thrombosis of one or both vertebral arteries which had propagated up the basilar artery into the posterior inferior cerebellar vessels, with infarction of one or both calcarine gyri (Fig. 14–57). Another explanation, since she had a previous history of cardiac difficulties, might have been embolization to one or both calcarine gyri (Fig. 14–58).

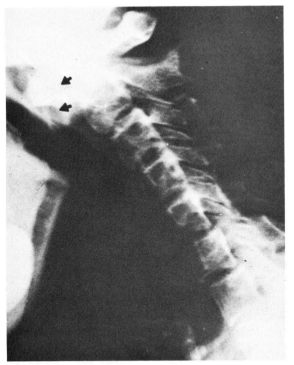

Figure 14–54. A 56-year-old woman with weakness in both hands and spasticity in lower extremities, with a longstanding history of rheumatoid arthritis, showing a subluxation of C1 on C2.

Such complications and occurrences of sudden death at the time of reduction and fusion merit caution in approaching these individuals. If atlantoaxial subluxation is present on x-ray examination and is unassociated with symptoms or signs of neurological impairment, surgical treatment does not seem warranted. In instances of the steplike dislocations, which are relatively uncommon, the author has not considered surgical intervention to be indicated.

Fractures and Dislocations of the Cervical Spine

Traumatic dislocations and fractures may occur in cervical spines already involved in rheumatoid arthritis or spondylitis rhizomélique. These are not common but do present a challenge in treatment. They can result in disastrous consequences including sudden death. In 1956, while associated with Wadsworth Veterans Hospital in Los Angeles, California, the author became acquainted with a young man so severely involved with spondy-

litis rhizomélique that in order to enter his automobile he had to have it modified. On the driver's side of the car, when the door was opened, the roof over the driver would also open in order for this individual to enter it. One day this young man turned onto a highway from a side road after having stopped for a traffic light. In the process of turning onto the highway, he misjudged the turn and struck the curb while traveling at about 10 mph. As the car struck the curb the driver died instantly. His death was witnessed by the author's surgical scrub nurse, who was in the right front seat of the automobile. At autopsy, traumatic dislocation of the atlantoaxial joint was found with transection of the spinal cord at the level. Before this injury, this young man's entire cervical spine had already appeared solidly ankylosed radiographically, due to ankylosing spondylitis.

Chin on Chest Deformity in Ankylosing Spondylitis

Intense interest at the University of Michigan Medical Center has developed recently

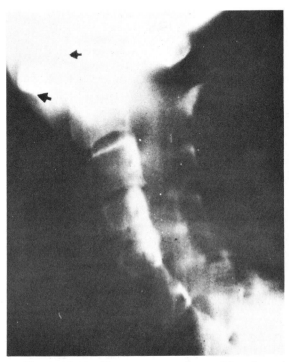

Figure 14–55. Tomograms confirm subluxation of C1 on C2.

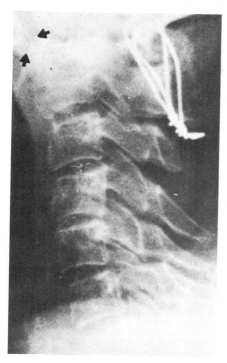

Figure 14–56. Following preoperative Vinke tong traction, fusion of C1 on C2 was performed without difficulty.

The following case presentations are illustrative of the problem and outline our approaches to management. The deformities usually seen in ankylosing spondylitis are quite readily recognized.

CASE 1. A 54-year-old man with a history of longstanding ankylosing spondylitis had fallen six weeks prior to the time he was seen with pain occurring in the cervical area with increased motion over his stiff-necked attitude and a very rapidly progressing chin-on-chest deformity (Fig. 14–59, *A* and *B*). No neurological abnormalities were found, but x-rays were interpreted as showing a dislocation of C-1 on C-2. Tomograms showed the dislocation more clearly (Fig. 14–60). He was placed in Vinke tong traction in bed with prompt improvement in his clinical and x-ray appearance (Fig. 14–61). A cervical occipital fusion was performed and he was immobilized in a Minerva jacket into which were incorporated the Vinke tongs. No internal fixation was used. The fusion appeared secure seven months postoperatively and immobilization was discontinued. After one year following the fusion he had regained nearly normal posture (Fig. 14–62).

in a group of individuals with ankylosing spondylitis who have a typical history of difficulties and who developed what we have termed the "chin on chest deformity." This should not be mistaken as a part of the natural history of ankylosis, it is the result of a specific defect. The various treatment programs the author and his colleagues have used with these individuals represent a departure from contemporary thought.

These patients had a long-standing history of ankylosing spondylitis with generalized stiffening of the entire spine including the cervical area. They were mostly over 50 years of age. There was a history of an apparently trivial injury followed by pain, increased motion of the neck, with the head and neck developing a rapid forward flexion attitude and the chin coming to rest near or on the chest over a period of two to eight weeks. Radiographic examination has been extremely difficult to obtain because of the combination of severe and sometimes bizarre flexion and rotational deformities in addition to ankylosis and osteoporosis.

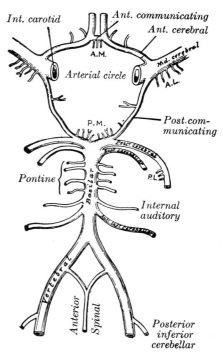

Figure 14–57. The arterial circle of Willis. (From Gray's Anatomy. Goss, C. N. (ed.), Philadelphia, Lea & Febiger, 1967.)

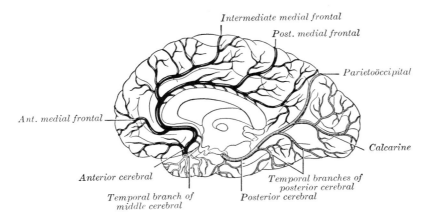

Figure 14–58. The calcarine gyrus. (From Gray's Anatomy. Goss, C. N. (ed.), Philadelphia, Lea & Febiger, 1967.)

CASE 2. A University professor of psychology with a long-standing history of spondylitis rhizomélique was involved in an auto accident and brought to the emergency room with severe neck pain and severe suboccipital headache. He complained of paresthesias in both hands and showed increased deep tendon responses in his lower extremities with a positive Babinski sign. Radiograms revealed a fracture through the area of the C5–C6 disc space (Fig. 14–63). He was placed in skull

tong traction on a Stryker frame and many efforts were made to effect reduction by altering the line of pull of traction and varying the amount of weight employed. Repeat x-ray examinations were not only difficult to obtain, but equally difficult to interpret. The first week saw deterioration of his neurological status, with progression of weakness in the hands. This man had a rather prominent goatee, and it was assumed by the attending surgeons that he had so much pre-injury flexion deformity

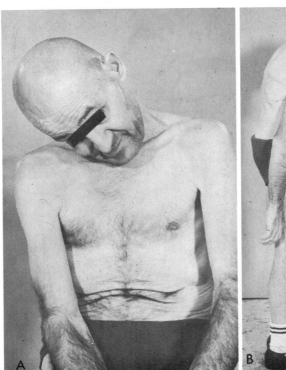
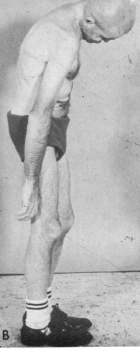

Figure 14–59. A 54-year-old male with a history of longstanding ankylosing spondylitis fell six weeks prior to these photographs and rapidly developed the chin-on-chest deformity. (Figs. 14–59 through 14–62 depict same patient.)

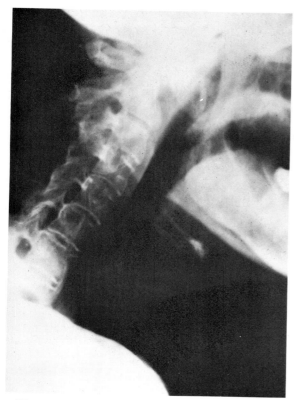

Figure 14–60. X-rays reveal subluxation of C1 on C2.

"re-ankylosis." One year post-injury his neurological status was much improved, although weakness in his hands and hypesthesia in the distribution of the sixth cervical nerve root was present bilaterally.

CASE 3. A 55-year-old male with long-standing ankylosing spondylitis had been followed at the Ann Arbor Veterans Hospital for many years (Fig. 14–66). He sustained a fall while hunting in the woods in Michigan's Upper Peninsula. He was transported from the scene of his fall in the back seat of an automobile and while en route to Ann Arbor, became quadriparetic and died a short time thereafter. At the time of autopsy a fracture was found through the arch of the spinous process of C5, with extensive damage to the spinal cord in this area (Fig. 14–67).

We have seen a number of other patients with the chin on chest deformity. It seems that the syndrome is quite clear and if properly recognized and appropriately treated, the deformity can be corrected and serious neurological complications avoided. The features of this syndrome are as follows: first, a history of longstanding ankylosing spondylitis with a fixed cervical spine, followed by some type of injury, usually not of great magnitude, most commonly a fall. After injury, the patient notices pain, increased cervical motion and pro-

that he was unable to properly shave his chin. There was extreme difficulty because of his broad shoulders in acquiring adequate roentgenograms. Because of increasing neurological involvement, it was thought the best hope would be to attempt reduction by manipulation under anesthesia. The author, in an attempt to determine the physical appearance of this man prior to injury, inquired if he had recent photographs. One month before his accident he fortunately had had a photograph taken for his driver's license. This showed no chin on chest deformity, and his wife and his friends said that his goatee had been simply a tonsorial adornment. Reduction by manipulation was carried out using the patient's photograph as a guide (Fig. 14–64). Post-manipulation he was immobilized for four months in a plaster bed on a Stryker frame. Subsequent immobilization consisted of a Forster collar with a dorsal extension (Fig. 14–65). One year post-injury he showed evidence of solid healing radiographically and

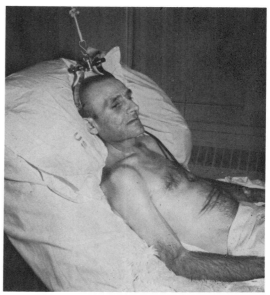

Figure 14–61. Patient in skull tong traction in bed shows marked improvement in the chin-on-chest deformity.

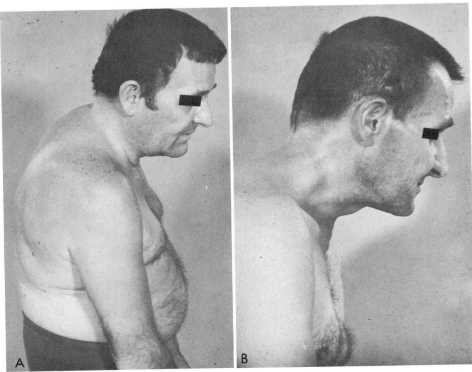

Figure 14–62.   One year postoperative fusion of C1 on C2. There has been marked improvement in the position of the cervical spine in addition to weight gain and improvement in the patient's well-being.

gressive forward displacement of the head on the trunk, to the point where the flexion is so great that the chin comes to rest on the chest. In this series of "chin on chest deformity" patients anesthesia was difficult to administer, and in almost every instance a tracheotomy was considered to facilitate the administration of anesthesia, but did not prove necessary. In more recent cases, endotracheal anesthesia has been facilitated, using a fiberoptic endotracheal tube (Fig. 14–68). To date, a halo traction has not been used, but might be an attractive alternative to a Minerva jacket. Postoperative traction could be retained with a halo traction, using an outrigger-type jury rig attached to a body jacket.

Atlanto-axial Fusion

In certain dislocations and fracture dislocations of traumatic origin or secondary to rheumatoid arthritis, fusion of the atlantoaxial joint is sometimes necessary. Kahn and Yglesias (in 1935) were among the first to report on cervico-occipital fusion. With the passage of time, fusion of the occiput has been shown to be difficult to achieve and usually unnecessary, since there is no derangement of the atlanto-occipital joint. Fusion of the occiput also imposes an unnecessary and undesirable restriction of motion, especially rotation. In most instances the patient is placed in skull tong traction on a frame; anesthesia is induced with the patient supine; and an endotracheal tube is inserted. It is important to protect the eyes by applying a small amount of moist cotton over the closed lids and sealing these pads in place with tape. Care must be exercised by the anesthesiologist during the surgical procedure to avoid any pressure on the orbs when the patient is placed in the prone position, since the pressure may produce blindness. The surgeon should be well advised to question the anesthesiologist from time to time about this as the operative procedure proceeds.

With the patient prone and after the occipital and cervical areas have been prepared and draped, an incision is made at the anatom-

Figure 14–63. A 53-year-old man with longstanding spondylitis rhizomélique was involved in an automobile accident and brought to the emergency room with severe neck pain and severe suboccipital headache. He complained of paresthesias in both hands and showed hyperreflexia in the lower extremities. X-rays revealed a fracture through the area of the C5-C6 disc space. (Figs. 14–63 through 14–65 depict same patient.)

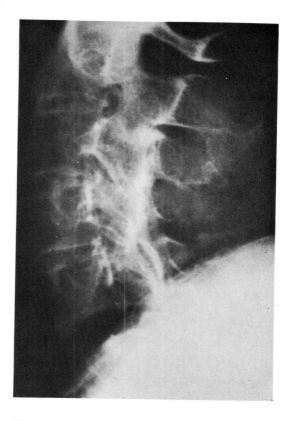

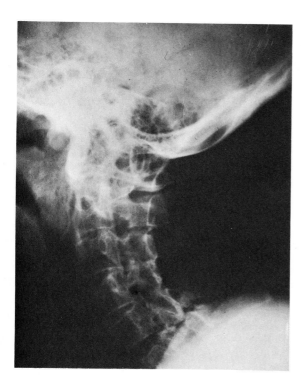

Figure 14–64. Four months following manipulative reduction, normal anatomical restoration has been achieved.

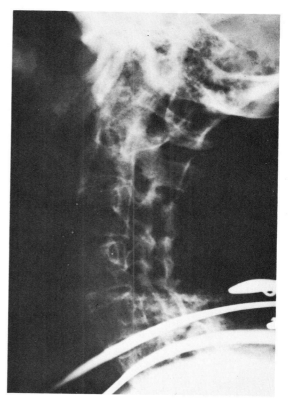

Figure 14–65. Patient was immobilized in a Förster collar.

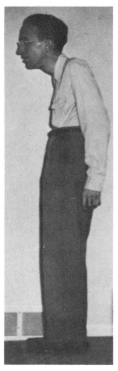

Figure 14–66. A 55-year-old male with longstanding ankylosing spondylitis sustained a fall while hunting in the woods of northern Michigan. He was transported to the University of Michigan Medical Center by automobile, some 700 miles. In transit, he noted progressive evidence of ascending paralysis beginning in his leg and extending up, to involve his trunk and then his arms. On arrival to the hospital he was totally paretic and died a short time after hospital entry.

ical midline from the external occipital protuberance down to the midcervical area. The ligamentum nuchae and posterior neck musculature are stripped from the spinous processes of the second vertebra and the lower portion of the occipital bone. As the dissection is deepened, it is important to palpate for the neural arch of the atlas, to know its whereabouts and to assess the degree of instability of the atlantoaxial articulation. In those individuals with rheumatoid arthritis, there is a high degree of instability and a tendency of the neural arch of the atlas to subluxate anteriorly.

As the neural arch of the atlas is being exposed, it is extremely important to proceed from the midline laterally. A portion of the vertebral artery leaves the foramen on the medial side of the rectus capitis lateralis and curves around the superior articular process

of the atlas (Fig. 14–69). The vertebral artery then comes to lie in the groove on the cranial surface of the posterior arch of the atlas and enters the vertebral canal by passing under the posterior atlanto-occipital membrane (Fig. 14–70). This portion of the artery is covered by the semispinalis capitis and is contained in the suboccipital triangle. In keeping the dissection closely on the posterior bony surface of the arch of the atlas, damage to the vertebral artery can be avoided. In this area there is a posterior vertebral venous plexus which should be avoided. This was described by Zalnai of Budapest. Should this plexus be entered, bleeding can be quite readily controlled by electrocoagulation. After exposure of the posterior neural arches of the atlas and axis, the posterior atlantoaxial ligament and posterior atlanto-occipital membrane must be mobilized from the neural arch of the axis. This can be done using a curved dura elevator, proceeding from the midline laterally (Fig. 14–71). If the dislocation or fracture dislocation has been due to flexion, that is, forward displacement of

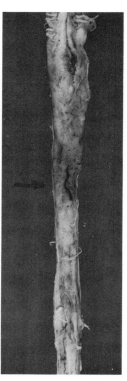

Figure 14–67. Autopsy on patient depicted in Figure 14–66 reveals fracture through the arch of the fifth cervical vertebra with extensive damage to the spinal cord.

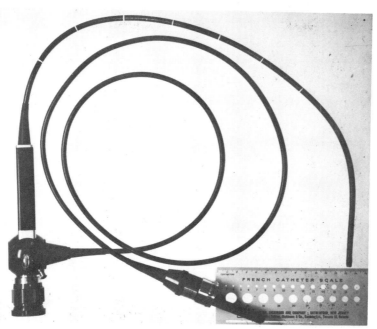

Figure 14–68. Endotracheal anesthesia has been facilitated by use of a fiberoptic endotracheal tube.

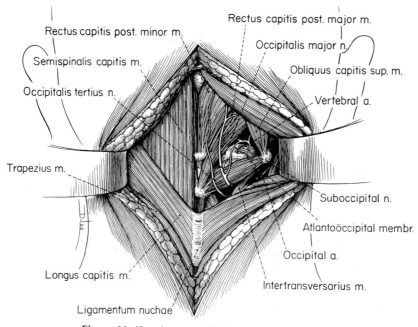

Figure 14–69. Anatomy of the suboccipital triangle.

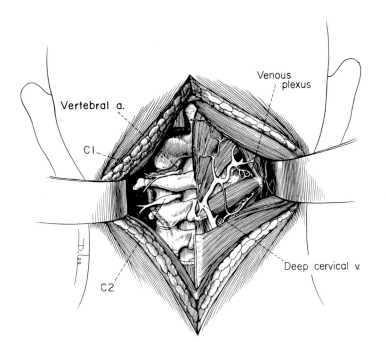

Figure 14–70. Exposure of the posterior neural arches of C1-C2.

the atlas on the axis, it is desirable to use an internal fixation to gain some stability. We found the following technique to be very satisfactory.

A piece of stainless steel wire of 18 or 20 gauge and about 10 to 12 inches in length, is bent at its midpoint to resemble the letter **U**.

The **U**-shaped end is next bent into a rather sharp curve, almost a right-angle. The **U**-shaped end is carefully fed beneath the arch of the atlas and its **U**-end picked up just below the occiput. The **U**-end is then drawn through and placed around the barest spinous process of the second cervical vertebra, to take hold of

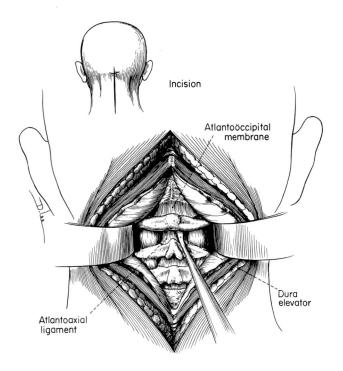

Figure 14–71. The posterior atlantoaxial ligament and posterior atlanto-occipital membrane are mobilized from the neural arch of the axis, using a curved dura elevator.

the base of that process on its caudal side. A hole is made superficial to the **U**-end of the wire in the base of the spinous process of the second cervical vertebra. The hole should be large enough to allow the passage of one of the free ends of the wire. The hole can be made by using a large towel clip, a Lewin bone clamp or a similar device. After the free end of the wire is threaded through the hole, the two free ends of the wire are then tightened to approximate the first and second cervical vertebrae. We have used the Shifrin wire tautener, but other types of wire tauteners are quite helpful, and when such a device is not available the free ends of the wire can be clasped with heavy pliers and the wire tautened. The wire is next twisted and if one is using the tautener of the Shifrin type, it is wise to decrease the tension on the wire as the twists are being made to avoid breakage of the wire. Three or four twists are sufficient (Fig. 14–72). The excess wire is then cut off and discarded. We have found this method of wire fixation to be superior to all others that we have tried. On some

occasions a hole was made through the posterior neural arch of the first cervical vertebra and the wire passed between the two cortices. This has a great mechanical disadvantage of having only one cortex against which the wire is offering stress. When the wire has been placed about the neural arch of the first cervical vertebra, there appears to be a double mechanical advantage. In some instances it is virtually impossible to make a hole in the first cervical vertebra through which a wire could be threaded without the wire pulling through the posterior cortex of the neural arch.

After internal fixation has been performed, the fusion bed is prepared with great care, using either an air drill or a rongeur (Fig. 14–73). We have avoided the use of osteotomes and mallet, preferring to decorticate the posterior neural arch of the first and second cervical vertebrae by using a rongeur. A bone graft is next obtained from the posterior iliac crest, the incision beginning at the posterior iliac spine and going forward about three inches. The bone graft usually consists of one-

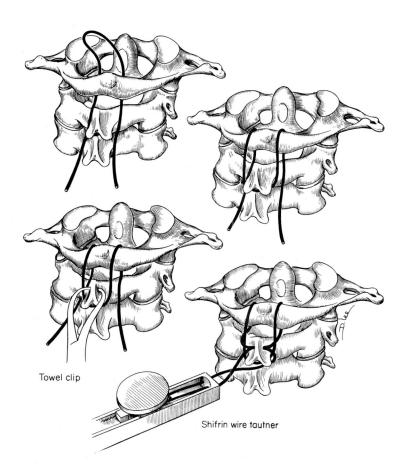

Figure 14–72. The technique of wire immobilization in performance of fusion of the atlas to the axis.

Towel clip

Shifrin wire tautner

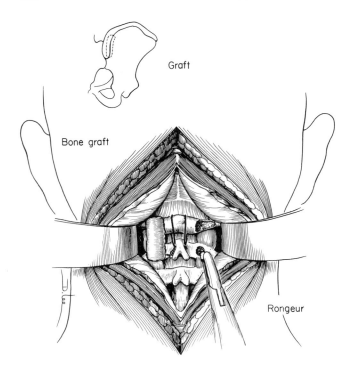

Figure 14–73. The neural arches of C1 and C2 are decorticated, using either rongeur or air drill. A bone graft is obtained from the iliac crest and placed in the prepared bed. Wire fixation of this type is not used in hyperextension dislocation.

half of the thickness of the ilium; the outer half is used. This is split into strips and placed in the recipient fusion beds between the first and second cervical vertebrae.

In hyperextension dislocations of the cervical spine, which occur less frequently, an internal fixing wire should not be used, since the tightening of the wire may serve only to produce a hyperextension deformity. In these instances we prefer preoperative reduction with a halo cast combination, and perform the operation with the patient so immobilized. In these instances the neural arches of the first and second cervical vertebrae are simply decorticated and the bone graft placed in the bed.

References

1. Adson, A. W.: Fixation of the spine for dislocation following removal of a high-lying tumor of the cervical portion of the spinal cord. Proc. Staff Meet. Mayo Clin. 8:1933.
2. Badgley, C. E., and Bailey, R. W.: Stabilization of the cervical spine by anterior fusion. J. Bone Joint Surg. 42A:565, 1960.
3. Bette, H., and Engelhardt, H.: Folgezustande von Laminektomien au der Halswirbelsaule. Zeitsch Orthopadie 85:564, 1955.
4. Cattell, H. S., and Clark, G. L., Jr.: Cervical kyphosis and instability following multiple laminec-

tomies in children. J. Bone Joint Surg. 49A:713, 1967.
5. Denny-Brown, D.: Neurological conditions resulting from prolonged and severe dietary restriction: case reports on prisoners-of-war, and general reviews. Medicine 26:41, 1947.
6. Freund, H. A., Steiner, G., Leichtentritt, B., and Price, A. E.: Peripheral nerves in chronic atrophic arthritis. Am. J. Pathol. 18:865, 1942.
7. Kahn, E. A.: Personal communication.
8. Kahn, E. A.: The role of the dentate ligaments in spinal cord compression and the syndrome of lateral sclerosis. J. Neurosurg. 4:191, 1947.
9. Macnab, I.: Anterior occipitocervical fusion. J. Bone Joint Surg. 49A:1010, 1967.
10. Martel, W., and Abell, M. R.: Fatal atlanto-axial luxation in rheumatoid arthritis. Arthritis Rheum. 6:224, 1963.
11. Martel, W.: Cervical spondylitis in rheumatoid disease: comment on neurological significance and pathogenesis Am. J. Med. 44:441, 1968.
12. Martel, W., Holt, J. E., and Cassidy, J. T.: Roentgenologic manifestations of juvenile rheumatoid arthritis. Amer. J. Roentgenol. 88:400, 1962.
13. Martel, W.: Occipito-atlanto-axial joints in rheumatoid arthritis. In Radiological Aspects of Rheumatoid Arthritis. Proceedings of an International Symposium. International Congress Series No. 61. Amsterdam, Excerpta Medica Foundation, 1963.
14. Schneider, R. C., and Crosby, E. C.: Vascular insufficiency of brain stem and spinal cord in spinal trauma. Neurology 9:643, 1959.
15. Stevenson, G. C., Stoney, R. J., Perkins, R. K., and Adams, J. R.: A transcervical transclival approach to the ventral surface of the brain stem for removal of a clivus cordoma. J. Neurosurg. 24:544, 1966.

OSTEOTOMY OF THE SPINE FOR FIXED FLEXION DEFORMITY

PAUL E. McMASTER, M.D.

Beverly Hills, California

Osteotomy of the spine for correction of severe fixed flexion deformity has proved to be a very satisfactory procedure.

There are different stages in the treatment of ankylosing spondylitis (rheumatoid arthritis of the spine; Marie-Strumpell arthritis). The early stages of the disease with inflammation and pain require medical therapy and instruction in proper postural positions of standing, sitting and lying, to prevent or overcome any tendency to flexion deformity of the spine. Hyperextension exercises are useful and braces may be necessary. The final stage, however, with severe fixed flexion deformity (bony ankylosis), can be corrected only with spinal osteotomy. This procedure offers the patient not only dramatic improvement in appearance but also the opportunity to look ahead and see the horizon, as well as improvement in general well being. Thus, it affords him an important psychological lift.

Credit for the first described osteotomy of the spine goes to Smith-Petersen, Larson, and Aufranc.[1] They described and reported the results of six cases in 1945. Since then a number of successful cases have been reported by various authors.

Severe fixed flexion deformity, in which the patient has difficulty in seeing ahead, requires operation. Spine osteotomy also may improve the function of thoracic and abdominal structures, afford the patient a better chance of returning to gainful occupation, and increase his chances of returning to, and being more acceptable in, general society. One patient in our series had been refused a baby by an adoption agency because of his deformity, but after operation, because of improved appearance, he and his wife were awarded a baby.

Most patients who are seen for correction are in the fourth and fifth decades of life. Occasionally, patients are seen in later decades but often they have rather well accommodated to the physical, psychological and social aspects of life. Also, the older patient with beginning senile changes presents an increased medical hazard to osteotomy. One patient in his middle fifties had calcification of his abdominal aorta, and was at first refused for fear that with the forcible extension and correction the aorta might rupture. He was finally operated, however, after considerable pressure and, fortunately, a good correction without aorta complications was obtained. Another patient, of sixty-seven, was refused an osteotomy because of her general senility changes, but she persisted for several months and offered affidavits absolving all involved of blame for any untoward results. Osteotomy was finally done and good correction obtained, but she expired within 24 hours, probably from cerebral anoxia. An autopsy was not obtained.

Thus, senility changes or certain serious medical problems are considered to be contraindications. Another contraindication to osteotomy is associated severe fixed flexion deformity of one or both hips. Previously, for correction of this deformity, cup arthroplasty was tried but without much success. Also, in some of these cases resection of head and neck of femurs (Girdlestone) was done, but with only fair success in some. Now these associated hip flexion deformities can be quite well treated with total hip joint replacement arthropasty. Such correction, incidentally, may obviate the later need for spinal osteotomy.

The optimum site of osteotomy is in the lumbar spine. Ankylosis of the costal vertebral joints would make correction in the thoracic spine difficult and not advised. Cervical spine osteotomy occasionally is indicated, and successful cases have been reported.

Two patients seen by the author had pronounced fixed flexion deformities of both thoracolumbar and cervical spine. Cervical osteotomy might have been indicated in both, but, after some thought, lumbar osteotomy was done and generally satisfactory correction was achieved in each. Both patients were pleased with the result, and cervical osteotomy (which was considered probably necessary as a second procedure) was not done.

The operative technique was well described by Smith-Petersen and his associates. Painstaking attention to the technical details is important. The wedge of bone to be removed has a posterior base, the apex lies at the anterior margins of the intervertebral foramina and the fulcrum of corrective motion is at the posterior vertebral body margin. An osteotomy at either one or two levels may be done; but almost invariably, if two are done, most of the correction occurs at only one level; hence now usually only one level is done and this mostly at the level of L2-L3. The angle of spine correction obtained corresponds in general to the angle of the wedge or wedges, and an average good correction should range from 40 to 55 degrees.

Intubation anesthesia is used, and great care is taken, as careless manipulation of head and neck could conceivably cause a fracture of the ankylosed cervical spine.

Operative Technique

A prone position is used for operation. In severe deformities and in older patients a "side" rather than prone position may be considered preferable. Adequate padding of the down-knee in side position is important to prevent footdrop, and for arms and armpits in the prone position to prevent wrist-drop. The incision spans at least four spinous processes and has its center at the elected osteotomy site. If there is a question as to the exact level, a lead marker placed over the spine and a preoperative roentgenogram will be helpful. The wound is deepened, and the erector spinae muscles are reflected subperiosteally and widely. Partial or complete ossification of intraspinous ligaments, as well as ligamentum flavum, will be noted. The ossified intraspinous ligament is removed with rongeurs and osteotomes at the selected site of osteotomy. The two adjacent spinous processes are removed in slivers which are used later in the fusion procedure. A window is then made in the ossified ligamentum flavum with a narrow osteotome, using much care because the underlying dura is likely to be thickened and adherent. The dura should be carefully stripped away to avoid tearing or puncturing; the flow of spinal fluid into the wound adds an additional operative problem, although not too serious. Rents in the dura should, of course, be repaired if possible. A few such rents have occurred but no evident complications have resulted.

Through the window, up-biting forceps are used to remove the remainder of the os-

sified ligamentum flavum. A blunt probe is then inserted through each intervertebral foramen, from each lateral portion of the exposed spinal canal in an upward, outward and forward direction. Its point, which then can be seen laterally, serves as a guide for unroofing the foramen, which is done bilaterally. Osteotomes, rongeurs and up-biting forceps are used for this stage. Unroofing the foramen may be easy, but often the inflammatory process which caused the articular destruction has led to fibrous and osseous proliferation, with encroachment on the foramen. This condition adds to the technical difficulties, and much care must be taken not to traumatize nerve roots.

Correction of the deformity after completion of the wedge, or wedges, is accomplished by raising the head and foot of the table, thereby hopefully approximating the opposing oblique surfaces of the osteotomy but, more often than not, careful manual pressure downward at the osteotomy site is required for closure. An audible and often "sickening" snap may be heard during the correction, which indicates anterior separation. No untoward result or complication has been noted by adding this manual forcible correction. Further, in none of my cases has correction not been obtained; hence, there has been no need for a second anterior incision. The locking of the osteotomized surfaces and the integrity of the posterior longitudinal ligament should ensure against any serious displacement. At times, the approximation of the opposing osteotomy surfaces is not completely accurate, or the amount of correction seems inadequate. In case of either or both, the head and foot of the table are lowered, thus opening the wedge or wedges again. Then the necessary revision can be done.

When a satisfactory correction and closure of the wedge or wedges, is obtained, a spine fusion is done. Surfaces of opposing laminae are bared, bone chips are raised, and the slivers cut previously from the spinous processes are laid across the prepared bed. Routine closure of soft tissues is then done and a heavy posterior body plaster shell, extending to one or both knees, is applied on the operating table. When this shell hardens the patient is turned over on it, and an anterior shell is made. The patient should be turned often postoperatively to prevent pressure sores and the top half of the shell removed for skin care.

Stitches are removed at about two weeks and a body cast applied, without extension to one or both knees as was done in the early cases, because such hip immobilization appeared to allow increased stiffness in an arthritic hip. The cast is applied with the patient on Goldthwait irons (Fig. 14–74) and relaxed with a sedative or light anaesthesia. This procedure allows recovery of any correction lost during the two weeks after operation (occasionally from 10 to 20 degrees) by simply increasing the hyperextension of the irons (Fig. 14–75 A and B). The patient is kept at bed rest for a period of about one month post-surgery, and then permitted to stand and walk but discouraged from sitting, (Fig. 14–76 A, B and C). It is considered advisable to wear a body cast for at least six months, with an interval change if necessary. In some earlier cases a hyperextension back brace was applied at four months' post-surgery, but patients were not always faithful in wearing it and some definite loss of correction resulted.

Careful observation of both patient and roentgenograms is necessary to prevent loss of correction. Such loss has been observed as late as six to 12 months after surgery, (Fig. 14–77 A and B.) Should significant loss of correction occur during this time, the patient should be placed either back at bed rest on a hyperextended frame, or again on the Goldthwait irons under anaesthesia. When correction or improvement is obtained, another body cast is applied. It is estimated that at least one year is necessary for sufficient solid bone union to occur to prevent loss of correction. During this time support must be worn.

Roentgenograms are made a few days after surgery to determine the amount of correction and any abnormal displacement. Three different types of correction have been noted; the first and most common type occurs with rupture of the anterior ligaments and anterior separation of two intact vertebral bodies, (Fig. 14–75 A and B). The second correction is one with intact anterior ligaments, but with fracture or dehiscence transversely or obliquely through a vertebral body. The superior body fragment is displaced backward and tilted downward posteriorly and upward anteriorly, (Fig. 14–78 A, B and C.) The third type, noted in one patient, showed the posterior aspect of the vertebral body to be crushed down and compressed and with increased anterior body height; ossified anterior ligaments remained intact, (Fig. 14–79 A and B).

Complications

The author has done forty spinal osteotomies, and several non-fatal complications

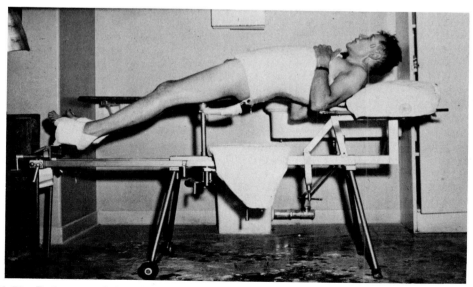

Figure 14–74.   Patient extended on Goldthwait irons and body cast applied. Note head and neck position (cervical ankylosis).

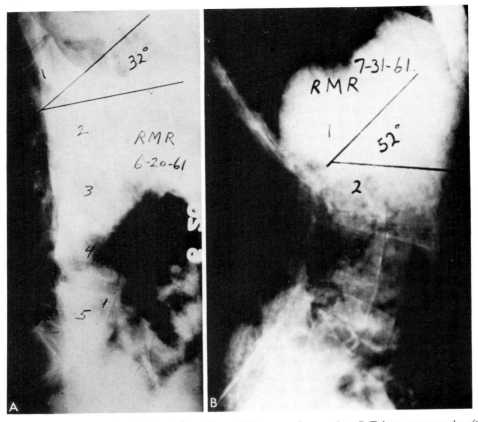

Figure 14–75. *A,* Postoperative roentgenogram shows 32 degrees of correction. *B,* Taken seven weeks after surgery and after hyperextension on Goldthwait irons shows 52 degrees of correction.

and two fatal ones have occurred. The latter included a 67-year-old female (above described), who expired within twenty-four hours, probably from cerebral anoxia, and who should not have been done. The other was a 51-year-old male, who was alert, mentally responsive, with stable pulse and blood pressure and with intact neurological status for sixteen hours and suddenly developed a cardiac arrest and expired.

Non-fatal complication included temporary ileus and paresthesias of extremities. There was one foot-drop from inadequate padding of a "down-knee" and one wrist-drop from inadequate padding of an arm in the prone position, both of which recovered. Another patient with a single level osteotomy and just over 60 degrees of correction developed paraplegia within 24 hours and required emergency laminectomy. Recovery, but not complete, occurred. Thrombophlebitis has oc-

curred, and pulmonary infarct in two cases. There was one case with a non-fatal cardiac arrest. One developed a recurrence of nephrolithiasis, and in the first case done in 1948, a sacral pressure sore developed but healed although slowly.

Often in ankylosing spondylitis there are associated hip and shoulder rheumatoid arthritic changes. Such have been noted to progress after osteotomy despite anti-rheumatic medication and physiotherapy measures (Fig. 14–80 *A, B* and *C.*) One patient at a year and a half had a severe flareup of arthritis of a knee which required synovectomy.

Summary

Forty lumbar spinal osteotomies have been done by the author since 1948. The results have been in general most rewarding.

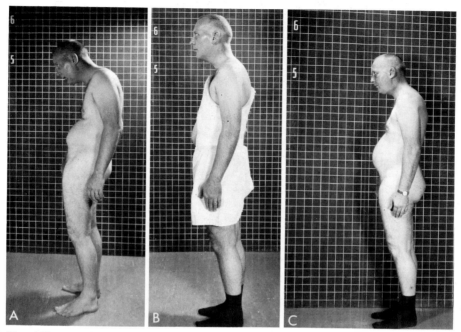

Figure 14–76. *A,* Preoperative photo. *B,* Six weeks postoperative, patient standing with body cast. *C,* Appearance one and a half years post-surgery.

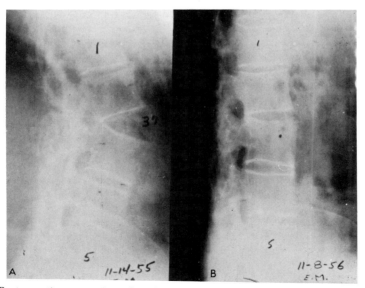

Figure 14–77. *A,* Postoperative correction of 37 degrees. *B,* One year later, much loss of correction. Patient was lost track of after six months, did not report back and was not faithful in wearing his brace.

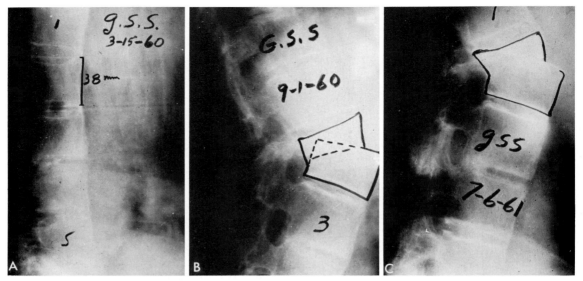

Figure 14–78. *A,* Preoperative roentgenogram. *B,* Two months postoperative, showing transverse split through vertebral body. Anterior intervertebral ligaments remain intact. *C,* One year postoperative, good correction and solid bony fusion of the L2 body fragments.

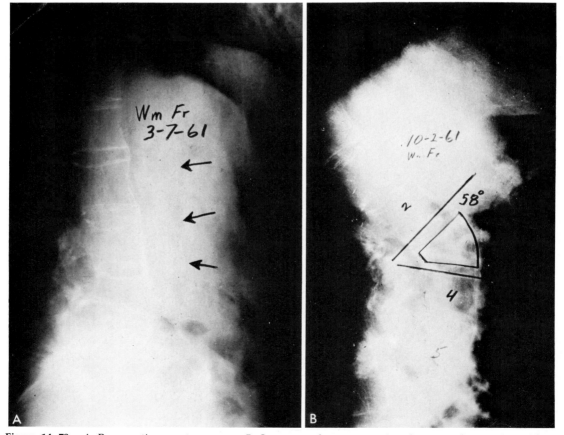

Figure 14–79. *A,* Preoperative roentgenogram. *B,* Seven months postoperative shows good correction with posterior body markedly crushed down and some increased anterior body height.

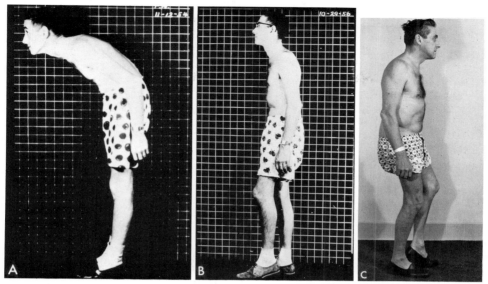

Figure 14–80. *A,* Preoperative photo in 1954, 31 years old. *B,* Photo one and a half years postoperative; note some flexion contracture of left hip. *C,* Photo of same patient 19 years post-surgery; note that spinal osteotomy correction has held up well. Left hip, because of pain and increasing deformity, has since required total hip-joint replacement, and so far he is doing well.

Careful selection of patients, with attention to indications, contraindications and surgical technique as well as to post-operative management will usually give satisfactory results. Specific contraindications to osteotomy are the older patient with already beginning senility changes and the patient with serious medical problems, either of which would offer a serious risk to the major surgical procedure. Also, correction of one or both marked hip flexion contractures should be done with total hip joint replacement arthroplasty before spinal osteotomy and conceivably could obviate the later need for spinal osteotomy.

Complications are not uncommon but, fortunately, most are non-fatal and temporary and, with careful attention to details, even some of these can be avoided.

Loss of initial surgical correction may occur, but this should be avoided by adequate and prolonged support by both body cast and brace for a minimal period of one year.

Reference

1. Smith-Petersen, M. N., Larson, C. B., and Aufranc, O. E.: Osteotomy of spine for correction of flexion deformity in rheumatoid arthritis. J. Bone Joint Surg. *27*:1–11, 1945.

CHAPTER 15

Tumors of the Spine

KENNETH C. FRANCIS, M.D.
New York University

INTRODUCTION

Neoplastic disease of the spine can be a most difficult and perplexing problem. The spine is a vast and most complicated segment of human anatomy and can be the source of practically any pathological process. It can be either the primary site of these conditions or, and frequently, the most important secondary anatomic manifestation of disease originating in other areas of the body. The problem is further magnified by the fact that the "organ not only is osseous in nature but is also the protector of a vital vascular and neurologic constituency. The problem is further complicated when one considers the many degenerative processes that commonly afflict the spine. The alert clinician, therefore, must be aware that neoplastic disease of the spine does exist, and must, at the very least, be suspicious of its existence. There are a number of clinical signs and symptoms that should make the clinician aware that a tumor may be the basic problem.

GENERAL CONSIDERATIONS

Primary tumors of the osseous spine are unusual, both benign and malignant. Benign tumors predominate in the child and young adult. It is extremely unusual to encounter a benign tumor of the spine in an adult over 30 years of age. Primary malignant tumors, however, are more common in the adult, and are an important segment of the problem.

The situation is completely reversed when consideration is focused upon metastatic disease. Certain malignant tumors of childhood can occasionally metastasize to the spine; however, the situation is vastly magnified in the adult. The author would emphasize that *any* tumor can metastasize to the osseous spine from any organ.[1] In the adult, this problem assumes major proportions related intimately to diagnosis and therapy.

DIAGNOSIS

Since the axial skeleton of a human being is prone to many non-neoplastic conditions, the orthopedic surgeon quite understandably may be lulled into a false sense of security. Nevertheless, there are certain signals that should make the clinician suspect that he may be confronted with a patient whose complaints do not conform to those of the common spine problem. These complaints frequently are subtle in nature and easily ignored. One purpose of this chapter is to elaborate the pitfalls the clinician may encounter. Accurate history, complete physical examination and adequate laboratory investigation, and intelligent interpretation of these results still remain the bases for excellent diagnosis, irrespective of the anatomical region involved.

HISTORY

A patient who is suffering from a neoplasm of the spine experiences pain. Pain patterns related to the spine can be most perplexing when compared with pain patterns arising in other areas of the osseous skeleton. The astute clinician must recognize that the spine is in reality only the "caretaker" of an immensely complicated anatomical, neurological and vascular community. The situation is further complicated by the integral "closeness" of the anatomy. Unless one recognizes these facts, symptoms may be considered inconsequential and thus ignored initially, only to become consequential at a later date. Neoplasms of the spine produce varying but *persistent* pain. The pain is not of a mechanical type; i.e., it is not relieved totally by rest, heat or massage. A thorough history is mandatory, since many patients who complain of recent neck or back pain may be unable to associate a significant history with the relevant problem at hand.

PHYSICAL EXAMINATION

It is impossible to enumerate all of the basic clinical findings relative to examination of a patient suffering from neoplastic disease of the spine. The manifestations are variable and perplexing, depending upon the region involved, the anatomic segment of the vertebra or vertebrae involved, and the specific etiology. Obviously, examination of a patient suffering from an isolated lesion in the pedicle of L4 with nerve root symptoms will differ from that of a patient suffering from widespread spinal disease secondary to breast carcinoma. There are, however, certain basic clinical findings that should at least alert the clinician to the possibility of neoplastic disease.[1] Regardless of the segment of spine involved, tenderness, in the author's experience, is practically always present. There may be little or no muscle spasm. One of the most important physical findings is the relative absence of positive straight leg raising in many patients with severe involvement of the spine from metastatic disease. When confronted with a patient suffering from severe back pain in whom the straight leg raising test is negative bilaterally, one should become keenly aware that the problem might be a tumor.

X-RAY DIAGNOSIS

The author cannot overemphasize the importance of adequate x-ray examination for any patient complaining of back or sacral pain. The examination should include anteroposterior lateral and oblique views of the area in question. If the patient's symptoms persist, another examination should be performed four to six weeks later. If any type of lesion is suspected on routine films, cone-down views should be obtained of the area, and tomography, if necessary, can be of great benefit. Phosphate bone scans have become quite accurate and are extremely useful to demonstrate lesions that may be completely invisible on routine x-rays. This technique is employed by the author for all types of particularly malignant tumors of bone. An example of a benign tumor for which bone scanning is important in the diagnosis is esosinophilic granuloma. Although only one vertebra might be involved, the scan can demonstrate other lesions, if present, in other areas of the skeleton.

BIOPSY

As in the management of any tumor in any location, the first necessity is to obtain a histologic diagnosis. This is most important in the treatment of the patient. It is obvious that one cannot treat a patient intelligently without a definite diagnosis. and blind dependence upon laboratory and roetgenographic findings results in less than optimal treatment for the patient under any circumstance. Therefore, it is the author's belief that, after thorough history, physical examination and laboratory data, a histologic diagnosis definitely must be obtained.

The common objective of all biopsy procedures is to obtain an actual tissue specimen for histologic study. In recent years, a number of methods for obtaining biopsy specimens without open surgical procedures have been developed. A most important procedure is the trocar biopsy of the spine, for which a number of different instruments have been designed. The specimen obtained actually is a core of tissue from within the trocar. Trocar biopsy of the spine has definite usefulness; however, the insertion of a large trocar under local anesthesia can be fraught with pain and disaster and in a not infrequent number of cases a definite diagnosis cannot be established. Those tumors of the spine most suitable for trocar biopsy involve the lower lumbar segments and the sacrum. The procedure should be performed under fluoroscopic and radiographic control, which is absolutely necessary in order to determine the exact position of the trocar. The use of general anesthesia has been beneficial to relieve the pain of this procedure and may well provide impetus for more extensive employment of this technique.

Open surgical biopsy of the spine has many advantages. The area to be biopsied and the pathological process involved can be visualized thoroughly and the exact type and extent of the disease process determined, which often cannot be done by x-ray alone. In addition, a satisfactory and diagnostic tissue specimen can be obtained. It is the author's practice to obtain a frozen section at the time of surgery, not for diagnosis but in order to be certain that the pathologist has been supplied with definitely representative tissue and not necrotic debris. If the latter is the case, further tissue can be obtained before the wound is closed.

Open surgical biopsy of the spine is the procedure of choice for relatively localized spinal tumors, particularly when the vertebral bodies are involved. A posterior surgical approach to tumors involving the posterior elements is best. The laminae are well visualized, and specimens can be easily obtained. If necessary, a laminectomy can be performed. Every vertebral body can be approached surgically. Of course, the technique varies with the segment under consideration. The exact technique and approaches available are fully presented in Chapter 4. Tumors of the lumbar and lower dorsal spine are best approached through a retroperitoneal kidney incision, making certain that the approach is anterior to the psoas muscle. This approach provides excellent exposure of the vertebral bodies and of the entire diseased process. The lower lumbar spine is best approached by performing a retroperitoneal incision just above and parallel to the inguinal ligament. The peritoneum can be retracted medially, the retroperitoneal space opened, and the entire lower three lumbar vertebrae easily biopsied. The sacrum is best approached surgically through a very small incision in the midline in order to make certain that any further surgical procedure that might be indicated has not been compromised. Biopsy of vertebral bodies in the dorsal area can be easily performed through a costotransversectomy, and representative tissue can be obtained. The cervical spine can be approached through an incision which parallels the anterior border of the sternocleidomastoid muscle, and the approach to

the vertebral bodies is made through the anterior triangle of the neck.

Obviously, the decision as to whether to perform a trocar or an open surgical biopsy depends upon the specific situation. In the author's opinion, the majority of localized and solitary tumors of the spine are best approached through the open surgical technique, which is safer and provides a far wider appreciation of the pathological situation existing at the time.

PRIMARY BENIGN TUMORS

Primary bone tumors of the vertebrae are infrequent. The common bone lesions of the extremities are not encountered in the same proportion in the spine. Whether this is in some way related to the embryonic mechanism is an intriguing question. For instance, 70 per cent of osteogenic sarcomas arise in the metaphysis of the distal femur and proximal tibia; rarely do we encounter such a tumor in the spine. Although we are discussing benign vertebral tumors, such a discrepancy is interesting.

OSTEOCHONDROMA. Both multiple and solitary osteochondromas occur, but are unusual, in the spine; however, when multiple osteochondromatosis exists, the spine can be affected. These tumors usually produce no significant clinical symptoms, and the x-ray is diagnostic (Fig. 15–1). They can be pedunculated or sessile, with the usual cartilaginous cap being present. Treatment is usually unnecessary unless there is nerve root compression due to the location of the lesion in the vertebra. If such is the case, surgical resection is indicated.

OSTEOID OSTEOMA. This lesion may be considered a benign neoplastic entity. Although its occurrence in the spine is unusual, the astute clinician should consider this possibility when a patient complains of persistent back pain relieved only by aspirin.[2] If the patient is a child or young adult with such symptoms and the x-ray is essentially negative, a trial of salicylates for a short time is certainly indicated. The lesion can produce a clinical scoliosis. If the typical complete response is present, radiographic investigation is indicated. The lesion invariably involves the facets and can be detected only with adequate radiographic examination. When this lesion is located in the spine the zone of sclerosis

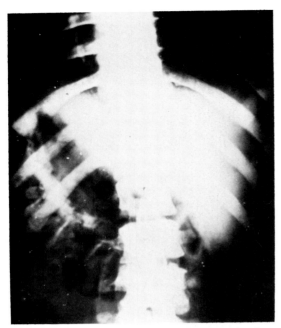

Figure 15–1. A patient with multiple osteochondromata and spine involvement.

around the nidus is not as dramatic as when the lesion is located in a long bone (Fig. 15–2). Occasionally, with adequate x-ray examination, the nidus can be detected. If the x-rays demonstrate sclerosis and some thickening in the region of the pedicle, further study is indicated. The treatment of osteoid osteoma is strictly surgical and consists of resection of the nidus.

ANEURYSMAL BONE CYST. This tumor was described by Jaffe and distinguished from the true giant cell tumor of bone. It can produce pain and can occur in the spine, usually involving the body. The characteristic "blowout" pattern on x-ray may not be present when this lesion is located in the spine, since the vertebral body may be collapsed, confusing the issue. Radiographically, the lesion is destructive, with a thin shell of bone which produces the characteristic x-ray appearance (Fig. 15–3). Surgical biopsy is mandatory. In the author's experience, x-ray therapy is the treatment of choice when the spine is the site of origin of this lesion. The tumor is radiosensitive with relatively small doses of radiation therapy, i.e., 2000 to 3000 rads. Surgery has little to offer. Bleeding can be considerable and makes surgical resection impossible.

OSTEOBLASTOMA. This tumor was reported by Dahlin as "giant osteoid osteoma" and by Jaffe as "osteoblastoma." Histologically it is closely related to the nidus of an osteoid osteoma, but on a much larger scale. The most frequent site of origin of this tumor is the axial skeleton. Radiographic characteristics can be variable, although usually the tumor is dense (Fig. 15–4). Experience in recent years has led the author to doubt that such tumors are basically benign. Although the rate of periph-

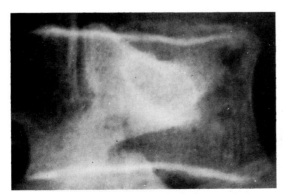

Figure 15–2. Osteoid osteoma involving the pedicle of a lumbar vertebra. Note minimal new bone production.

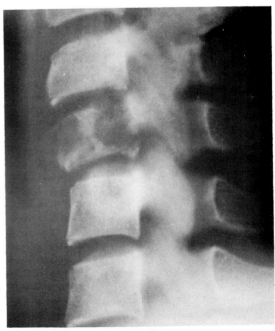

Figure 15–3. Aneurysmal bone cyst arising in the fourth cervical vertebra.

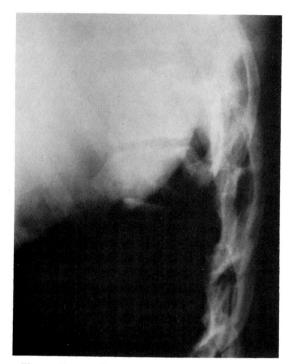

Figure 15–11. Osteogenic sarcoma, probably multi-centric in body of D12.

sive (Fig. 15–13). The diagnosis can be easily missed. Rectal examination usually reveals a somewhat lobulated and resilient posterior rectal mass. The rectum may be pushed anteriorly. For some reason anterior breakthrough from the sacrum occurs much earlier than breakthrough posteriorly.

The literature records only four cases of longterm survivals without recurrence among 180 cases of sacral chordomas.[3] Distant metastases may occur, but in no more than 10 per cent. Since the disease is slowly progressive and indolent, inadequate surgery has frequently been performed. The only treatment of a chordoma is total surgical resection. Obviously, this is almost always impossible when the spine itself is involved. Occasionally, removal of as much of the tumor as possi-

tumors progress at a leisurely pace, there may be a history of many years of discomfort.

Symptoms most often are produced by displacement phenomena rather than by rapid bony destruction. Pain, as previously mentioned, is the most frequent initial symptom. The pain may be mild and has often been ascribed to arthritis or some other degenerative process. X-rays disclose purely lytic destruction of the bone involved, be it the body of a vertebra or the sacrum. Unfortunately, these tumors are always more extensive than the x-ray would suggest. When these tumors arise in the vertebrae, as mentioned previously, symptoms are due to compression of structures in their vicinity. When the sacrum is involved, as the tumor progresses, nerve root neuropathies and bladder and rectal incompetence become evident. The most frequent and important physical finding is a presacral mass which may be felt only by rectal examination. The importance of an adequate rectal examination cannot be overemphasized, since the lesion in the sacrum may be small on the x-ray; however, the breakthrough anteriorly can be quite exten-

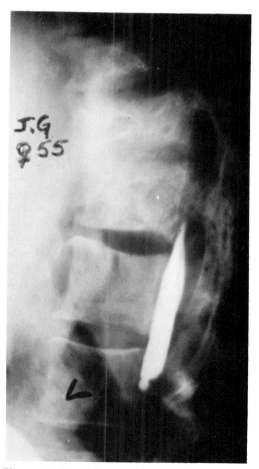

Figure 15–12. Collapse of body of D12 caused by Paget's disease. Such collapse is indicative of malignant change.

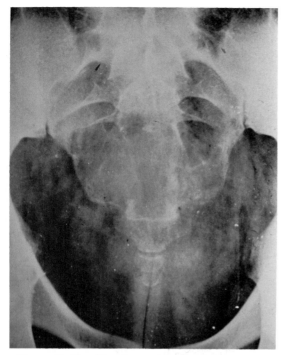

Figure 15–13. Chordoma of sacrum. A large anterior mass was present.

ble to relieve complications from pressure may provide the patient with a period of comfort; however, the author knows of no long-term survivors in this situation. In the past, sacral chordomas were resected using the posterior approach only. This approach to these tumors has been almost totally useless. It is impossible totally to remove a chordoma of the sacrum using the posterior approach, since the anterior mass, which is almost always present, cannot be appreciated, and the margin of resection is severely compromised. The combined abdominal-sacral approach has proved to be a more satisfactory technique for radical resection of these tumors.[3] The patient is placed on his side on the operating table. A laparotomy is performed by the surgeon, who mobilizes all of the vital structures anterior to the presacral mass. In addition, the actual extent of the anterior mass can then be easily appreciated. The tumor is approached posteriorly and resected, with all of the anterior structures mobilized and protected. It is felt by the author that only in this manner can these tumors be satisfactorily removed. It must be stated that if a sacral chordoma ex-

tends into the first or second sacral segment, the tumor is most often inoperable.

METASTATIC TUMORS

It should be emphasized at the outset that any malignant tumor can metastasize to bone, and the spine is no exception. Indeed, in adults over 50 years of age metastatic involvement of the spine is not at all infrequent and is a major problem for the orthopedic surgeon. Although, as mentioned earlier in the text, primary malignant tumors arising in the spine, other than multiple myeloma, are rare, metastatic disease involving the spine is not.[1] Since the majority of these patients are adults or older adults the diagnosis of a metastatic lesion is often both difficult and elusive. An adequate history is of prime importance when a patient complains of vague neck or back pain. If an adequate history is not obtained and the presence of a previous malignancy is not indicated, many patients are relegated to treatment for arthritis or other degenerative disabilities so common in our population today (Fig. 15–14 and 15–15). Therefore, a high index of suspicion is of paramount importance.

As mentioned previously, the most important symptom is pain. The pain pattern is definitely different when compared to nonneoplastic conditions. Pain frequently is variable and usually not relieved completely by rest. Findings on physical examination are variable, of course, depending upon the site of disease. In the author's experience, metastatic disease involving the cervical spine does not produce tilting of the neck as in the classic torticollis. Traction rarely relieves the pain, and most often increases it. Radicular symptoms may or may not be present. Metastatic disease involving the dorsal spine may manifest itself as radicular pain, and frequently there are few objective findings. Patients suffering from metastatic disease of the lumbar spine most commonly present with pain increased by motion. It is the author's experience that very frequently in a patient with severe low-back pain from metastatic disease the straight leg raising test is completely negative. This finding has been extremely important in producing the index of suspicion. Radiographic findings most commonly are those of destruction, with varying amounts of new bone formation.

Metastatic cancer of the prostate frequently involves the spine and is typified by

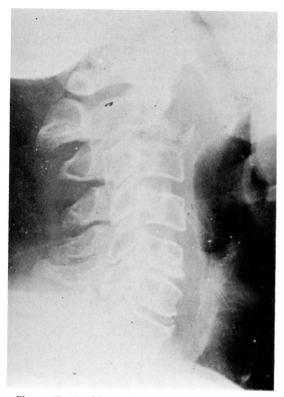

Figure 15–14. Metastatic carcinoma of second cervical vertebra. Severe pain was present. There was no neurologic complication.

tial diagnosis is that of multiple myeloma. Both conditions can be radiographically identical. As discussed previously, pertinent laboratory data frequently will rule out one or the other. Establishing a histologic diagnosis is important. If a patient presents with no evidence of disease other than a lesion in the spine, a biopsy should be performed to establish the exact diagnosis. Since patients suffering from metastatic disease are being more effectively palliated at the present time, such a factual diagnosis is extremely important. Obviously, treatment of a patient with a metastatic lesion from the breast will be medically different from that for a patient suffering from a lymphoma. This is also true of metastatic prostate cancer. Obviously, if there is disease in the spine and there are other lesions elsewhere in the skeleton, biopsy of a more simply approached lesion would certainly be indicated.

Treatment

The treatment of metastatic disease in the spine is a complicated problem and depends upon the individual situation present. In general, localized lesions in the spine should be treated with x-ray therapy. Symptomatically, many patients respond to such therapy, despite the origin of the tumor. If there is wide-

the common purely osteoblastic lesions. Any segment of a vertebra may be involved, including the lamina. Pathological fractures occur frequently, the typical fracture being that of collapse of the vertebra in varying degrees. It is important to differentiate the type of collapse caused by metastatic cancer from the typical osteoporotic wedge compression fracture and traumatic wedge compression. The discs are, at least initially, more resistant to the disease process than bone. For this reason very often the disc spaces are completely intact. This is not always the situation, however, since a diseased vertebra can actually collapse around the disc, producing the radiographic appearance of a loss or decrease in the disc space. It is extremely important to examine the pedicles, since not infrequently one or both pedicles of a vertebra may be totally absent on the AP x-ray, owing to destruction. Not infrequently, one observes destruction of the pedicles with no abnormality of the vertebal bodies. The most important differen-

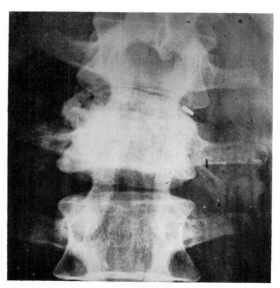

Figure 15–15. Metastatic carcinoma of second lumbar vertebra, postlaminectomy. Note absence of pedicles.

spread involvement of the spine, only the most symptomatic area should be treated with x-ray therapy. In the author's experience, these patients do not tolerate large, heavy and bulky braces. Some type of light support is sometimes of great symptomatic benefit to the patient. As mentioned previously, appropriate medical treatment for individual tumors is of extreme importance. Complications of metastatic disease of the spine, other than pain, are neurological. It is important to emphasize that paraplegia which may occur in the presence of metastatic disease of a vertebra is the result of pressure from the tumor itself upon the spinal cord. The paraplegia is *not* the result of a mechanical injury to the spinal cord, such as traumatic fracture. For this reason stabilization of vertebrae with attempted fusion is illogical. How can one expect a spinal fusion in the lumbar area to stabilize a vertebra when it requires at least six months for the fusion to become solid? Obviously, the disease progresses and the fusion is useless. The use of methylmethacrylate cement to stabilize vertebrae in the presence of metastatic disease is also illogical. One must always remember that the disease process progresses even while being treated, and that we are not dealing with a stable situation, as when treating a traumatic problem.

References

1. Francis, K. C., and Hutter, V. P.: Neoplasms of the spine in the aged. Clin. Orthop. 26:54–66, 1963.
2. Greiberger, R. H.: Osteoid osteoma of the spine. Radiology 75:232–236, 1960.
3. Localio, A., Francis, K. C., and Rossano, P. G.: Abdomino-sacral resection of sacrococcygeal chordoma. Ann. Surg. 166:394–402, 1967.
4. Gorji, J. and Francis, K. C.: Multiple myeloma. Clin. Orthop. 38:106–119, 1965.
5. Meyer, J. E., and Schulz, M. D.: "Solitary" myeloma of bone. Cancer 34:438–440, 1974.
6. Francis, K. C., Higinbotham, N. L., and Coleg, B. L.: Primary reticulum cell sarcoma of bone. Surg. Gynec. Obstet. 99:142–146, 1954.
7. Dahlin, D. C.: Bone Tumors. Springfield, Charles C Thomas Co., 1957.

CHAPTER 16

Intraspinal Neoplasms

FREDERICK A. SIMEONE, M.D.
Pennsylvania Hospital and University of Pennsylvania

There are only a few kinds of cells within the spinal canal which can become neoplastic. Metastases to the spinal cord itself are extremely rare. When metastatic malignancy does enter the spinal column, it usually spreads from the marrow of the vertebral structures or by direct extension from a nearby viscus. Metastatic tumors within the spinal canal, therefore, are principally extradural, since the dura mater seems to form a natural barrier through which malignant extension is most rare. The extradural venous plexus is rarely involved in tumor formation, but it may be a site for hematogenous metastatic spread. The remaining contents of the spinal canal are the cord, meninges and spinal nerve roots. As such, intraspinal neoplasms lend themselves to a convenient classification, based on their relation to the dura and the spinal cord. Considered in order of frequency this includes: (1) extradural, (2) intradural-extramedullary, (3) intramedullary.

LOCATION AND CLINICAL CORRELATION

Extradural Tumors

These are by far the commonest tumors of the spinal canal. As mentioned above, they invade the intraspinal space from contiguous structures (Fig. 16–1). Therefore, they are virtually all metastatic. Their mode of presentation and the evolution of subsequent neurologic

signs can alert the wary diagnostician from history alone. Pain is the hallmark of a metastatic extradural tumor, although symptoms of cord and nerve root compression occasionally predominate.

PAIN. Axial pain, which is often accurately localized by the patient to the site of the tumor, is commonly the first symptom. Occasionally a nerve root may be involved so that more remote radicular symptoms are present. Thoracic spinal metastases are most common. This is likely explained by the higher number of thoracic vertebrae, and further by the proximity of the thoracic cord to the lung and breast, which are the commonest organs of origin of spinal metastases.

The initial complaint may be gnawing pain in the middle of the spine. The discomfort is usually unrelenting and aggravated by activity. As the symptoms progress the pain becomes less tolerable and is refractory to non-narcotic medication. The patient must lie on his side in order to sleep. Radiating pain may be sufficient to mislead the physician along alternative paths. Discomfort in the distribution of the seventh to ninth thoracic nerve roots on the right side is often mistaken for gall bladder disease. When lower nerve roots are involved, other gastrointestinal disorders are implicated. The axial pain usually supersedes radiating pain in severity. As the neoplasm increases in size specific neurologic deficit can result. The rapidity of development of subsequent neurologic findings after the onset of the axial pain differentiates this tumor from

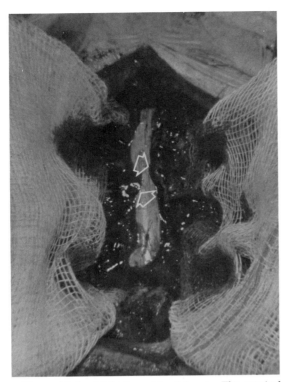

Figure 16–1. Metastic epidural tumor. The cervical laminae, C4 through C7, have been removed. The central area shows normal dura mater which is being invaded, from either side, by projections of beefy adenocarcinoma (arrows). The tumor could be dissected easily from the dura, but it extended into the vertebral bodies anteriorly.

intradural neoplasms. A few weeks after the onset of the spine pain, the patient may describe symptoms of spinal cord or specific nerve root pressure.

CORD COMPRESSION SYMPTOMS. At first the patient has difficulty in maintaining balance. His gait may become wide based. It may be more difficult to walk at night than during the day. He will find that his legs tire after a short walk. The spinal cord symptoms usually develop bilaterally or, if one leg is affected first, the difference in time is ordinarily a matter of days.

Urinary symptoms develop simultaneously or just after leg weakness. The patient will experience urgency, dribbling incontinence and, finally, lower abdominal distention with retention. Sensory symptoms appear late and are rarely troublesome. He may notice a numb or "unreal" feeling in his lower extremities. Occasionally a patient will volunteer that

he is unable to test the temperature of the bath water with his toes. Despite marked loss in pain and temperature sensation, however, patients rarely complain of these. Incidental injury in the painless segment is rare.

RADICULAR SYMPTOMS. Pain is the principal symptom of nerve root compression within the spinal canal. It invariably precedes symptomatic weakness. Some time after the development of pain, the patient may experience numbness in the extremities or the torso. The distribution of pain and numbness can accurately localize the affected nerve root. Rarely, root pain is present in the absence of spine discomfort, particularly with laterally placed tumors. The patient will frequently seek relief by the application of heat or ointments; it is not uncommon to see permanent skin changes resulting from vigorous use of these remedies. Because nerve root compression can be aggravated by movement, the extremity may present the smooth, waxy skin of disuse.

The motor projection of thoracic nerve roots into intercostal nerves produces no noticeable weakness when affected. In an extremity, however, motor radiculopathy soon becomes noticeable. Focal weakness, fasciculations, and atrophy evolve in that order.

Intradural-Extramedullary Tumors

Because these tumors frequently grow in relation to a nerve root, radicular and spine pain are common (Fig. 16–2). They frequently precede by months or years the development of signs of spinal cord compression. For reasons which are not understood, a patient may suffer pain at night yet be totally asymptomatic during the day. A syndrome of spinal or radicular night pain, therefore, can lead the suspecting examiner to further studies early in the course of the tumor. Since the vast majority of intradural-extramedullary tumors are meningiomas or neurofibromas, the neurological clinical syndrome often progresses very slowly. The symptoms of difficulty with gait, urinary retention and radiculopathy proceed in variable order depending on the location of the tumor (Fig. 16–3). The predilection of intraspinal meningiomas for middle-aged women might sharpen slightly the index of suspicion. Often the slowly evolving neurologic syndrome is attributed to other causes, such as diabetic neuropathy, primary

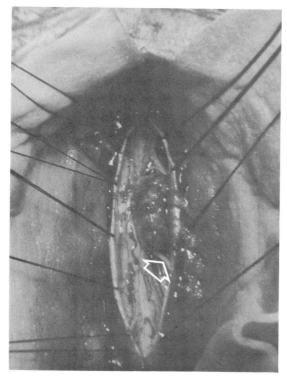

Figure 16–2. A dorsally placed meningioma compresses and deviates the spinal cord. Note the stretching of the nerve root which was responsible for radicular symptoms (arrow). The entire tumor could be removed without damage to the spinal cord.

cend ipsilaterally in the posterior columns of the cord. Therefore, it is possible for a centrally placed lesion to affect pain and temperature only, in segmental fashion, without altering light touch or position sense. This "segmental differential sensory deficit" is characteristic of an intramedullary tumor. Careful examination will outline a bandlike area of reduced pain and temperature extending several segments below the tumor. In their most common location, the cervical cord, this annoying deficit will present in the hands and can lead to an early diagnosis. Subsequently, long tract signs, weakness and incontinence develop. The evolution of these symptoms is almost invariably slow, and this fact, associated with the absence of pain, is responsible for misdiagnoses such as multiple sclerosis and cervical spondylosis. Extensive intramedullary gliomas, involving the entire length of the spinal cord, have been successfully removed.[9]

lateral sclerosis or cervical spondylosis. The clinician may thus accept the lesion as incurable. Despite this, the possibilities for excellent recovery even in the face of advanced myelopathy following removal of the tumor are so great that the examiner is obligated to consider these tumors whenever feasible.

Intramedullary Tumors

The rarest of the three basic types, intramedullary tumors can progress insidiously and are often painless. The characteristic feature of these lesions, though not always present, relates to their anatomic location within the center of the spinal cord. Fibers which control pain and temperature cross in the spinal cord several dermatomes above their point of entry. Nerve fibers subserving light touch and proprioception, however, as-

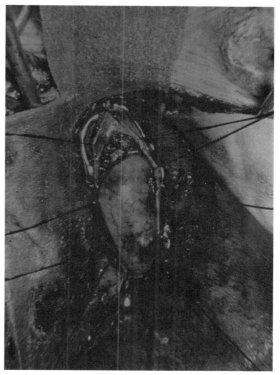

Figure 16–3. A high lumbar laminectomy with open dura retracted by traction sutures. There is a huge intraspinal neurofibroma which completely blocks the canal. Immediately above the tumor distended veins are further evidence of compression.

HISTOLOGIC TYPES OF INTRASPINAL NEOPLASMS

Extradural

As mentioned earlier, extradural tumors are principally metastatic. The commonest sites of origin of these lesions are from carcinoma of the lung in males and carcinoma of the breast in females. Prostatic carcinoma and tumors of the gastrointestinal tract, as well as thyroid carcinomas, are commonly seen. Occasionally tissue of reticuloendothelial origin may present in the spinal canal, and epidural lesions are not uncommon in patients with lymphomas, multiple myeloma, etc.

Intradural-Extramedullary Tumors

Fortunately, the vast majority of tumors in this location are either meningiomas or neurofibromas (the latter tumors are also called neurilemmomas, schwannomas, etc.) Both of these tumor types are benign, well encapsulated, and separate easily from the spinal cord. They are usually small, rounded tumors which produce neurological signs relatively late in their course, because of their very slow growth. Meningiomas are far more common in the thoracic region (81 per cent) than in the cervical (16 per cent) or the lumbar (3 per cent) regions. Sacral meningiomas are extremely unusual. Neurofibromas, on the other hand, are relatively evenly distributed in the cervical, thoracic, and lumbar areas, and sacral neurofibromas are occasionally demonstrated. Thoracic neurofibromas comprise 39 per cent of the total, lumbar 32 per cent and cervical 23 per cent.[7] Neurofibromas can originate from Schwann cells along nerves near the nerve-nerve root junction, which is in the intervertebral foramen. Consequently, they may present both as intradural-extramedullary tumors and as extradural masses within and without the spinal canal (so-called "dumbbell tumor").

Occasionally, malignant tumors which "seed" from other sites in the central nervous system will be found in an intradural-extramedullary location. They are generally classified by the location of the cell of origin, rather than the site of the intraspinal metastasis. Similarly, ependymomas, which begin within the substance of the spinal cord, can grow outside as well but are also classified with intramedullary tumors because of the location of the original cells.

Intramedullary Tumors

Intramedullary tumors are the least common of the three types. Their distribution includes 17.5 per cent in the cervical region, 32.5 per cent in the thoracic region and 47.5 per cent in the lumbar region.[7]

These tumors are usually derived from one of the types of glial cells, and, therefore, are broadly called gliomas. Glial cells make up the supporting structure of the substance of the central nervous system. Ependymomas, from cells which line the ventricular system, and astrocytomas, from cells which seem important in structural and biochemical support of the central nervous system, are the commonest intramedullary tumors and occur with about equal frequency. Other intramedullary tumors are rare. Metastatic tumors to the substance of the spinal cord are, surprisingly, most unusual.

Less Common Neoplasms

CHORDOMA. Chordomas of the spinal canal take origin from the verterbral bodies or sacrum. The cell of origin is common with that which ultimately differentiates into the cartilaginous component of the spinal canal. These tumors, therefore, tend to destroy adjacent bone, and typical roentgenographic findings are usually present by the time symptoms develop. Spinal chordomas can be relatively slow growing, encapsulated, and susceptible to complete removal when accessible. As sacrococcygeal tumors in children they can lead to destruction of the cauda equina and its roots if left untreated. More malignant versions of this tumor can progress fairly rapidly and produce symptomatic and myelographic signs appropriate for the diagnosis of metastatic epidural disease.[11]

ANGIOBLASTOMA. Angioblastomas can develop as true neoplasms of the vascular structures of the spinal cord. They are fairly well encapsulated masses of abundant capillaries lined by endothelial cells. Central degeneration can lead to cystlike changes in these tumors.

HEMANGIOMA. These are ordinarily present from birth and may not change significantly in size. Both angioblastomas and hemangiomas are subject to spontaneous internal hemorrhage with attendant spinal cord damage. These lesions may be seen together. Both are seen with increased frequency in patients who have other evidence of vascular tumor formation in the eye (von Hippel-Lindau disease) or skin (Wyburn-Mason disease). Elective surgical intervention is considered only when there is evidence of progressive neurologic deficit. Occasionally, emergency surgery may be required to evacuate an intraneoplastic hemorrhage.

LIPOMA. Intraspinal lipomas may become symptomatic at any age, though they are thought to be present from birth. One might expect, then, that they would be more prevalent in childhood. These masses are usually extensions of subcutaneous lipomas for which visible evidence on the skin of the back is often available. A defect in the adjacent lamina through which the lipoma extends into the spinal canal is frequently seen. If first treated in adulthood, surgical correction of this lesion may be attended with significant risk of increased neurologic deficit.

TUMORS OF BLOOD-FORMING ORGANS. Leukemias, sarcomas and lymphomas can present as extradural tumors in the spinal canal. A relatively rapid, painful course with progressive neurologic deficit may be expected if they are not treated. Although there is no lymphatic tissue in the spinal canal, lymphomas are frequently found here. Metastatic spread from the marrow of adjacent bone or viscus is the source of the lesion. Their course follows the lines of other metastatic tumors, but they are separated here to emphasize their radiosensitivity, a factor to be discussed with treatment of cord tumors.

EPIDERMOID TUMORS. Epidermoid tumors of the spinal canal are seen with greater frequency in the lumbar region, overlying the cauda equina. They are also seen with greater frequency in patients who have had a lumbar puncture performed at some time in the past. Some theorize, with good statistical substantiation, that these tumors originate from clusters of skin which are deposited in the lumbar theca incident to puncture with a hollow needle. They are well-circumscribed tumors whose contents are of a cheesy nature, consistent with desquamated epithelial cells.[8]

AGE DISTRIBUTION

The age distribution of Elsberg's 275 original cases was as follows:[3]

10 years or less	5 cases
11 to 20 years	28 cases
21 to 30 years	41 cases
31 to 40 years	60 cases
41 to 50 years	70 cases
51 to 60 years	47 cases
61 to 70 years	24 cases

This pattern would follow today, though increased longevity has mirrored the discovery of more tumors in older age groups. This same longevity factor has increased the incidence of metastatic spinal cord tumors in comparison with other types whose incidence has remained the same.

Intraspinal tumors in children are rare. Ford found three cases of spinal cord tumors among 70,000 patient records reviewed from the Pediatrics Department of the Johns Hopkins Hospital.[4] In 1942, Hamby was able to collect 214 cases from the literature.[8] In 1960, Rand and Rand reported 72 personal cases in a series which remains the most detailed analysis of intraspinal tumors of childhood.[12] In adulthood the ratio between intraspinal and intracranial tumors is roughly 1 to 4, whereas in childhood this ratio can be expected to be around 1 to 20.

RELATIVE INCIDENCE OF SPINAL CORD TUMORS

Under ordinary circumstances the neurosurgical practice will yield 10 brain tumors for every spinal cord tumor. Distribution of tumors by location in relation to the dura is as follows:

Intraspinal Tumors
A. *Extradural.* Over 50 per cent of all spinal cord tumors; most are metastatic.
B. *Intradural.* 50 per cent or less of all spinal tumors.
   1. *Extramedullary* (71 per cent of all intradural tumors).
     a. Neurofibroma   27%
     b. Meningioma   23%
     c. Sarcoma   10%
     d. Other forms cell-type (each less than 2%)   11%
       Lymphoma, epidermoid, lipoma, melanoma, neuroblastoma, etc.
   2. *Intramedullary* (29 per cent of all intradural tumors)
     a. Ependymoma   8%
     b. Astrocytoma   9%
     c. Others (each less than 2%)   12%

These include lipoma, epidermoid, teratoma, dermoid, carcinoma, melanoma, hemangioblastoma, etc.

LABORATORY STUDIES

PROTEIN DETERMINATION. With the exception of roentgenographic studies, laboratory data frequently add little to the diagnosis of spinal cord tumors. Elevations in spinal fluid protein may be expected if a partial or complete block is present. Similarly, neurofibromas in the spinal subarachnoid space are capable of producing phenomenal elevations in spinal fluid protein. When the diagnosis of spinal cord tumors is seriously considered, however, the lumbar puncture may best be performed in conjunction with myelography. Because the myelogram is the last word in the diagnosis of these tumors, protein determinations rarely suffice as the sole indication for lumbar puncture. The same is true of manometric studies (Queckenstedt test), which may be attended with some risk when the tumor is firmly impacted against the spinal cord.

ELECTROMYOGRAPHY is rarely of value in the diagnosis of spinal cord tumors, though it may isolate a single nerve root compression syndrome if fibrillation is present.

RADIOLOGICAL ASPECTS. Spinal cord tumors may be suspected on plain X-rays because of the propensity of some to erode adjacent bone. Calcification within the tumor, or other direct evidence of an intraspinal mass, is rarely seen.

The secondary effects of pressure erosion are of several types:

Erosion of the Pedicle. Because of the effects of chronic intraspinal pressure, the pedicle immediately adjacent to the tumor can be thinned. Under these circumstances, the pedicle on the anteroposterior view is frequently of smaller dimensions than its neighbors, but its bony cortical margin is usually preserved. The preservation of this cortical margin is a sign of chronicity, in contradistinction to actual destruction of the architecture of the pedicle as seen in metastatic disease.

Destruction of Vertebral Architecture. Malignant tumors which metastasize to the vertebral bone marrow or otherwise extend from paraspinal organs can destroy any portion of the spine. With significant destruction, the portions of bone become radiolucent and the cortical margin is lost. This is a sign of

a rapidly progressive malignant tumor. In contrast to pressure erosion of the pedicle, as mentioned above, in this situation the entire pedicle is frequently absent on routine films. Secondary collapse of the vertebral body often follows such destruction (Fig. 16–4).

Widening of the Intervertebral Foramen. This is a specific abnormality generally restricted to neurofibromas which leave the spinal canal along a nerve root. In the oblique view the affected intervertebral foramen appears uniformly dilated when compared to the adjacent foramina.

Myelographic Changes in Intraspinal Tumors

Tumors in the three characteristic locations described above have very specific myelographic appearances. With high accuracy, the examiner can combine a myelographic appearance with the clinical pattern of presentation, as described above, and predict benign or malignant neoplasm. Virtually all extradural tumors are malignant, most extramedullary-intradural tumors are benign, and solid intramedullary mass lesions are mostly malignant. A myelogram which can delineate these loci has important therapeutic implications.

EXTRADURAL TUMORS. Most patients on whom a symptomatic extradural tumor is found will show a complete myelographic block. Initially, the back pain is usually insufficient to warrant myelographic study. With the onset of neurologic deficit, the spinal cord is grossly compressed and the myelographic contrast material may not pass this point. When a complete block is expected, the myelogram must be performed with minimal alteration of cerebrospinal fluid dynamics. Fluid should only be removed if subsequent chemical or bacteriological studies are expected to have therapeutic implications.

Extradural tumors usually produce a "paint brush" myelographic block (Fig. 16–4). The dura on one side of the cord is pushed up against the spinal cord itself, which is, in turn, compressed against the contralateral dura. These combined points of compression form the irregular edges of the myelographic block and will have different radiographical densities. The spinal cord shadow is usually deviated from the margins of the spinal canal in one view. This is because the tumor comes from the vertebral body, pedicle or lamina. If

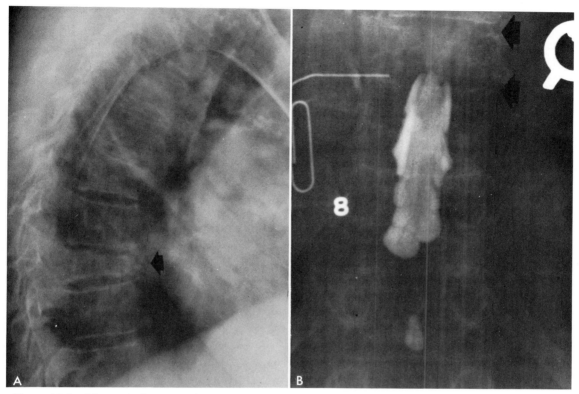

Figure 16–4. Metastatic disease to thoracic vertebrae, with collapse and spinal cord compression.
A demonstrates marked loss of stature of the T10 vertebral body in a patient with a known carcinoma of the breast.
B is a myelogram which indicates a complete epidural block with typical "paint brush" appearance. The paper clip marks the site of the block for ease of surgical identification of the appropriate level. The large arrows are placed at the superior and inferior limits of the collapsed vertebra.

surgical correction is contemplated, it is important to determine the relationship between the tumor mass and the spinal cord itself. Extradural tumors which do not produce a complete block often appear as smooth, broad-based defects, impinging on one side of the myelographic column.

INTRADURAL-EXTRAMEDULLARY TUMORS. These tumors also frequently produce a complete block by the time of myelography. Margins of the block are frequently smooth or lobulated. One gets the impression that the contrast material is in direct contact with the tumor, which is distinct from the myelographic appearance of extradural tumors. Edges of the tumor mass can be outlined as it impinges against and deviates the spinal cord. The spinal cord shadow itself is often pushed over to one side of the spinal column and, frequently, stretched nerve roots are visible above or below the tumor shadow.

Figure 16–5 demonstrates the characteristic appearance of a thoracic meningioma. Because of the complete block only the lower margin of the tumor is shown. The true "outlining" effect is possible when the tumor does not produce complete block, as seen in Figure 16–6. This high cervical meningioma is completely surrounded by contrast material and its lobulations are easily demonstrable. Not opposite the spinal cord, but lying free in the subarachnoid space, cauda equina intradural extramedullary tumors produce a caplike defect (Fig. 16–7). Virtually all tumors in this location are benign, though in younger patients one may see ependymomas of the cauda equina which produce a defect myelographically indistinguishable from benign tumors. These tumors connect to the substance of the cord and are thus classified with intramedullary neoplasms.

INTRAMEDULLARY TUMORS. A vast ma-

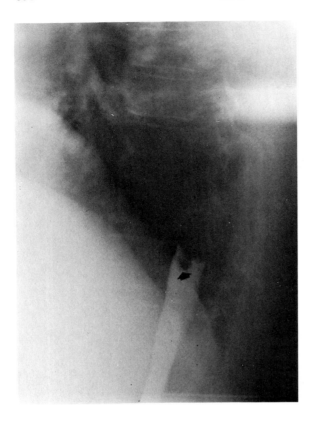

Figure 16–5. Intradural-extramedullary tumor (meningioma). The myelogram outlines a smooth, rounded block with a typical "cap" effect often seen with intradural-extramedullary tumors. In addition, the arrow indicates a separate lobular projection of the tumor mass.

jority of intramedullary spinal cord tumors are gliomas, which indicates that they arise from cells which support and nourish neural tissue. Most are glioma subtypes, astrocytoma or ependymoma, though other neoplasms of gliomatous origin such as oligodendroglioma, and medulloblastoma, are found. Ependymomas most frequently originate at the conus medullaris and grow into the lumbar theca. As described above, ependymomas in this location can have the myelographic appearance of intradural-extramedullary tumors. Spinal cord gliomas elsewhere, however, simply produce a fusiform dilatation of the spinal cord shadow which has a characteristic myelographic appearance (Fig. 16–8). Not infrequently an extradural mass lesion, immediately anterior or posterior to the spinal cord can deviate the cord against the dura and widen it in such a fashion that on a single anterior-posterior view, one might suspect an intramedullary lesion. Carefully performed lateral myelographic views, however, make this important distinction.

One cannot discuss intramedullary spinal cord tumors without mention of syringomyelia. This entity is characterized by the development of a fluid-filled intramedullary cavity which is myelographically indistinguishable from a spinal cord tumor. Cavities most commonly occur in the cervical region and are basically of two types. In the first, the cavity is filled with spinal fluid which may communicate with the intracranial ventricular system. This lesion is confusingly called hydromyelia. It is considered a developmental abnormality and, although it produces a symmetric dilatation of the spinal cord, it is rarely associated with a complete myelographic block. The second form of syringomyelia contains a yellow, proteinaceous material within a gliotic cavity. It is frequently found in direct contact with, and occasionally in the same spinal cord but remote from, an intramedullary glioma. Myelographic distinction between syringomyelia and an intramedullary spinal cord tumor is often impossible, and surgical exploration is usually required. Occasionally it is possible to manipulate the contrast material into the ventricular system then down into the "hydromyelic" cavity, thereby confirming the diagnosis of a cystic intramedullary lesion filled with spinal fluid.

Important Factors in the Performance of a Myelogram

Myelography in spinal cord tumors is not a routine procedure. Maximum information can be gained with minimum injury to the patient, and specific steps during the procedure must be tailored to the information required. The following points must be reemphasized to avoid neurologic disasters associated with myelography in the face of spinal cord tumor, and to provide the surgeon with maximum information he may need to attack the mass:

1. If a complete block is suspected, remove no spinal fluid and insert a minimum amount of contrast material (1 ml) initially. More contrast material may be added later if the block is not present.

2. Do not remove the contrast material if a complete block is present, or if a partial block is present in the face of advanced neurologic deficit.

3. Place a radiopaque marker over the lesion and make a permanent x-ray film which shows the relationship of the two. Then scratch the skin under the marker. In certain patients whose skin might be expected to move signficantly, it is not extreme to insert a hypodermic needle into a spinous process over the block then cut the needle flush with the skin. This needle, of course, will be removed at surgery.

4. If the point of myelographic block does not correlate with the neurologic syndrome, one might assume that more than one lesion is present. Contrast material must then be injected into the cisterna magna at the base of the skull so that it may outline a higher lesion. A cisternal injection is frequently required when the upper extent of a long tumor must be visualized.

5. Any significant change in the patient's neurologic status following myelography indicates that an emergency decompres-

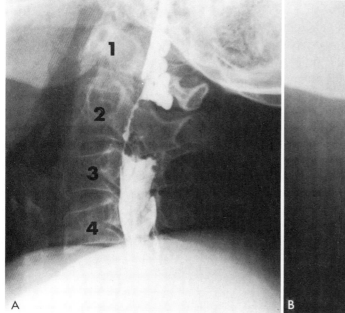 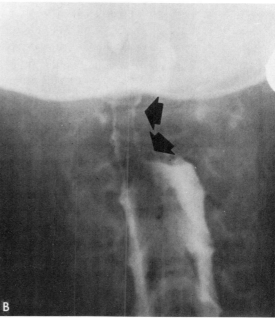

Figure 16–6. Laterally placed high cervical meningioma.
A clearly outlines a globular tumor mass in an intradural-extramedullary location opposite the second cervical vertebra. The typical appearance of an intradural lesion is emphasized by the quality with which the tumor is outlined because the contrast material comes in direct contact with the mass itself. *B,* Anterior-posterior view of the same myelogram indicating contrast material between the tumor mass itself and the spinal cord. The myelogram, in its inferior portion, indicates that the spinal cord is deviated away from the tumor.

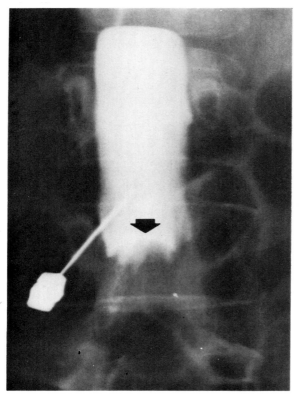

Figure 16–7. Intradural-extramedullary tumor with confusing myelogram. The myelogram indicates a complete block opposite L4 in a patient with a long-standing history of back and radicular pain. The block essentially has a "paint brush" appearance and initially might be confused with an extradural lesion. Careful inspection of the nature of the block, however, indicates that there is a smooth "cap"-shaped defect whose apex is opposite the arrow. Multiple views indicated that the irregular effect was due to contrast material streaming around the sides of the tumor mass.

sion might be required. This is particularly true when a complete block is present.

6. Visualize the tumor from several aspects, and do not omit the lateral view. This is particularly true with symmetric dilatations of the spinal cord in which an intramedullary tumor is suspected in the anteroposterior film.

SURGICAL TREATMENT OF INTRASPINAL TUMORS

Surgical treatment of spinal cord tumors was not considered seriously until the end of the nineteenth century. Although a few cases

with operation on the spine to alleviate compression from injured vertebrae had been reported, it was not until 1887 when Charles Gowers diagnosed neoplastic compression of the spinal cord, and Sir Victor Horsley successfully removed a cord tumor for the first time.[5] Twenty-four years later, C. A. Elsberg published his classic *Tumors of the Spinal Cord*. By the time of his final revision of this book (1941) this author had performed surgery on 275 intraspinal tumors.[3]

The treatment of intradural-extramedullary tumors is complete removal, utilizing the gentlest possible technique. The surgeon is encouraged to exenterate the center of the tumor prior to its excision, to facilitate gentle manipulation of its mass and the adjacent spinal

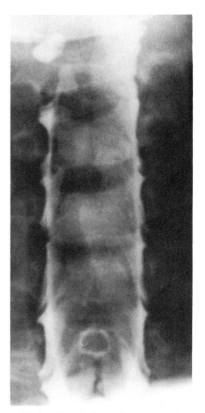

Figure 16–8. Cervical myelogram with intramedullary spinal cord tumor. Note that the subarachnoid space on the lateral surfaces of the spinal cord is extremely thin. The spinal cord shadow occupies almost the entire spinal canal. The subarachnoid space widens at the lower cervical level, which indicates the bottommost extent of the tumor mass. The mass itself occupies most of the cervical spinal cord superiorly. Plain anterior-posterior x-rays indicated widening of the interpedunculate distances.

cord. Remarkable improvement in neurologic deficit can be expected to follow a meticulously performed operation. Unfortunately, this is not true of extradural tumors. Because the neurologic deficit proceeds rapidly and is often advanced at the time of surgery, operation will not in many cases alter the neurologic status. Despite isolated instances of dramatic recovery following removal of extradural tumor which had produced complete paralysis for several days, experienced neurosurgeons feel that complete paralysis for greater than 48 hours is not likely to be altered surgically. The surgeon is frequently faced with complete paralysis of borderline duration in which a fuzzy history makes the decision to operate even more difficult. Under pressure from the patient's family and physicians, he will be asked to decompress a permanently damaged spinal cord.

The decision to operate is usually based on logical criteria. Clearly, if the patient has diffuse metastases incompatible with life of a few months duration, a nonoperative approach is suggested. Factors which lean to surgery include good general health, youth, an undiagnosed primary tumor, a short neurologic history, and the preservation of some useful spinal cord function (such as sensation or bladder control). The ultimate decision, however, is usually based on a variety of medical, psychological and social factors. The patient and family must understand that if complete paralysis has been present for forty-eight hours or more, or if the patient has been unable to walk for several days, the surgical procedure will likely yield no useful alteration in neurologic function.

Intramedullary spinal cord tumors offer the neurosurgeon one of his greatest challenges. Growing slowly within the substance of the cord, they leave at their margins a plane of cleavage from which they can be gently teased without apparent damage. Intramedullary ependymomas and astrocytomas extending the entire length of the cervical or thoracic spinal cord have been excised without producing neurological deficit.

Many neurosurgeons prefer a technique described by Elsberg in 1916.[2] With this procedure, the intramedullary tumor is attacked in two operations. At the first, the dura is opened and sutured back. A midline incision in the spinal cord over the tumor may be performed. At this point the procedure is terminated and, one week later, reoperation is performed. In some cases, the tumor had become extruded by the time of the second surgery, making a dissection from the substance of the cord much easier. Such a staged approach is particularly useful in gliomas extending for great distances throughout the spinal cord. Metallic clips, placed along and parallel to the margins of the incised cord, can serve as radiopaque guides. When subsequent x-rays indicate separation of the clips, a tumor recurrence can be suspected.

Surgical exploration is indicated in intramedullary tumors to differentiate a mass lesion from a syrinx. Even with partial removal, an intramedullary tumor may respond to radiation therapy, a form of treatment which may likely be useless for syringomyelia. Although evacuation and permanent drainage in syringomyelia may not alter the progression of the disease, most feel this form of treatment is worthy of trial. Recent efforts to "tap" the mass with a percutaneous needle might afford diagnosis without laminectomy.

RADIOTHERAPY IN TREATMENT OF SPINAL CORD COMPRESSION DUE TO METASTATIC TUMOR

One of the few recent developments in the treatment of spinal cord tumor is an increased awareness of the possibilities of radiotherapy as the initial and only form of treatment. Decompression of the spinal cord for malignant (usually metastatic) tumor, followed by x-ray therapy, has been standard, yet emergency radiation promptly after demonstration of a myelographic block is now advanced by some as the initial and only therapeutic modality in selected cases. Because this concept has generated much controversy, it is worthy of more detailed discussion.

Little experimental work in the role of radiation therapy in spinal cord tumors is available. Rubin, an aggressive advocate for x-ray therapy in a wide variety of spinal tumors, placed Murphy-Sturm lymphoma in the necks of a series of rats and correlated biological recovery with the forms of treatment.[13] In general, neurologic recovery was related to the degree of presenting impairment and to the daily dosage schedule (the higher the initial daily dose, the greater the recovery). Rubin also reported 100 per cent recovery in five patients treated for spinal

TABLE 16–1

| Type Tumor | Response | | | |
	Excellent	Fair	Poor	None
Breast	5	3	12	2
Hodgkin's Disease	2	4	1	–
Lymphosarcoma	2	1	6	6
Reticulum Cell Sarcoma	4	2	4	4

cord compression secondary to Hodgkin's lymphoma. Only two of five patients with carcinomatous cord compression, however, seemed to respond satisfactorily to x-ray treatment.

In a larger series, Kahn et al. radiated 82 patients with evidence of spinal cord compression from extradural metastases.[10] Thirty-six of these patients had malignant lymphomas, and 22 had carcinoma of the breast. The results for this group are given in Table 16–1.

The table indicates that even with radiosensitive tumors of reticuloendothelial origin, excellent results are not guaranteed. In metastatic carcinoma, the outcome is particularly poor. It is noteworthy that the above does not include over 100 patients who presented to this clinic in the same interval with metastatic spinal cord compression due to carcinoma of the lung. This represents a particularly common cause of spinal cord compression which, if irradiated and included in the above overall figures, would likely reduce enthusiasm for unselected irradiation of the spinal cord for metastatic tumors.

The series also shows, as expected, that the patients with advanced neurologic deficit did far worse. Dosages used in the series were 2500 rads in 20 days. Extension of dosage above 3000 rads did not improve the chances of success.

We feel that removal of an intramedullary

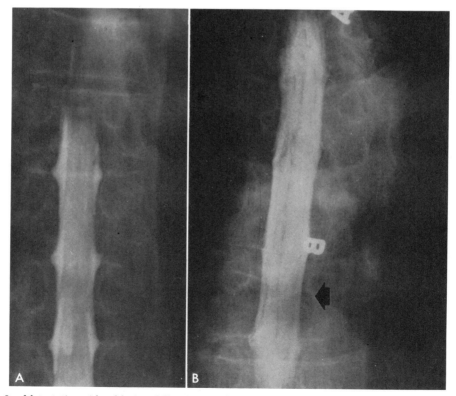

Figure 16–9. Metastatic epidural lesion following irradiation. A, The complete myelographic block secondary to metastatic epidural lymphoma. The leading edge of the block has a typical "paint brush" appearance. Emergency x-irradiation was started at this level because the patient had known primary lymphoma elsewhere. B, Two weeks later and after considerable neurologic improvement, repeat myelography indicates the complete disappearance of the block and no evidence of residual epidural tumor.

glioma should be followed by x-ray therapy extending above and below the site of the lesion. When a nonresectable mass is found, because of the risk of seeding throughout the spinal canal from this tumor, which tends to metastasize within the central nervous system, irradiation of the whole spinal axis is often advised. Radiation doses are again taken to tolerance, which is commonly considered 4000 rads in five weeks.[14]

Malignant reticuloendothelial tumors with cord compression but with evidence of incomplete neurological deficit can be treated with aggressive emergency irradiation after myelography. Irradiation is particularly safe when a partial myelographic block is demonstrated. When the tumor produces rapid severe myelopathy, which at the time of the initial examination is near complete, surgical decompression followed by irradiation is considered safer. Little enthusiasm is generated by the results of irradiation alone in advanced carcinomatous cord compression. Figure 16–9 indicates, however, remarkable myelographic clearing in a case of lymphomatous block.

RECENT DEVELOPMENTS IN THE CARE OF SPINAL CORD TUMORS

The role of radiation therapy in cord compression secondary to radicular endothelial tumors, and needle aspiration of intramedullary spinal cord masses have been alluded to. The role of microsurgery in surgical incision of these lesions, particularly the intramedullary type, cannot be overemphasized. The enhanced appreciation of fine structures delineation of color differences between normal and abnormal tissue, and better illumination have rendered safer the removal of such lesions. Greenwood's perfection of the bipolar coagulator has made a focused hemostasis in and on the cord safer.[6]

Newer and highly specified angiographic techniques, which involve the insertion of a catheter near the fine vessels which leave the aorta to supply the spinal cord, have been perfected by Di Chiro.[1] These angiograms, combined with subtraction techniques to soften the images of the overlying vertebra, have been effective in the preoperative diagnosis of vascular spinal cord tumors.

References

1. Di Chiro, G., and Doppman, J. L.: Differential angiographic features of hemangioblastomas and arteriovenous malformations of the spinal cord. Radiology 93:25–30, 1969.
2. Elsberg, C. A., and Beer, E.: The operability of intramedullary tumors of the spinal cord. Remarks upon the extrusion of intraspinal tumors. Amer. J. Med. Sci. 142:636–647, 1911.
3. Elsberg, C. A.: Diagnosis and Treatment of Surgical Diseases of the Spinal Cord and Its Membranes. Philadelphia, W. B. Saunders Co., 1916. (Second ed. 1941)
4. Ford, F. R.: Diseases of the Nervous System in Infancy, Childhood and Adolescence. Ed. 2, Springfield, Ill., Charles C Thomas, Publisher, 1960.
5. Gowers, W. R., and Horsley, V. A.: A case of tumor of the spinal cord. Removal, recovery. Med. Chir. Trans. (S.2), 53:379–428, 1888.
6. Greenwood, J.: Surgical removal of intramedullary tumors. J. Neurosurg. 26:275–282, 1967.
7. Greenwood, J.: Spinal cord tumors. In Neurological Surgery. J. R. Youmans (ed.). Philadelphia, W. B. Saunders Co., 1973. Vol. 3, p. 1514–1534.
8. Hamby, W. B.: Tumors in the spinal canal in childhood: Analysis of the literature of a subsequent decade (1933–1942); report of a case of meningitis due to an intramedullary epidermoid communicating with a dermal sinus. J. Neuropath. Exper. Neurol. 3:397–412 (Oct.) 1944.
9. Horrax, G., and Anderson, D. G.: Encapsulated intramedullary tumor—whole spinal cord from medulla to conus. Surg. Gynec. Obstet. 68:814–819, 1939.
10. Kahn, F. R., Glicksman, A. S., Chu, F. C. H., and Nickson, J. J.: Treatment by radiotherapy of spinal cord compression due to extradural metastases. Radiology 89:895–900, 1967.
11. Kamrin, R. P., Potanos, J. N., and Pool, J. L.: An evaluation of the diagnosis and treatment of chordoma. J. Neurosurg. Psychiat. 27:157–165, 1964.
12. Rand, R. W., and Rand, C. W.: Intraspinal Tumors of Childhood. Springfield, Ill., Charles C Thomas, Publisher, 1960.
13. Rubin, P.: Extradural spinal cord compression by tumor. Radiology 93:1243–1248, 1969.
14. Editorial: Radiation myelopathy. Brit. Med. J. 1:469, 1965.

CHAPTER 17

The Management of Chronic Pain of Spinal Origin

JOHN H. HUBBARD M.D.

University of Pennsylvania School of Medicine

"The phenomena of pain belong to that borderland between the body and the soul about which it is so delightful to speculate from the comfort of an armchair, but which offers such formidable obstacles to scientific inquiry."

Kellgren[34]

"It is disgraceful in every art and more especially in medicine after much trouble, much display, and much talk, to do no good at all."

Hippocrates[27]

The final common pathway to the operating table is frequently the fate of patients with spinal pain. Results are so tenuous in some categories that surgeons must reassess their therapeutic logic. The psychic, social and economic consequences of traditional approaches to the "pain complaint" seem, often, to be the product of insular thinking and a pragmatic viewpoint conditioned by a surgical philosophy. Certainly "he who operates only to take away pain will be disappointed in not being able to find it." Nearly all of us have won evanescent victories over pain in patients who presented no convincing pathologic findings on exploration of the spinal canal. Many of these successes are placebo effects which sadly wear off during the following months.

Furthermore, one may subdue his patients with contrived diagnoses (e.g., perineural fibrosis, focal arachnoiditis) when evidence is meager. Patients and their physicians become constrained to find a definitive cure, given the dignity of a "diagnosis." The complex interaction of a person and his pain over several months or years clouds the physician's insight as to both the structural and psychogenic basis for a patient's suffering. There is little doubt that most persons with intractable pain who consult a physician are seeking help. However, what they attempt to say is frequently misinterpreted, and their subconscious motives for seeking therapy are often kept from "surfacing" by our special ability to pigeonhole all their problems into one monolithic category or another. This penchant for compartmentalization may be a holdover from our earlier days in medical training, when we doggedly sought to arrive at a single diagnosis based on some ghastly array of symptoms. In regard to the general inadequacy of training in the pain arena, John Bonica has said, ". . . hundreds of thousands of suffering patients are not given relief they need, others are mistreated and become addicted to narcotics, still others incur a prolonged disability because of chronic pain, and some are even mutilated."[5]

The evaluation of persons with prolonged painful states must begin with an attempt to define organic lesions which might explain the distress; whenever possible, an anatomic diagnosis should be made. Thereafter, contributing emotional and psychosocial factors should be rigorously sought out and weighed against structural body derangements as the cause of the patient's suffering. Early childhood and adolescent experiences are clearly of great importance. Weir Mitchell noted nearly a century ago that children react to pain as their parents do, and it is wise to teach a hurt child silent, patient endurance in "the face of pain"; this self-conquest of restrained emotion would likely be carried over into adult life.[59] I am convinced that early memory engrams of painful experiences profoundly affect behavior in subsequent illnesses.

One young woman described the pain of chronic low-back strain as exactly like the "terrible pain I had for two weeks with meningitis when I was nine years old." Another young lady, a college student, had back and hip pains for several years. She was eventually evaluated by myelography which was normal. Her symptoms began within a few months following the death of her brother from acute leukemia. She and her family had developed denial patterns to deal with their loss. The patient admitted that she and her family had never experienced the appropriate grief reaction to the loss of someone so close, "her best friend." This admission, with the help of an understanding psychotherapist, is helping her cope with tremendously charged unresolved emotional stresses. Her pain complaint is diminishing as she emotionally readjusts. No one has intimated that her suffering is imaginary. It certainly is not!

Walters has splendidly described the attributes of "psychogenic regional pain."[95] Although pain in this condition is a socially acceptable form of suffering, it is quite real to the patient and is probably developed from "remembered" early pain experiences. This pattern of behavior insulates the patient and helps him avoid even more stressful influences in his daily life. It is no surprise that one should "choose" to communicate his anxieties by means so socially acceptable and evocative of such genuine sympathy from others. On the premise that subconscious mechanisms are at work to produce dissociative and conversion symptoms accompanied by somatic hallucinations, these patients should never be labeled as frauds or malingerers. Hysteria, on the other hand, which is little different from psychogenic regional pain, evokes the worst prejudices in some physicians, with an emphasis on therapeutic nihilism. Mennell, the author of a widely read monograph on back pain, states, "it is my experience that no man, woman or child ever complains of back pain without some pathological cause or physical reason. It there is such a thing as psychosomatic backache, symptoms are vague, and of course, the signs which are elicited from an adequate physical examination will not fit into any pattern which is normally expected when a pathological basis is present."[58] Few would take issue with his first statement. However, because the pain tolerance of individuals varies so much, so will the resultant disability and

complaint behavior evoked by a given pathologic process. Herein lies the issue in therapy of chronic pain—not whether pain is real or imaginary, but rather whether the emotional manifestations are out of proportion to the intensity of physical stimulus. Mennell's second observation suggests that distribution of pain dramatically differs in psychogenic versus organic states, which is definitely not the case. Although pain distribution and sensory impairment are not strictly radicular in psychogenic syndromes, they are rarely confined to the distribution of a single nerve root in most chronic low back problems, with the exception of a classical lumbar disc protrusion. Symptoms of psychogenic back pain are not often vague, as he suggests, but graphic and elaborate at times. "I feel as if there is a dog biting at my buttocks," or "The pressure builds up so much through my thigh that I believe it will burst open." "There is a stabbing sensation on the outside of my calf that feels as if someone is turning a knife in the bone."

The way in which patients describe their pain should be carefully recorded, verbatim if possible. Subtle gestures and mannerisms along with the nuances of pain description will depend upon the intelligence, linguistic abilities and theatrical style of each patient. We tend to reduce these responses to conform with our preconceived notion of pain quality (e.g. aching, shooting, tingling, throbbing), while the English language has innumerable adjectives which may amplify description of pain and help us to understand its pathologic basis.[56] Familial patterns of pain behavior should be kept in mind. Ethnic influences also have been shown to determine how one or another group of people with differing national origins may be expected to respond when in pain. Naturally, these norms are punctuated with exceptions, but help to establish guidelines in diagnosis. "Augmenters" and "reducers" in psychologic testing situations show contrasting behavioral patterns when in pain. Athletes and nonathletes similarly differ in their mean ability to tolerate painful stimulation.[73, 92]

Routine psychologic testing is seldom helpful in differentiating psychogenic from somatogenic pain states. The MMPI (Minnesota Multiphasic Personality Inventory) reveals significant elevations of the hypochrondiasis, depression, and hysteria scales in over 75 per cent of all patients suffering chronic pain. Indeed, it is rare to observe a completely

normal psychologic profile in any patient suffering from prolonged painful disability. Satisfactory control of pain in the "organic" segment of this population is reflected by
improved (normalized) MMPI scores. The
draw-a-person test may be very helpful in
bringing out fantasies and delusional systems
in the patient's pain complaint. He is given
free rein to draw-in and graphically illustrate
his painful areas on a standard silhouette of a
person. Use of psychogalvanic skin responses[2]
and other psychophysiologic reactions in evaluating response to experimental pain holds
promise in triage of patients for appropriate
therapy, but is yet poorly standardized.

When discomfort causes limitation of motion, or is associated with marked guarding on
passive movements, the Pentothal test is an
appropriate diagnostic tool. The patient is first
instructed to respond by limb withdrawal or
forcing the examiner's hand away when
Achilles tendon pressure or trapezius pinch
becomes unbearably painful. He is then subjected to the limb motion which approximates
his worst spontaneous discomfort. Pentothal
is slowly administered intravenously to barely
achieve disappearance of the eyelid reflex. As
the patient gradually comes around, the *test*
pain and *clinical* pain are alternately elicited.
If the maneuver causing clinical pain is now
tolerated better than trapezius pinch or tendon
pressure, it can be assumed that the patient
has a low threshold for pain complaint. In
such a case there is probably a significant
psychogenic component.

Differential anesthetic block of the cauda
equina has been advocated to differentiate between real and imagined pain, as well as between sympathetic dystrophies and pain resulting from compression of dorsal root fibers.
The short-term and placebo relief of pain with
this procedure makes its interpretation difficult. Furthermore, by the time anesthetic concentration is sufficient to block sensory conduction in the nerve root, the patient feels
segmental numbness and, except when frankly
delusional, is likely to acknowledge pain
relief.

I have found that lumbar myelography is
a valuable tool for deciding where to operate
rather than when to operate. There is a high
incidence of lumbar myelographic abnormalities in patients undergoing study of the posterior cranial fossa.[30] Nearly all of these patients
were asymptomatic in so far as low back
complaints were concerned.

PAIN GAMES

Some patients become inextricably
trapped into playing a role. The pain complaint empowers them to achieve so many
subconscious objectives productive of secondary gain that the most skillful psychotherapist frequently is frustrated in attempting to treat these manipulative people. They
are Szasz's "Nobel laureates of pain."[86]
Physicians' attempts to help such individuals
often reinforce their pain behavior and cause
the constellation of symptoms they manifest
to become even more elaborate.

The pain "professional" frequently views
himself or herself as a colleague of the
therapist. What thereafter develops may be
destructive to their relationship unless this
kind of transaction is quickly thwarted. However, the dilemma may be compounded if
such a patient is forced by the wary physician
into a totally passive role in curing his pain.

Particularly in the case of psychogenic
regional pain, the therapist's failures become
patient victories; physician challenge and defeat are the perpetuating forces in this bizarre
life-style. The patient who plays little active
part in his getting well remains guiltless when
his doctors' efforts fail. If, as Thomas Jefferson said, "the art of life is the art of avoiding
pain," then these unfortunate patients have
stifled pleasurable senses which can enrich
one's life while heightening their awareness of
stimuli which condition avoidance behavior.

The manipulative pain patient creates
havoc when treated by two physicians simultaneously. Among those most often inveigled
while treating chronic low back pain are the
orthopedist, physiatrist, family physician, psychiatrist and neurosurgeon. Therapists can be
pitted against one another, and conflicts can
be generated by 1) quotes out of context, 2)
misinterpretation of instructions, 3) fact giving
way to fantasy, 4) polypharmacy, and 5) seeking advice from the physician outside his special area of competence. A case in point of the
latter is the patient who, being cared for by a
physiatrist and neurosurgeon concurrently,
seeks the surgeon's advice on back-bracing,
while at the physiatrist's office later the same
day, inquires exhaustively about the merits of
cordotomy with no mention of his thoughts
regarding the use of a brace.

A source of further therapeutic pitfall is
the attitude that "continued pain (which) cannot be treated by other means is a valid reason

for the continued use of narcotic analgesics."[33] The irrevocable state of chronic addiction and personality disintegration are too often the consequence of this attitude. In a study of 400 pain-prone patients, it is notable that drug addiction was viewed as an expression of hostility to society.[20] In each case, the physician symbolized the authority structure. The patients were generally angry, hostile and aggressive toward their physicians. There were no positive relationships. We must realize that a sense of urgency communicated by intensity of the "pain complaint" may be magnified far out of proportion to both the patient's anxiety and physical pain. Emotional support, tolerance and understanding are important in controlling the patient's overaction. Further, the physician is given an opportunity to assess the genuine irritative component of the pain, which provides the only sound basis for use of analgesics. In many situations, muscle relaxants, psychotropic agents, or placebos may be far more appropriate.

The surgeon's prerogative can be usurped by an exceedingly demanding patient. Most orthopedists and neurosurgeons have accumulated a bevy of patients in whom they wish foresight could have predicted the miserable outcome of surgery. Too late, as events unfold in the postoperative period, we observe behavioral characteristics or motivational factors which clearly preclude a good result. Moreover, about a third of patients with chronic pain experience a transitory placebo effect from a variety of operative procedures.[39] Several months, occasionally a year or more, may be required to ferret out real from imaginary benefits of therapy. Surgeons should bear this fact in mind when they recommend procedures with a relatively low yield of satisfactory results. It is far too easy for us to over-rate the short-term good results and forget delayed failures in these cases. In recommending a "high risk" procedure (i.e., one having a meager chance of success) we abrogate our responsibility to the patient. For when it fails, we can say "I told you so!" The patient assumes responsibility for having harassed the surgeon into performing a useless operation, and the latter's conscience remains clear.

Surgeon's "solitaire" involves rationalizing each unexplained poor operative result by the diagnosis of a potentially overlooked spinal condition. This ploy presupposes that every pain manifestation goes *pari passu* with some tangible musculoskeletal derangement comparable in magnitude to the patient's complaint. To justify the need for reoperation on the grounds that something was handled incorrectly, the first (second, third, etc.) time around, explanations such as *pedicular kinking* of the nerve root from descent of the pedicle related to disc collapse, intervertebral *foraminal migration* of a disc fragment, facet *impingement* on the nerve root causing compression from behind, instability of the *motor unit*, nerve root fibrosis, and pseudoarthrosis are currently in vogue.[46] Granted that these conditions do occasionally occur, it becomes essential to exclude them as contributory factors at the time of the *initial* operation. In the absence of an obvious lesion to explain the patient's symptoms and physical findings, the intervertebral foramina should be thoroughly explored and mobility of the nerve root demonstrated before abandoning the search. Often an intact disc or two may be curetted away when the surgeon is driven by desperation to perform some clinical ritual to help the patient.

Excessive bleeding is commonplace during laminectomy in the hands of those who pay little attention to hemodynamics in the positioning of the patient. Supporting an even mildly overweight individual on flank bolsters can invite compression of abdominal veins and markedly increase the epidural venous pressure. Blood loss from the spinal canal may exceed 1000 cc, and so badly obscure the field that no one could carry out a competent exploration. A number of alternative positioning techniques are available to circumvent this problem (Fig. 17–1). The effectiveness of

Figure 17–1.   Several postures for surgery of the lumbar spine under reduced abdominal pressure.[11] A, Salaam position, Mohammedan praying position or buttock seat position.[17] B, Georgia prone position.[78] C, Hastings frame.[24] D, Tuck position,[96] modified knee chest position. E, Semi-prone position. Myoglobinuria and post-operative hypotension (1) have been encountered when too much weight is born on the calves. Proper positioning avoids this difficulty. The author prefers the "salaam position" for laminectomy. The semi-prone position is quite satisfactory for inter-laminar removal of a laterally placed herniated disc. All of the illustrated positioning techniques significantly reduce epidural venous bleeding.

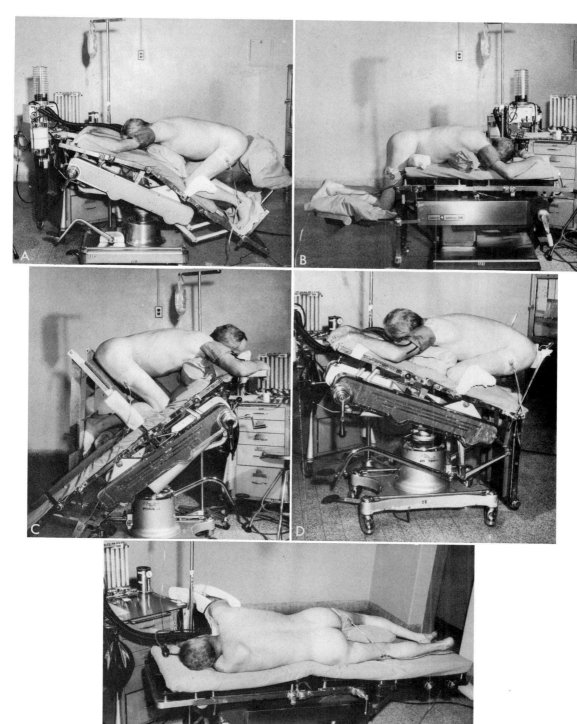

Figure 17–1. *See opposite page for legend.*

these positions in reducing vena cava pressure has been amply demonstrated.

McNab reported 80 per cent satisfactory results in first operations for "facet impingement" syndrome, while only 25 per cent were helped when treated for the same disorder after having undergone an earlier unsuccessful laminectomy.[46] The same series revealed that only 16 per cent of patients without convincing abnormalities were benefited by operation, even fewer than one might expect from placebo surgery. DePalma and Rothman reviewed the results of lumbar spinal surgery in 517 patients. Of this group, 150 had undergone reoperation and 70 were available for followup.[9] They seem to have had remarkable success in finding a plausible etiology for persistent or recurrent pain in *every case*. Extensive canal and disc space exploration and posterolateral fusion were performed. About half of the initial results were satisfactory. The fact that 87 per cent of the patients deemed the operation "worthwhile" deserves comment. Having been a partner with his surgeon in the decision to operate, it is fitting that the patient rationalize the value of his judgment as long as the procedure did not further compromise his coping mechanisms. Should paralysis or sensory impairment result, he would have cause for displeasure. Similarly, a clash of personalities between the patient and an unsympathetic physician may nullify the benefit of a neutral surgical procedure. In another category are patients who seek out invasive treatments; often they have placidly undergone sundry operations, frequently eight or more. These individuals inflate our good results if the "patient's acceptance" of surgery becomes the yardstick by which to measure the effectiveness of therapy. We should, therefore, adhere to the objective criteria of increased functional capacity and independent appraisals by family and employers as the basis for extolling our restorative skills.

Pain and the Family

One's life setting can be conducive to illness. Psychogenic factors may continue to perpetuate pain states long after the organic nidus becomes quiescent. The family unit or its threatened disintegration has an important role to play as a reinforcer in this maladaptive state. Verbal reports of suffering or pain behavior can have immense conditioning effects on those closest to the patient, with a minimal expenditure of effort to communicate on his part. One's spouse may unwittingly strengthen deleterious interactions. He or she may be barely aware of the relentless course of this corrosive process and totally ineffectual in modifying it.

E. J., a 46-year-old metallurgist-engineer, and part-time musician, fell asleep while driving home, having played trumpet until 2:00 a.m. with a jazz combo. He shattered his right femoral head and acetabulum, requiring hip arthrodesis, after five operations in the intervening six years gave him no relief of his chronic pain on walking. He had six children and a haggard young wife, who made ends meet on very little income. A percutaneous cervical cordotomy which caused analgesia to the T10 level dramatically relieved his pain, and the patient remained ecstatic about his "new life" while in the hospital for the next few days. His friends said that they considered the result truly a miracle. When he failed to return for a postoperative visit three weeks later, the author discovered, in a phone conversation with his wife, that Ed had been lying in bed staring at the ceiling for most of the time since returning home. He complained bitterly of pain over his left eye and got up only to use the bathroom and to eat. When he was finally reexamined, the patient admitted to complete relief of hip pain, which incidentally has not recurred in the subsequent two years. During that visit he was very unhappy with his misfortune of having had one pain mysteriously replaced by another. In the past year, supportive psychotherapy has been instrumental in permitting him to ventilate his hostility toward both his wife and a brother-in-law. The supraorbital pain complaint disappears for several weeks when his emotional seas are tranquil, to return instantly with the most trivial squall. We sought to explain why he should "choose" head pain to replace that which had been relieved. During percutaneous cordotomy there is frequently very transient sharp pain radiating to the scalp and rarely to the supraorbital region as the result of heating C2 nerve fibers with radiofrequency current. It was concluded that the epoch of pain produced in creating the spinal cord lesion may have conveniently generated a memory engram to replace the now interrupted input from his hip which had reverberated through those circuits for so many years.

Not infrequently a person with a long and illustrious pain history finds a compatible individual whom he or she marries with the implicit understanding by both partners that sick behavior is to be part of that lifelong contract. The dependency structure cultivated thereafter can be undermined by attempts from outside to promote well behavior in the patient. Subconscious resistance can be expected from the dominant partner in considering any change which would threaten dissolution of their "harmonious" relationship.

Compensation: The Adversary Game

No stratagem could have been developed with a greater bias against a person's getting well than the system which so generously rewards a man for staying ill. Sick behavior is the *sine qua non* for continuation of most disability insurance. Compounding this social malfeasance are those vast refuges of human anonymity, production lines. With so little room at the top, few high school educated, middle aged men or women can rise above the monotony of tasks performed by rote to attain positions requiring imagination and ingenuity. When faced with a major illness or injury which temporarily removes them from the frenetic workaday world, some of these individuals subconsciously develop a pain defense which protects them from returning to menial servitude. It often simply takes on the characteristics of the original "legitimately" painful condition, which had only temporarily incapacitated the worker. With children now independent and mortgages paid off, both the subconsciously motivated and opportunistic individual can be content to retire with life-time compensation amounting to the majority of his income. He need no longer risk the continued loss of self-esteem and the gradual buildup of restlessness and hostility inevitable in returning to his former job. While his physicians and representatives of insurance carriers try desperately to vocationally rehabilitate him, the patient stays in strong contention by making demands on his employer to assign him to duties which are outside the scope of his abilities, either trivial tasks or a supervisory role. Such patients must be identified early because analgesics and psychotropic medication, classical psychotherapy and surgery have no place in their treatment. Vocational retraining based on the individual's current aspirations and aptitude, along with intensive use of psychologic methods, including *behavioral modification,* offer the only hope of getting many of these people back to work. When immediate forfeiture of compensation threatens every attempt of the individual to seek gainful employment, such a program is doomed to failure. First, insurance carriers must develop equitable and ingenious plans to subsidize some "good risk" workers in their efforts to make a comeback. Reinforced by a few successes and feeling once again worthwhile, these men and women may remain productive for many years.

INTERDISCIPLINARY PAIN CONTROL CLINICS—AN EFFORT BY MANY TO HELP A FEW

Chronic intractable pain arising from non-malignant disease seldom has a wholly organic or psychogenic etiology. Even those patients capable of achieving good results from surgery must undergo major emotional readjustment after so many years of psychic disability. A surgeon who views the pain and suffering process too mechanistically will inevitably have many poor results. On the other hand, psychiatrists who treat patients with chronic pain using classical psychotherapeutic techniques and hypnosis only rarely achieve a cure and frequently become discouraged by their inability to break the patient's cycle of somatization. In a psychiatric setting, the patient may feel that he has been abandoned by "his doctor"; that nobody believes he has "unbearable pain"; that "it's all in his head." The patient returns to "his" surgeon or someone else, demanding, "Fix me."

The concept of a pain clinic is a relatively new one. Specialists in anesthesia, orthopedics, neurologic surgery, physical medicine, psychiatry, psychology and social work, along with nurse clinicians and paramedical personnel, contribute to an eclectic approach to the evaluation and treatment of patients with chronic pain. General practitioners or family physicians, well trained in "dolorology," may assume the responsibility of being the patient's "manager." These physicians often provide the continuity of care which is so desirable, while the clinic provides support to both patient and therapist that seldom is attained within the more loose framework of community medical practice. The clinic serves as an authority figure for the patient, and the verdicts given by its pain specialists often dissuade him from continued "shopping." Frequent therapy conferences bring together all physicians involved in the patient's care, which enhances everyone's understanding of the problems that arise in the course of therapy.

Moreover, they help to minimize conflicts and inconsistencies in approaching these matters.

Some critics of pain clinics view them as graduate schools for professional pain patients. Admittedly, there is a certain small group of individuals who have made a career of pain, and regard each defeat of a physician's efforts to help them as a personal victory—the more skilled a physician is in the pain game, the more stimulating the challenge. These passive-aggressive adversaries insinuate by their actions and reactions "poor me, dumb you!" The vast majority are not social derelicts, however, and are sincere in wanting to be relieved of their suffering.

A number of comparatively unorthodox and variably effective treatment modalities may be incorporated into a center for pain control. Combinations of therapeutic techniques can be used to advantage in this close knit multidisciplinary environment, while their use alone would be doomed to failure. For example, few patients in pain would be willing to participate in group or family therapy sessions without the concurrent support of physical modes of therapy (e.g., medications, electrical stimulation, biofeedback, nerve block). Yet, much of the patient's maladaptive behavior may have at its roots poor interpersonal and family relationships which magnify the pain complaint far out of proportion to any known organic basis for his suffering. As he learns to deal more effectively with anxiety-provoking life situations, his dependence on drugs and paraphernalia will diminish. Hypnosis, biofeedback conditioning, and even transcendental meditation are advocated to help patients control their outward manifestations of pain. While each has proven effective as an adjunct to therapy, none of these methods alone is likely to have prolonged usefulness without relearning on the part of the patient. *Operant conditioning* is one such program for modifying behavior and redirecting the patient's psychic energies into productive encounters. This method, also termed "behavioral modification," utilizes a controlled environment wherein trained technicians and nurses supervised by a clinical psychologist reward the individual for non-pain behavior. Negative reinforcers, such as the "gift" of medication in response to a complaint of pain, are strictly avoided by delivering medication at a slightly more frequent interval than the patient would ordinarily request. The dose of drug is gradually reduced while the volume of vehicle remains the same. Similarly, physical therapy and reconditioning exercises are prescribed to tolerance just short of incapacitating pain. The therapist, therefore, does not need to respond to the patient's discomfort by "giving" him a respite from work. Gradually, tolerance is built up over several weeks, with the patient charting and otherwise graphically documenting his own progress. Negative interactions with his therapist are completely avoided by structuring the environment to circumvent every opportunity for "help me, I hurt" behavior. The hospital or rehabilitation center provides an artificial setting for such "brainwashing" techniques. Upon returning to his home surroundings, one is certain to be confronted by stresses which cannot be simulated in the therapeutic milieu. Therefore, it is essential that such a program be conducted with the cooperation, understanding and education of the family and closest friends, to assure maximum benefits to the patient. Pilot projects of this type have interested insurance carriers and promise to be expanded in order to handle large numbers of individuals disabled by chronic pain. The considerable cost of these programs can be justified by the extravagant economic burden of the alternatives (i.e., multiple operations, re-evaluations, and interminable disability payments).

CONSERVATIVE THERAPY FOR SUBACUTE NECK AND LOW-BACK PAIN

Non-surgical and *conservative* are adjectives called upon interchangeably to describe temporizing remedies for pain. Yet, some very radical therapy is advocated "cloaked in the trappings of conservatism" (Fig. 17–2). Prolonged treatment with stupefying medications, enforced immobility, applications of heat and ultrasound, along with use of devices which pull the skeleton in one direction or another can demoralize the patient who perceives no benefit from weeks of undaunted adherence to the rigors of a program his doctor implied would make him well.

There is certainly no virtue in saving the patient an operation when surgery offers an appreciably better chance of early return to full activity than periods of rest and reconditioning which fail to attack the cause of his problem. If the indications for spinal surgery

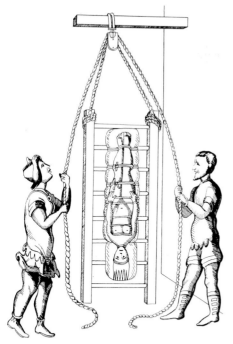

Figure 17–2. Representation of the ancient mode of performing succussion, as described by Hippocrates, given by Vidius Vidius in the Venetian edition of Galen's Works (Cl. vi, p. 271). "The ladder is placed on the ground. The ankles are fastened securely to the ladder and in like manner, he is further secured both above and below the knee and also at the nates. The trunk is not secured because to do so would interfere with the effect of the succussion. The arms are to be fastened along his sides to his own body and not to the ladder. When matters have been arranged thus the ladder is hoisted up and succussion (i.e. shaking the spine) is applied." Copied from a plate reproduced in *Backache from Occiput to Coccyx* by G. L. Burke, W. E. G. MacDonald Publisher, Vancourver, B. C., 1964.

are unequivocal, results are phenomenally good in persons motivated to get well. Confronted by objective and progressive neurological impairment, the surgeon can be fairly confident of obtaining satisfactory results. Similarly, when motion aggravates pain related to radiographically visible spinal instability, fusion is likely to relieve the discomfort. By contrast, anterior cervical spinal fusions and lateral lumbar fusions performed for symptomatic treatment of neck pain and "lumbago" in the absence of demonstrable instability or hypermobility, are destined to eventual failure in the majority of patients.

PATIENT EDUCATION

Much depends on the patient's understanding and acceptance of instructions from his physician regarding posture, graded activity schedules, use of appliances, and steps to be taken in the gradual reconditioning process. The use of a bed board, cervical pillow, limitations placed on exertion, weight reduction, rest periods, and a program for restoration to limited duty all play an essential part in the reeducation of persons with recurring spinal pain. Even the careful explanation of how to get into or out of an automobile is not to be overlooked as trivial. A realistic estimate of recovery time should be given the patient to avoid his becoming disappointed by expecting too much, too fast. The approach to rehabilitation should highlight what *is* permitted rather than what *is not* at each stage in the reconditioning process.

PHYSIOTHERAPY

Massage, hydrotherapy and ultrasound application each have their champions. These ancillary measures potentiate pharmacotherapy and graded exercise programs. Inquiry into the objective scientific criteria for their use is outside the scope of this discussion.

Sir Robert Jones, in commenting on treatment by manipulation nearly a century ago, stated that "we should mend our ways rather than abuse the unqualified. Dramatic success at their hands should cause us to inquire as to the reason; it is not wise or dignified to waste time denouncing their mistakes for we cannot hide the fact that their successes are our failures."[23] Certainly, few of us who have witnessed the harm such jostling of the spine can cause, both by delay in diagnosis and by direct injury, could possibly bestow such an unqualified accolade on this practice. Nevertheless, there has to be some merit in its use by trained physicians when applied with specific indications as an adjunct to therapy.

The author recalls an experience in his own childhood, at the age of ten, when sharp relentless rib cage pain immediately followed the upstroke of a gargantuan swing at a golf ball, while the object remained perched impertinently on the tee. Thereafter, each breath was like "the devil's grip." An agonizing half hour later, he was delivered to the office of an ancient and frail gentleman skilled in the art of manipulation. His office was bare aside from the adjustment table along with a few pillows and sandbags piled on a shelf at the end of the quaint room. As instructed, the pallid and diaphoretic little patient lay supine on the table with his forearms folded upon a pillow placed over his chest. The old man grasped the patient's wrists quite firmly and with an abrupt downward thrust, the pain was made to miraculously vanish.

What had so dramatically occurred in realigning the costovertebral articulation was an experience foreign to most physicians. Our modern treatment of this disorder would have included rib cage taping, local anesthestic block and analgesics with gradual resolution of the discomfort over a few days or weeks. Advocates of spinal manipulation have written extensively on the subject and some of these authorities include physicians. These techniques, along with intermittent traction, can be beneficial if judiciously applied. However, they will intensify the patient's distress if employed in disregard of the underlying pathology. In several series, about half of all patients with subacute or chronic low-back pain are helped for a while by manipulation of the spine. A far smaller number of those with demonstrable plain film and radiographic abnormalities are made comfortable as compared with those lacking objective findings.

PHARMACOTHERAPY OF SPINAL PAIN

ANALGESICS

The mild pain killers which have both anti-inflammatory and antipyretic qualities are particularly effective in the treatment of chronic spinal complaints when combined with sedatives and muscle relaxants. Acetaminophen (Tylenol) is equianalgesic with aspirin and causes less gastrointestinal discomfort. However, aspirin is much more efficacious than acetaminophen in the control of rheumatoid pain.

Dextropropoxyphene (Darvon) is more acceptable than aspirin to many patients with mild chronic pain. Certainly, there is some placebo effect of prescription drugs compared with over-the-counter remedies. Dextropropoxyphene combined with aspirin or acetaminophen has a greater analgesic effect than when used alone. Sixty mg of codeine has equal or slightly greater analgesic potency than 65 mg of dextropropoxyphene. Higher

doses can be more effective. Neither of these drugs has a serious addiction potential.

Pentazocine (Talwin) is a benzomorphan derivative which has been known to precipitate withdrawal symptoms in patients dependent on narcotics. An intramuscular dose of 30 to 50 mg is equianalgesic to 10 mg of morphine. The drug is definitely a better analgesic when given intramuscularly than when taken by mouth. The author has been disappointed by the tolerance patients develop when given this compound orally. The intramuscular route, while more effective, has minimal appeal in long term outpatient management of intractable pain.

Methadone (Dolophine) has experienced recent popularity in the control of chronic pain. The drug produces negligible euphoria and few abstinence symptoms. It is prescribed orally, dissolved in a masking vehicle, starting with 5 to 10 mg every 4 to 6 hours with gradual reduction in dosage, as part of a behavior modification program.

Oxycodone combined with aspirin, phenacetin and caffeine (Percodan) is a semisynthetic narcotic analgesic having a sedative quality and capacity to control pain of moderate severity. Both psychic and physical dependence may develop with its prolonged use. In some of our patients temporarily weaned from this drug by use of other measures to control pain (e.g., acupuncture, hypnosis or electrical stimulation) abrupt crises have occurred during which the patient became anxious and demanded to receive the drug again. After a few days or weeks, supportive therapy could be effectively substituted for the drug.

ANTI-INFLAMMATORY COMPOUNDS

Phenylbutazone (Butazolidin) and oxyphenylbutazone (Tandearil) are specifically useful in treatment of inflammatory arthritides. They are not indicated for general purpose analgesia. Agranulocytosis, thrombocytopenia and aplastic anemia occasionally result from their use. Reversible but distressing side effects, especially gastrointestinal irritation, occur quite frequently. These compounds or indomethacin (Indocin) cannot be recommended for the treatment of chronic cervical or lumbar pain.

MEMBRANE STABILIZING AGENTS

Diphenylhydantoin (Dilantin) and carbamazepine (Tegretol) are chemically dissimilar compounds with anticonvulsant properties. Both diminish post-tetanic potentiation of synaptic transmission in the central nervous system. Additionally, diphenylhydantoin has a direct effect on neuromuscular transmission by producing membrane stabilization. This drug causes inhibition of repetitive firing upon depolarization of a motor nerve by high extracellular potassium concentrations.[83] Unfortunately, the effect of these drugs in eradicating the agony of tic douloureux is not apparent in spinal pain. We have observed prolonged dramatic effects in fewer than 10 per cent of such patients, and then only when significant radicular dysesthesias or hyperpathia dominated the clinical picture.

MUSCLE RELAXANTS

Sixty years ago, mephenesin was investigated as an internuncial neuron blocking agent. Its action in reducing experimentally produced spasticity led to moderate success in patient trials. Mephenesin carbamate (Tolseram) had a more prolonged action, and enjoyed some popularity in the treatment of muscle spasm for several years. A chemically similar substance, methocarbamol (Robaxin) was discovered to be even more effective and better tolerated; lightheadedness and dizziness are occasional side effects in the usual dosage of 500 mg four times daily. Muscle relaxants have sedative side effects in doses which dramatically reduce spasm, and could be more aptly termed "people relaxants." The U.S. Food and Drug Administration has declared them as "possibly effective" inhibitors of reflex muscle spasm based on available experimental and clinical evidence. Their pri-

mary neurophysiologic effect is one of defacilitation both in the brainstem reticular activating system and in the spinal interneuron pool. Drugs in this category are outlined in Table 1.

Diazepam (Valium) is a compound similar in configuration to chlordiazepoxide (Librium). However, diazepam calms and more effectively reduces tension and anxiety. It blocks rigidity of the truncal musculature in the "stiff man syndrome" and reduces adventitious movement in Huntington's chorea. The drug causes fatigue, drowsiness, ataxia, slowing of reflex responses and impairment of coordination. It may aggravate depression and should not be used in suicidal patients. Doses which are effective in reducing skeletal muscle spasm make operation of a motor vehicle hazardous. Diazepam should be used in the treatment of chronic spinal pain only when reflex irritability of the neuromuscular unit can be demonstrated or is strongly suspected based upon the patient's symptoms. When bed rest is indicated, the following dosage schedule will be beneficial in overcoming both spasm and anxiety:

10 mg. four times daily for two weeks (bed rest and bathroom privileges)
10 mg. three times daily for four weeks (three hour daytime rest period)
5 mg. four times a day for two weeks (climbing, lifting, and driving an automobile restricted).

In fully ambulatory patients, lower doses are usually mandatory. To combat anxiety in the absence of significant spasm, meprobamate or phenobarbital may be prescribed. The abuse potential of the latter compound, espe-

TABLE 17–1. DRUGS USED SPECIFICALLY AS MUSCLE RELAXANTS

Generic Name	Trade Name	Dosage	Side Effects
Carisoprodol	Rela, Soma	350 mg 4 times daily	Possible mild analgesic action, drowsiness, dizziness, transient MS-like state, brainstem dysfunction
Orphenadrine citrate	Norflex	100 mg twice daily	First used for Parkinson rigidity, anticholinergic properties, with Darvon may cause confusion
Chlorzoxazone	Paraflex	500 mg 4 times daily	Marketed with acetaminophen (Parafon-Forte). GI disturbances, dizziness, lethargy

cially by psychoneurotic individuals, limits its usefulness in chronic pain–anxiety states.

ANTIDEPRESSANTS AND PSYCHOTROPIC DRUGS

Amitriptyline hydrochloride (Elavil) and imipramine hydrochloride (Tofranil) are widely used tricyclic antidepressants with striking chemical similarity to phenothiazines but with relatively little effect in quieting agitated psychotic patients. Individuals with endogenous depression syndromes characterized by regression and inactivity are dramatically helped by these drugs, their beneficial effects having been discovered quite accidentally. Perhaps these medications work by dulling depressive ideation rather than by causing euphoria. Indirect evidence for this contention is the fact that normal persons do not become psychically stimulated. On the contrary, fatigue and difficulty concentrating characterize the action of these compounds in volunteers. In animals, the slowing of motor activity is the rule, but both imipramine and amitriptyline have been shown to potentiate the augmentation in rate produced by amphetamine or methylphenidate (Ritalin) in operant conditioning experiments. Such findings suggest that these drugs produce some kind of sensitization within the central nervous system to the effects of adrenergic compounds.

The author's experience with tricyclic antidepressants in treatment of chronic pain is limited to amitriptyline, which may cause slightly more drowsiness than imipramine. The drug may be given in a single daily dose of up to 150 mg at bedtime to avoid some of the excessive lethargy encountered during the day. Even in the absence of clinical depression or elevation in the "depression scale," the MMPI, we have frequently observed good results with this drug in postherpetic neuralgia, post-thoracotomy dysesthesias and other kinds of somatic pain with a disagreeable quality. This drug is potentiated by addition of promethazine (Phenergan) or fluphenazine (Prolixin) when anxiety and agitation contribute to the clinical syndrome. Depressed older patients with chronic spinal pain routinely do well after taking amitriptyline for two or three weeks. If asked directly whether the pain is gone, their usual answer is "no." However, the pain *complaint* threshold is markedly elevated, and the patient's return to nearly unrestricted activity graphically conveys the favorable outlook.

RADIOTHERAPY FOR BENIGN MUSCULOSKELETAL PAIN

A group of Swedish workers studied the effect of radiotherapy for relief of cervical and lumbar spondylosis and in chronically painful musculoskeletal conditions.[21] Earlier reports of longterm good effects in half of all patients treated for these disorders prompted their investigation. A double blind study was designed in which alternate patients were given placebo exposure to the equipment without radiation while the others received three treatments (300 to 600 rads, 170KV-HVL); in the case of spinal pain, exposure was divided between two dorsal portals. Radiotherapy brought major relief of neck pain in 14 of 34 patients with cervical spondylosis (41 per cent) while 20 of 47 receiving placebo therapy were made appreciably more comfortable (42 per cent). Good results of either type of intervention show impressively how the therapist's commitment and support, along with the elaborate trappings of his trade, may favorably condition the patient's response to treatment.

ACUOLOGY – INTERVENTIONS WITH THE NEEDLE

Acupuncture

The oldest of these methods is acupuncture (Latin: *pricking with needles*), which had its origin nearly 3000 years ago in eastern Asia. Although in less favor during the early part of this century, the Cultural Revolution within the People's Republic of China fostered renewed interest in this ancient skill, and stimulated resurgence of its practice for both anesthesia and control of pain. Neither Meridian Theory, upon which acupuncture points are based, nor pulse diagnosis for localization of disease processes can be reconciled with modern neuroanatomical and physiological concepts. Further frustrating a scientific approach to appraisal of these phenomena are the adherents to either of two divergent philosophies. The first group awkwardly tries to "dignify" this art by tailoring it to the Gate Theory of Pain or some other Western set of logic.[47] A second group perpetuates our ignorance by warning that Occidentals do not have the temperament to effectively use traditional Chinese acupuncture.[89] These latter individuals make a plea for entrusting these ancient skills only to Oriental practitioners.

Taub recently stated that "there has been no controlled statistical evidence from Chinese or from the many Western European practitioners of acupuncture that it is in any way superior to a placebo in treatment of chronic pain."[88] He cautions that a scientific inquiry into its cross-cultural effectiveness must depend upon controlled studies carried out in western lands by physicians fluent in the Chinese language and well-schooled in modern medicine, who have traveled to China to study the acupuncture art.

Some investigators suggest that acupuncture may be a form of hypnosis. Critics of this viewpoint argue that while 80 per cent of the Chinese can be brought to levels of surgical analgesia with acupuncture, fewer than 20 per cent of North Americans are hypnotizable to a comparable analgesic state. They vehemently deny that the mechanism in each case could be similar. The fallacy in this conclusion lies in the overlooked fact that susceptibility to hypnosis in a population reflects its penchant for unerring obedience to authority. Could results similar to those of acupuncture be obtained simply by hypnosis in Chinese patients?

The fact that animals can be made immobile in the face of severe pain following acupuncture has been proposed as evidence for a physiological effect. In most studies the animal had been so painfully stimulated in the "control" period that its subsequent immobility when challenged by intense pain, in all probability, reflects a complete disintegration of escape-defense behavior in an emotionally bankrupt creature.

In a series of 25 patients, residents of an eastern U.S. city, who were recently treated by acupuncture for chronic low back pain, one third were significantly improved after four or more treatments. A larger percentage of those who had not undergone previous back surgery were helped, but most of this latter group had negative myelograms. In the same clinic, five of 11 patients with neck pain related to degenerative cervical arthritis had significant improvement in their condition. Admittedly, the number is small and followup is of too short a duration to yield definite conclusions. Most acupuncturists claim only very modest results in patients with longterm pain and in those who have previously undergone neurolytic procedures (e.g., chemical and surgical rhizotomies).

Paraspinal and Epidural Nerve Block

Blockade of sensory fibers emanating from the paraspinous tissues, and the injection of local anesthetics into the epidural space are worthwhile diagnostic measures and afford temporary pain control in many conditions. In certain instances, relief persists days or weeks after injection of relatively short-lasting local anesthetics. Another example of valuable short-term treatment by infiltration is the injection of myofascial trigger points.[90]

Cutaneous Infiltration for Musculoskeletal Pain

Injection of procaine and caffeine into scars has been advocated to relieve pain at remote locations in the body. These cutaneous disturbance emitting fields (DEF) supposedly set up pain patterns referred to deep tissues.[18] This technique is not new; René Leriche apparently successfully injected an appendectomy scar to relieve a frozen shoulder. In a recent series of 51 patients, 39 achieved instant relief of pain in one or another part of the body upon injection of an obvious scar. Much like acupuncture sites, these scars were noted to have an impedance different from the surrounding tissues. Most patients were free of pain for up to 24 hours; when it recurred, another injection brought about an equally dramatic result.

Analgesic Effects of Peri-articular, Epidural, and Intrathecal Steroids

There is little to suggest that steroids have analgesic properties; on the contrary, their effectiveness in controlling pain is well correlated with the anti-inflammatory action of these drugs. Epidural injection of hydrocortisone acetate dissolved in 30 ml of 1 per cent procaine was carried out by Gardner and his colleagues in 239 patients with chronic spinal pain.[16] Fifty-seven per cent of this group achieved fair to excellent relief of symptoms.

However, there is no long term followup report on the fate of these individuals.

Eighty mg of methylprednisolone acetate (Depo-medrol) and forty mg of procaine were mixed with cerebrospinal fluid and instilled into the subarachnoid space in 75 patients with various causes of spinal pain including arachnoiditis. Forty of the group were significantly helped; two of these patients had failed to respond to epidural steroid injection earlier.

Quite recently, a group of patients with chronic low back trouble have been given injections of steroid-procaine mixtures into the articular facets in order to assess the likelihood of producing long-term relief from electrolytic destruction of nerve twigs innervating these joints[60] (vide infra). When relief of pain lasts two or more weeks following facet injection and should it then recur, these investigators seek to denervate the facet joints unilaterally or bilaterally by x-ray controlled radiofrequency coagulation.

Intrathecal Use of Ethanol and Phenol

Both ethyl alcohol and phenol attained meteoric popularity nearly two decades ago for the control of painful spasms associated with paraplegia. Each of these substances in relatively low concentrations can destroy nervous tissue. Today, they retain definite but limited usefulness for treating chronic pain in patients with non-malignant disease. Intrathecal instillation of either compound can be disastrous if the distribution of the drug is not controlled by proper positioning of the patient. Bladder dysfunction is the most frequent disabling sequela. In the opinion of many surgeons, indications for use of these compounds is restricted to patients already without appreciable voluntary control of urination.

Because alcohol is hypobaric with respect to cerebrospinal fluid, the patient should be placed in a semiprone position, with his lumbar spine flexed. This position is easier to achieve using an operating table rather than the patient's bed or an examining table. In this position, the dorsal roots to be blocked are located uppermost. Needle puncture of the subarachnoid space is carried out at the spinal level corresponding to the roots to be blocked. Alcohol is injected in increments of 0.5 ml at intervals of 5 minutes until the desired radicular analgesia is obtained. A flushing sensation is frequently reported. No more than 3 ml of drug should be injected at any one "sitting."

The patient must remain completely immobile for 45 minutes after the last injection. If more than one level is to be blocked, the head or foot of the table can be raised to accomplish that objective. The L2, L3 and L4 nerve roots are easily blocked without much risk of bladder difficulty, but chemical rhizotomy of L5 and S1 is more frequently complicated by vesical hypotonia because other sacral fibers are invariably damaged.[87] Irregularities in the thecal sac because of epidural scarring, along with cysts and adhesions in the subarachnoid space, make results of this procedure even more unpredictable in the patient who has undergone multiple back operations.

Phenol solutions are hyperbaric, which necessitates positioning of the patient so that the dorsal roots to be blocked are located most dependent within the spinal canal. By dissolving 225 mg of phenol in 3 ml of Pantopaque (7.5 per cent phenol solution), one can radiographically control the flow of the mixture, bathing only desired nerve roots in the drug. We have been encouraged by the pain relief afforded individuals with pelvic cancer following this procedure but cannot enthusiastically recommend its use in ambulatory patients with intact bladder function.

Paraspinous Rhizotomy with Ammonia Sulfate

In his revival of *Labat's Textbook of Anesthesia*, Adriani mentions the use of ammonium salts as neurolytic agents. He was disappointed by their transient effect, except in high concentrations, and claims that ammonium chloride works equally as well as the sulfate. Others have recently begun using these compounds for treatment of intercostal and postthoracotomy neuralgia with encouraging initial success.[74] It appears that the commercially available 0.75 per cent ammonium sulfate solution is nearly useless, and that 10 per cent is the minimum effective concentration for producing analgesia of long duration in the distribution of intercostal nerves. There is evidence that a 20 per cent solution may be even more effective. The compound is very irritating and should be injected only after procaine localization and blockade of the nerve. To my knowledge, this compound has not been used for chemical rhizotomy of nerves innervating the limbs. I doubt that the ammonium ion confirms any special neurolytic properties on the solution. Its action may be primarily "osmolytic," a topic to be discussed in the following section.

Salt, and Water, and Slush—A Subarachnoid "Space Odyssey"

Another curious epoch in pain treatment began in 1967 when Hitchcock reported having favorable results with injection of iced normal saline into the lumbar sac for relief of intractable pain.[28] Since cold saline rapidly warms to body temperature within one to three minutes after instilling a 20 ml bolus into the subarachnoid space, destruction of fibers by induced hypothermia could not conceivably be its mode of action.[32] It was reasoned by others that the instilled supernate, or slush, must also be hypertonic because the solution had been frozen and allowed to thaw.

Several workers began to treat patients by intrathecal hypertonic saline infusion for both benign and malignant conditions. Their success was quite variable, but few doubted the existence of an objective benefit from the procedure in many patients. Those of us who have instilled 5 per cent sodium chloride solutions (about 1700 mOsm/L) have been impressed with an initial yield of good results which fade over several days up to a month or more.

In an attempt to explain the analgesic action of hypertonic salt solutions, King and co-workers studied the effects of various salt solutions on the compound action potential using cat dorsal roots in vivo.[35] C-fiber activity was markedly diminished by hypertonic solutions containing chloride (total osmolarity 500 to 2500 mOsm/L), including choline chloride, while other sodium salts were ineffective. They postulated that high concentrations of chloride ion would selectively cross the axon membrane and block propagation of an action potential for an indefinite period. Unmyelinated pain fibers, because of their disproportionately large surface area to volume ratio, might be blocked irreversibly. Differential block of C-fibers was even more impressive when *hypotonic* saline or distilled water was circulated in the subarachnoid space of monkeys. Further studies are being carried out to explain and evaluate these observations, and clinical trials are planned.

It is difficult for us to reconcile these experimental facts with our failure to elicit any change in sensory function, whether or not the patient obtained pain relief. However, careful mapping of two-point discrimination and quantitative pain threshold measurements were not performed. For the treatment of occipital, cervical and thoracic pain, cisterno-lumbar perfusion has been carried out using a pair of needles, one at each end of the spinal canal.[49]

The author prefers to perform the procedure with the patient under general anesthesia and in the sitting position. Early attempts to instill hypertonic saline into the lumbar sac using only sedative-analgesic combinations were stressful procedures for both patient and physician. Muscle rigidity in the limbs becomes intense and painful in spite of large intravenous doses of diazepam. Anxiety, hypertension and hyperventilation were the rule. After lumbar puncture, all obtainable CSF is exchanged with oxygen, following which the spinal subarachnoid space is "filled up" with hypertonic saline (5 to 10 per cent) to a level corresponding to the upper limit of the patient's pain. Estimation is necessary because the volume of the thecal sac is variable; usually 30 to 50 ml is instilled. The patient is allowed to remain in the sitting position for an hour before being taken to the recovery room. The time course for return of subarachnoid fluid osmolarity to normal is demonstrated in Figure 17–3. Hyperventilation and hypertension during this procedure can be minimized by buffering the saline solution to pH 7.35 to 7.40 before injection.

There has been no complication of any significance in performing 22 saline infusions. Transient hesitancy of urination lasting up to a day occurred in eight patients; a single bladder catheterization was required in two patients. Pain was relieved in six cancer patients for one week to two months but eventually returned in all. Four patients got no relief. Infusion was again very helpful in one of three patients in which it was repeated. In benign conditions, primarily chronic low back pain with or without arachnoiditis, results have been very disappointing; only two of eight patients achieved relief symptoms of more than three months. One man, a 46-year-old laborer with severe diffuse lumbar arachnoiditis is working regularly and is now asymptomatic after having experienced severe radicular pain and spasms for many months prior to the infusion. The fact that steroids were also instilled at the same time certainly makes this result uninterpretable.

Patient M.C. 4/72

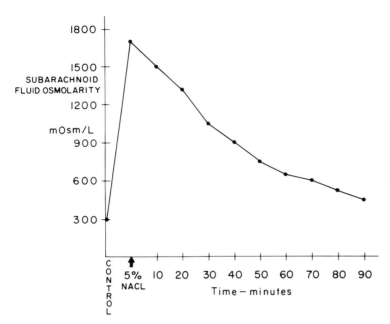

Figure 17–3. The time course for return of CSF osmolarity toward normal after complete O_2-CSF exchange and instillation of 50 ml of 5 per cent sodium chloride solution into the spinal subarachnoid space for the treatment of chronic pain (see text).

Hitchcock recently has reported better results with 10 per cent sodium chloride solutions.[29] Eighty-six per cent of 116 cancer patients noted initial pain relief with subarachnoid instillation of hypertonic saline; 50 per cent had persistent good results three months later. Muscle weakness developed in 3 per cent and sphincter problems in 8 per cent. The degree of objective sensory loss was not described, but results are very encouraging and suggest that the more concentrated solution might be tried in patients with chronic benign pain. Others have instilled concentrations in excess of 20 per cent with resultant severe bladder and motor strength impairment.

To confound the issue a little further, good relief for one to three months has been obtained in nine of 14 individuals with painful malignancies by simple "to and fro" barbotage of their cerebrospinal fluid for several minutes.[42] A study in monkeys has impressively demonstrated lumbar nerve root demyelination following this procedure.

Radiofrequency Percutaneous Rhizotomy of the Articular Nerve to the Facet Joint

In 1971 Rees, an Australian surgeon, first reported on 1000 operations that he performed during a 10-year period for relief of low back pain.[68] His procedure consists of inserting a long scalpel through a paraspinous stab wound and thrusting it into the intertransverse ligament. The blade is then swept up and down, purportedly to sever dorsal twigs of segmental nerves just before their entry into the apophyseal joint capsules between the articular facets. It intrigues me that the tissue trauma and hemorrhage caused by such a maneuver could be compatible with the splendid results Rees claims.

Later in the same year, Shealy began to make radiofrequency lesions for the purpose of interrupting facet joint innervation with the help of both electrical stimulation and radiographic control.[76] Stimulation of paraspinous nerve filaments terminating around the articular facet reproduces the patient's pain and in many cases provides assurance that the anterior primary division of the spinal nerve root is outside the lesion zone. If the electrode is too close to the root, severe radicular pain in a dermatomal distribution occurs with 25 to 50 Hz stimulation at less than 1 volt; muscle contraction results at 1 to 2 volts. An RF lesion is produced gradually after x-ray confirmation of the needle position; the tissue temperature is raised to about 70°C for 90 seconds. The procedure is performed bilaterally at levels corresponding to the patient's pain. After several hours of bedrest, he is permitted to carry out "mobilizing" spinal exercises. Most patients leave the hospital on the following day.

In the first 180 patients to undergo RF rhizolysis, good to excellent results are reported in 87 per cent of previously unoperated patients (71 of 81), in 65 per cent of those with previous lumbar surgery but no fusion (25 of 38) and in 34 per cent of patients with spinal fusions (21 of 61).[77] About 25 per cent of the patients with good initial results had recurrence of pain within one week. Shealy cautions that results will be poor in previously operated patients when symptoms have changed in character or distribution (such as in psychogenic pain or arachnoiditis). One is on more secure ground making these lesions in persons with very transient or no relief from their *original* symptoms following laminectomy. His followup period is as yet too brief for important conclusions to be drawn in this innovative study.

It is not surprising that failure to relieve pain was common in individuals with fused spines, but rather that any significant success was achieved in as many as a third of these patients. The dissection inherent in a lateral approach to lumbar spine fusion should strip the nerve supply to facet joints; furthermore,

grafted bone would be expected to bridge the axilla between the superior facet and transverse process, making needle penetration difficult. Placebo effects contribute significantly to the results of any treatment for pain, and only careful long-term followup of these "cured individuals" can put to rest any doubts. Several papers have dealt with innervation of the apophyseal joint and the nature of nerve endings in and about its capsule.[3, 67, 82] Based upon these anatomic studies, one can postulate the ideal lesion site (Fig. 17-4). There is concern, however, that such lesions actually destroy the entire medial division of the posterior primary ramus and significantly denervate the intrinsic paraspinous muscles. Electromyographic studies will be necessary to test this hypothesis.

NEUROANATOMIC FACTS AND PHYSIOLOGIC HYPOTHESES RELEVANT TO THE CONTROL OF PAIN BY ELECTRICAL STIMULATION AND ABLATIVE SURGERY

Everyone has a unique way of looking at the pain problem, depending on his training

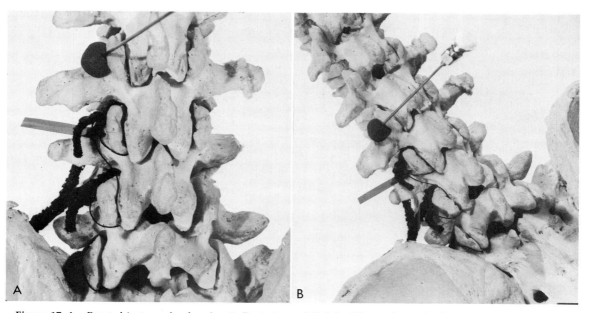

Figure 17–4. Facet rhizotomy landmarks. *A*, Posterior and *B*, left oblique views of a "mock-up" which illustrates the course of nerve twigs innervating the facet joints. The celluloid marker points to the junction of superior facet border and base of the transverse process; the needle is inserted into a plasticine moulage which simulates the ideal lesion. Note the twig of the L3 posterior primary division which courses downward to enter the L4–L5 articulation.

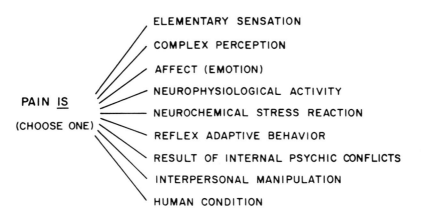

Figure 17–5. Current ways of viewing pain. (From Sternbach, R. A.: Strategies and tactics in the treatment of patients with pain. In B. L. Crue, Jr. (Ed.): *Pain and Suffering—Selected Aspects.* Charles C Thomas, Springfield, p. 177, with permission, 1970.)

and experience (Fig. 17–5). Regardless of one's outlook, there are numerous experimental facts that each of us must weigh in his concept of pain. Classical teaching about peripheral receptors and exteroceptive sensory pathways has undergone little metamorphosis in the past two decades. There is more doubt, perhaps, that specific pain receptors are ubiquitous in the dermis, since most stimuli which produce pain initially evoke the sensation of touch, temperature, or pressure. The *modality specific* theory of sensation has been shaken by more appealing hypotheses which emphasize the importance of patterned sensory input in determining just what the organism perceives. Excessive peripheral stimulation of any type might be expected to cause pain.

Stimuli which exceed receptor threshold will cause propagation of action potentials in the axons of peripheral nerves whose afferent fibers enter the spinal cord through the dorsal root. These signals are integrated in the dorsal gray matter, producing both excitation and inhibition in as many as six adjacent spinal segments in man. Purposeful local responses, such as limb withdrawal to pain, have a segmental origin. Naturally, important descending tracts carry supraspinal impulses which modify reflex behavior at the spinal level.

Most temperature and nociceptor fibers travel for a few segments after entering the tract of Lissauer, then synapse in the substantia gelatinosa Rolandi as well as deeper in the posterior horn upon central transmission "T" cells. The axons of the "T" cells cross to the opposite anterolateral quadrant of the spinal cord and ascend to the brainstem and thalamus as the lateral spinothalamic tract. Some fibers remain ipsilateral, while others contribute bilaterally to the spinoreticular, spinotectal and ventral spinothalamic tracts. Although some spinothalamic tract fibers enter the specific sensory nucleus of the thalamus (VPL), many more are destined to synapse in the bulbar and midbrain reticular formation, or upon cells of the diffuse thalamic projection system. These latter fibers make up the paleospinothalamic tract. Activation of this system is characterized by appreciable conduction delays and strikingly prolonged afterdischarge, suggesting multisynaptic reinforcement in reverberating neuronal circuits. The cellular aggregates composing this primitive part of the thalamus are found near the midline (CM—centrum median, Pf—parafascicularis, DM—dorsalis medialis). Repetitive electrical stimulation of these nuclei causes diffuse cortical activation, the recruiting response. These so-called *intralaminar nuclei* probably have much to do with the affective component of pain perception. Roughly 60 per cent of the cells in this region respond only to intense peripheral stimulation which would be expected to have a noxious quality. Neospinothalamic fibers share with the lemniscal (proprioceptive) system a more specific somatotopic pattern of termination in the nucleus VPL, the direct stimulation of which evokes a discrete cortical response in the parietal lobe. Each neuron in the VPL which responds to mechanical stimulation at the periphery has a restricted receptive field on the opposite side of the body and is modality specific.

In 1965, Melzack and Wall proposed the "gate theory" of pain transmission which has won broad support among sensory physiologists.[52] They suggested that a reciprocal and dynamic state of activity exists between the spinal cord inputs from myelinated (A delta) fibers and small, unmyelinated C fibers which modulates T (central transmission) cells in the dorsal horn. The so-called "gate" can be variably open, permitting cephalad conduction of incoming signals, or closed, thus blocking transmission in ascending pathways. On the basis of evidence from extracellular recordings in the dorsal gray matter, the authors concluded that intermediate cells in the substantia gelatinosa modulate the gate mechanism; these cells are activated by incoming A delta fibers to produce a spike which causes presynaptic inhibition in axons which would otherwise fire the T cells. On the contrary, C fiber activity (conducting "slow pain") would "turn off" SG cells and, therefore, abolish the inhibitory block of fibers ending on the T cells. The gate would then be open, and transfer of information could proceed unimpeded to centers for conscious perception by the animal.

Malfunction in this encoding operation at the level of transition from first to second order sensory neuron could explain a number of pathologic conditions associated with chronic pain. Many neuropathies, because of myelin loss in peripheral nerves, would logically be characterized by dysesthesias and diffuse pain resulting from unchecked C fiber activity. The relief of discomfort by mechanical stimulation (e.g., vibration, massage) in the victim of "painful phantom limb" might, similarly, be explained in terms of gate theory. Peripheral stimulation of mechanoreceptor fibers (actually larger in diameter than the A delta type) would close the gate by activating the inhibitory SG cells in the dorsal input zone of the spinal cord.

It has been more recently demonstrated that a number of subcortical descending fibers and brainstem reticular inputs end on the gating system and exert inhibitory controls.[55, 57] Conceivably, these fibers directly hyperpolarize the spinal sensory neurons. The latter terminals may be part of a feedback circuit set into action by fast-conducting lemniscal afferents. The "inhibitory surround" created by such activity would lead to precise patterns of T cell discharge ascending to orderly conscious interpretation. The abolition of these refined modulators of T cell output would lead to diffuse repetitive discharge in many dorsal horn cells. If the balance of peripheral large and small fiber inputs were simultaneously upset, a phenomenal spectrum of sensory distortion might ensue with myriad, grotesque qualities, all of which the patient communicates as "pain."

Most cells in laminae I and V of the dorsal horn respond exclusively to damaging or near-damaging stimuli. This observation implies that these neurons are alerting cells which lack modality specificity. Other neurons respond only to simultaneous thermal and mechanical stimulation. Such convergence demonstrates an "intensity function" of these neurons, with little evidence that they possess any qualitative discriminatory capacity. Does chronic deafferentation of these cells following spinal cord or peripheral nerve injury remove inhibitory controls and permit them to discharge spontaneously?[43] This mechanism may explain the "central pain state" which sometimes follows injuries of the brachial plexus and spinal cord.

Old Magic – New Magicians

"Electricity is winning victories over pain every day . . . electrical instruments have become part of the armamentarium of every physician." When Spendler wrote these words one hundred years ago (1874),[80] Galvanism was just about as popular as the "electrical inhibition" of pain is becoming today. Physiatrists, neurosurgeons, chiropractors and acupuncturists have all hopped on the bandwagon to prescribe or implant a variety of electrical gadgets for the treatment of intractable pain. Some wag summed up the particular problem confronting us. "Novel remedies for the suffering temporarily help so many folks with pain, that one need only be constantly inventive to cure these folks again . . . again and again."

A battery-operated inductorium has been marketed for 55 years without specific claims being made for its beneficial effects. Many types of vibrators and stimulators are currently available as relaxers and for the treatment of musculoskeletal aches and pains, not to mention the possible erogenous applications of these devices.

Encouraged by their studies of "gate" theory in animals, a clinical trial of peripheral nerve stimulation was reported in 1967 by Wall and Sweet.[94] It was postulated that stimulation of low threshold myelinated fibers in peripheral nerves might inhibit spontaneous C fiber pain by closing the overly facilitated gate.

Results were encouraging. In 1970, Shealy reported on dorsal column electrostimulation with the same objective.[75] Only three of six patients implanted with these devices had been followed for longer than six months; one successful implant provided excellent relief of pain for over one year after a seven year epoch of back and leg pain. Another individual with endometrial carcinoma claimed good relief with the device "half the time." A third patient with paraplegia and multiple sclerosis achieved good relief of pain for several months, and afterward had no pain *in spite of* not using the dorsal column stimulator (DCS). It is difficult to reach a conclusion from these data. Nashold and Friedman have reported their experience with DCS implantation in 30 patients, 11 of whom had chronic low back pain and a history of unsuccessful spinal fusion or surgery for lumbar disc.[63] Results were excellent in only two patients, good in one and fair to poor in eight. Of the latter group, four patients underwent repeat operation for removal of the device.

Naturally, the preoperative selection process should ferret out some of those individuals who are unlikely to benefit from electrohypalgesia. Hosobuchi and his associates have devised a means to test patients for both pain relief and tolerance to the alternative sensation (i.e., buzzing, humming, vibrating) before implantation of the DCS unit.[31] Using a lateral approach to the spinal cord between C1 and C2 on the side of the major clinical pain, a stimulating electrode is inserted into the dorsal column under radiographic control. A small amount of iophendylate (Pantopaque) is instilled into the subarachnoid space to outline the dentate ligament, after which the needle is withdrawn a bit and angulated to penetrate the cord three to four mm posterior to the ligament. Short-term stimulation in a group of 34 patients turned up nine who found the sensation intolerable. Two patients admitted finding the sensation pleasurable. Of 24 who underwent DCS implantation (including none of those finding the stimulation unpleasant), there were good to excellent results in 75 per cent. The nature of their pain and length of followup were not stated in the report. Hosobuchi and Shealy have emphasized the psychoneurotic, hysterical and depressed features of the illness in patients who are intolerant of the vibratory sensation. However, the author hastens to add that prolonged transcutaneous electrical stimulation, from personal experience and that of colleagues, produces an unpleasant sensation in anyone free of pain. Whether a patient's pain disrupts his psychic "economy" to such an extent that he opts for a lesser form of sensory perturbation must be a very individual matter.

Some surgeons rely upon the MMPI scores to accept or reject patients for surgery. Others, including most psychiatrists, discount the value of MMPI profiles, since most patients with chronic pain score high in hypochondriasis, depression and hysteria categories. However, elevations to the right of the scale (reflecting characterologic, or psychotic, traits) portend an unsatisfactory outcome of surgery.

Of the initial 95 DCS implants performed at several different institutions by members of the Dorsal Column Stimulator Study Group the results, unselected as to etiology of pain, were as follows: good to excellent in 55 patients (58 per cent) and fair to poor in 40 patients (42 per cent).[76] Although poor results are likely to become apparent within a few months, late failures of the DCS system or accommodation of nervous tissue with markedly increased thresholds for stimulation will eventually reduce the yield of good results significantly below those quoted.

Technique of DCS (Neuro-Pacemaker) Implantation

The patient is operated upon in the sitting position, precautions having been taken to avoid air embolism. A bilateral laminectomy is performed from the T3 through T6 level in most cases of lower extremity or back pain. The small size of the spinal canal makes lower placement of the electrodes inadvisable. Next, a 3-inch transverse incision is made just below the clavicle; a subcutaneous tunnel is then created running over the shoulder from the clavicle to the laminectomy site.

The electrode (Fig. 17–6) must be delivered from the subclavicular incision to the laminectomy site. This can be accomplished by passing it within a 1/4" Penrose drain. A small, subcutaneous pocket, just large enough to accommodate the receiver, is developed beneath the lower flap of the clavicular incision. The pocket must be far enough below the clavicle to permit placement of the antenna (Fig. 17–6) over the receiver postoperatively.

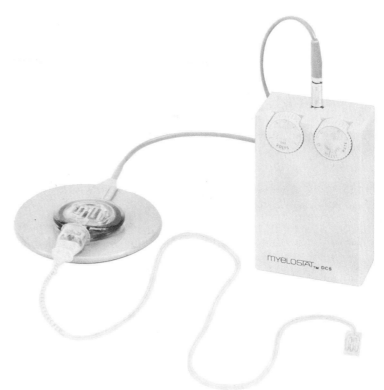

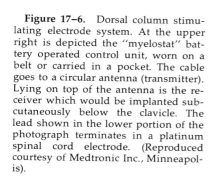

Figure 17–6. Dorsal column stimulating electrode system. At the upper right is depicted the "myelostat" battery operated control unit, worn on a belt or carried in a pocket. The cable goes to a circular antenna (transmitter). Lying on top of the antenna is the receiver which would be implanted subcutaneously below the clavicle. The lead shown in the lower portion of the photograph terminates in a platinum spinal cord electrode. (Reproduced courtesy of Medtronic Inc., Minneapolis).

The receiver cannot be implanted at a depth greater than 1 to 2 cm beneath the epidermis if adequate RF coupling is to be achieved.

The dura is carefully opened in the midline *leaving the arachnoid intact.* If the pain is unilateral, the dural incision is placed toward the side of the pain. Number 4–0 mersilene or silk sutures are used to anchor the electrode subdurally at each of its four corners. Proper placement of the sutures to avoid buckling of the electrode is essential to prevent cord compression. The dura is then closed watertight. Both the laminectomy site and the subclavicular incision are closed in a standard fashion.

Debate exists concerning the advisability of using monopolar versus bipolar electrodes. Bipolar electrodes permit better localization of stimulating current and are more predictable in their function. Controversy exists as to whether subdural extra-arachnoid or intradural placement (i.e., insertion between the layers of the dura using microsurgical techniques) is the preferable means of implantation. In either case, the electrodes may lie 1 to 3 mm from the pial surface of the spinal cord. In order to achieve a good result, the patient must perceive tingling in the area of his pain with proper stimulation parameters.

Three case histories illustrate how one can be misled by equating the patient's acceptance of this device with a good result insofar as pain relief. Each of these individuals had no regrets about having submitted to DCS implantation and was pleased with the result.

CASE 1

B.D., a 60-year-old woman, who had suffered aching right thoracic paraspinal pain, progressively more severe for three years, underwent myelography which revealed no abnormality. Neurologic examination was normal and there was minimal tenderness upon pressure over the ninth and tenth ribs. Psychologic evaluation demonstrated no personality characteristic which would presage a bad result from stimulator implant. The patient has been taking four to six 50 mg Demerol tablets daily for the past year. She was referred to a neurosurgeon with considerable experience in DCS implantation. For the first week following operation, the patient had total relief of pain using the stimulator. Thereafter, the pain did not recur despite her no longer using the device. Three months later, she had a flareup of intercostal pain while anxious; the stimulator brought the discomfort under control. By the next morning, the pain had disappeared, and she has not had to rely upon electrical stimulation again in over five months. When I expressed my delight over her pain relief, the patient explained,

"Oh yes, that terrible pain is gone, but now there is an aching in my shoulder where the wire goes and burning next to the incision Doctor_____ made to put the stimulator in my back." Undaunted, I replied, "But it must be satisfying not to be so dependent upon all that medication to relieve your pain." Whereupon she admitted that the new pain required as much Demerol for its relief as did the old discomfort in her chest.

CASE 2

A.F., a 45-year-old rug weaver, had undergone laminectomy in another hospital three years earlier for treatment of neck pain associated with cervical spondylosis. Soon afterward, he began to experience burning dysesthesias in both hands. Because these sensory abnormalities progressively limited his ability to work for more than a few minutes at a time, he became depressed and agitated. Analgesics, antidepressants, and intrathecal steroids gave him no relief. Physiotherapy aggravated his symptoms. When a resident physician told him to "learn to live with it," he became discouraged and sought an opinion elsewhere. After orthopedic consultation at a large eastern medical center, the patient underwent posterior cervical fusion with considerable relief of these symptoms for three months. Thereafter, his discomfort was accentuated. A DCS unit was implanted in the high cervical region; he was discharged after three additional weeks of hospitalization. According to the operating surgeon, the result was gratifying. When I contacted A.F. by phone six months later, he explained with disdain, "I'm surprised you people would be interested in what happened to me." Asked how he was getting along, the patient replied, "Just great! I'm about halfway back . . . don't know if I'm going to make it, but I'm halfway back. You remember when I was in your hospital . . . I couldn't even hold a pen to write my name. Now I can write three or four lines before those horrible cramps come on." In the meantime, he sold his home, abandoned his work and moved to Florida in order to avoid the possibility that "the cold weather this winter might start up that trouble in my hands."

CASE 3

V.F. is a 34-year-old man who had undergone eight operations for leg and back pain since the age of 17. The first procedure was carried out to excise a herniated lumbar disc. Subsequently, he underwent a fusion, two rhizotomies, lysis of adhesions, a unilateral cordotomy, hypertonic saline infusion and, finally, implantation of a dorsal column stimulator. The patient had been taking ten injections of Talwin daily in order to continue college studies. His absenteeism increased proportionate to a reduction in medication. An RF cordotomy performed two years prior to DCS implant had been the only procedure to give him significant relief of his pain. This short-lived reprieve from suffering coincided with divorce from his first wife and the beginning of a second marriage. The "chronically ill role" appeared to play an important part in this pa-

tient's new relationship; the author suggested psychiatric and family counseling for the couple. Over the next two months tensions grew and feelings had to be communicated. The emotional stress on the patient became overwhelming and he sought an escape. When we temporarily declined to consider DCS implant, he consulted another neurosurgeon who agreed to perform the operation. Initially, the patient had no relief of his symptoms despite adequate stimulation in the pain distribution. During the past four months, however, he has gotten 40 to 50 per cent relief, provided that physical exertion is limited. He requires less Talwin, but also is taking promethazine and diazepam to maintain his marginal status.

Fox has tabulated the incidence of complications encountered by 10 neurosurgeons in connection with DCS implantation.[15] His survey represents a collectively large experience in performing this operation. Common complications were classified as those with an incidence greater than 5 per cent; these include: 1) irritating thoracic dermatome stimulation with intradural electrode placement; 2) stimulation of incorrect dorsal colum fibers with little stimulation of correct ones; 3) change in posture causing a change in current strength to the dorsal columns; and 4) leakage of CSF when implant lay in the subdural location. About half of the patients were unable to achieve adequate levels of pain control for technical or psychologic reasons. Fox believes, as do many other surgeons involved in implantation of these devices, that patients with chronic pain are unlikely to make successful readjustment after DCS implantation without supportive psychotherapy. Like the "cardiac cripple" who is cured of his physical disability by heart valve replacement, role reversal in a society which has viewed him so long as an invalid becomes a stressful endeavor in which the patient cannot succeed without the support and understanding of his family, friends and physicians. Finally, paraparesis resulting from angulation of the electrode causing compression of the spinal cord has been a significant complication because of its severity; the incidence is quite low, however, and the deficit is partly or completely reversed by immediate reoperation.

Transcutaneous Nerve Stimulation

In order to predict a patient's response to dorsal column stimulation, his tolerance for a sensory alternative to pain can be tested using

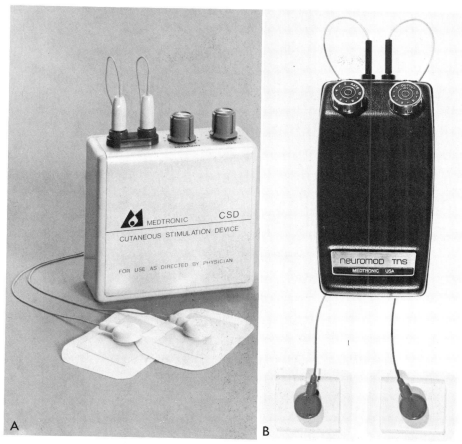

Figure 17–7. Examples of two models of transcutaneous nerve stimulators with cutaneous electrode pairs. The newer, more compact device is shown at the right. Both have fixed pulse width, but rate and voltage are variable (see text). (Reproduced with permission of Medtronic Inc., Minneapolis.)

a transcutaneous electrical stimulator (Fig. 17–7). As a result of the dramatic relief of certain locally painful conditions (e.g., surgical scars, herpes zoster and painful joints) the transcutaneous units have gained popularity as the *primary* therapy for some types of chronic pain and are no longer relegated to the category of "screening devices." The cumbersome task of affixing the electrodes with conductive paste and tape, as well as the variable electrode-to-skin resistance, which depends upon the patient's position, are major drawbacks for which solutions must be found.

In patients without feasible alternatives for definitive treatment of their pain, we have found that 40 to 50 per cent of individuals with intractable sciatic pain have good relief. The patient is permitted to use the TNS device in his home environment. In those who experi-

ence initially satisfactory results (two to three weeks of 90 to 100 per cent relief of their pain) a followup period of six to 12 months will confirm the persistence of relief in most instances. Skin irritation has forced temporary discontinuance of stimulation for one to three days, but is not a serious problem. Encouraging but checkered results have been obtained in patients with brachial plexus injuries, phantom limb pain, penetrating trauma of the cauda equina, lower extremity causalgia,[61] and paraplegia.[10] There is far too little uniformity in these patients' psychological backgrounds or in anatomy of their lesions to allow an objective assessment of these preliminary observations. Long has published a preliminary report of his experience with a large group of patients who have undergone prolonged transcutaneous nerve stimulation.[45]

Implanted Peripheral Nerve Stimulators

Experience with peripheral nerve stimulators, which have been implanted primarily around the sciatic or ulnar nerve for pain control, is limited to fewer than 100 operations performed by a half dozen investigators. Results have been encouraging, although certainly not spectacular, and the opportunity to further refine this technique of "pain blockade" is spurring the interest of several neurosurgeons. Pain arising in the distribution of a single peripheral nerve trunk is often relieved provided the alternative tingling and buzzing sensations are tolerated by the patient.[45b] Wall and Sweet who pioneered in these efforts demonstrated that about half of their patients were free of pain for over 30 minutes after only two minutes of percutaneous or transcutaneous stimulation.[94] Within several months the effects were diminished considerably. To eliminate the possibility that distraction influenced the good results, they stimulated neighboring nerves without an effect on the individual's pain. Wepsic and Sweet, in 1968, reported on the ideal stimulus parameters.[85] Extremely short duration pulses (0.5 milliseconds) were found to cause "burning," while those of long duration (2 to 3 milliseconds) resulted in spread of the stimulus beyond the nerve distribution. Low frequency stimulation (less than 20 Hz) produced a throbbing sensation, and frequencies greater than 75 Hz instigated burning and itching in the skin adjacent to electrodes.[85, 93] Very high voltage (current) causes "cold numbness" to supervene. These authors' experience agrees with ours; optimal parameters for stimulation are the following: 0.1 to 0.4 milliamperes current, 1 to 2 millisecond pulse duration, and 30 to 60 Hz frequency.

Does Electrical Stimulation Really Control Pain?

It should be pointed out that electrical stimuli probably have no unique properties which interrupt painful stimuli, since mechanical vibrators can raise the threshold to perception of pain following application of heat to the skin,[84] just as they block the sensation of intolerable itch in human volunteers.[53] The most effective frequency is close to that for maximal relief of pain using electrical devices. Furthermore, vibratory stimuli block the intolerable "tickle" sensation which might otherwise be expected to build up when the lips are lightly brushed by a nylon thread.[54] Repeated rapid inflation and deflation of a sphygmomanometer cuff on the forearm, distal to the point at which a 60 Hz electrical shock is applied, significantly raises the threshold to pain.[26] In rats, probing of the vagina causes a powerful inhibition of the withdrawal response to concurrent painful stimulation of the leg, a "reflex" dependent upon segmental spinal mechanisms;[36] whether cephalad propagation of pain impulses is blocked was not studied. It is conceivable that each of these mechanical methods brings about activation of large myelinated A fibers which converge in the dorsal root entry zone and provide inhibitory control over the gating system. The pattern of impulses arriving in the spinal cord would, therefore, be little different from that achieved by electrical stimulation of the lowest threshold afferent fibers.

Campbell and Taub recently published evidence for pain relief based on *peripheral* depolarizing blockade.[8] They applied an electrical stimulus over the digital nerve of 11 subjects, proximal to a calibrated pin prick delivered to the fingertip. Moderate intensity (10 to 12 volts) bursts raised the touch threshold; higher intensity, continuous electrical stimulation (22 volts) caused elevation of both touch and pain thresholds. In the latter instance, the A delta wave (purported to conduct epicritic pain sensation) was greatly diminished in tracings obtained by averaging the median nerve sensory compound action potential recorded transcutaneously at the wrist. The hypothesis put forth by these workers does not explain the prolonged elevation of pain threshold observed by others after brief peripheral nerve stimulation. The techniques employed necessitate many assumptions about the relative contributions of A alpha and A delta blockade to the results obtained. Both peaks are suppressed during continous stimulation, and dissonant firing patterns in either "species" of fibers could cause the amplitude of the compound action potential to diminish without necessarily reflecting the "dropping out" of any fiber group.

Electrical stimulation may block pain impulse transmission or, alternatively, provide a pleasurable sensation which subverts anxiety, agitation, and the "pain complaint." The latter effect has been observed innumerable times in both man[25] and animals. Olds demonstrated that animals with hypothalamic electrodes would shock themselves by pressing a bar thousands of times daily to the point of exhaustion.[65] An identical bar which delivered food or water was rarely touched. Mayer and his associates have been able to produce analgesia in *one quadrant* of a rat's body by midbrain stimulation, while not altering position or light touch threshold, and without disturbing the level for perception of pain elsewhere.[51] Most of the effective loci for stimulation were located near the midline in the periaqueductal or interpeduncular gray substance, far from specific sensory pathways. While being stimulated, one animal stood for several minutes waist deep in ice water as he ate some pellets, only to jump out in displeasure 30 seconds after the current was turned off.

In four out of five conscious patients undergoing thalamotomy for relief of pain, stimulation in the nucleus parafascicularis of the thalamus and midbrain tegmentum brought about inhibition of experimentally induced pain in addition to relief of their chronic painful symptoms.[69] These observations are contradicted by earlier stimulation trials during thalamotomy in humans, which elicited paresthesias, terror, intense anxiety, ocular motor dysfunction, a sense of suffocation and numerous other stressful symptoms without elevation of clinical or experimental pain threshold.[22, 62] It should be noted, however, that stimulation parameters differ significantly among these studies. It *is* possible to diminish patient suffering by stimulation in the specific thalamic nuclei (nVPL, nVPM); one pays the price, however, of creating paresthesias which simply mask clinical pain.

The ultimate prosthesis for electrical stimulation to relieve chronic pain should meet the following criteria. It should:

1. provide for low current stimulation of a locus in brain or spinal cord which totally inhibits pain without causing *any* alternative sensation;
2. block conscious perception of pain arising from pathologic tissue without interfering with mental processes or level of awareness;
3. consist of a self-contained, completely implantable safe device with chemically inert electrodes and a subcutaneous energy source which would rarely if ever have to

be replaced or which could be recharged transcutaneously;

4. have tunable stimulus parameters which could be adjusted or turned off by some brief externally applied electromagnetic, radiofrequency, or other type signal delivered from a miniature transmitter.

Although these stipulations might someday be met, and "droves" of patients achieve lasting pain relief with such a device, there surely will be a few who loudly denounce both engineers and surgeons for their contribution to the behaviorally controlled society described by George Orwell in his classic, *1984*. I suppose it could be argued that behavioral modification and other "non-invasive" methods of pain control have a similar potential for abuse in the hands of the unscrupulous.

Most neurophysiologists would agree that our knowledge of precise function in sensory pathways and in their intervening neuronal pools is fragmentary. Any effort to formulate a new conceptual framework in one's observation of pain problems, either in the clinic or in the laboratory, could make an important heuristic contribution to solving the dilemmas confronting us. Our present crude concepts of pain pathophysiology should be viewed only as working hypotheses for the future.

Ablation of Neural Pathways for Pain Relief

The terms ablation (L. *to carry away*), interruption (L. *to make a break in continuity*), and destruction (L. *to ruin the structure of*) all convey a sense of permanent loss. Nevertheless, the two former terms are frequently substituted euphemisms for the latter one. No neurosurgeon ever doubts that the insertion of a knife or radiofrequency probe to alleviate pain is a *destructive* operation. Because of the irreversibility of lesions produced by these procedures, one must weigh the risks of significant neurological complications, eventual annoying dysesthesias and anesthesia dolorosa against the prospect of long term success in relieving the individual's pain. With this admonition to keynote the remarks which follow, and a plea that the reader bear in mind that none of these procedures offers even a two-out-of-three chance for pain relief lasting more than two years, I shall summarize the status of several neurosurgical operations carried out primarily for the control of pain.

DORSAL ROOT RHIZOTOMY
(NEURECTOMY, NEUROLYSIS)

"Neurectomy is the desparing resource of the Physician when he hands a case over to the final mercies of the surgeon." Despite the taint of exaggeration in this plaintive statement, it is as pertinent today as it was a century ago. The results of posterior rhizotomy for chronic spinal pain reflect only modest success in treating a difficult problem. White has described the outcome of sectioning lumbar dorsal roots for intractable sciatic pain after unsuccessful disc surgery or because of focal arachnoiditis.[97] Of 20 patients with this symptom, 14 were initially much better. Three individuals had been followed only four months or less. Therefore, 11 of 17 patients had good results during a followup period of longer than six months (65 per cent). White expressed enthusiasm for the procedure and suggests its use for the treatment of patients with unilateral pain in the distribution of one or two nerve roots, and in the absence of significant low backache. Furthermore, he states that dysesthesias, motor deficits, and a high failure rate (40 per cent at one year, 50 per cent at five years) make cordotomy an inferior operation in this specific group of patients. However, should even two additional patients in White's rhizotomy series fail to maintain relief at five years, a likely possibility, the long term success rate for root section would be nearly identical to that for cordotomy (50 vs 53 per cent). Echols claims that 60 per cent of his patients have achieved good results from rhizotomy, but details of individual cases and followup periods are not reported.[12] Onofrio and Campa, in a review of 12 years' experience with 286 rhizotomies performed at the Mayo Clinic, comment on the results of root section in 78 patients with "discogenic" pain who had previous unsuccessful spinal surgery.[66] Followup evaluations were adequate in 72 individuals, of which 32 were improved (43 per cent). They conclude that "rhizotomy has a poor to fair chance of success." Loeser surveyed the experience of a group of seven neurosurgeons associated with the University of Washington Pain Clinic in their performance of 45 rhizotomies; while short-term operative success (less than three months) in this group of patients was 63 per cent, long-term good results quickly dwindled to 28 per cent.[44]

Because the nerve roots to be severed usually cannot be identified with much confidence using paraspinal nerve blocks, the surgeon must be guided by the radicular distribution of the patient's pain. In performing this operation, one often finds that the dorsal roots are encased in scar and difficult to isolate. Subarachnoid adhesions frequently make separation of the nerve root trunks difficult, with damage to their blood supply and frank hemorrhage resulting from too vigorous a dissection. It may be desirable to awaken the patient momentarily after sectioning the suspect nerve roots in order to determine adequacy of fiber interruption before completing the operation.

SPINOTHALAMIC TRACTOTOMY (OPEN AND PERCUTANEOUS CORDOTOMY)

Spiller's postmortem observation of tuberculomas symmetrically placed in the anterolateral quadrants of the spinal cord in a man with bilateral lower extremity analgesia prompted Martin to perform the first cordotomy for relief of pain in 1911.[81] Since that auspicious beginning, many thousands of operations have been carried out for a variety of painful somatic conditions. The largest experience and greatest success with cordotomy has been in the alleviation of pain in terminal malignancy. A recurrence rate in excess of 50 per cent and high incidence of troublesome dysesthesias in patients with benign neuralgias and chronic radiculopathy should dissuade the wise physician from recommending this operation enthusiastically for persons with long life expectancy.

The development of percutaneous radiofrequency cordotomy with the patient awake has placed at the disposal of the neurosurgeon a simple effective method for control of pain. Rosomoff has stated that cramping, throbbing and aching pain are most often relieved by the operation, but that burning sensations and paresthesias are much less likely to be abolished.[72] The unilateral procedure will provide total contralateral analgesia, the level of which can be very well controlled from the sacral dermatomes up to C4 segment. However, it is rarely possible to obtain upper extremity analgesia and spare pain sensation in the trunk and lower extremity. It must be stressed that low backache and pain of diffuse lumbar arachnoiditis fail to respond to the unilateral procedure. The risks of weakness, bladder dysfunction, impotence, and respiratory paralysis, in the author's opinion, contraindicate bi-

lateral high cervical cordotomy for midline pain associated with benign disease. The alternative, open thoracic cordotomy, obviates the risk of respiratory failure. However, complications are just as frequent, and the incidence of postoperative dysesthesias is somewhat higher than with the percutaneous procedure.

Technique of Percutaneous Cordotomy

The patient is pre-medicated with phenobarbital, promethazine and diazepam to attain a relaxed, cooperative state. He is placed on a standard x-ray table for polaroid film control of needle placement, or on a special-studies carriage if the C arm image intensifier monitoring unit is to be employed. His head is supported by the padded Rosomoff head holder, and his shoulders are elevated, using an inflatable pillow to attain a gentle cervical curve with upward convexity (Fig. 17–8). An open mouth AP film of the odontoid and a lateral upper cervical radiograph are taken; if exposures are optimal, the skin over the mastoid process opposite the side of clinical pain is prepared with antiseptic solution and a No. 18 thin-walled, short bevel spinal needle is inserted in line with a point 5 mm behind the

posterior longitudinal ligament at the level of C1 and C2. One per cent lidocaine (xylocaine) is injected as the needle is advanced, with care being taken to avoid intravasation of anesthetic. Resistance is encountered when the ligamentum flavum is reached. If the needle is not about to enter the spinal cord in the optimal location to produce a lesion, as determined by the lateral TV image or radiograph, it should be partially withdrawn and reinserted, taking into account the previous error. As the resistance of ligamentum flavum is overcome, one enters the epidural space. At this point 2 to 3 ml of local anesthetic should be injected to block the C2 sensory root following preliminary aspiration to ascertain that the needle is neither in a vein nor in the subarachnoid space. The dura is then penetrated, and the needle is attached to a manipulator for fine control of positioning. After forewarning the patient that he may experience a slight headache, 10 cc of air is injected to outline the surface of the spinal cord; 0.5 to 1 ml of contrast medium (Pantopaque) may be instilled after mixing with a small volume of cerebrospinal fluid to delineate the dentate ligament. The author prefers the latter maneuver over air injection because it seems to improve the accuracy

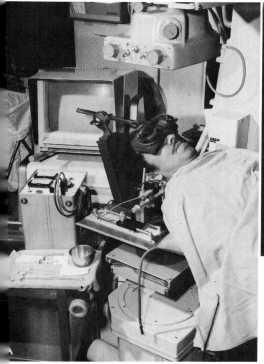
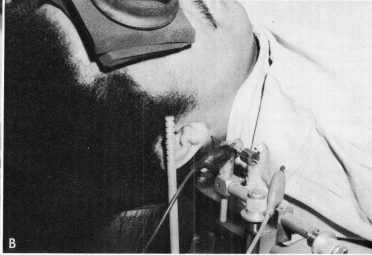

Figure 17–8. *A,* Arrangement for percutaneous radiofrequency cordotomy demonstrating the use of a Rosomoff head-holder and manipulator; a C-arm image intensifier unit permits excellent radiographic control of needle placement. *B,* Closeup to demonstrate site of needle insertion and the manipulator used to accurately guide the electrode into the spinal cord.

of needle placement within the cord. The tip of the spinal needle is adjusted under x-ray control to lie in line with the lateral border of the odontoid process in the AP projection, and 2 mm anterior to the dentate ligament (for lower extremity pain) on the lateral view. A teflon-insulated wire electrode is then inserted through the needle to project 4 mm from the needle shaft. Calibration must have been carried out prior to beginning the operation to assure that the electrode, firmly set in the sizer clamp, will project the proper distance from the spinal needle with a 2-mm length of Teflon insulation between the needle bevel and the exposed electrode tip. An impedance monitor is a valuable adjunct to assure that the cord has been penetrated. Stimulation can be carried out before generating the lesion to determine whether the needle is situated dangerously close to motor fibers. The use of electrical stimulation to cause paresthesias in specific contralateral dermatomes to more accurately localize the electrode has been disappointing.

A 5-second burst of RF current (60 to 80 mA, 25 to 30 RF volts) is delivered, after which the patient is checked for development of a sensory level to pinprick. Strength in the ipsilateral limbs is also tested after each attempt to create a lesion. The duration of current passage is gradually increased to 30 seconds in 5-second increments, or until a solid analgesic zone develops. The needle is then removed, and the patient is returned to his room. Codeine or dextropropoxyphene and aspirin are occasionally required for relief of a mild suboccipital heachache which persists from one to four days after the procedure.

An alternative approach for producing an RF lesion in the spinothalamic tract involves needle insertion medial to the carotid artery and into the C5 – C6 disc.[41] After passing through the intervertebral disc, the needle enters the anterior quadrant of the spinal cord. This freehand method permits little adjustment of the needle after entry into the spinal cord, and it is frustrating to perform in patients with significant cervical spondylosis. In spite of its lack of esthetic appeal, the author acknowledges the good results of this technique in the hands of those who have developed it. It does have a significant advantage in circumventing the risk of respiratory paralysis when one must make bilateral lesions.

Twelve of Rosomoff's 100 bilateral percutaneous cordotomies were performed for benign radicular pain.[70] Early results were encouraging and death occurred in only two cases (2 per cent). Tidal volume was decreased by 36 per cent; however, an increased respiratory rate somewhat compensated for the change, resulting in an overall decrease in minute respiratory volume (MRV) of only 13 per cent.[71]

Because the initial results of cordotomy for chronic pain are quite favorable, it would be instructive if we could learn why so many late failures occur, and devise means to prevent some of them.

All available evidence confirms that functional regeneration of the coagulated or severed pathways does not occur. However, as early as a few hours following cordotomy, the nerve endings in the analgesic skin can be demonstrated to convey an uncomfortable sensation on repetitive electrical stimulation. Cutaneous pinprick or testicular pressure in the "insensitive" region may evoke the feeling of stinging pain or cramping in a symmetrical point on the opposite side (allechesthesia).

Uncrossed direct ventral spinothalamic fibers may help to explain these observations. It is also well known that dorsal column fibers carry information relative to the quality of tactile sensation and serve as intensity detectors for low frequency stimuli. Progressive facilitation in these pathways could theoretically bring about renewed cephalad transmission of previously blocked impulse patterns interpreted consciously as pain.

A disturbingly common finding in patients immediately after unilateral cordotomy, or a few days later, is the emergence of pain on the contralateral side. The classical explanation for this phenomenon in patients with malignant disease has been the *unmasking* of a lesser source of pain by alleviation of the "primary hurt." A more appealing mechanistic hypothesis would be that cordotomy had resulted in switching of the same pain inputs to remaining sensory pathways. Therefore, the appearance of pain in the previously uninvolved side could be construed as referred discomfort from the original site of pathology.[64] Unfortunately, only inferential evidence presently supports this viewpoint.

LONGITUDINAL COMMISSURAL MYELOTOMY

This operation gained popularity throughout France and Germany 20 years ago for relief of bilateral pain in the lumbosacral region, but has never sparked much enthusiasm on the North American continent. In this procedure, the spinal cord is split vertically along its axis somewhat reminiscent of cutting a hot dog roll nearly in two. Great care must be taken to avoid lacerating the anterior spinal artery by extending the incision too deeply. However, thorough midline separation of the cord substance is essential to interrupt crisscrossing axons of the T cells on either side destined to form the lateral spinothalamic tracts.

Since crossing of these fibers may take place as much as three segments rostral to the level of the corresponding dorsal root, one must take this fact into account when planning the longitudinal extent of the incision. Laminectomy is carried out from D9 through D12 for pain in the L3–S1 distribution. Using the binocular operating microscope, a 3 to 5 cm midline incision is made along the exposed spinal cord after coagulating and reflecting the dorsal spinal vein. When possible, a short-acting anesthetic should be employed to permit testing the patient for an adequate sensory level; if necessary, the cord incision is extended prior to wound closure. Sourek's experience with myelotomy in 25 patients, three of whom had chronic spinal pain, demonstrates how limited analgesia can be even after "generous" incision of the cord.[79] The remarkable observation in this series was the gross disparity between the relatively extensive area of pain relief and the restricted dermatomal distribution of analgesia to pinprick. It was shown that sensory conduction was impaired below the level of the lesion even though pinprick sensation was not altered. We have performed only two lumbar commissural myelotomies, both in patients with malignant disease. In each case, the result was satisfactory for over three months; bowel and bladder functions were very transiently impaired. Sourek reported that most of his patients complained of unpleasant burning sensations in the most distal dermatomes which disappeared within a few days following surgery. Hypesthesia and some loss of position and vibration sense suggested damage to the dorsal columns in these patients.

The indications are poorly defined for performing myelotomy in individuals with bilateral lumbosacral pain resulting from arachnoiditis or epidural scarring. It is perhaps a better operation than open bilateral thoracic cordotomy, but the incidence of impotence, dysesthesias, and later recurrence of pain must first be documented. The rather limited number of dermatomes which can be rendered totally analgesic, even by an extended cord incision, may presage a disappointingly high rate of pain recurrence.

CEREBRAL STEREOTAXY FOR RELIEF OF THE "PAIN COMPLAINT"

There is not a single report in the medical literature published in the English language which stresses the results of cerebral lesions made in more than a "handful" of patients for treatment of benign painful disorders. Because the author has never performed a psychosurgical operation for relief of "suffering," the discussion which follows provides the reader with only a studied opinion regarding the virtues of "disconnection" operations in the control of chronic pain.

Most workers in this field agree that in order to attain satisfactory pain relief and lessen the patient's suffering, both family and physician must accept behavioral and personality change as a "necessary evil." More refined operative techniques have replaced the crude frontal lobotomy; these newer operations diminish affective feeling tone but without devastating the individual's ability to remain socially responsible and reflect upon the future consequences of his behavior. Intelligence also appears to be intact when challenged by the usual testing methods. Several investigators have been impressed by a high correlation between degree of psychoneurosis, freefloating anxiety with agitation, or overreaction and the favorable results from cerebral stereotactic operations for pain.

The only currently important categories of cerebral surgery for pain are 1) thalamotomy and 2) cingulumotomy, along with their modifications. Theoretically, each of these operations is a logical and scientifically valid application of our knowledge concerning emotion modifying pathways to the solution of an impelling clinical problem.

Early experience with lesions in the specific thalamic nuclei (nVPL and nVPM of the ventrobasal thalamus) demonstrated that pain relief was seldom satisfactory even with production of profound sensory loss in the painful region. In animal experiments, a considerable number of sensory fibers were shown to synapse in the reticular system and in the paramedian (intralaminar) thalamic nuclei. To make the prospect of interrupting these diffuse projections even more intriguing was the fact that these nuclei had long been suspected to be vital "way stations" for modulating input to the limbic system. In the followup of six patients with chronic spinal pain who underwent either lateral mesencephalotomy (three) or mesencephalotomy plus medial thalamotomy (three), one in each group attained satisfactory relief of pain while the other two had little or no prolonged relief.[99]

Mark and Ervin published their experience with medial thalamic lesions.[48] An updated report of their results appears in a monograph by White and Sweet on neurosurgical relief of pain.[98] Thirty-eight patients underwent thalamotomy, nine of whom experienced chronic intractable pain with a benign cause. Of these nine individuals, none had a good result for over one year. Even more important, the *initial* result was fair to poor in all but one patient, a lady who had multiple sclerosis. She died 10 months later.

Cingulumotomy involves cutting the large fiber bundle which connects the medial frontal lobe with the hippocampus via a circuitous route over, around, and down behind the corpus callosum. Lesions are made in this pathway about 3.5 to 5 cm behind the tip of the frontal horn of the lateral ventricle. LeBeau carried out some of the pioneering studies on effects of "anterior cingulectomy" in man.[40] These early operations were performed through a unilateral craniotomy, with cutting of the tract under direct vision. He concluded that there was little effect on intelligence, and he denied adverse psychological reactions in these patients. One should be aware, however, that 60 per cent of his patients had severe retardation, epilepsy with violent outbursts and retardation, or were unmanageable psychotics. It was concluded that "results are bad with introversion, chronic anxiety and pain, also in psychopathics . . . good in extroversion with irritability and violence." Foltz and White performed 16 cingulumotomies for pain, with the goal of reducing both fear and anxiety.[14] Five of their patients had psychogenic pain disorders; four of these individuals were greatly improved. In another five, with clear cut organic pathology and significant contributing emotional factors, two experienced a good result. None of these patients had chronic spinal pain of benign origin. The authors state that they realized the patient

would be "a different person after the operation." Results of bilateral incisions in the cingulum bundles were superior to those after the unilateral operation. Using Köhler's kinesthetic figural aftereffect test, it was possible to predict those who would be most helped by the procedure; "augmenters" had an unmistakably better outcome than did "moderates" or "reducers." Ballantine and his collaborators reported on a large series of cingulumotomies for psychiatric disorders; included in this population were 12 interspersed procedures carried out for pain of malignancy.[4] They give no details of the outcome in the pain group. Brown and Lighthill tabulated the results in 110 patients undergoing bilateral cingulumotomy for a variety of psychiatric disorders.[7] Although their data sample includes no painful states, the results of surgery are pertinent to this discussion. There were no deaths. Postoperative confusion and urinary incontinence persisted less than a week in the vast majority of patients. Eighty-seven per cent of the results were considered to be "very satisfactory"; 71 per cent of this group were "well," while the remaining 16 per cent were "greatly improved." Intractable psychoneurotics, obsessive-compulsive neurotics, manic-depressive psychotics, and individuals with affective psychoses made up the majority of the population. Others suggest that obsessive-compulsive neurotics, especially, can be restored to a completely normal life-style following cingulumotomy.

Many surgeons who embark upon interruption of the limbic system, with pain relief as their objective, defend the operation as a maneuver producing "no change in intelligence and no objectionable personality traits." It is my opinion that a conduction bundle so large, which interconnects diverse and dynamic information processing stations, must make some major contribution to the individual's behavior. Therefore, its destruction should be manifested by a detectable change in that behavior. Faillace et al. investigated nine patients who had undergone cingulumotomy for pain.[13] The four individuals initially benefited by the procedure demonstrated abnormalities of "non-verbal ordering," and in the "tapping test." It was implied that repetitive tasks (e.g., knitting, shifting gears in an automobile) might be made more difficult by cingulum ablation. This would be a small sacrifice for pain relief; unfortunately, only one of the original nine patients maintained his freedom from pain for over three months. Since seven of the nine had cancer, projection of these results to benign states is impossible. The recent series of Turnbull, in which he combined midbrain and bilateral cingulate lesions, demonstrates only 50 per cent good results in patients with "benign" pain (three of six) in relatively short-term followup.[91] In contrast, nine of his 10 patients with malignant disease have been significantly relieved for over one month.

The initially satisfactory but transient good results in many patients undergoing cingulumotomy should encourage modifications in technique. Unfortunately, there are two important factors which severely impede progress in stereotaxic surgery: 1) the limited applicability of pain research in lower animals to human pathologic behavior, and 2) the capriciousness of empirically lesioning the human brain.

References

1. Alexander, J. P.: Problems associated with the use of the knee chest position for operations on lumbar intervertebral discs, J. Bone Joint Surg. *55B*:279–284, 1973.
2. Alexander, L.: Differential diagnosis between psychogenic and physical pain: The conditional psychogalvanic reflex as an aid, J.A.M.A. *181*:855–861, 1962.
3. Badgley, C. E.: The articular facets in relation to low back pain and sciatic radiation, J. Bone Joint Surg. *23*:481–496, 1941.
4. Ballantine, H. T., Cassidy, W. L., Flanagan, N. B., and Marino, R.: Stereotaxic anterior cingulotomy for neuropsychiatric illness and intractable pain, J. Neurosurg. *26*:488–495, 1967.
5. Bonica, J.: Pain. U.S. National Institute of General Medical Sciences, Bethesda, Maryland, U.S. National Institutes of Health, 1968, p. 13.
6. Brody, H.: Chinese versus American acupuncture. New Eng. J. Med. *287*:724–725, 1972.
7. Brown, M. H., and Lighthill, J.A.: Selective anterior cingulotomy: A psychosurgical evaluation. J. Neurosurg. *29*:513–519, 1968.
8. Campbell, J. N., and Taub, A.: Local analgesia from percutaneous stimulation: A peripheral mechanism. Arch. Neurol. *28*:347–350, 1973.
9. DePalma, A. F., and Rothman, R. H.: Surgery of the lumbar spine. Clin. Orthop. *63*:162–170, 1969.
10. Davis, R.: Personal communication.
11. DiStefano, V. J., Klein, K. S., Nixon, J. E., and Andrews, E. T.: Intra-operative analysis of the effects of position and body hiatus on surgery of the low back: A preliminary report. Clin. Orthop. *99*:51–56, 1974.
12. Echols, D. H.: Sensory rhizotomy following operation for ruptured intervertebral disc: Review of 62 cases. J. Neurosurg. *31*:335–338, 1969.
13. Faillace, L. A., Allen, R. P., McQueen, J. D., and Northrup, B.: Cognitive deficits from bilateral cingulotomy for intractable pain in man. Dis. Nerv. Syst. *32*:171–175, 1971.
14. Foltz, E. L., and White, L. E.: Pain "relief" by frontal cingulumotomy. J. Neurosurg. *19*:89–100, 1962.
15. Fox, J. L.: Dorsal column stimulation for relief of intractable pain: Problems encountered with neuropacemakers. Surg. Neurol. *2*:59–64, 1974.
16. Gardner, W. J., Wasmuth, C. E., Goebert, H. W., and Sehgal, A. D.: Effects of intrathecal and epidural steroids, as communicated to F. A. Alexander and quoted in Hale, D. E. (ed.): Anesthesiology. Philadelphia, F. A. Davis, 1963, p. 836.
17. Gardner, R. C.: A safe, time-tested durable brace support system for precise spinal surgery: A method utilizing well tolerated pressure points and proper positioning, Orth. Review *11*:43–45, 1972.
18. Gerzner, L. F.: Management of intractable pain by neural therapy. Med. J. Aust. *1*:1051–1054, 1970.
19. Gillman, J.: Pain relief and other effects following barbotage, Lancet *1*:746, 1972.
20. Glaser, F. B.: Narcotic addiction in the pain prone female patient. I. A comparison with addict controls, Int. J. Addict. *1*:47, 1966.
21. Goldie, I., Rosengren, B., Moberg, E., and Hedelin, E.: Evaluation of radiation treatment of painful conditions of the locomotor system. A double blind study. Acta Radiol. (Ther.) Stockholm *9*:311–322, 1970.
22. Gybels, J., Peluso, F., and Cosyns, P.: Modification of sensation evoked by skin stimulation during central nervous system stimulation. Electroencephalogr. Clin. Neurophysiol. *27*:657–658, 1969.
23. Haggard, H. W.: Devils, Drugs and Doctors. New York, Harper and Bros. 1929.
24. Hastings, D. E.: A simple frame for operations on the lumbar spine, Canad. J. Surg. *12*:251–253, 1969.
25. Heath, R. G., and Mickle, W. S.: Evaluation of seven years experience with depth electrode studies in human patients, *In* E. R. Ramey and D. S. O'Doherty (eds.) Electrical Studies of the Unanesthetized Brain. New York, Haber, 1960.
26. Higgins, J. D., Tursky, B., and Schwartz, G. E.: Shock elicited pain and its reduction by concurrent tactile stimulation. Science *172*:766–767, 1971.
27. Hippocrates: The Genuine Works of Hippocrates, London, Sydenham Society, 1859.
28. Hitchcock, E.: Hypothermic subarachnoid irrigation for intractable pain. Lancet *1*:1133–1135, 1967.
29. Hitchcock, E., and Prandini, M. N.: Hypertonic saline in the management of intractable pain. Lancet *1*:310–312, 1973.
30. Hitselberger, W. E., and Witten, R. M.: Abnormal myelograms in asymptomatic patients, J. Neurosurg. *28*:204–206, 1968.
31. Hosobuchi, Y., Adams, J. E., and Weinstein, P. R.: Preliminary percutaneous dorsal column stimulation prior to permanent implantation: Technical note, J. Neurosurg. *37*:242–245, 1972.
32. Hubbard, J. H.: Unpublished observations.
33. Jaffe, J. H.: Narcotics in the treatment of pain. Med. Clin. N. Amer. *52*:33–46, 1968.
34. Kellgren, J. H.: Deep pain sensibility. Lancet *1*:943, 1949.
35. King, J. S., Jewett, D. L., and Sundberg, H. R.: Differential blockade of cat dorsal root C fibers by various chloride solutions, J. Neurosurg. *36*:569–583, 1972.

36. Komisaruk, B. R., and Larson, K.: Suppression of a spinal and a cranial nerve reflex by vaginal or rectal probing in rats. Brain Res. *35*:231–235, 1971.

37. Kroger, W. S.: Hypnotism and acupuncture. J.A.M.A. *220*:1012–1013, 1972.

38. Krumperman, L. W.: Personal communication.

39. Lasagna, L., and Werner, G.: Conjoint clinic on pain and analgesia. J. Chron. Dis. *19*:695–709, 1966.

40. LeBeau, J.: Anterior cingulectomy in man. J. Neurosurg. *11*:268, 1954.

41. Lin, P. M., Gildenberg, P. L., and Polakoff, P. P.: An anterior approach to percutaneous lower cervical cordotomy. J. Neurosurg. *25*:553–560, 1966.

42. Lloyd, J. W., Hughes, J. T., and Davies-Jones, G. A.: Relief of severe intractable pain by barbotage of cerebrospinal fluid. Lancet *1*:354–355, 1972.

43. Loeser, J. D., Ward, A. A., and White, L. E.: Chronic deafferentation of human spinal cord neurons. J. Neurosurg. *29*:48–50, 1968.

44. Loeser, J. D.: Dorsal rhizotomy for relief of chronic pain, J. Neurosurg. *36*:745–750, 1972.

45a. Long, D. M.: External electrical stimulation as a treatment for chronic pain. Minn. Med. *57*:195–198, 1974.

45b. Long, D. M.: Electrical stimulation for relief of pain from chronic nerve injury. J. Neurosurg. *39*:718–722, 1974.

46. McNab, I.: Negative disc exploration. An analysis of the causes of nerve root involvement in 68 patients. J. Bone Joint Surg. *53A*:891–903, 1971.

47. Man, P. L.: Mechanism of acupunctural anesthesia: The two gate control theory, Dis. Nerv. Syst. *33*:730–735, 1972.

48. Mark, V. H., and Ervin, F. R.: Role of thalamotomy in treatment of chronic severe pain. Postgrad. Med. *37*:563–571, 1965.

49. Mathews, G. J., Ambruso, V. T., and Osterholm, J. L.: Hypothermic, hyperosmolar saline irrigation of cisterna magna, a new method for relief of pain. Surg. Forum *21*:445–447, 1970.

50. Matsumoto, T., and Hayes, M. F.: Acupuncture, electric phenomenon of the skin, and post-vagotomy gastrointestinal atony. Am. J. Surg. *125*:176–180, 1973.

51. Mayer, D. J., Wolfle, T. L., Akil, H., Carder, B., and Liebeskind, J. C.: Analgesia from electrical stimulation in the brainstem of the rat. Science *174*:1351–1354, 1971.

52. Melzack, R., and Wall, P.: Pain mechanisms: A new theory. Science *150*:971–997, 1965.

53. Melzack, R., and Schecter, B.: Itch and vibration. Science *147*:1047–1048, 1965.

54. Melzack, R., and Eisenberg, H.: Skin sensory afterglow. Science *159*:445–447, 1968.

55. Melzack, R., and Wall, P., Psychophysiology of pain. Int. Anesthesiol. Clin. *8*:3–34, 1970.

56. Melzack, R.: On the language of pain. Anesthesiology. *34*:50–59, 1971.

57. Melzack, R.: Phantom limb pain: Concept of a central biasing mechanism. Clin. Neurosurg. *18*:188–207, 1971.

58. Mennell, J. M.: Back Pain: Diagnosis and treatment using manipulative techniques. Boston, Little-Brown and Co., 1960.

59. Mitchell, S. Weir: Doctor and Patient. Philadelphia, J. B. Lippincott, 1904.

60. Mooney, V.: Personal communication.

61. Myer, G. A., and Fields, H. L.: Causalgia treated by selective large fiber stimulation of peripheral nerve. Brain *95*:163–168, 1972.

62. Nashold, B. S., Wilson, W. P., and Slaughter, G.: Sensations evoked by stimulation in the midbrain of man. J. Neurosurg. *30*:14–24, 1969.

63. Nashold, B. S., and Friedman, H.: Dorsal column stimulation for control of pain. Preliminary report on 30 patients. J. Neurosurg. *36*:590–597, 1972.

64. Nathan, P. W., Reference of sensation at the spinal level. J. Neurol. Neurosurg. Psychiat. *19*:88–100, 1956.

65. Olds, J., and Milner, P.: Positive reinforcement produced by electrical stimulation of septal area and other regions of rat brain. J. Comp. Physiol. Psychol. *47*:419–427, 1954.

66. Onofrio, B. M., and Campa, H. K., Evaluation of rhizotomy: Review of 12 years' experience. J. Neurosurg. *36*:751–755, 1972.

67. Pedersen, H. E., Blunck, C., and Gardner, E.: The anatomy of lumbosacral posterior rami and meningeal branches of spinal nerves (sinu-vertebral nerves), with an experimental study of their functions. J. Bone Joint Surg. *38A*:377–391, 1956.

68. Rees, W. E. S.: Multiple bilateral subcutaneous rhizolysis of segmental nerves in the treatment of the intervertebral disc syndrome. Ann. Gen. Prac. (Australia) *16*:126–127, 1971.

69. Richardson, D. E., and Akil, H.: Acute relief of intractable pain by brain stimulation in human patients. Presented at the American Association of Neurological Surgeons annual meeting, Los Angeles, April 1973.

70. Rosomoff, H. L.: Bilateral percutaneous cervical radiofrequency cordotomy. J. Neurosurg. *31*:41–46, 1969.

71. Rosomoff, H. L., Krieger, A. J., and Kuperman, A. S.: Effects of percutaneous cervical cordotomy on pulmonary function. J. Neurosurg. *31*:620–627, 1969.

72. Rosomoff, H. L.: Personal communication.

73. Ryan, E. D., and Kovacic, C. R.: Pain tolerance and athletic participation. Percept. Mot. Skills *22*:383–390, 1966.

74. Sarot, I. A.: Ammonium sulfate in chest wall pain. Ann. Thorac. Surg. *10*:479–480, 1970.

75. Shealy, C. N., Mortimer, J. T., and Hagfors, N. R.: Dorsal column electroanalgesia, J. Neurosurg. *32*:560–564, 1970.

76. Shealy, C. N.: Discussion presented at the *Seminar on Dorsal Column Stimulation*, Temple University Health Sciences Center, Philadelphia, September 1972.

77. Shealy, C. N., Prieto, A., Burton, C., and Long, D. M.: Articular nerve of Luschka rhizotomy for relief of back and leg pain. (Submitted for publication.)

78. Smith, R. H., Grambling, Z. W., and Volpitto, P. P.: Problems related to the prone position for surgical operations. Anesthesiology *22*:189–193, 1961.

79. Sourek, K.: Commissural myelotomy. J. Neurosurg. *31*:524–527, 1969.

80. Spender, J. K.: Therapeutic Means for the Relief of Pain. London, Macmillan, 1874.

81. Spiller, W. G., and Martin, E.: The treatment of persistent pain of organic origin in the lower part of the body by division of the anterolateral column of the spinal cord. J.A.M.A. *58*:1489–1490, 1912.

82. Stillwell, D. L.: Overlapping segmental capsular innervation by adjacent roots. Anat. Rec. *125*:139–162, 1956.

83. Su, P. C., and Feldman, D. S.: Motor nerve terminal and muscle membrane stabilization by diphenylhydantoin administration. Arch. Neurol. *28*:376–379, 1973.

84. Sullivan, R.: Effect of different frequencies of vibration on pain threshold detection. Exp. Neurol. *20*:135–142, 1968.

85. Sweet, W. H., and Wepsic, J. G.: Treatment of chronic pain by stimulation of fibers of primary afferent neurons. Trans. Am. Neurol. Assoc. *93*:103–107, 1968.

86. Szasz, T. S.: The painful person. J. Lancet *88*:18–22, 1968.

87. Tank, T., Dohn, D. F., and Gardner, W. J.: Intrathecal injections of alcohol or phenol for relief of intractable pain. Cleve. Clin. Quart. *30*:111–117, 1963.

88. Taub, A.: Acupuncture, Science *178*:9, 1972.

89. Toyama, P. M.: Acupuncture: Its use in control of pain. Presented at a Symposium, Functional Methods for Treating Pain, LaCrosse, Wisconsin, September 1972.

90. Travell, J.: Basis for multiple uses of local block of somatic trigger areas (procaine infiltration and ethyl chloride spray). Mississippi Valley Med. J. *71*:13–20, 1949.

91. Turnbull, I. M.: Bilateral cingulumotomy combined with thalamotomy or mesencephalic tractotomy for pain. Presented at the American Association of Neurological Surgeons annual meeting, Los Angeles, April 1973.

92. Walker, J.: Pain and distraction in athletes and non-athletes. Percept. Mot. Skills *33*:1187–1190, 1971.

93. Wall, P. D., and Cronly-Dillon, J. R.: Pain, itch and vibration. Arch. Neurol. *2*:365–375, 1960.

94. Wall, P. D., and Sweet, W. H.: Temporary abolition of pain in man. Science *155*:108–109, 1967.

95. Walters, A.: Psychogenic regional pain, alias hysterical pain. Brain *84*:1–18, 1961.

96. Wayne, S. J.: The tuck position for lumbar disc surgery. J. Bone Joint Surg. *49A*:1195–1198, 1967.

97. White, J. C.: Posterior rhizotomy: A possible substitute for cordotomy in otherwise intractable neuralgias of the trunk and extremities of non-malignant origin. Clin. Neurosurg. *13*:20–41, 1966.

98. White, J. C., and Sweet, W. H.: Pain and the Neurosurgeon: A Forty Years' Experience. Springfield, Ill., Charles C Thomas, 1969, pp. 843–887.

99. Wycis, H. T., and Speigel, E. A.: Long range results in the treatment of intractable pain by stereotaxic midbrain surgery, J. Neurosurg. *19*:101–107, 1962.

CHAPTER 18

Psychiatric Considerations in Pain

DIETRICH BLUMER, M.D.
Harvard University

INTRODUCTION

There is ample evidence for the role of higher neural or psychological processes in pain. In clinical practice, the chief problem relates to the often suspected, sometimes appreciated, but little understood role of psychological factors in chronic pain of supposed spinal or more peripheral origin. The characteristic psychiatric and psychological traits are reported for an initial series of patients referred by surgeons because of their chronic atypical (functional) pain. A method of psychiatric and psychological evaluation, gradually developed over the past 12 years, is described. Based on the study of 383 patients with chronic atypical pain, most of them referred by neurosurgeons or orthopedic surgeons, the clinical psychiatric and the psychodynamic profile of the patient with pain-neurosis is further documented and elaborated upon. The important role of the surgeon, whose help is as much sought after as the psychiatrist's is shunned, and the various therapeutic approaches are discussed.

THE ROLE OF HIGHER NEURAL OR PSYCHOLOGICAL PROCESSES IN PAIN

Pain can be measured in the laboratory, yet as a clinical symptom it remains a highly subjective event. Beecher pointed out that the *meaning* of pain and anxiety constitute

basic elements in the pain process; he cautioned that we are not likely to make an effective attack on the psychophysics of pain experienced in disease until a host of elusive variables have been brought under control.[2]

While physical pain may begin as a relatively simple peripheral neural event, we learn about it only *after* this event has been processed through the higher segments of the central nervous system, in a complex and only partly understood process of facilitation and inhibition. Melzack and Wall have introduced a new concept of neural mechanisms for pain, postulating a gate-control system effective at the spinal cord level as modulator of sensory input.[12] Melzack and Casey have further proposed a complex conceptual model of the sensory, motivational-affective, and central-control determinants of pain.[11] In this model the neospinothalamic projection system, the reticular and limbic structures (via the paramedial ascending system), and the neocortical centers all interact with one another and project to the motor system. There is good clinical evidence of the role of higher cerebral levels in pain from the observations of a profound change in suffering from severe incapacitating pain toward relative indifference, following posteromedial orbital tractotomy or cingulotomy. Physical pain is invariably in part a higher neural or "psychological" phenomenon.

Pain threshold and pain tolerance are clearly affected by a number of psychological factors. *Early conditioning*, whether personal or cultural, exerts a commanding influence on the response to pain. One may compare the traditional Japanese obliviousness to pain with the much freer pain response acceptable in some Mediterranean cultures. Various significant *situational* factors can be influential. The extreme excitement of a soldier in battle tends to preclude awareness of severe injury. The presence of others who can bring comfort alleviates pain, while loneliness tends to intensify it. The degree of trust in the dentist influences our suffering at his hands, and depending on who stepped on my foot, the resulting pain may be acute or easily negligible. The *individual meaning* of the pain sensation determines the suffering from it to a remarkable degree: a severe injury can be welcome and no pain relief may be demanded in the case of the soldier to whom it means rescue to safety from front line battle;[1] conversely, a slight substernal pain may be felt very acutely by a person to whom it signals the threat of a heart attack.

Thus, pain cannot be understood as the mere excitatory effect of a peripheral lesion on a number of pain fibers. Moreover, pain occurs without involvement of peripheral pain receptors, such as in cases of painful phantom limb or of transection of the spinal cord. And with certain focal epileptic seizures, in dreams, upon hypnosis, or on a mere suggestion pain is experienced entirely as a higher neural or psychological event. We all carry a repertory of pain experiences—the faded memories of our own and of witnessed painful injuries and ailments. It is not improbable that these memories may be rekindled for psychological reasons, under certain circumstances, and may last, intractable to physical intervention. In addition, a well-understood, acute pain may become a chronic, atypical pain.

Aristotle and Plato classed pain with pleasure as a "passion of the soul." While it is evident that physical pain cannot be regarded independently of the emotional state of an individual, and that pain can be a sensation so emotionally charged that it may indeed assume the quality of an emotion, we should not include purely mental pain, the anguish of the mind, in our considerations. Yet under certain conditions mental anguish manifests itself as "physical" pain which ultimately may be recognized as "psychogenic" pain. Merskey's definition of pain as "an unpleasant experience which we primarily associate with tissue damage or describe in terms of tissue damage or both" is highly practical.[13] It includes both the pain of (chiefly) somatic and the pain of (chiefly) psychic origin. The former is variously referred to as physical, bodily, or organic pain, the latter as psychogenic, atypical or functional pain. Use of the label "imaginary" for atypical pains should be avoided; they are just as real to the patient as the medically more legitimate organic pains.

"SOMATOGENIC" OR "PSYCHOGENIC" INTRACTABLE PAIN

Pain is never a purely somatic event, but it may be more or less clearly related to a somatic lesion or disease. The psychic component of an organic pain, however, may be predominant and may mislead an observer. Thus a "somatogenic" pain *occasionally* may become manifest upon emotional stress, may be described in exaggerated dramatic terms, or may vanish upon administration of placebos or psychotherapy.[19] "Psychogenic" pain, on the other hand, *often* dates its onset back to some physical trauma, may be associated with lesions, may be described without dramatization, and *often* responds, albeit temporarily, to operations or lesser physical procedures.

While we have a fair general understanding of the kinds of injuries and ailments that tend to be associated with pain, there is very little agreement about the psychological conditions favoring pain.

Acute pain has various psychological facets, but it is the chronic, intractable pain of uncertain origin which represents by far the greatest challenge to the psychiatrist or psychologist who investigates clinical pain syndromes. We all know of cases in which a longstanding obscure pain was finally related to a somatic lesion. Such cases, however, are as rare as the chronic sufferer with psychogenic pain is common.

The mental effects of *physical* pain vary with duration and intensity of the pain on the one hand and the personality of the sufferer on the other hand.[5] The individual may become totally preoccupied with his pain, withdrawn and depressed. He may become irritable and demanding, or anxious and agitated. Or he may keep active and productive, with admirable stoicism. The patient with chronic psychogenic pain seems to hold up surprisingly well "with all that pain." His emotional problems antedate the pain and in point of fact are alleviated by it.

Walters classifies psychogenic pain into three groups.[23] *Tissue tension pains* arise when muscular or mucosal tissue becomes tense and painful during emotion. *Regional pain* is the class of functional pain for which no physical cause is found—a somatic hallucination of pain in a regional distribution which does not follow an anatomical pattern but is mapped out by past or present life experience, and occurs when a patient feels threatened, hurt, injured, or bereft. Walters states that regional pain is found not only in hysteria but also throughout the whole range of neuroses, psychoses, situational states, and minor reactions of everyday life. *Psychogenic magnification,* finally, refers to the "functional overlay" with pain in the presence of a physical lesion.

Merskey and Spear describe the following characteristics of pain of psychological origin:[14] it tends to last continuously from day to day without disturbing sleep, frequently involves several areas with predilection for the head and, most importantly, occurs with valid evidence of psychiatric illness.

Engel, in a classic paper, discussed pain as a psychological phenomenon.[7] He listed the following features as characteristic for pain-prone individuals, i.e., individuals who use pain as a psychic regulator, whether the pain includes a peripheral source of stimulation or not:

1. A prominence of conscious and unconscious guilt, with pain serving as a relatively satisfactory means of atonement.
2. A background that tends to predispose to the use of pain for such purposes.
3. A history of suffering and defeat and intolerance of success (masochistic character structure). A propensity to solicit pain, as evidenced by the large number of painful injuries, operations and treatments.
4. A strong aggressive drive which is not fulfilled, pain being experienced instead.
5. Development of pain as a replacement for a loss at times when a relationship is threatened or lost.
6. A tendency toward a sado-masochistic type of sexual development, with some episodes of pain occurring in settings of conflict over sexual impulses.
7. A location of pain determined by unconscious identification with a love object, the pain being either one suffered by the patient himself when in some conflict with the object, or a pain suffered by the object in fact or in the patient's fantasy.
8. Psychiatric diagnoses include conversion hysteria, depression, hypochondriasis and paranoid schizophrenia, or mixtures of these. Some patients with pain do not fit into any distinct nosologic category.

Sternbach et al. report that, on psychological examination by means of MMPI, patients with chronic pain related to clearly documented and well-understood lesions, and whose complaints seem appropriate to the physical findings, were practically indistinguishable from the neurotic patient with chronic "psychogenic" pain.[20] Hypochondriasis, reactive depression, dependency, and denial of emotional or interpersonal difficulties were found in all chronic pain patients; and both groups of pain patients were found to be similar as far as doctor-patient interactions were concerned.

Patients with chronic "intractable" pain are little known to psychiatrists. They seek help from other physicians and, above all, from surgeons. Thus, Freud treated patients with the complaint of pain in his early career only, as long as he was known as a neurologist. Patients with ulcers, headaches, arthritis, and chest pain may be referred by internists, but nowadays, most pain patients reach a psychiatrist or psychologist through the surgeon who insists on a very comprehensive evaluation.

The use of psychological testing is of particular value in the study of patients who may somatize their psychological conflicts. Over the past twelve years we have studied close to 400 patients whose pain was not adequately explained by their physical findings, most of them referred by a neurosurgeon or orthopedic surgeon. We have regularly employed psychological testing and have developed a questionnaire which reflects characteristic traits of the pain-prone patient and could serve as the expedient basis for a psychiatric interview. We have followed a small group of patients over a brief period of time, and in several cases we have undertaken prolonged psychotherapeutic and psychopharmacological efforts.

Before describing the details of our present method of psychiatric and psychological evaluation of patients with pain, and elaborating more fully on our findings and conclusions, we present our findings on an initial series of 27 patients with chronic "atypical" pain.

CHARACTERISTIC TRAITS IN A SERIES OF SURGICAL PATIENTS WITH CHRONIC PAIN

The Sample of Patients

Over a period of two and a half years, 52 patients with the chief complaint of pain were referred from the Neurosurgical Division of the Johns Hopkins Hospital for psychiatric evaluation. From this total, 27 patients were included in the study. They represent a relatively homogeneous group, suffering from long-standing severe pain in the absence of related physical findings. The other 25 were excluded for the following reasons:

1. Organic disease appeared plausibly related to the pain (nine patients).
2. Headache of various etiologies was the leading symptom (eight patients).
3. Compensation appeared to be a chief factor (two patients).
4. Duration of the pain was less than six months (two patients).
5. Only one psychiatric interview had taken place (four patients).

The study group consisted of nine men and 18 women. Five were referrals from the ward, 22 from private service. The age span ranged from 16 to 68; the average age was 45.5. Fourteen patients suffered from neck pain, or back pain, or both, with additional pain in the extremities; five complained of pain in the extremities alone; and two suffered from facial pain. The remaining six patients complained of painful sensations in the jaw, chest, or groin; along a surgical scar; and in the sublingual, or retroauricular area. In two patients pain occurred paroxysmally, in two others it was intermittent and in all others it was practically continuous. Duration of the symptoms varied from a half year to 30 years, averaging about seven years.

In spite of the chronicity of the complaint, these patients invariably presented with an acute problem. More than half of them (17) had come from distant areas to seek help from the neurosurgeon.

Method of Study

The patients were referred by the neurosurgeon after completion of studies for an organic cause of their pain, or while such studies were still in progress but were expected to be negative. They were told by the neurosurgeon that they were going to be seen by a psychiatrist who was part of the team investigating their ailment and the effects of the ailment on their lives. If necessary, they were reassured that this did not imply that their pain was thought to be imaginary. Each patient was studied through psychiatric interviews, and was seen for an average of four sessions during his hospital stay. Gaining cooperation was the initial, and often very difficult, task for the interviewer because the patient felt his pain was not taken for real and resented the appearance of a psychiatrist. It was usually explained that in his case it had been impossible so far to pinpoint the cause of pain, that emotional factors could be important in many illnesses, and that we were trying to help him by looking at his problem from all possible angles. The history of present illness, general past history, and family history were then obtained. Particular attention was given to the nature of the patient's pertinent relationships to others, and to his working habits. Whenever possible, a close relative was interviewed (15 cases). In addition, nine patients were seen in psychotherapy following discharge and were studied more intensively. Profiles of the Szondi Test were obtained from 20 patients.

The Clinical Findings

A number of traits were typically present in the group studied.

1. Marked denial of emotional conflict was strikingly evident in all but one case. Patients maintained that they had no problems at all—that family and job were wonderful—if only they could get rid of that pain, then everything would be all right. In other words, such patients might claim that their life circumstances were much more fortunate than could possibly be true. This denial was not surprising upon first contact of a "surgical patient" with a psychiatrist. However, it was impressive in its degree and was maintained throughout subsequent interviews even though a fairly good rapport had been established.

2. In contrast to their assertions, it was evident that the majority of these patients were living in intensely conflicting relationships with either the spouse or a close relative,

where resentment and hostility were never openly expressed. As a rule, the partner would share the patient's denial of any emotional conflict and attend to the sufferer with excessive concern. This type of relationship was positively identified in 16 patients (13 female, 3 males). Its existence was suspected in the remaining patients as well, but could not be substantiated, owing to lack of clear information about the family picture. The predominance of females among these 16 patients results from the fact they were more often accompanied by relatives who could be interviewed.

3. A surprising finding was that nearly half of the patients (eight females, five males) had a close relative who was crippled or deformed. We counted four relatives crippled by polio, and one each by osteomyelitis, diabetic gangrene, injury, cancer of the leg, and tuberculosis of the hip. One relative was paralyzed following a back operation. In addition, we found two relatives with facial deformities (by cancer and Bell's palsy) and one with an accidentally severed breast. The mutilated relative was the spouse in four cases, a parent in four, the only child in three, and a sibling in two (Cases 5 and 6). Two female patients had married men who were already crippled. In every case this relative played a very significant role in the patient's life. In all cases, the presence of injury or deformity in the relative preceded the onset of pain in the patient.

4. In 14 patients (eight female, six male) the experience of "organic" pain had preceded the "psychogenic" pain. In eight cases the pain experienced by a close relative appeared of importance in connection with the presenting symptom.

5. All but five of the patients (four female, one male) clearly wanted surgery. The average number of past operations was four per patient, for females and males alike. It is, of course, not surprising to find a patient on a surgical ward who wants surgery. The striking fact here was that these patients continued to seek readmission to a surgical service despite repeated negative checkups and unsuccessful operations.

6. Three patients (two females, one male) had made nearly successful suicide attempts, two had been subsequently admitted to a psychiatric hospital. No other incidence of "nervous breakdown" requiring hospitalization occurred in the group studied.

7. A final trait may also be considered characteristic. Fourteen patients (10 female, four male) had been excessively active, working relentlessly, often from a very early age, without taking vacations, until the pain set in. Such a patient might say: "If only I could get on the go again, everything would be all right."

Only nine of the 27 patients (six female, three male) studied would accept psychiatric help—and even these did so with marked reluctance. A good followup (over a period of nine months to two years) on six of these nine patients showed that three became symptom free, two improved markedly, and only one remained unimproved.

The Test Findings

For psychodiagnostic purposes, Szondi Test profiles were obtained on 20 of the patients. The results of blind evaluations done by A. Beeli, Ph.D., in Lucerne, Switzerland, are summarized. Szondi's "experimental diagnostics of drives" test method is seldom employed in the U.S. How and why the test functions, as well as the more recent refinements of the test's interpretation, are almost entirely unknown here (see section on methods of psychological evaluation).[22]

From the Szondi Test profiles, it was impossible to make positive diagnoses of known psychopathological categories. The profiles indicated that one probably had to deal with a neurosis, but not with any of the known and well-described neurotic reactions. Traits of inhibition, hypochondriasis and conversion hysteria (the latter particularly in females) were predominant. Beeli writes: "The psychodynamics can be well described, because this group obtained strikingly uniform test results. It must be emphasized that, not only certain factorial and vectorial reactions largely predominate, but almost every case presents the signs which are typical for the group." In the foreground, one finds "the dependent, good-hearted, passive and inhibited child who suffers from feelings of guilt and the tendency toward self punishment." There is a rigorous defense against aggressive-vengeful-dependent strivings. Beeli states that the behavior of this group may be characterized by a "strong tendency toward (sado-) masochistic ties with family, spouses, friends, etc., where the oral needs of being accepted, spoiled and catered to may be quite excessive."

Illustrative Cases

Case I. Crippled daughter—denial of marital conflict—suicide attempt prompted by abrupt confrontation with psychogenicity of pain.

A 50-year-old housewife had suffered from back pain for the past seven years. Medical and surgical treatment, including three operations on her back, had failed to help. Her only child, a daughter, had been afflicted by polio, but regained full strength of her legs after seven years. The patient's complaint started shortly before the daughter left home. She claimed to lead a happy life with many hobbies, and felt that her bad back was the one and only problem. When she was asked about her husband, she said that he was "not a weakling" and denied any marital difficulties, saying: "How could I have trouble with him? I am away from home in hospitals for so much of the time." She was very hostile toward the interviewer and accused him of advocating divorce when he inquired about possible marital difficulties again.

Her pain responded well to the injection of saline. It was repeatedly noticed that she could move around rather freely when she believed that she was not observed, but visits by her husband accentuated her agony. He would anticipate her wishes, rub her back, and soothe her any way he could.

When there was no indication for an operation, neither patient nor husband knew where to go. Against the patient's will, she was referred to a psychiatrist. The husband was advised not to be so anxious about her pains. Immediately following her discharge, she made a suicide attempt by taking a large number of sleeping pills.

Case II. Crippled spouse and mother—denial of any emotional conflict—desperate desire for surgery.

This 58-year-old housewife with no children came from the West Coast. With the exception of an appendectomy and a gall bladder operation, she had been well in the past. One and a half years ago an operation for diaphragmatic hernia was performed. Soon she begain to suffer from pain along the site of the incision. Her husband now had to help out with the housework. She had a second operation for "relapse of the diaphragmatic hernia" but her chief complaint remained unaltered and she felt that she could not go on any longer.

Two years ago her mother suffered a pathological fracture of the left hip and had been an invalid ever since. Also, the patient's husband had lost his right hip joint in boyhood, due to tuberculosis. Eight years following their marriage he underwent an operation for rehabilitation of the hip—only to become more of an invalid, unable to work.

She presented herself as a tense, stern, but ra-tional woman, with no signs of acute distress. She insisted that her only concern was physical pain, and that she definitely wanted to have an operation. When she was finally told by the neurosurgeon that no operation was indicated, she began to cry helplessly. When the husband was told the same, he began to hyperventilate and slumped over in his chair. The neurosurgeon had the impression, from a few utterances, that the husband harbored a wish that she would die during surgery.

Case III. Sadistic mother—sado-masochistic marital relationship—persistence on physical nature of pain after psychotherapy—remission of pain upon improvement of marriage.

A 33-year-old housewife suffered from severe headaches and an excruciating facial pain. In order to get away from a sadistic and alcoholic mother, she had married young and had three children before the marriage failed due to her husband's unfaithfulness. Years later she remarried, thereby providing her children with a fine home. But she had to deal with a difficult mother-in-law, terminally sick with cancer. In this setting the pain began: she got up one morning, stood in front of the mirror combing her hair, and was suddenly seized with intense pain on the right side of her face. In connection with this mode of onset, some significance may be attached to the fact that she used to comb the sick mother-in-law's hair. Following the death of the mother-in-law she entered the hospital. When all studies were negative, she agreed to begin psychotherapy. The total dissatisfaction she felt toward her husband soon became the main theme of discussions. He was irresponsible and showed no signs of love toward her, but she thought of her children and was afraid of a separation. Only on occasion could she relate the intensity of her resentment towards him and the almost irresistible impulse to hit him. The pain was at times better, at other times worse. She kept insisting that something organic was wrong and discontinued psychotherapy after one year of irregular visits. One year later she wrote a letter to her psychotherapist. She said that she had become pregnant for the first time in her second marriage, and that her health had improved greatly. Sometime after she had given birth to a healthy baby, it was learned that her husband was now much more responsible and happy, and that she felt "great." Only occasionally would she feel some pain, but when this occurred she would continue what she was doing and would soon feel better.

Case IV. Maintenance of a physical pain for marked secondary gain—disappearance of pain upon inpatient psychiatric treatment which combined ignoring the pain and focusing on psychological issues.

A 16-year-old high school student had suffered a

compound fracture of his left wrist and continued to experience over the following two years a "murderous" pain at the site of the injury. When he arrived in the hospital, the family was "at the end of the rope." Against his protests, he soon was transferred to the psychiatric service. There his display of extreme suffering was completely ignored, and he was taken off analgesics. In therapy, he realized that he had many aggressive feelings, initially directed towards the therapist who refused him all medication, but mainly directed towards his parents.

This boy had been spoiled greatly by his parents, but had never been allowed to express any resentment. He wanted to be liked and would hold back the anger he felt towards parents who were constantly arguing and who expected a lot from him. Following the injury, he found that whenever he had pain, his parents would stop fighting, comfort him, and desist from making any demands on him. His "murderous" pain served him as a safe means to get revenge on his parents; therefore, he had maintained it. After he began to verbalize his annoyance, the pain in the wrist soon disappeared, and he was discharged after six weeks of psychiatric hospitalization. He received weekly outpatient psychiatric care for several months from a therapist closer to home, and has remained symptom-free.

The two following cases exemplify the importance of the role of the crippled relative in the only instances where this was not a parent or spouse.

Case V. Crippled sister—promiscuous husband—persistent denial of role of psychological issues.

A 27-year-old woman had been raised in an orphanage with her sister, six years her senior. They were inseparable until the sister was struck by polio at the age of 14. She was unable to walk for a full year, and became totally indifferent toward the patient, her healthy little sister. She rejected the opportunity to be adopted by parents who would have taken her little sister as well, and chose to be adopted alone by a lady whose husband had died from polio. The patient stated: "I had more heartache than it takes to fill a book. But it doesn't help to think about these things."

She complained of pain in the left side of her back for five years' duration. She had married ten years ago. We learned that her husband was erratically employed and frequently involved with very young girls. Following her discharge she discontinued psychotherapy after two sessions.

Case VI. Crippled sister—relentless activity since early adolescence—denial of any psychological conflict.

A 35-year-old man had had a sister two years younger than himself who had developed cancer of the leg at age nine. The father had remained at home, because he felt he was the only person capable of soothing the girl, and the patient had to leave high school at the age of fourteen to do the farming during the father's frequent absence from work. The sister died when he was 16, after five years of prolonged suffering.

The patient felt a constant pain in the right shoulder and arm, dating back to an accident eight years ago and unrelieved by two surgical procedures. It was remarkable that he kept working relentlessly in spite of his complaint. He owned a service station, worked all week and every Sunday, often for sixteen hours a day. When off work he was busy with various societies, or he was hunting. He stated he got along well with everybody—including his wife—and that his only problem was the pain.

The next two cases stand out diagnostically from the other patients.

Case VII. Bizarre pain in a schizophrenic woman—persistent demand for surgery.

A 58-year-old woman had a bizarre complaint about "a jagged object" causing her intolerable pain in the sublingual area. She complained pathetically, and demanded surgery as her only salvation. The pain dated back nineteen years, but had only become constant two years ago. She had undergone a total of seven surgical procedures for this complaint. On two occasions, she was scheduled for radical surgery on the floor of her mouth, but each time developed an excruciating pain in her neck and shoulder which led to cancellation of the procedure. She lived together with a sister and brother-in-law whom she loathed but towards whom she could never express any true feelings. She had to be committed to a psychiatric hospital when she became convinced that everybody was conspiring against her. With body hallucinations and pathetic-extravagant, erratic behavior she could best be classified as having a schizophrenic reaction of the hebephrenic type.

Case VIII. Demand for surgery in a peregrinating patient of the "Munchausen type."

A 58-year-old man complained of constant pain in his left chest area, following a left thoracotomy for aneurysm four years ago. He was gloomy, sullen, and totally preoccupied with his pain. He described this pain as "setting in every morning as a muscle-spasm and becoming constant—it's like a wheel starts to turn." He had been hospitalized many times for this complaint, and as far as could be established, had undergone four operations: a posterior rhizotomy, two explorations of the chest, and a high cervical cordotomy. He demanded surgery as the only cure for his pain. He stated that he would commit suicide if he lost the hope of getting well. When surgery was refused he left the hospital in anger, saying he would seek help from another medical center. He could be best termed a case of "Munchausen's syndrome."

Comments

INTERPRETATION OF OUTSTANDING CLINICAL FEATURES

The outstanding clinical features of the above cases may be interpreted as follows:

1. *Denial of emotional conflict,* particularly denial of unsatisfactory relationships, is a direct measure of the degree of disturbance in the patient's relationship with others.

2. As a rule, there exists *one critical relationship* in the present life situation of the patient. In this relationship pain plays a central role. Pain is an agonizing experience not only for the patient but also for the observer. The patient not only tortures and punishes himself but also inflicts torture on those close to him. The partner shares the ambivalence: while he secretly enjoys the suffering, he feels very guilty and bends over backward in anxious concern. Recognition of the mutual infliction of pain in the relationships of our patients leads us to term their crucial conflict as *sado-masochistic.*

In these persons the *masochistic need* prevails over the sadistic tendencies. Any direct expression of aggression may lead to loss of love. In our patients any outward aggression is hidden and rigidly inhibited; masked as pain, it serves to secure and solicit acceptance and affection. This handsome secondary gain may render the condition intractable.

3. Experience with a *mutilated close relative* may stimulate the reaction of "psychogenic" pain. The patient identifies with the victim and begins to suffer all the tortures he has inflicted on the other in his fantasy. He expiates the guilt for his aggressive feelings according to the old *lex talionis.* In his monograph The Painful Phantom, L. C. Kolb reports: "Indeed, of twenty-one patients with the syndrome of painful phantom limb, fourteen gave information indicating a close and significant emotional attachment to another amputee in the past."[10] The choice of an already crippled spouse appears indicative of the patient's sado-masochistic personality structure.

4. The *memory of a close relative's pain* is used in the neurosis the same way the experience with mutilation is used. *The memory of somatic pain experienced by the patient himself* also serves the neurosis. However, it may not be the same pain. Typically, it does not follow any neurological pattern but is de-termined by its usefulness within the psychological pattern of maladaptation in which the patient is trapped.

5. The *great desire for surgical procedure* is indicative of a strongly masochistic need to be mutilated. Again there is a marked secondary gain involved. The type of patient we have studied does not become addicted to drugs, but may be addicted to the knife. The desperate request for surgical intervention represents an exacerbation in the course of the pain-neurosis.

6. The actual *attempt of suicide* is but a step beyond seeking surgery. Rigorous removal of any secondary gain should be undertaken only in the psychiatric hospital (Case I).

7. It is our impression that the *excessive activity* displayed by many patients represents an attempt to channel strong aggressive drives in a socially acceptable direction. But they work themselves "to death"—into a state of constant pain. Again, this trait bears a self-destructive note.

THE DIAGNOSTIC PROBLEM

Diagnostically, these patients do not fall into any well-defined categories. Marked guilt and need for punishment, with turning of aggression against oneself, are, of course, characteristic of the depressive reaction. Unawareness of emotional conflict and display of a physical impairment for secondary gain are typically found in the hysteric patient. A curious mixture of these traits is present in patients with longstanding "psychogenic" pain, together with the other distinct characteristics described. They are neither basically "depressed" nor basically "hysteric," but are, in the majority, in a psychopathological class of their own. They represent a conversion reaction in infantile-dependent, inhibited sado-masochistic personalities. This reaction may be best referred to as "pain-neurosis." Two patients who appeared to be somewhat different from the group were briefly described in Cases VII and VIII.

METHOD OF PSYCHIATRIC AND PSYCHOLOGICAL EVALUATION

The patient with atypical pain will see a psychiatrist almost exclusively after referral from another physician. If the patient is "somatizing," i.e., if his pain serves as the veiled expression of psychological needs and conflicts, he looks upon the psychiatrist or the psychological evaluation as an unwelcome intrusion, and his resistance tends to be much more marked than that of a patient with organic pain. He may protest that his pain is not imaginary or that he is not crazy. Some patients will act conciliatory, and say that they do not care how they are being helped, even though they are indeed firmly committed to the physical approach. Very few patients, however, will be unwilling to cooperate at all or will refuse to complete the evaluation, if the need for such is firmly stated by the primary physician.

The patient with chronic pain of uncertain origin should be advised by his physician that psychiatric evaluation or psychological testing, or both, are required. In medical centers for chronic pain problems such an evaluation is, in general, routinely performed and the patient is informed about this fact. He may be advised that the evaluation is necessary because psychological factors tend to influence pain for better or for worse, and also because the effect of chronic painful suffering on his emotional well-being and daily life needs to be assessed. The psychiatrist or psychologist may then restate the same rationale. A matter-of-fact, but courteous or even friendly approach should be pursued; some gentle persuasion may have to be employed to get all the testing done.

The evaluation may be carried out either by a psychiatrist, who will conduct a more or less extended clinical interview, or by a well-trained clinical psychologist, who may choose to supplement his test battery by a clinical interview. An occasional patient who is judged a suicide risk or who may display bizarreness suggestive of a schizophrenic condition will definitely require the attention of a psychiatrist.

Engel has pointed out that many patients who are pain prone for psychological reasons very readily pour out the significant facts of their life's story.[7] This is true in our own experience. On the other hand, many patients give a rather bland account of their past history and may conceal significant facts. Moreover, a trait universally present in atypical pain patients is marked denial of any emotional or interpersonal conflict. The conflicts are somatized and concealed, yet may be made apparent by psychological testing procedures.

Our current method of evaluation has been developed over the past 12 years. It consists of the administration of a questionnaire, followed by a psychiatric interview which clarifies and, if necessary, develops the answers to the questionnaire, and by the concurrent administration of a psychological testing battery.

The Questionnaire (See Table 18–1)

The questionnaire begins with an inquiry centering on the present physical complaint, and attempts to establish duration, mode of onset and type of pain, surgical procedures and their results, dependence on medication, past history of pain, and accident proneness (questions 1 to 15).

Pain-prone patients usually describe their pain as continuous, perhaps with exacerbations (question 5). A few surgical procedures usually have been performed on the chronic case, characteristically with the relief from pain after each operation gradually diminishing to zero (question 8 and 9).

Questions 16 through 22 deal with personal habits. Sleep may frequently be disturbed; although in many patients who complain of continuous pain, sleep may remain surprisingly undisturbed. Appetite is usually good. Smoking and alcohol consumption may at times be excessive. Sex life is frequently impaired, in the first place or after onset of the pain.

A number of items in the questionnaire cover family history and current living situation (questions 23 through 34). People closely involved with the patient are usually described as being very concerned and considerate (24). A crippled or deformed close relative is frequently present (31); this item is often erroneously answered in the negative.

Important questions pertaining to emotional and interpersonal conflicts follow (35 through 60). Tenseness, nervousness (35), depression (52), or even despair (54) may be admitted to, but are blamed on the pain. Problems in getting along with other people (40) are almost invariably denied, even though abuse suffered at the hands of a parent or spouse may be recorded (51). Highly characteristic of pain-prone patients is their appraisal of their relationships to spouse, children, and often parents as "wonderful" (questions 41 through 44). Grave disappointments in other relationships may be listed (45), and may refer to episodes in which the patient passively

TABLE 18–1. QUESTIONNAIRE FOR PAIN SYNDROME*
(Not to be included in Medical Chart)

Please try to answer all the questions. Use extra sheets or the back of the page if necessary.

Name: Birthdate:

Address: History No.:

Years of Education: Date:

Occupation: Physician:
     Your own:
                                             Hospital Room:
     Your spouse's:

Your Illness: (If you have more than one kind of pain, list more than one answer to each of the questions 1–8 below.)

  1. When did your pain first begin?
  2. What were the circumstances of this first onset of pain?
  3. Where is your pain localized?
  4. How does your pain feel to you?
  5. Is the pain continuous, or does it come and go? (If it comes and goes, please indicate how often and how long it lasts; if it is continuous, describe whether or not it changes.)
  6. What makes your pain worse?
  7. Have you found any methods of lessening your painful suffering?
  8. What operations have you had for your pain? (Please list with dates.)
  9. Was your pain helped by the operations? For how long did you feel relief after the operations?
 10. What other operations have you had? (Please list.)
 11. What other physical complaints do you have? (Please list.)
 12. What medications do you need for pain?
 13. How often do you take these medications?
 14. Did you ever suffer from severe pain over a period of time before the present illness? (Please give dates if applicable.)
 15. Have you ever been hurt in accidents? (Please list incidents, giving year.)

Your Habits:
 16. In general, how well do you sleep?
 17. How often in a week do you need sleeping pills?
 18. How is your appetite?
 19. How much alcohol do you drink? How often?
 20. How much do you smoke per day?
 21. Has sex been important to you in your life?
 22. What effect does your illness have on your sex life?

Your Family:
 23. List the names and relation to you of all people who live with you.
 24. What is their reaction to your illness?
 25. When did you get married? (Please note period(s) of previous marriage(s), if applicable.)
 26. List your children's names, ages, and sex. List your brothers and sisters and their ages. Where are they living now?
 27. What type of work did your parents do?
     Mother:
     Father:
 28. What kinds of difficulties did your parents have in their marriage?
 29. What are or have been the illnesses among —
     Mother: Sisters:

     Father: Brothers:

     Spouse: Children:

*The actual questionnaire is spaced out over seven pages. The responses characteristic for pain-neurotics are described in the text.

TABLE 18–1.   QUESTIONNAIRE FOR PAIN SYNDROME* (*Continued*)

30. Who among these close relatives is deceased? (Please give year and cause of death.)
31. Among your relatives or close friends, who has (or had) any crippling condition, deformity, or chronic physical handicap? (Please describe.)
32. Did (or does) anyone else in your family suffer from severe pain over a period of time?
33. Who among your relatives has (or had) any mental or nervous condition?
34. Has there been any divorce or separation in your family? (Please list year of divorce or separation.)

Your Emotional Life:
35. Do you consider yourself tense or nervous?
36. What emotional difficulties do you have?
37. Did you have any emotional difficulties in the past?
38. Did you ever see a psychiatrist? If yes, when and for what reason?
39. With whom do you discuss your feelings, or do you tend to keep them to yourself?
40. What problems do you have in getting along with other people?
41. How did you get on with your mother?
42. How did you get on with your father?
43. How is your relationship with your spouse?
44. How is your relationship with your children?
45. Have you ever been badly disappointed in others? (Please specify.)
46. Do you have much patience?   Yes_____   No_____
47. How often do you get angry? (Per day? Per week? Per month?)
48. Have you ever really lost control over your temper?
49. Have you ever felt like hurting someone else?
50. What was the most angry thing you ever did?
51. Have you ever suffered physical abuse from someone else? (If so, please specify.)
52. How often do you get depressed?
    all the time _____   every few days _____   every few weeks _____
    every few months _____   rarely _____   never _____
53. How often do you cry?
    all the time _____   every few days _____   every few weeks _____
    every few months _____   rarely _____   never _____
54. Have you ever felt despair?
55. Have you ever wished you were dead?
56. Have you ever thought about harming yourself?
57. Have you ever done anything to harm yourself?
58. Has your illness made you more irritable or has it taught you more patience?
59. Are you a religious person?
60. Do you go to religious services regularly?

Your Activities:
61. List all different types of employment, with approximate duration (e.g., salesman 1965–68; clerk 1968–present.)
62. What were your working hours before your illness?
63. When did you last work regularly?
64. How steadily had you been working?
65. What are your working hours now?
66. At what age did you start to work for the first time?
67. Do you have good friends?   3 or more _____   1 or 2 _____   None _____
68. What effects does your painful illness now have on your social life?
69. How did it affect your social life in the past?
70. Do you think you are basically more active and energetic than the average person?
    Yes _____   No _____   Average _____
71. Do you like to enjoy as much leisure time as possible?
    Yes _____   No _____
72. What have been your hobbies?
73. Which hobbies can you still pursue?

allowed others to take advantage of him. Problems with anger and aggression (questions 47 through 50) are only rarely listed, while suicidal intent may or may not be reported (56 and 57). The wish to be dead would not be unusual, at least in a fleeting form, in patients with chronic pain, and a negative answer to such a question (55) may be indicative of denial.

The final section of the questionnaire deals with the range of activities, past and present, performed by the patient (questions 61 through 73). The history of work activities is important for rehabilitation planning (61). Excessive work habits, including, sometimes, a history of steady work since early adolescence, are characteristically present in pain-neurotics (questions 62, 64 and 66), who tend to be more active than the average person and may abhor leisure time (questions 70 and 71). In the same vein, they often have many hobbies which require physical exertion; this is particularly striking in female patients (72).

The Interview

The interview consists of clarification and elaboration of the areas covered in the questionnaire. With many patients, the interview will not add much to the information obtained by the questionnaire, nor will it determine type and degree of underlying psychopathology as well as can be done through psychological testing procedures. The degree of resistance to the psychiatric inquiry can be fairly easily established; it tends to be commensurate with the degree of denial of existing psychological conflicts. The presence of schizophrenic traits may occasionally be observed. Of great importance in some patients is the assessment of suicidal potential—in particular, if any sort of confrontation with the psychological nature of the presenting problem is planned.

The interview should further establish an estimate of the patient's need and readiness for a psychotherapeutic intervention. Special problems concerning psychiatric treatment of the pain-neurotic are discussed in a later section.

Psychological Testing

In stark contrast to the superficial mental well-being projected by the pain-neurotic, the presence of deep-seated psychological conflicts can be established through psychological testing. These conflicts invariably are denied on the questionnaire and in the interview. Indeed, a naive observer will be impressed by the patient's apparent maintenance of a solid mental attitude "in spite of all the suffering." He may further take at face value the patient's characteristic statement that "everything would be just wonderful if it weren't for that pain." Therefore, the use of a sensitive psychological test battery in the evaluation of patients with atypical pain is highly desirable.

The choice of tests to be administered for clinical purposes depends on the particular skills and preferences of the individual psychologist. Our own experience has been primarily with the Szondi Test and, to a lesser degree, with the MMPI. Our current battery of tests includes, in addition to the Szondi, the following: TAT, Rorschach, WAIS, Draw-a-Person, and Sentence Completion. We believe that any of the well-established projective testing procedures can provide useful information concerning the psychopathology of patients with atypical pain, as long as they are employed by a skillful psychologist. The use of five or six selected cards of the TAT may be particularly revealing in patients who use a stark denial of aggressive and dependent strivings. We do not, however, have sufficient data at present either to state a preference for any one of these tests or to report findings of particular significance on any individual test among them.

The Szondi Test is, in our experience, a highly useful instrument for the evaluation of patients with pain. The test findings in our initial series of pain-neurotics have been summarized above, and some further findings will be reported below. The Szondi Test, however, is little used (except in some European countries), and the literature available on it in English does not deal sufficiently with its rationale, its methods of interpretation, or the conditions proper for its validation.[6, 21]

The MMPI, on the other hand, is in wide use. It is very easily administered, and the test results reported show characteristic findings in groups of patients with chronic pain. However, a negative MMPI score, in our experience, does not exclude the presence of psychogenic factors in a given patient. Like all inventory-type tests, the MMPI score is based on how the patient sees himself, and does not necessarily reflect the more unconscious instinctive conflicts of the individual.

THE PSYCHOPATHOLOGY OF PATIENTS WITH CHRONIC ATYPICAL PAIN (PAIN-NEUROSIS)

It was evident from our first series of patients with obscure pain that a brief but in-depth study of such patients could document a rather specific and coherent psychopathology. We discovered that on the psychological level the pain is *not* obscure but, instead, is associated with and determined by a number of significant personality and behavioral traits. These traits form a relatively unique pattern when compared with other groups of psychiatric cases. Further controlled studies are needed, however, to differentiate more clearly pain-neurotics from other psychosomatic conditions and to differentiate subgroups among the pain-neurotics.

Our further experience with a much larger group of patients suffering from chronic atypical pain confirmed the significance of the characteristic traits determined in our first series; it permitted a clearer focus on some of these traits and led to the consideration of a few additional traits judged significant for pain-neurotics. A sharpened and slightly broadened view of the psychopathology of pain-neurosis based on our study of a total of 383 patients with chronic atypical pain is now presented. Most of these patients were referred by neurosurgeons and orthopedic surgeons.

The *denial of emotional and interpersonal conflicts* is a primary finding in pain-neurotics. More prolonged psychiatric exploration and psychological testing specifically point to the *denial of infantile needs to be dependent, to be spoiled and physically catered to on the one hand, and of hostile, sado-masochistic strivings on the other.* With the advent of pain, the patient becomes securely dependent, obtains constant physical care and simultaneously satisfies his aggressive strivings by making life difficult for his family, while suffering the punishment of pain and thereby atoning for guilt. Thus, pain may bring about so much secondary gain that its intractability becomes very understandable. There is not only a denial but also an inability to identify and verbalize feelings. Psychotherapy is ignored, then, for good reason.

A *passive(-aggressive) or (sado-) masochistic life style* is apparent in most cases: history of past abuse; choice of an abusive spouse; failure to assert oneself at work or

at home; and finally, the persistent pursuit of surgical procedures.

Relentless activity at work (and often with hobbies) is a trait that seems to begin early, and that tends to bear the masochistic note of sacrifice for others. While such efforts are pursued for others, there seems to be a constant hidden wish to be rewarded and, finally, to be taken care of by others. These patients tend to be performers in a muscular-physical sense; leisure and reflection are strange to them.

These characteristic traits are present in various combinations in individual patients. They may be clearly present, or become apparent only upon psychological testing. Experience from our first patient series indicated time and again the presence of a *crippled relative* in the lives of these patients. In addition, we became impressed with the frequency of *alcoholism* and *promiscuity* among significant next-of-kin. The following cases are chosen to illustrate these various aspects of the pain-neurotics chiefly from the clinical angle. The next section will then give further psychological test findings.

Clinical Findings

DENIAL

Some patients will present an utterly bland life history and allege an excellent marital relationship. Yet the test findings will indicate denial, a need to suffer and marked dependency needs.

Case 1. A 47-year-old housewife, married for 31 years, complains of a multitude of pains: facial pain of 22 years' duration, which has spread to the side of head and neck; chest and arm pain for 11 years; occasional upper back pain for three years; and further back pain following an accident six months earlier. A growth was removed from her sinus 16 years ago, but the pain remains unchanged. The only other operation was a hysterectomy eight years ago. She recalls having suffered from pains in her legs as a young child.

She has two married sons and a single daughter. Her husband has deformed kidneys and "too much urea in his blood." She describes her relationship with him as "one of the best" and says he is most considerate of her.

Her father and mother both died of heart attacks, eight years and one year ago, respectively. She was very close to her father, and came to regard her mother more as she matured.

The patient becomes emotional when her head pain is severe and tends to get a little depressed "with the change in weather"—she dislikes rain.

She finds that she no longer enjoys being around her children, yet claims no other emotional or interpersonal difficulties. She rarely gets angry, has felt despair only on a few occasions and denies any suicidal ideation.

Four Szondi Test profiles showed excessive marked dependency needs, neurotic inhibition, guilt feelings, and a hypochondriacal attitude.

The MMPI indicated that the patient focused her attention on bodily functions, showed extreme denial of emotional problems, lacked confidence and had difficulty making decisions.

Arrangements were made to see her psychiatrically at the times of her return visits to the neurologist. She showed marked reluctance to see the psychiatrist and did not return after the first followup visit, though her hypochondriacal preoccupation had not been challenged.

One wonders what a further inquiry might have revealed about the nature of relationships in the patient's family of origin. She had hinted about problems in her relationship with her mother. Of specific significance was the information that the sister had married an alcoholic and brutal husband; while the patient herself, saddled (sic!) with "a very understanding husband," had to satisfy her masochism by suffering constant pain.

This particular patient is one of the few in our series referred by a neurologist rather than a surgeon. She seemed less intense with her pain complaint than most patients, and had only undergone a single surgical procedure during her 22 year career as a pain patient.

Case 2. A 37-year-old housewife and former physiotherapist has suffered from episodic but daily dull aching in a spot above the left eyebrow for seven years. After a time the pain also occurred in the left neck. Two operations (sections of cervical nerves and posterior roots) in the past year had brought no relief. She used to be very active at home, in church, and with hobbies (swimming, knitting, bridge). She describes her relationships with parents, husband and children as very good. Her father had just died six months prior to her evaluation. He had walked on crutches since suffering from polio at age 15, and had been confined to a wheelchair for the last several years of his life. On two occasions the patient had been treated by a psychiatrist because of her pain but without any success. She was "slightly disappointed" nine years ago when her husband accepted a job which required frequent travel away from home.

Four Szondi Test profiles indicated very marked passive-masochistic tendencies, infantile needs to be taken care of, a strong ethical sense, and a proneness to use of neurotic denial.

There is no hint of any overt aggressiveness in this history. Yet, one wonders about the more deep-seated reaction of this very dependent woman to her husband's decision to spend most of the time away from home. The presence of the crippled father appears a significant factor, favoring identifica-

tion with the role of a victim and self-punishment. The unusual factor here is her willingness to see a psychiatrist.

Case 3. A 46-year-old production foreman, highly intelligent, with continuous back pain and episodic leg pain since an accident at work six years ago. Six surgical procedures had, at best, given relief for a couple of weeks on two occasions. He had also undergone two procedures for nasal septum deviation. He depends on the use of Demerol every few hours, with additional doses of Talwin, and admits to past periods of addiction to morphine.

He sleeps poorly, eats well, and smokes two and a half packs of cigarettes daily. Because of his pain and all those analgesics, his sexual activity is now reduced to a few episodes per year.

He has not worked now for almost three years, but was a very hard worker, working overtime, often working on weekends, and hardly ever missing a day in fourteen years. He has also given up his hobbies of hunting, fishing, gardening and landscaping, and stays in bed most of the time, reading when he can concentrate.

He describes his late parents, his wife and his children as fantastic people, adding: "I just can't understand about separations and divorces." He denies any emotional or interpersonal difficulties, but admits to getting depressed a few days per month when he feels sorry for himself. His father, dead for nine years, had been confined to a wheelchair for the last six years of his life because of emphysema. The patient had nursed several relatives without complaining and found it difficult to have the roles reversed.

Four Szondi Test profiles revealed marked aggressive tendencies which were kept strictly concealed, infantile dependency needs, a marked need for tender physical care, and neurotic denial. The findings on TAT, Rorschach, Figure Drawings and Cole Animal Tests were summarized as follows: He attempts to repress most feelings. He particularly defends against angry, aggressive feelings with denial and reaction formation. He aspires to a rugged, domineering, masculine identity, yet his test responses also show considerable passivity and unmet narcissism. He may use pain as a passive-aggressive means of dominating others.

The contrast between the alleged fantastic family relations and lack of emotional conflicts on the one hand, and the test findings on the other, is highly characteristic. It results from the marked denial of, or inability to appreciate, feelings, needs and conflicts. Aggressiveness, not masochism, is the predominant problem here, but it is strictly concealed and denied, with pain as the symptom. Again there is the presence of a crippled parent.

Case 4. A 52-year-old woman, married since age 19, had hurt her back 14 years ago while working as a nurse's aide, when she tried to save a patient from falling out of bed. A lumbar fusion was performed a couple of months later, and she had been free from pain for at least seven years when pain in the small of the back and in the left leg occurred. A second operation three years ago gave relief for about one year. A third operation one and a half years ago gave relief for about one year. When she returned home from the hospital that time, she discovered that her husband had become involved with her best girl friend and had deserted her. Since then he has not asked her for a divorce, yet she said he was "dead" as far as she was concerned. When asked how she would describe their relationship prior to the unexpected desertion, she said, "He was perfect—a wonderful husband and father."

She similarly describes her mother as wonderful and great, and spoke of a very loving relationship with her father ("I was his favorite"). Yet, the parents had been divorced for thirty years and she had not seen her remarried father for many years. She denied difficulties in getting along with people and any emotional conflicts in the past.

In view of the characteristic inability to perceive needs, feelings and conflicts, it is not so surprising that a "perfect marriage" suddenly is on the rocks.

Case 5. A 71-year-old woman, married since age 30, had suffered from continuous and gradually increasing pain in the rectal area over the past eight years. Four local surgical procedures had not given any relief. The pain started shortly after her husband had undergone successful surgery for a cancerous lesion. The couple had never had any children.

When the patient was 15, her mother became psychotic and remained mute. Around the same time her only sibling, a brother, was killed in the war. Although she felt terribly sorry for her father, she too left him and had seen him rarely since. Prior to meeting her husband, she had had a child whom she gave up for adoption. In the face of all these very painful events, she asserted that she had never experienced any emotional or interpersonal difficulties. She described her husband as very sympathetic toward her and alleged an excellent relationship between them.

Case 6. A 39-year-old unemployed engineer had experienced, over the past six years, an agonizing pain at the base of the spine that awoke him in the middle of the night every month or two and lasted for half an hour. He had suffered injury to the base of the spine on three occasions between the ages of seventeen and thirty.

His wife of three years, whom he had met through a computer match-up, also has pain "from phlebitis," dating back to the time when they met. The patient had been in psychotherapy for some two years prior to their marriage, because of feelings of depression and impotency, and had been helped.

We learned that his father was bad-tempered and would beat the mother, the brother and the patient for little reason, sometimes every day. (The patient was beaten the least of the three.) He had not seen the father for twenty years. When in high school he was "literally shoved around," and later would be struck by strangers who got angry with him. In spite of an obviously high intelligence, he was unsuccessful in his occupation, had not worked for two years, and had considered driving a bus for a living. Four Szondi Test profiles revealed a feminine-passive sexual orientation, infantile needs to depend and to be cared for, and predominant neurotic denial.

Because of these clear-cut findings and the lack of any physical explanation for the pain, he was told in the second session that his symptoms undoubtedly had emotional roots. After all, he had previously been in psychotherapy for over two years, and had been helped for depression and impotence. But he adamantly rejected the idea of the psychogenicity of his pain, and refused to seek psychiatric help. He admitted to being prone to worry. He also admitted to being able to elicit pain in his finger within minutes. But he was convinced that the pain at the base of the spine was physical.

OVERT SADO-MASOCHISM

The following cases document the propensity of pain-neurotics to choose brutal spouses. Their pain often occurs or intensifies only after physical abuse has ended or has lessened. Very typically, the pain begins following remarriage to a wonderful spouse, when "everything is just perfect."

The twenty cases with overt sadomasochistic ties to a spouse (or lover) listed here are from the series of 288 pain patients evaluated at the Johns Hopkins Hospital. The patterns described appear to be present in 5 to 10 per cent of patients with chronic atypical pain.

In the following patients, no actual separation from the brutal partner had occurred.

Case 7. A 32-year-old nurse's aide and housewife with pain in stomach and head of one year's duration. Husband is verbally and physically abusive when he drinks. She lives unhappily at her in-laws' house.

Case 8. The 38-year-old wife of a dentist with "migraine" history of thirteen years' duration and with continuous headaches for one year. Parents were "perfect," but husband is jealous and has at times choked her.

Case 9. A 42-year-old female with chronic low back pain since her twenties. Since her divorce from first husband, she has associated for six years with a boyfriend who beats her occasionally, when either drunk or sober. She has suffered three accidents and has undergone one back operation.

Case 10.   A 49-year-old housewife with pains in stomach for about eight years and headaches for about two years. The husband used to beat her, but she refused to talk about it. More recently there have been only verbal arguments. About nine years ago she helplessly looked on while her sister was beaten to death by the husband. Three stomach operations, five other operations, including one back operation.

Case 11.   A 36-year-old farmer's wife with low back and left hip pain for nine months. Husband beat her until a year ago. He was also cruel to the children. Pain stems from injuries which were suspected as being the result of her husband's cruelty, but she states she can cope with everything and has "a wonderful family." Had two hip operations, nine and five years ago.

Case 12.   A 41-year-old housewife with neck, shoulder and arm pain of two years' duration when first seen. Two neck operations failed to help. Finally, after two psychiatric hospitalizations for depression, she revealed that her husband got drunk episodically and would then abuse her verbally and physically. Her neck trouble started after her husband threw her down a flight of stairs. (He claimed amnesia for his acts.) She never really accepted psychiatric help and finally committed suicide.

In the following fourteen cases, separation from a brutal partner had taken place. The pain would typically occur or intensify after the patient remarried a kind and considerate spouse, when "everything would be wonderful if it were not for that pain."

Case 13.   A 33-year-old wife of a farmer has had neck pain for 10 years. Onset of pain coincided with divorce from a verbally and, at times, physically abusive first husband and remarriage to a "wonderful" second husband. Practices horseback riding and shooting. Has had two neck operations.

Case 14.   The 48-year-old wife of an officer has had right-sided pain in back and leg for one year. First husband was a sadist when drunk (which was most of the time) and sexually demanding. Remarried 12 years ago; second husband "just the opposite," never demanding, very considerate, a "beautiful relationship." Three back operations in one year.

Case 15.   A 46-year-old housewife and shipping clerk with pain in left back and leg of one year's duration. Divorced her first husband after 23 years. He had turned out to be an alcoholic who beat and cursed her. Remarried for two years to a husband who is kind and patient but who has a back problem himself.

Case 16.   37-year-old housewife with back pain of seven years' duration. First husband would beat her, choke her, take knives to bed, and threaten to kill her. "I finally had to leave (after three years) when he beat me so bad." Current husband of 11 years treats her "like a queen," but spends too

much money. One back operation and five other operations.

Case 17.   38-year-old divorcee with low back pain of four years' duration. She had been married until seven years ago to a man who "beat her all the time" and was unfaithful. Later, lived with a common-law husband, who was kind but saw other women and deserted her promptly after they were lawfully married. She has had rhinoplasty and a back operation.

Case 18.   60-year-old housewife with back pain of 20 years' duration and intense rectal pain of four years' duration. When young, had been married for several years to a man with violent temper who constantly beat her. Remarried 32 years ago to a fine second husband who is always at her side. Three back operations and two other operations.

Case 19.   40-year-old woman with back pain of many years' duration. She had been much abused by a first husband of 18 years. Current husband is a kind man. Her pain had abated some but recurred on the third day of their honeymoon. She is still afraid that her first husband might sexually abuse their daughters. Five back operations and 10 various other operations.

Case 20.   57-year-old housewife with headache and leg pains of one year's duration. She was married a first time for nine years to a sadistic and alcoholic surgeon ("You don't give up on people, they may be just confused."). She describes her relationship to her second husband of 17 years as "wonderful, very stable, a heaven."

Case 21.   45-year-old telephone operator and housewife with backache following four relatively minor accidents over the past nine years, relieved by surgery the first three times. She had been married for 17 years to a brutal man who drank and ran around, was sexually rough and demanding, was jealous, and beat her often. The pain problem started just before her divorce from this husband and increased over the following eight years after she married an "opposite" second husband, a policeman, whom she describes as very devoted, gentle, affectionate and extremely satisfying sexually. The only problem is the pain!

Case 22.   A 45-year-old woman, highly intelligent, married currently for the third time. She has had six back operations over the past 19 years. Since her second operation 18 years ago, she has suffered from headaches which became constant following the last successful back operation three years ago. The first husband, of five and a half years, was an alcoholic, very jealous and violent, and had once almost choked her to death. The second husband, of four years, was very nice at first but later proved to be more jealous than the first and had sadistic quirks: he would tie her up, bring her to near-orgasm, but then walk away and go to sleep. He also used various self-made electrical contraptions on her. He ultimately died from an MI. The third husband is not sadistic, but did run around initially. Lately, he has chosen separate bedrooms, treating her like a mother and companion while constantly professing deeper love. He would lock her out of the house if she even mentioned seeing a psychiatrist. She has constantly bent over backwards for others: parents, husbands, children. Her own father has been an alcoholic for the past 25 years, and beats her mother regularly.

Case 23. A 45-year-old carpenter who has suffered from pain in back, inguinal areas, and legs over the past eight years. His wife had suffered from "insane spells" during which she would hit him over the head. Six years ago a fusion gave him relief, but two years later the wife "broke his back" in a fight. She left him finally for another man, taking their four children and threatening to kill him if he ever came for them. Four years ago she had actually taken a shot at him. He obtained a court order to see his children, but never tried to have it enforced. Two years ago he married a church woman nine years his senior. He lives with her and his sickly mother. He describes the pain as if his back were being "crushed by a truck." He denies any anger or grudge against his brutal first wife, who had also beaten the children cruelly.

Case 24. A 59-year-old female teacher with pain to the right temple of five years' duration. This pain began one year after the death of her husband, who had been a "Jekyll and Hyde," physically abusing her at times. On one occasion he had broken her arm. A right supraorbital nerve avulsion one year ago brought her no relief.

Case 25. A 41-year-old housewife with spasms and pains in both legs dating back to a car accident four years ago and persistent in nature for one year. Describes wonderful relations with parents and children and states that her husband had been very good to her. Yet, she also states that her husband had tried to kill her several times, and finally left her for another woman after the car accident. She divorced him six months ago.

Case 26. A 39-year-old mother with back and leg pains following a car accident suffered a year and a half ago. Over the opposition of her parents, she separated from her husband two years ago after staying with him for 11 years. For all but the first two years of their marriage he was verbally and physically abusive toward her whenever he was intoxicated. Her father was an alcoholic, but she got along famously with her mother. A spinal fusion a year ago gave her relief from the pain for seven months only, and she is now hoping for a second operation.

The patients listed so far readily told us about their sado-masochistic relations, although a few of them refused to divulge any details. The following two cases exemplify that such pathological liaisons may be carefully concealed by the patient, only to be revealed fortuitously by a concerned spouse or after prolonged acquaintance with the patient through an unusual chain of events.

Case 27. A 55-year-old woman had suffered from angina pectoris for more than three years. An angiography performed before bypass procedure for the angina left her with pain in the right arm, which became intense after the heart surgery abolished most of the anginal pains, one year ago. She told us she had been married a first time at age 24, and described a very good relationship for 27 years, until the husband died four years ago. She had remained very devoted to him through more than three years of his terminal illness (cancer), and had spent 16 hours daily in the hospital during his last three months. After his death, a bitter disappointment to her was the refusal of her two stepsons to let her have her share of the inheritance. She had totally failed to look out for herself prior to her husband's death. Three years ago, she married a wealthy man who had suffered through a prolonged unhappy first marriage to an alcoholic woman, who had finally committed suicide. They expected to lead a very happy life but the pain intervened. She was very friendly and cooperative during the psychiatric evaluation, but seemed relieved when it was completed. Four Szondi Test profiles revealed presence of intense dependency needs, some depressive traits, and marked passive-masochistic strivings.

The husband then asked to speak with the psychiatrist privately. He was concerned about the role that past events played in his wife's pain. He revealed that her former husband of fifteen years had been less than ideal; he was domineering, and nice to people only when they did things exactly his way. Moreover, there had been a first marriage to a soldier who turned out to be a monster: a bigamist, drinker, and sadist who had often threatened to kill her. A divorce was finally arranged, after nine years, through legal pressures exerted by the man who then became her second husband.

Case 28. This patient, a government employee prior to his illness, was first seen at age 55 and then occasionally over the next six years. At age 31, while at work, he had suffered the sudden onset of a severe pain in both hips "as if someone had come with an axe and hit me." He had to be carried home. A cordotomy three years later brought some relief over the next 16 years, during which time he had kept working. At age 50, however, he was disabled. A repeat cordotomy, three surgical procedures on the left hip, exploration for lumbar disc, exploration of the sciatic nerve, and some other procedures, had not relieved the pain. The operations had impaired his walking and bladder control. At age 38 and again at age 51 he saw a psychiatrist for a few visits. ("My nerves were bad."... "I was at odds with the world.") At age 41 he lost his wife, from a complication following surgery for peptic ulcer–a disorder she had contracted since the onset of his pain. He then lived with his mother-in-law for eight years until she died, and finally moved in with his sister and her husband. Both his brother and his sister had suffered nervous breakdowns. The patient was always a great sports fan and kept active in church work for as long as he was able.

At the time of his first visit, the patient claimed he got along well with everybody, had sarcastic remarks for the psychiatric approach, and maintained that his only problem was the pain. Szondi Test profiles were characteristic for pain-neurosis. He was persuaded that further surgery was not indicated, and agreed to take antidepressant drugs and return for supportive visits with the psychiatrist every two months. While taking Tofranil he did a little better, but would still bemoan his fate and frequently express the wish to be in heaven with his dear late wife. With the exception of a pilgrimage to the Mayo Clinic, the course remained uneventful for a year and a half, after which time he had to be hospitalized for a severe bout of ulcerative colitis. As soon as the colitis was under control, he developed a psychotic depression with suicidal utterances and torpor, during which he would lie in his own excrement. In this highly regressed state he indicated that (for the first time in over 25 years) his hip pains were completely gone. The pain returned upon his transfer to the psychiatric wing. He was slowly regaining the ability to care for himself when another flare-up of the colitis required a total colectomy. His excessive need to be physically cared for was apparent during this entire hospitalization. He still required a stay in a nursing home before he could return to live with his sister.

What had brought on the crisis? A young woman from his church, for reasons of her own, had pursued him, wanting to marry him. As he was torn between accepting or rejecting the offer, the colitis flared up. While he was in the hospital, the preacher from their church appeared and asked for a confidential talk with the psychiatrist. He revealed the following: When the patient's wife was alive, she would leave a sealed letter with the preacher whenever she went away with her husband, with the instruction that the letter be opened only in the event that she did not return from their trip. The wife finally revealed the reason for all this: The patient had the persistent habit of putting his hands around her throat when they were in bed, threatening to kill her and then commit suicide. The preacher had promised the wife not to reveal this secret to anybody, but was now compelled to break his silence, out of concern for his other parishioner, the young woman who was about to marry this man so sadly unfit for marriage.

The patient readily abandoned these wedding plans. Over the following five years he returned to the psychiatrist whenever he felt more downcast than usual, was treated with antidepressants and did a little better. He required another operation, this time for his urinary difficulties. The old pain remained his constant companion.

As was previously pointed out by Engel, one parent of the pain-neurotic patient frequently turns out to be overtly sadistic. The following examples are listed from our series.

Case 29. A 43-year-old housewife suffered from head and neck aches for nine years and from low back and leg pains for eight years. Two back operations and insertion of electrodes for dorsal column stimulation had not given relief but had only changed the location of the pain. The father, a dentist, used to punish the patient with stick and fist, keeping her and her mother in a state of total submission. The patient lived in constant fear of him. Her husband of 11 years had, likewise, been totally dominated by his mother, and suffered from outbursts of rage during the early years of their marriage, during which he would beat her. The patient now fears that the mother-in-law may come to live with them. Communication between patient and husband is limited.

The patient had a fair insight into her difficulties. She related her "upper pains" to psychological stress, but firmly believed her "lower pains" were due to physical irritation.

Case 30. A 39-year-old woman with episodic pain in her paralyzed left arm, a pain which became constant over the past one and a half years. She had injured the arm at age 22 when she had "frozen on train tracks" and was only partially pulled away from the oncoming train. A cervical rhizotomy one year ago had not helped the pain.

Her father was an alcoholic who would "beat mother to death." Mother had fled from him when the patient was six years old, and married an amputee. The patient herself was divorced from her first husband because of incompatibility five years ago, and one and a half years ago married an extremely kind and understanding widower. She denies any emotional difficulties, except tension and depression because of her pain, and states she gets along with everybody very well. She works with amputees.

Case 31. The 60-year-old wife of a retired colonel with constant right arm and neck pain, and headaches for two years. Two surgical procedures had not given relief. Her father was described as a cruel individual with an uncontrollable temper, who was physically abusive of his wife. Patient had been married a first time to a man who shunned work and was a thief. Never had any children. She denied any emotional or interpersonal difficulties other than those she attributed to the pain.

Case 32. A 38-year-old black housewife with headache and left facial pain of one year's duration. The current complaint occurred after a disc operation for back pain and inability to walk for several weeks. She related a fantastic story: She and a sister were the out-of-wedlock children of their mother and a white physician. This father was "mad and wealthy" and, so she believed, had killed both his white wife and his black mistress (her mother). He pursued the patient and her sister sexually and would beat them brutally. She does relate her head pain to a scar suffered at her father's hands. On one occasion, after a severe beating from her father, she attempted to kill herself but he saved her. Sixteen years ago he died from a heart attack before her eyes, and she feels guilty because she was deliberately slow in calling for assistance. She loves her own husband, but is not sexually responsive. She is a good mother.

Whether truth or fantasy, her story is significant. Her Szondi profiles indicated marked masochistic and projective-paranoid tendencies. Because of marked agitation over her pain, a fear of losing her mind, and suicidal intent, she was admitted to the psychiatric unit, which she left shortly when she felt bothered by a black male patient. Chlorpromazine calmed her agitation and mitigated the pain.

Case 33. A 31-year-old housewife with continuous right-sided pain in neck, ear, face, shoulder, arm and hand of more than three years' duration. She no longer is able to relax for sex, but sleep and appetite are satisfactory. The husband is a hard worker and good family man. They have two boys. Initially, he had no sympathy for her ailments, but since a tumor (benign and unrelated to the pain) was removed from her thyroid three years ago, he has been very understanding.

The patient is very involved with her parents. For the past seven years the father has been drinking daily, and often to excess. He is a "wonderful man when sober," but when drunk he tends to abuse mother both verbally and physically. The mother calls the patient daily during such bad times. The patient has talked to her father "until I was blue in the face," but to no avail.

Case 34. A 48-year-old housewife with pain at the back of her head and in her left arm for one and a half years, and with pain in her left lower back and buttock for a half year. A brief first marriage ended with the death of the husband during World War II. Two daughters from a second marriage are now out of high school. The marital relationship is said to be very good, though she admits to not being interested in sex because of her pain.

Her father married in his forties, after having many affairs. He mistreated the mother very badly. Mother is a victim of arthritis, having walked with a limp as long as the patient can remember, and later always on crutches. Her father would often knock her mother off her crutches, as well as beat the patient for little or no reason, using sticks he kept for just that purpose in the cupboard. Her mother finally left the father, after 20 years, and has vegetated in a nursing home for the past 15 years. Her father died nine years ago.

TIES WITH THE ALCOHOLIC AND THE PROMISCUOUS

In pain-neurotics, the exposure to abuse between and from parents, and the propensity to choose a spouse who will also be abusive includes other than physical abuse. While brutal behavior in the histories we obtained is often associated with alcohol abuse, life with an alcoholic who may never become violent is miserable and degrading enough. The pain-prone patient has often witnessed alcoholism in parents and/or has chosen an alcoholic spouse. Highly promiscuous behavior appears with surprising frequency among parents or spouses of pain-neurotics. As in the case of overt brutality, more subtle abuse may have been witnessed early in life, preceding the pain; sometimes the pain is concomitant with the abuse, but typically it begins or intensifies when the abusive behavior does not have to be endured anymore — when everything could be just fine.

Case 35. A 39-year-old nurse suffered seven years of pain in the left leg until a laminectomy eight years ago. Neck pain began four years ago and became continuous last year. She denied any emotional or interpersonal difficulties. She had separated from her husband after 15 years, the first five of which were fine, while they gradually achieved a decent standard of living. Then he "became an animal." He worked as a television repairman and had sex with any woman who was interested. He always had at least two women at hand who sometimes would phone the patient. Toward the end of the marriage, he began to beat her. Understandably, the patient did not want sex anymore. Following the separation, the husband wanted her back.

Case 36. A 37-year-old truckdriver had fallen at work six years ago and has suffered from continuous low back pain ever since. Three back operations brought no relief. He has worked since age eight, working 60 to 70 hours a week, with time off only between his trips. He has not worked since the fall, but still goes hunting and fishing, and does leather tooling. He was married first at age 18 for one year, then at 23 for five years, and both times discovered his wife was running around. He himself was faithful when married, but "in between I made up for it." He remarried at age 31 and alleges a very good relationship with his wife. However, his accident occurred one month after his third wedding.

Case 37. A 53-year-old surgeon has had episodic pains in his hands for the past three years. A laminectomy helped temporarily. Father died from a crippling neurological disease when patient was a young child; a stepfather was alcoholic. His first wife, of 20 years, was an alcoholic and committed suicide (after several unsuccessful attempts) three years before onset of his pains. He remarried one year after her death. During his difficult first marriage he drank and was in psychotherapy for five years. Currently he denies any psychiatric difficulties.

Case 38. A 45-year-old housewife with low

back pain of eleven years' duration. Five back operations had left her worse off each time. On Demerol for two years. Her illness started shortly after her first husband, who was an alcoholic, deserted her. A second husband of four years is very concerned and spoils her.

Case 39. A 52-year-old divorced woman with continuous pain in the back of the neck, dating back to a fall on the occiput five years ago. Eight local surgical procedures had helped only temporarily. She used to be a vigorous worker, often putting in 16 hours a day as a machine weaver, only to go fishing afterward. She still works eight hours daily, but had to give up her more athletic activities (tennis, golf, swimming) owing to her pain. Her father, a blacksmith and fireman, used to run around with other women, while mother loved her beer and often neglected to cook meals. The parents divorced about 14 years ago. Father also drank much and was an alcoholic until two years ago, when he married a girl six years younger than the patient. The patient married at age 22 and separated at 36, as her husband was insanely jealous. She had always been faithful, and sex was never important to her. Her husband then married a rich woman who turned out to be an alcoholic; he died from a coronary four years ago. She has three children and three grandchildren from the oldest daughter, who is divorced. Her youngest child and the grandchildren are cared for by the patient's mother, while the patient lives with an adopted mother (sic!) who cares for her pains. Any emotional or interpersonal difficulties were denied. Everybody congregates and gets along well—patient, children, grandchildren, adopted mother, mother, father, and his young wife. "We are all a big happy family," she stated. If it weren't for that pain . . . which made her say, "I am like a drowning rat now, holding onto a piece of wood or anything!" The unusual story was confirmed by the adopted mother who came with the patient to the hospital.

Case 40. A 26-year-old housewife with continuous pain at the base of the skull, affecting shoulders and radiating into arms, of four years' duration—"like a nail being driven into that area would feel like." A first cervical fusion had given her about 50 per cent relief, a second procedure, none. Her father has been highly promiscuous and gets drunk every night. He always had "one pain or the other" and had two neck fusions over the past three years himself; in addition, he had an intestinal operation for cancer, and has been depressed, hypochondriacal and indifferent. However, he continues to run around with women. Mother lives the role of a martyr, taking much verbal abuse from father once he starts drinking, and serving him hand and foot—"opening his whiskey bottles and cutting his toenails." Mother recently began seeing a psychiatrist, while father is openly hostile to such ideas. The patient married a young army officer less than one year after onset of the pain. She describes their relationship as wonderful, yet she is unable to

relax having sex. After she was persuaded to start psychotherapy, she was able to talk about her sexual inhibitions: they had always joked about her father's running around, but she thinks she cannot let herself enjoy a sexual relationship because that would put her in the same category as her father's whores. That is why, when she got married, her neck trouble was a "godsend." But, she wanted to be able to have sex for her husband's sake . . . After this confession she discontinued seeing the psychiatrist, stating that she had to travel to see more neck specialists.

MASOCHISTIC LIFE-STYLE

Masochism, dependency and denial of conflict in the pain-neurotic tend to center on various individuals, preferably one person. In some patients, however, the masochism is most apparent in their general life-style, as in a subservience to many people, in a proneness to be taken advantage of by others, a failure in one's undertakings, or in accident-proneness.

Case 41. A 36-year-old black nurse's aide and housewife with episodic severe pain in left ear and left side of the head. No serious problems are burdening her, she states, because her six children are almost all grown up. She married at age 15. After they had their second child, her husband would go out drinking while she stayed home with the children without complaint. For several years now, he has stayed at home after work, but does a lot of nagging and fussing. She cannot talk back to him. He is always buying things for himself, but will not let her buy anything for herself. She never brings any girl friends home because he would be critical of them, though she often had all the children from the neighborhood at her house because many of them were left on their own. She works full-time to clean the house, unable to get her now adolescent daughters to do much work. She visits her aging parents daily, to look after them. She never tells others when she is distressed, "because everybody tends to baby me too much." She showed perception when she complained: "My only problem is I try to treat everybody right, but I am the one who takes the hard knocks."

Case 42. A 37-year-old former construction worker with left-sided pains in limbs, shoulder, back, hips and genitals, dating back to a diving accident in the service at age twenty. A fusion five years ago was beginning to help him when he fell in the cellar and had back pains again. Two years ago he had another spinal operation and another accident. He had been a hard worker since age 11, preferred to work 55 hours per week, and still continued to work in spite of his pains (and a 100 per cent V.A. disability allowance) until five years ago. Married for 15 years, denies emotional or interpersonal difficulties other than grouchiness as a result of his pains.

CRIPPLED OR SICK SPOUSE

The presence of a crippled or deformed close relative is found so often in the history of pain-neurotics that there can be little doubt concerning its significance. Four cases of pain-neurotics with a crippled spouse have been noted in the early series (see Case I). While early exposure to a crippled parent or sibling may prompt, in the predisposed, sado-masochistic fantasies, a tendency to suffer the pains of the victim and to become crippled oneself, there also appears to be an attraction to crippled individuals on the part of those prone toward sado-masochistic ties.

Another variation is found in couples in whom an interdependence (presumably intense) is disturbed when one partner becomes chronically sick or crippled. The still healthy spouse is frustrated in his own dependency needs but cannot be openly vengeful. He may develop pains "to get even." Such couples exchange groans of distress not unlike the angry shouts or physical blows shared by more able-bodied couples. They may vie for surgical procedures.

Case 43. A 44-year-old woman with superior intelligence has suffered from back pain and right leg pain since a car accident two years ago. She has not been helped by three laminectomies and a sympathectomy. Her brother had lost part of his right arm during the war, and her fiance had been killed. She then married, at age 26, a man with a urogenital malformation for which he had had multiple operations. She was hesitant to divulge her husband's condition, and refused to describe it accurately. She had known about his condition when they married but she did not talk about it even to her father, who was a physician. In fact, she had never revealed this condition to anybody. Though her husband was able to have intercourse, they had not had sex for years. This abstinence was vaguely blamed on his further kidney operations, but it was also apparent that sex did not seem important to her. She kept very active: teaching, working toward an advanced degree, performing all the secretarial work in her husband's business, taking care of the home, reading, knitting, sewing, horseback riding, swimming and dancing. For several months prior to the accident she had also given daily care, after her regular work, to her mother-in-law, who suffered from thrombosis of her legs and a pain in her right foot, even though they could have afforded to hire help. Any emotional or interpersonal conflicts were denied, and the patient was firmly opposed to any further psychiatric intervention. She had taken tranquilizers only once in her life, when her husband underwent surgery for kidney stones ten years ago. It was also noted that her back pain got worse a short time after the accident, when her husband underwent surgery for a hernia.

Case 44. A 50-year-old woman has suffered from continuous low back pain and pain in both legs since straining herself while moving her washing machine five months ago. She had had four operations for various conditions in the past, but none for her present ailment. She divorced her first husband who had been an alcoholic. On the questionnaire, she gave a negative answer to the question regarding a crippling condition, deformity, or chronic physical handicap among relatives or close friends. Yet, when the psychiatrist came to her room for an interview he met a dwarf with deformed hands at her bedside. This was the woman's second husband, who "freaked out" the interviewer by baring a set of odd teeth and dropping sarcastic remarks about the psychiatric profession. The patient apologized for her husband's behavior but actually seemed to enjoy the spectacle.

Case 45. An 81-year-old retired theologian and educator complained of continuous pain in his left big toe of five years' duration — "like a rat is pulling and yanking and jerking on the toe." Consultations with many specialists throughout the country had not brought any help. In the year prior to the onset of pain, the patient's wife developed cerebral arteriosclerosis with constant dizziness, rendering her a cripple. In addition, their daughter had been operated on for pelvic cancer 12 years before, and their son died when he crashed in his own plane two years before. The old man denied any emotional difficulties and stated: "Of course, I am greatly concerned about my wife. But I have a philosophy that trouble comes to all of us. I believe profoundly in God's leadership, therefore I don't let myself get depressed." At the time of his son's death, he required an operation for a bleeding ulcer. He still served as a consultant to a college.

Case 46. A 49-year-old farmer's wife had been unable to work for the past five months, owing to pain in her neck and low back after slipping and landing on her buttocks. The pain was there all the time; she felt desperate and cried at least twice a day. Since having a partial hysterectomy 16 years ago, she had not felt well, suffering from hot flushes, irritability, and low spirits. Her husband was half-paralyzed and unable to work after a back operation six years ago. The patient carried the heavy burden of supporting the family. At first, she took care of their chicken farm, then did "a man's work" by laboring in a paper mill for the four and a half years before her accident. She obviously felt entitled to now retire with compensation.

RELENTLESS ACTIVITY

Hyperactivity is a very common, and frequently dominant, trait of the pain-neurotic. Usually it takes the form of relentless work habits, often starting in early adolescence — sometimes in childhood. The individual sacrifices play and leisure time for the good of the family. This self-sacrifice bears a strongly masochistic note. The relentless activity is necessary in order to be accepted, to atone for guilt feelings and to maintain a fragile self-esteem. Moreover, a reward is hoped for: the patient wishes to be taken care of in return by others. But this reward does not come. Children grow and leave home, and the spouse continues to take the hard working for granted. Then an injury intervenes and, in a sudden reversal of roles, the relentless worker turns into a helpless, needy sufferer who demands constant care. Many patients try to keep working as long as they can and become invalids only gradually. The words are often sighingly uttered, "If only I could get going again."

With many patients this work activity is physical labor, such as carpentering or welding. Even females may choose "muscular" work activities. Characteristic preferences, particularly for some females, are for activities such as swimming, horseback riding and tennis.

Case 47. A 54-year-old woman has suffered from pain in the head, neck and left arm since an accident two years ago. She has had six operations in the past, but none for her pain. As a child of immigrant parents, she began working at age eight in the small family plant. She would work from 7 to 10 A.M., before school, and from 2:30 to supper time, after school. Upon graduation from high school, she married outside her religion (a fact denied by her mother), had two daughters, and worked with her husband in his business. She now works as needed, anywhere from a few to 18 hours a day, sews clothing for the entire family, bakes, writes, does metal enameling, and goes camping and fishing. Both patient and husband are "perfectionists," and excellent family relations are alleged. It is not coincidental that the car accident which brought on her pain occurred on the very day the husband, after 24 years, gave up his traveling position to work full-time at home. He would call her every night during his travels. She now finally admits that he is hard to live with and jokes that she will pack his bags again. The children are both married and live far from home.

It is also significant that the patient's father had a leg amputated some 15 years ago for circulatory failure, and suffered from a painful phantom limb for the last three months of his life. The patient was with him almost constantly during this difficult period — "I could not leave his room."

Case 48. A 50-year-old welder unable to work for the past two years because of increasing distress from a left foot pain which began five years ago. The foot feels as if "it's being crushed in a vise." He has had eight operations, two for the foot pain. This pain appeared after he tried to stand and walk following a long recuperative period for an aorta graft. He has worked since age 16, working 50 to 65 hours per week, or more (and without vacations) when he had his own welding business for 10 years. Any emotional or interpersonal difficulties are denied, and a great relationship with wife and two daughters is alleged. He had a wonderful mother who died from cancer when he was 15 years old. The father was a drinker, very argumentative when intoxicated, who was abusive to the children, spanking them with pieces of wood. He died six years ago. One brother committed suicide after the death of his wife four years ago.

ATYPICAL PATIENTS WITH PAIN

The following patients with chronic pain vary sufficiently from the ordinary mold of pain-neurotics to be listed separately.

THE ADDICTED. It may seem surprising that the typical pain-neurotic does not more often become addicted to analgesics. One must remember, however, that most of our patients sought help from the surgeon, ostensibly to have their distress surgically relieved, but perhaps they also did so to undergo more suffering. In any case, to seek constant relief from pain by drugs is not the chief desire of these patients. Some do get addicted accidentally, but they manage to get off the particular drug without much difficulty. We have observed only five patients in whom the addiction seemed to be the main problem, and they usually did not seriously desire surgery.

Case 49. A 57-year-old former preacher, building manager and cabinet maker, suffered the sudden onset of low back pain four years ago. A lumbar laminectomy helped for one year, then the pain returned, became unremitting and rendered him unable to work. Alcoholism had interfered earlier with his career as a preacher and he was now dependent on Demerol. He married 14 years ago and his wife, a government worker in a responsible position, had become the sole support because of his illness. In the hospital he was belligerent, at times demanding injections and threatening to leave if he didn't get immediate satisfaction. At other times, he was contrite and apologetic. He was given Demerol in decreasing doses, as well as saline injections (which were entirely effective for the pain). When a pleural biopsy, necessary for an intercurrent condition, was scheduled, he angrily signed out against medical advice. He later called to apologize and explained he just couldn't take the additional pain of the procedure.

THE LONELY. It is most unusual to find a pain-neurotic suffering by himself. The marked dependency needs of the pain-neurotic almost invariably lead to an intense relationship, preferably to one partner, in which the need to cling as well as the hostility are denied, but do come through in a powerful form as pain. The following patient is the only one known to us who has kept on living by himself. One is inclined to doubt the role of psychological factors in his pain, but the patient appeared very markedly dependent in spite of his lonely life-style, and various traits characteristic of a pain-neurotic were present.

Case 50. A 73-year-old retired machinist suffering from a continuous pain around the right shoulder blade which developed very gradually over the past one and a half years. His history of eight operations for various conditions was remarkable. Darvon and Tylenol were now just as effective as Demerol had been. Married at 25, he left his wife and three children 22 years ago, "because of a lot of things, nothing big . . . things got out of hand." When pressed for specifics, he mentioned that he left when his wife asked him to do her job (cleaning the house) on a Saturday once too often, but he denied any grudge . . . "no time for that." He then lived with his parents and later by himself, keeping in touch with his two brothers, but with few friends. He does have a woman friend whom he sees on weekends. He denied any emotional or interpersonal difficulties. He had been a very steady worker, from age 16 until retirement. His only hobby now is reading, but the pain makes it difficult for him to concentrate.

THE SCHIZOPHRENIC. The schizophrenic with the chief complaint of pain is usually well recognizable. His physical complaints tend to be bizarre (see Case VII) and other signs of his mental illness are usually present. Case 32 did reveal a paranoid trait but was not diagnosed as schizophrenic.

Case 51. A 52-year-old divorcee who had flown in from Germany to be seen for a persistent facial pain related an unshakable belief that the nerves in both sides of her head were torn, resulting in muscular weakness. She stated that her brain would be poisoned and that she would lose her sanity unless a drastic surgical procedure was undertaken. Whenever doubt was expressed to her, she would repeat, "Just pull my scalp down, and you will see!" She was firmly convinced that she was doomed to die in Germany, because no German physician would do anything for her. She had worked as a medical secretary until she was forced to retire six months previously. Her complaints dated back 15 years, and had gradually intensified. Two years prior to onset, her only son had developed, at age eight, difficulties with his bite. She still carried documents of her son's oral-surgical problem with her and feels deeply dissatisfied with the medical help her son received.

THE MANIC. A single patient in the series was diagnosed as manic. The neurosurgeon thought this patient was psychotic, and the psychopathology was indeed well in evidence at the time of hospitalization.

Case 52. A 57-year-old widow with right facial pain, as well as "pain of the whole body." She talked constantly, with a marked flight of ideas, allowing someone else a word from time to time. She was somewhat grandiose, talking loosely about several boyfriends, and was very easily angered. She referred to psychiatrists as "a pain in the pocketbook" and wanted no part of them.

THE BRAIN DAMAGED. In the presence of a cerebral lesion, the relatively rare and characteristic syndrome of central pain must be considered. True central pain tends to flare up easily during emotional stress. Cerebral lesions, which are associated with a "frontal lobe syndrome," are characterized by a certain indifference to emotional tension, and an actual pain will have a much diminished impact.

In other patients, the cerebral impairment may disturb the customary emotional adjustment of the individual, and in some cases may lead to a "secondary pain-neurosis." We have observed three such cases in our series. The following is exemplary.

Case 53. A very active and successful high school principal was forced into retirement at age 62, following a series of minor cerebrovascular accidents. He complained now of chronic headache, as well as of a lack of ambition and strength. His recent memory had been mildly impaired, some concreteness of thought was present, and his speech and motions were markedly slowed. Depression was denied, but the frustration over his failings appeared significantly related to his pain.

Desire for monetary compensation is a well-known and important reinforcer of pain. In our series of surgery-seeking pain-neurotics, surprisingly, financial gain seemed to play either a subordinate role or no role at all.

THE PREVALENCE OF FEMALES AMONG PAIN-NEUROTICS

Based on his experience with almost 400 cases, Walters gives a ratio of seven females to three males among psychogenic ("regional") pain patients.[23] Our own figures for patients with atypical pain or pain-neurosis are comparable: At the Johns Hopkins Hospital we saw 194 females and 94 males; at the Massachusetts General Hospital, 60 females and 35 males. Our total ratio (254 females, 129 males) approximates two females to one male.

The reasons for this consistent and significant female prevalence are not clear. A number of factors may be of importance, either individually or, more probably, in combination. Biological factors (chromosomal or endocrine) on the one hand, and cultural factors (rearing practices, prevalent attitudes in society) on the other may favor passive-masochistic and dependent needs in females. Cultural factors may favor the tendency to use pain as an expression of conflict and distress in females. Males, by the same token, may be more inclined to become alcoholic or promiscuous, given the same basic conflicts familiar to us in pain-neurotics (self-sabotage and indirect aggressiveness, excessive dependency and show of false independence, inability to recognize and deal with emotional conflicts and denial). We have already noted the affinity of the pain-neurotic for the alcoholic and promiscuous. Finally, it is possible that women are more inclined to resort to pain as a defense against sexuality (see Case 40). The pain-neurosis in females appears to carry a more hysterical note than that in males; this is not surprising on general grounds, and is further supported by Szondi Test findings.

Psychological Test Findings

MMPI

Patients with the chief complaint of chronic pain tend to offer a profile of psychophysiologic reaction, with abnormally high scores on the Hs (Hypochondriasis) and Hy (Hysteria) scales. The D (Depression) scale score, however, is also often as elevated. Chronic pain patients thus may not show a clear "psychosomatic-V" (high Hs, low D, high Hy), but may score as psychophysiologic reactions with depression. It is possible that the high depression scores are only obtained with prolonged duration of pain, but we do not have sufficient data to support this view.

The MMPI, scored and interpreted for us by a computer (Roche Psychiatric Service Institute) gave the following clinically pertinent information about these patients with notable regularity.

Attention and concern is focused on bodily functions. There is marked denial of emotional problems. Such patients lack insight and have difficulty establishing mature interpersonal relationships. Motivation for psychotherapy is poor. Their condition appears to fall in the neurotic range. A number of patients are seen as somewhat overproductive in thought and action while others are seen as more depressed. Some patients reflect a strong tendency to see themselves, and to be seen by others, in a highly favorable light. They are prone to developing somatic symptoms in the face of emotional stress.

With a few patients, the interpretation indicated problems of suppressed hostility. A few women were described as overly feminine, with an almost masochistic willingness to assume burdens and to place themselves in situations in which they will be imposed upon.

Two typical profiles of this group, and their interpretations, are reproduced in Figures 18–1 and 18–2.

SZONDI TEST

FINDINGS AND CHARACTERISTIC PATTERNS IN PAIN-NEUROTICS. The Szondi Test has remained our preferred projective technique. In performing the test, a patient is required to make all the revealing choices while remaining unaware of the significance of his responses. The test not only assesses denial and concealment of conflict but also indicates the nature of the inhibited, repressed, or hidden tendencies. The Szondi Test scores give quantitative measures of the aggressive, passive-masochistic, affectionate, and dependent or independent needs which are so significant in patients with chronic atypical pain. Our clinical experience with the test has found it to be diagnostically precise and highly useful in evaluating pain patients, and we therefore summarize the findings even though the test is little known. A warning needs to be added. Although the Szondi Test seems simple and appealing in its quantitative measures, it requires an experienced interpreter who is aware of the variable qualitative aspects of the responses and can interpret them in context.

The findings of a blind evaluation of the Szondi Test profiles for 20 patients, performed by A. Beeli, were summarized in the earlier section detailing the characteristics of our initial series of pain-neurotics.

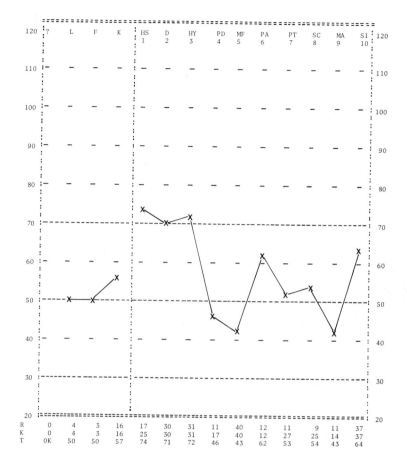

Figure 18–1. MMPI Profile of a 28-year-old pain-neurotic woman, with interpretation by computer. Profile is characteristic for psychophysiologic reaction with depression. Denial of emotional problems, resistance to psychotherapy, and neurotic range of condition are indicated.

The test results of this patient appear to be valid. She seems to have made an effort to answer the items truthfully and to follow the instructions accurately. To some extent this may be regarded as a favorable prognostic sign since it indicates that she is capable of following instructions and able to respond relevantly and truthfully to personal inquiry.

This patient may have a tendency to deny emotional problems, and to focus on numerous physical symptoms, such as pain, especially in the head, chest, or stomach. She also may exhibit problems associated with eating, including loss of appetite or over-eating. She lacks insight into her difficulties and may be expected to resist firmly any interpretation of her symptoms as psychogenic in nature. She may refuse psychiatric evaluation, and she would be difficult to motivate for psychotherapeutic treatment.

At present, she appears to be depressed. She views herself as unhappy and useless. Apathy, lack of interest, pessimism and worry may be expressed. If she denies depression and maintains a facade of cheerfulness, the possibility of suicide should be assessed carefully. It should be noted, however, that some patients apparently learn to live with a chronic depression and tend to view it without any great alarm.

She shows undue sensitiveness and suspicion of those around her. She may tend to misinterpret the motivations of others, leading to difficulties in her interpersonal relationships.

This patient's condition appears to fall within the neurotic range. She is using neurotic defenses in an effort to control her anxiety.

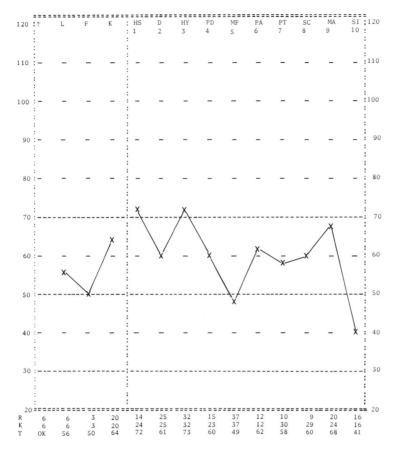

					HS	D	HY	PD	MF	PA	PT	SC	MA	SI	
	?	L	F	K	1	2	3	4	5	6	7	8	9	10	
R	6	6	3	20	14	25	32	15	37	12	10	9	20	16	
K	6	6	3	20	24	25	32	23	37	12	30	29	24	16	
T	OK	56	50	64	72	61	73	60	49	62	58	60	68	41	

Figure 18–2. MMPI Profile of a 52-year-old pain-neurotic woman, with interpretation by computer. Profile shows the "psychosomatic-V" (high Hs, low D, high Hy) and is characteristic for extreme denial of emotional problems, difficulty establishing mature interpersonal relationships, poor motivation for psychotherapy, and some overproductivity in thoughts and actions.

The unwillingness of this patient to admit to the relatively minor faults which most people have suggests that she is a person with strong needs to see herself, and to be seen by others, as an unusually virtuous person. Such people tend to be rigid, defensive, and uncompromising individuals who stress moral issues and emphasize their own integrity. They tend to be frustrated, insecure people who have little insight, and who are unaware of their own stimulus value. It is doubtful that these tendencies have invalidated the patient's test results, but they may have caused her to receive somewhat reduced scores on the clinical scales.

This patient may exhibit a variety of physical symptoms with an absence of overt anxiety and depression. It appears that this patient is focusing her attention and concern on bodily functions and showing extreme denial of emotional problems. Frequent symptoms are pain, especially in the head, chest or stomach, problems in eating such as loss of appetite or over-eating, and insomnia. Such patients lack insight and have difficulty establishing mature interpersonal relations. Although her prognosis in psychotherapy might be fairly good, considerable difficulty in motivating this patient for treatment may be anticipated.

She tends to be somewhat overproductive in thinking and action. She may be restless, over-talkative and, in the face of frustration, irritable, aggressive and impulsive. The normal expression of this trait is enthusiastic, energetic and persistent goal-direct activity.

She shows undue sensitiveness and suspicion of those around her. She may tend to misinterpret the motivations of others, leading to difficulties in her interpersonal relationships.

In the face of emotional stress and pressures, this patient may tend to develop somatic symptoms. If physical complaints exist for which no medical basis can be determined, attention should be focused on the relief of her emotional problems.

Characteristic test patterns are outlined in Table 18–2. Figures 18–3 and 18–4 show the Szondi Test profiles for two of the patients described earlier (Cases IV and 43).

COMPARISON OF TEST FINDINGS IN PAIN-NEUROTICS WITH A MATCHED GROUP OF HYPOCHONDRIACS. Twenty patients from a previously evaluated group of hypochondriacs were matched in age and sex with twenty pain-neurotics, and their test findings were compared. Each group was composed of seven males and 13 females. The mean age for the hypochondriacs was 44.6 years (males 43.3, females 45.3), ranging from 21 to 64 years; the mean age for the pain-neurotics was 43.9 years (males 41.6, females 45.2), ranging from 16 to 61 years. The first four Szondi Test profiles obtained were used in all the analyses.

TABLE 18–2.   SZONDI TEST PATTERNS CHARACTERISTIC FOR PAIN-NEUROTICS*

Vector Patterns

Sex vector (S)
S + −(!)
S 0 −   } Passive-masochistic sexuality
S + ±
Variation: s+! combined with hy−! Concealed aggressivity

Contact vector (C)
C − +(!)
C − 0   } Prolonged infantile contact needs
C 0 +
Variation: d + Depressive component

Affect vector (P)
P + −
P 0 −   } Conscientiousness, anxiety related to guilt,
P ± −   } need to conceal

Ego vector (Sch)
Sch − +   } Denial (inhibition or repression)
Sch − 0

Syndromes and Reaction Patterns

e hy k p   } Anxiety related to guilt and fear of punish-
+ − − +   } ment ("Hypochondriacal middle," but with-
± − − 0   } out projection [no p−])
Reaction pattern of sado-masochistic perversion; of inversion (lack of masculinity in males, masculine aggressiveness in females); of conversion hysteria in females.

Quantitative Tensions (ranked according to frequency of occurrence)

1. s −!   need to suffer (masochism)
   m +!   need to cling and to be accepted (orality)

2. h +!   need for physical closeness and care
   hy −! need to conceal conflicts

3. d −!   need to retain the old love object
   k −!   denial, despair

*The characteristic vector patterns, syndromes, reaction patterns, and quantitative tensions are listed and their principal meaning is indicated.

The hypochondriacs did not present with significant complaints of pain, but they did have excessive concern with their health which focused on the dread of various malfunctions and diseases in the absence of sufficient physical cause. This fear of illness and death is based on a subconscious anxiety related to guilt and fear of punishment, as was evidenced by their test patterns and with therapeutic intervention.[4] None of these patients was psychotic, but they all suffered from a hypochondriacal neurosis.

Hypochondriacs are an interesting control group for pain-neurotics because both groups somatize their psychological conflicts, with the central problem of guilt, resulting in the dread of disease in the former group and in excessive pain in the other. The hypochondriacs had all come to a clinic for internal medicine which specialized in treatment by diet, while the pain-neurotics had all come for surgery. There was, however, one significant difference: the hypochondriacs had maintained a generally satisfactory work adjustment, while the pain-neurotics were largely disabled.

Figure 18–5 shows the percentage of all vector patterns. The vector patterns are *ordered in psychologically related groups,* and the significant differences within the vector groups are indicated. The incidence of passive-masochistic sex patterns is significantly higher in the pain-neurotics (p < .02). Within the "ego patterns," pain-neurotics show a significantly higher incidence of neurotic patterns (p < .02) and a significantly lower incidence of "everyday" patterns (p < .001).*

The percentage of vector patterns for a very large group of normals is also charted in Figure 18–5, for comparison purposes. Most striking is the marked increase of dependent strivings (C −+, 0+) in *both* the pain-neurotics and the hypochondriacs over the values in the group of normals.

While both patient groups show an incidence of various vector patterns similar to

---

*The "everyday" pattern (Sch--) is characteristic for the average non-intellectual citizen who projects his needs onto the world around him but adjusts to the demands of reality. The unusually high incidence of the "everyday" pattern among hypochondriacs does not mean that they are more normal than the average citizen, since the patterns have to be interpreted within the context of the entire profile; their "everyday" pattern is related to the projection of excessive and ambivalent dependency needs onto various bodily organs.

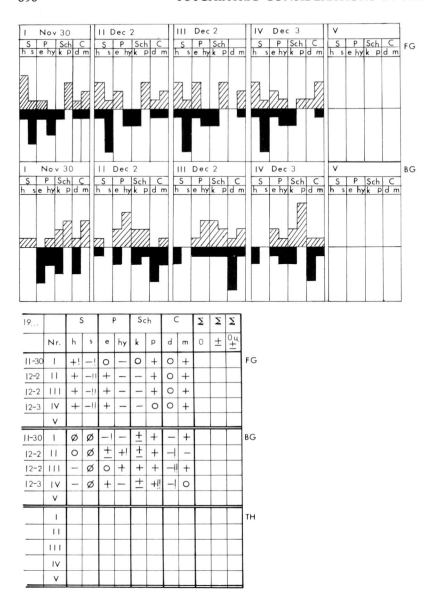

19...		S		P		Sch		C		Σ	Σ	Σ	
	Nr.	h	s	e	hy	k	p	d	m	0	±	0u/+	
11-30	I	+!	-!	o	-	o	+	o	+				FG
12-2	II	+	-!!	+	-	-	+	o	+				
12-2	III	+	-!!	+	-	-	+	o	+				
12-3	IV	+	-!!	+	-	-	o	o	+				
	V												
11-30	I	Ø	Ø	-!	-	±	+	-	+				BG
12-2	II	O	Ø	±	+!	±	+	-!	-				
12-2	III	-	Ø	o	+	+	+	-!!	+				
12-3	IV	-	Ø	+	-	±	+!!	-!	o				
	V												
	I												TH
	II												
	III												
	IV												
	V												

Figure 18–3. Four Szondi Test profiles of a 16-year-old male student with pain-neurosis (Case IV). With excessive masochistic tendencies (s-!!); infantile dependency needs (CO+,−!+); "hypochondriacal middle"

$$\begin{bmatrix} e & hy & k & p \\ + & - & - & + \\ + & - & - & 0 \end{bmatrix}$$

indicating guilt conflicts; and neurotic denial (Sch−+: inhibition; −0: repression); the test findings are highly characteristic for pain-neurosis.

normals, the pain-neurotics show a much higher incidence of quantitative tensions, indicating the presence of excessive needs. Figure 18–6 compares the incidence of quantitative tensions on each of the eight Szondi factors. Significant differences were obtained only on the factor s−, which indicates passive versus active strivings (in the normal range) or sado-masochistic strivings (in the abnormal range). There is a significantly higher incidence of quantitative tensions along the axis

s− in pain-neurotics, pointing to the marked masochism characteristic for this group. However, in the present sample this incidence is accounted for by the abnormally high masochism among the males only, with female pain-neurotics showing a significant lack of excessive aggressiveness when compared with the matched group of hypochondriacs. It must be emphasized that the scores of quantitative tensions in normals would approximate the zero line.

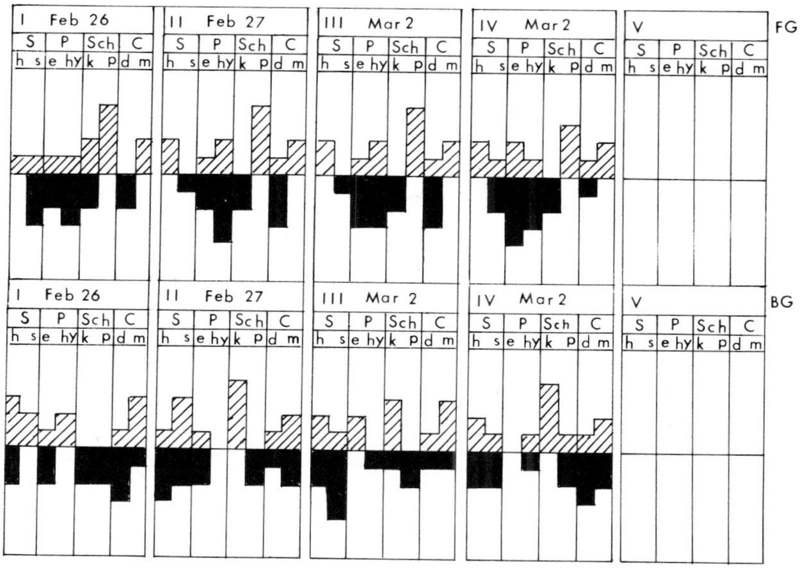

Figure 18–4. Four Szondi test profiles of a 44-year-old teacher and housewife with pain-neurosis (Case 43). Passive-masochistic tendencies (SO−, +−; s−!), infantile dependency needs (C−+) and neurotic inhibition (Sch−+) are characteristic for pain-neurosis. Guilt conflict with need to conceal is also

indicated $\begin{bmatrix} e & hy & k & p \\ \pm! & - & - & + \\ - & \pm! & - & + \end{bmatrix}$. S + O in-

dicates infantile sexual needs.

19...	Nr	S h	s	P e	hy	Sch k	p!	C d	m	Σ 0	Σ ±	Σ 0u/±	
2-26	I	O	−	−	−	±	+!	−	+				FG
2-27	II	+	O	−	±	−	+!	−	+				
3-2	III	+	O	−	±	−	+!	−	+				
3-2	IV	+	−	±	−	−	+	O	+				
	V												
2-26	I	±	+	−	+	−	−	−	+				BG
2-27	II	−	±	−	∅	+!	−	O	±				
3-2	III	±	−!	+	∅	+	−	O	+				
3-2	IV	±	−	∅	O	+!	−	−	±				
	V												
	I												TH
	II												
	III												
	IV												
	V												

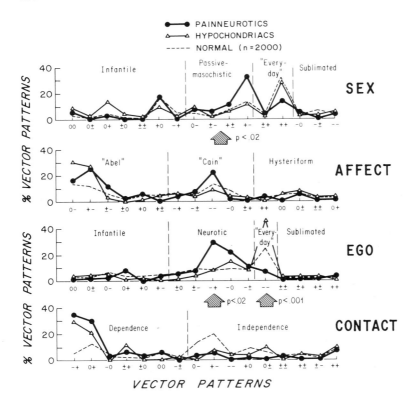

Figure 18–5. Szondi Test Patterns of pain-neurotics vs. hypochondriacs (7 males, 13 females: 4 profiles each = 80 profiles). The percentage of all vector patterns ordered in psychologically related groups are charted for 20 pain-neurotics, a matched group of 20 hypochondriacs and for a large group of normals (N = 2000). The following significant differences between the two patient groups are noted: higher incidence of masochistic sex patterns and neurotic ego patterns in pain-neurotics, and a higher incidence of "everyday"-ego-patterns in hypochondriacs. *Both* the "surgical group" with pain-neurosis and the "internal medical group" with hypochondriasis score much higher on "dependence" if compared with normals. The hypochondriacs (who have largely maintained their work adjustment) score closer to the normals on the sex and ego vectors, if compared with the (largely invalid) pain-neurotics.

Each of the four vectors (Sex, Affect, Ego, Contact) consists of two paired factors. Each factor is scored as either +, −, ±, or 0. All possible combinations are charted.

OTHER TESTS

We do not have sufficient data to report on the sensitivity of various other psychodiagnostic instruments in the assessment of pain-neurotics. We believe, however, that tests like the TAT, Rorschach, Draw-a-Person, Sentence Completion, as well as others, can be highly useful tools in the hands of the skilled psychologist for this purpose.

THE ROLE OF THE SURGEON OR OTHER PRIMARY PHYSICIAN

Patients with pain-neurosis are almost invariably drawn to a surgeon as their helper. They may first see their personal physician for referral to a surgeon, but, then, what the surgeon says will be of special importance. These patients prefer to have a surgeon as their primary physician—or at least to have one close at hand. As a result of their intractable condition they tend to go on to further specialists in the surgical field, either by their own

choice or encouraged by their physician. Every neurosurgeon or orthopedic surgeon will recognize the type of pain patients we have described in certain problem patients from his own practice. With widening reputation, a surgeon will invariably attract more such patients. Pain-neurotics abound among those who seek help from the surgeon who specializes in the relief of pain.

There are clear reasons why the pain-neurotic is so fixated on the surgeon. First, the surgeon enjoys the well-earned reputation of being able to cut out and clear up pain. The pain-neurotic denies any psychological conflict; he conceals, somatizes and encapsulates his distress; he then presents himself to the surgeon for relief. His characteristic belief that "everything would be all right if it were not for that pain" makes him intensify his plea. Second, patients who continue to suffer without physical cause fulfill their masochistic needs, which we have amply documented in the preceding chapter, by being instinctively attracted to surgical procedures, and the specter of more suffering, mutilation and even death.

Many experienced surgeons readily recognize such a problem patient; some state bluntly that they "will not touch her (him) with a ten-foot pole." Others get more involved with the pain-neurotic; they may feel challenged by or very compassionate toward the chronic sufferer. It is not incorrect to view surgery as a noble sublimation of man's natural aggressive instinct. It is probably less correct, however, to blame the excessive use of surgery performed on masochistic patients on a surgeon's over-aggressiveness. In our experience, unnecessary surgery is more likely to be undertaken because of the surgeon's lack of experience with these difficult patients and his resulting inability to remain objective in the face of their desperate pleas for help. Many surgeons will take a closer look, i.e., will operate, in a case with questionable findings. If, however, such a patient can be identified as a pain-prone patient and a candidate for a career as a pain-neurotic, there is much to be

argued in favor of a more conservative approach. We found that such patients usually experience relief from an initial operation for months, even years, only to return to the surgeon with renewed pain and the request for more operations which gradually lose their effectiveness. Surgery should not be performed for a placebo effect, not only because of the risk involved in every operation but also because it confirms the patient's belief that a cut in the right place might solve his problems—if earlier operations failed, there may just have to be a better cut. Moreover, previous operations tend to cloud a clinical picture that is already obscure; questions of scarring from the former procedure(s) etc., may trouble the patient and physician.

Clearly, the final decision for or against an operation is the surgeon's. It is also true that the type of patient we have described as the pain-neurotic may, indeed, have a lesion for which surgery must be performed. But

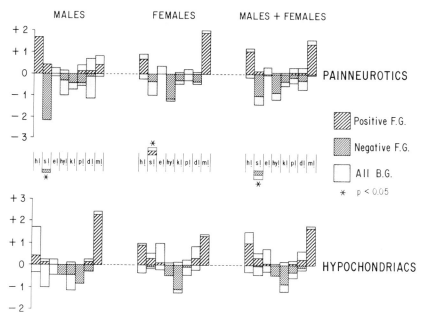

Figure 18–6. Szondi Test quantitative tensions of pain-neurotics vs. hypochondriacs (7 males and 13 females) The quantitative tensions (number of "exclamation marks" for each factor, in means over four profiles) are recorded separately for males and females as well as jointly for both; the scores on foreground (F.G.) and background (B.G.) profiles are differentiated but added in the same column.

Significant differences were obtained only on the factor s. Quantitative tensions in the factor s are indicative of sadistic (s+!) or masochistic (s–!) tendencies. Pain-neurotics show a significantly higher incidence of quantitative tensions in the s– direction, pointing to the marked masochism characteristic for this group. This incidence, however, is accounted for by the findings among the males, while female pain-neurotics show a significant lack of aggressiveness if compared with the female hypochondriacs. In normals, similar scores for quantitative tensions would approximate the zero level.

before performing surgery to relieve pain, the psychological issue must be weighed.

The surgeon should be alert to the problems posed by the seemingly solid citizen who may have been a tireless worker, who emphasizes that he has no problems, who alleges a very wonderful family life, for whom, perhaps after much suffering of abuse, everything may go just right—if it weren't for that pain—yet who has become more of an invalid since the onset of the pain than one would expect, and who may be very unconcerned about the risks posed by surgery. If this patient already has a history of surgical procedures, further caution will be needed.

The surgeon may wish to get the opinion of a psychiatric colleague or that of a psychologist. The more problem patients with pain he sees, the more desirable will be such an alliance. It must be kept well in mind that the very resistance to a psychiatric or psychological evaluation is frequently suggestive of a psychosomatic problem. It is more important to gain knowledge of the full clinical picture, and less important that a patient may feel "insulted" for having his sanity doubted.

Unfortunately, it may not be easy to gain the interest and steady cooperation of a psychiatric colleague or psychologist in dealing with pain patients. Nobody likes to run into a stone wall—to the chronic pain-patient, the invitation to talk about his feelings seems totally out of place. The evaluation of difficult pain patients, however, does represent an interesting challenge, particularly to a psychologist. Psychotherapy with a pain-neurotic tends to bear few rewards. More will be achieved if the surgeon is willing to stand by in a supportive role, just as a physician.

THERAPEUTIC APPROACHES

The notorious intractability of so many chronic pain patients cannot be simply explained by the persistence of these individuals in trying to find a physical solution to a basically psychological conflict, as if they were curable once they submitted to the treatment of their neurosis. In fact, this very insistence on a physical solution reflects their inability to sort out and deal with their conflicting psychological needs. We can conjecture that there must be milder forms of the pain-neurosis which may respond better to psychotherapy, or that at an early stage, perhaps before any

operation has taken place, these patients may be less intractable. Engel has indeed cited patients with "psychogenic" pain who responded to brief psychotherapeutic intervention.[7] In our experience, such cases appear to be decidedly rare among those pain patients referred to the psychiatrist by the surgeon.

We can describe a number of typical therapeutic engagements which occur with pain-neurotics, depending on the cooperation of patient and next-of-kin on the one hand, and availability of professional help on the other.

Primary Physician in Supportive Role

If psychiatric help either is not available or is not accepted by the patient, regularly scheduled visits to the primary physician may be an important help. Psychotropic drugs may be administered (see below) in preference to analgesics. The physical impairment must be de-emphasized, and resumption of an active life should be encouraged as much as possible. The pain should not be made light of, but the need for distraction through useful activity must be stressed. It may then be possible to arrest the vicious cycle of pain-less activity-more pain-more despair, or even to reverse it. The next-of-kin may need to be advised, together with the patient. Such an approach practiced by the non-psychiatric physician tends to carry more influence than if it came from a psychiatrist. Further unnecessary surgery should be advised against, regardless of the chance of a placebo effect. Consultations with other specialists may be unavoidable, and if so the consultant should be well informed of the rationale and importance of the treatment chosen.

Psychiatric Intervention

Referral to a psychiatrist may lead to a "flight into health." We have observed on several occasions patients who were willing to give up the pain, if the primary physician insisted on the need for psychiatric intervention. Sometimes the pain began to respond, for example, to a nerve block or even to a strictly diagnostic procedure, once the psychiatrist was in the picture. While such "flight into health" falls short of a cure and may be very temporary, it is nevertheless welcome to everybody involved. It tends to occur if the partner in the pain drama—spouse, next-of-kin or friend—is fed up with the pain and welcomes the psychiatric intervention.

PSYCHIATRIST IN SUPPORTIVE ROLE

This approach is feasible, and may bear a modicum of success if the spouse or other partner of the patient favors it. Tranquilizers and/or antidepressants may be prescribed. Stressful situations are discussed, with sympathy for the patient's hurt *feelings,* and self-assertiveness is encouraged. The pain, while not belittled, should not be discussed much. The partner-in-pain may be seen conjointly, albeit at the risk of doubling resistance, in an effort to air disputes and improve communications. The patient may sooner or later shop for more surgery, and the continued support of the primary physician will be very helpful.

PSYCHOTHERAPY

Intensive and protracted analytically oriented psychotherapy for several sessions a week, practiced by a skillful and firm therapist, has been successful in some cases. The therapist must be available to the patient as needed, must be able to handle a strong transference, and must be willing to take proper charge of the situation if the patient demands analgesics or seeks more surgery. Again, the patient's situation must be right for the success of such an approach, as may be the case after a patient's pathological (sado-masochistic) symbiosis has been dissolved by loss of the partner.

PSYCHIATRIC HOSPITALIZATION

Psychiatric hospitalization allows the patient to be removed from a home which fostered the pain-neurosis and permits well-planned attempts toward healthier ways of interacting with others. It has been demonstrated that with persistent lack of any response to atypical pain, this pain tends to become obsolete and expendable.[17] The entire staff must be trained to ignore the pain and, instead, to be tuned in to any manifestations of feelings. This approach precludes the use of any medication for pain, and few patients may be ready to undertake such a rigorous treatment program. Furthermore, because of the very human reflex to be sympathetic and

soothing toward one who is in pain, there tends to be marked hesitation on the part of a psychiatric staff to adopt such an approach. Finally, more permanent success would need to be assured by the proper education of those who will be near the patient after his discharge.

Conjoint Treatment in an Inpatient Pain Unit[8]

In such a Pain Unit, psychological assessment of the chronic pain patient is performed jointly with neurosurgical evaluation, permitting an evaluation of the relative proportion of organic and emotional causes of the pain. The psychological problems are treated by daily group therapy sessions consisting of frank discussions of how pain is used by each patient (e.g., for retaliation against spouse; to gain sympathy, narcotics, financial compensation, admiration for bravery, etc.) and how it interferes with rehabilitation. Certain interpersonal problems are dealt with in a few individual sessions by a directive and behavioral approach. Vocational and educational counseling, as well as social work assistance, is available, The staff is trained to forgo the traditional offerings of sympathy and concern for pain and to promote healthy behavior such as walking, socializing, or any other productive activity directed toward achievement of goals which were set upon admission. Despite the decrease of analgesic intake and the increase in activity level, the pain levels tend to decrease, and the patient's view of himself as a chronic invalid is effectively challenged. If surgery is felt to be warranted, a decision concerning operation is made only after clarification of the patient's psychological problems. The explanation by the *senior surgeon* to the patient of his physical *and* psychological status, and the feasibility of surgery, has proved to be the most critical point of the program.

This conjoint treatment takes into account very crucial issues presented by chronic pain patients: they listen more closely to their surgeon than to any psychiatrist or psychologist; they are not psychologically minded but action oriented; the enormous secondary gains secured by chronic pain must be undercut, and the old frail habit of marked activity must be reestablished and reinforced as much as possible. Therapeutic efforts of this conjoint type require an elaborate setting but appear to be among the most promising.

Hypnosis

The need for modest expectations in the treatment of pain-neurotics is still evident. Neither masochism nor excessive dependency can be eradicated, but a modification of these tendencies toward activity, gain of acceptance for productive performance, and an improved self-concept may be achieved. It also must be kept in mind that intractable pain in some patients is preferable, if a suicidal depression, other self-destructive behavior or psychosis is the only alternative.

The fact that chronic pain is needed by some patients, in whom it may be a substitute for a major mental disorder (see Case 28), represents a major reason for cautious use of the *hypnotic treatment of pain*. Though the pain may be safely transferred to another part of the body or lessened through hypnosis, complete removal of the pain by this means may precipitate a psychosis or suicidal act in a patient whose guilt and self-destructive urge had been satisfied by the chronic suffering. Beyond intrapsychic significance, the crucial role of the chronic atypical pain in the patient's interpersonal relationships further precludes simple removal through hypnosis. Thus, hypnosis is frequently ineffective in ameliorating functional pain, and it can lead to serious complications. Conversely, when the use of hypnosis is limited to the suppression of pain with a clear organic etiology, it is remarkably safe.[15] Hypnosis may be particularly helpful, however, for the exploration of the meaning of an atypical pain and as an auxiliary method in skillful psychotherapy.[18] The use of hypnosis is further limited, though, by the fact that while a great majority of individuals (over 90 per cent) have some degree of hypnotizability, only a small minority (about 10 to 15 per cent) respond to hypnotic suggestion with profound anesthesia.

Medication

The use of *psychotropic medication* is clearly indicated if a patient with chronic pain shows signs of an associated schizophrenic, depressive, or anxiety state; neuroleptic, antidepressant, or tranquilizing drug treatment is

then indicated.[9, 16] Even with more ordinary pain-neurotics, such drugs are frequently employed to lessen suffering.

Among the antidepressants, amitriptyline (Elavil), with its additional sedative effect, may be more effective tham imipramine (Tofranil). Chlorpromazine (Thorazine), thioridazine (Mellaril), and fluphenazine (Prolixin), among the neuroleptics, and chlordiazepoxide (Librium) and diazepam (Valium), among the minor tranquilizers, have all been reported to give a measure of relief in psychogenic pain. They may give better results than analgesics.

It is not sufficiently understood that opiates tend to have a marked tranquilizing effect which, rather than their analgesic effect, may explain their desirability to some chronic pain patients.

The *placebo effect* of various preparations can represent a useful adjuvant in the management of chronic pain patients.[3] The placebo effect of surgical procedures is difficult to establish but probably diminishes with increasing number of operations.

SUMMARY AND CONCLUSION

Pain is never a simple somatic experience. A "host of elusive variables" tend to be involved because invariably pain is an individual psychic experience. We must understand an individual's upbringing and cultural background, his needs and anxieties, and the personal meaning of a pain; only then does his pain experience become somewhat predictable. We know of no short-cut to the fuller understanding of pain.

Although patients in acute pain can be managed, regardless of the "functional overlay," with modern drugs and procedures, and old-fashioned reassurance, patients with chronic obscure and intractable pain are most difficult to manage. If they have not chosen to lead the life of invalids addicted to drugs, they seek out the surgeon and demand to be cured. We have described their problem as *the pain-neurosis of the surgery-seeking patient*. Behind an obscure pain is a concealed but not-so-obscure set of psychological difficulties which can be made clear by psychiatric interviews, special questionnaire, and psychological tests. The term "pain-neurosis" has been chosen to emphasize that we are dealing with a group of patients with a relatively homogeneous psychopathology. Most of these patients are not basically depressed or hysterical, anxious or schizophrenic; they represent a group of their own. The term "pain-neurosis" tells the surgeon that surgery will not cure the basic problem. But he must be able to recognize this type of patient.

The following *clinical-psychiatric profile for pain-neurotics* can be outlined. These patients may project a picture of rugged normalcy — if it weren't for that pain. Emotional difficulties are only admitted as a result of the pain, and interpersonal relationships are described as just fine, or unbelievably perfect. A history of mental and physical abuse may be given, but this is mostly a thing of the past, or "nothing I can't handle." Marked denial of psychological conflict goes hand-in-hand with the characteristic rejection of any psychiatric approach, but there is much urgency to have their problem removed by the surgeon's scalpel. Prior to onset of pain, they have characteristically led a life of relentless activity, often in a very physical sense and sometimes from an early age; the reversal to a dependent, demanding, invalid life-style seems very surprising. Close ties to a crippled or deformed next-of-kin are often detected, and an affinity with other "pseudo-independents" — alcoholic and/or promiscuous individuals — may be apparent in their history.

Psychological testing and in-depth psychiatric exploration establish the hidden *psychodynamic profile of the pain-neurotic* as an individual with marked conflicts and weaknesses who has lived above his means prior to onset of the pain. Sado-masochistic and infantile-dependent needs are prominent, but result in guilt and are strongly denied. The pain handily solves these conflicts, requiring dependency and providing atonement for guilt, while at the same time allowing a good measure of revenge toward the partner-in-pain, who has to keep bending over backward for the sufferer, swallowing his anger over the patient's constant agony and demands, and only secretly enjoying the suffering. This veiled intense sado-masochistic symbiosis in some cases replaces a previous overt sadomasochistic union.

The prevalent masochistic leanings result in desire for surgery, mutilation, or even death. Multiple surgical procedures speed the patient on the path to invalidism. Such patients should be recognized early, and the very first operation, unless there is a clear need, should be avoided. Pain-neurotics are not psy-chologically minded, and usually are not good candidates for psychotherapy. The surgeon who feels overly burdened by the patient's demands for a cure should not abruptly reject the patient via referral, but should remain available to help him back to a life offering rewards for activity instead of for pains — not pain-free probably, but with much less emphasis on pain. The modern pain clinics, guided by surgeons, yet psychologically oriented, are setting an important example.

References

1. Beecher, H. K.: Pain in man wounded in battle. Ann. Surg. *125*:96–105, 1946.
2. Beecher, H. K.: Quantification of the subjective pain experience. Proc. Amer. Psychopath. Assoc. *53*:111–128, 1965.
3. Beecher, H. K.: The placebo effect as a non-specific force surrounding disease and the treatment of disease. In Payne, J. P., Butt, R. A. P., Janzen, R., Keidel, W. D., Herz, A., and Steichele, C. (Eds.): Pain. Basic Principles–Pharmacology–Therapy. Baltimore, Williams & Wilkins, 1972, pp. 175–180.
4. Blumer, D.: Zur Psychologie der neurotischen Hypochondrie. Thesis, Zurich, 1957.
5. Bonica, J. J.: The Management of Pain. Philadelphia, Lea & Febiger, 1953.
6. Deri, S.: Introduction to the Szondi Test. New York, Grune and Stratton, 1949.
7. Engel, G. L.: "Psychogenic" pain and the pain-prone patient. Am. J. Med. *26*:899–918, 1959.
8. Greenhoot, J. H., and Sternbach, R. A.: Conjoint treatment of chronic pain. In Bonica, J. J. (Ed.): Advances in Neurology, Vol. 4, New York, Raven Press, 1974.
9. Kielholz, P.: Diagnosis and treatment of psychogenic pain. In Payne, J. P., et al. (Eds.): Pain. Basic Principles–Pharmacology–Therapy. Baltimore, Williams & Wilkins Co., 1972, pp. 172–174.
10. Kolb, L. C.: The Painful Phantom. Psychology, Physiology and Treatment. American Lecture Series. Springfield, The Charles C Thomas Co., 1954.
11. Melzack, R., and Casey, K. L.: In Kensalho, D. (Ed.): The Skin Senses. International Symposium on the Skin Senses — Florida State University. Springfield, The Charles C Thomas Co., 1968, p. 423.
12. Melzack, R., and Wall, P. D.: Pain mechanisms, a new theory. Science *155*:108–109, 1967.
13. Merskey, H.: An investigation of pain in psychological illness. D. M. Thesis, Oxford, 1964.
14. Merskey, H., and Spear, F. G.: Pain, Psychological and Psychiatric Aspects. London, Balliere, Tindall and Cassell, 1967.
15. Orne, M. T.: Pain suppression by hypnosis and related phenomena. In Bonica, J. J. (Ed.): Advances in Neurology. New York, Raven Press, 1974, pp. 563–572.
16. Reisner, H.: Psychotherapeutic drugs and the alleviation of pain. In Payne, J. P., et al. (Eds.): Pain.

Basic Principles–Pharmacology–Therapy. Baltimore, Williams & Wilkins, 1972, p. 174.

17. Rioch, D. McK.: The future of psychiatry from the standpoint of physiology. In Hoch, P. H., and Zubin, J.: The Future of Psychiatry. New York, Grune and Stratton, 1962, p. 41.

18. Rosen, H.: Hypnotherapy in Clinical Psychiatry. New York, The Julian Press, 1953.

19. Rosen, H.: Psychosomatic aspects of orthopedics (Discussion). In Cantor, A. J., and Fox, A. N. (Eds.): Psychosomatic Aspects of Surgery. New York, Grune and Stratton, 1956, pp. 145–158.

20. Sternbach, R. A., Wolfe, S. R., Murphy, R. W., and Akeson, W. H.: Traits of pain patients: The low-back "loser." Psychosomatics 14:226–229, 1973.

21. Szondi, L., Moser, U., and Webb, M. W.: The Szondi Test in Diagnosis, Prognosis and Treatment. Philadelphia, J. B. Lippincott, 1959.

22. Szondi, L.: Lehrbuch der Experimentellen Trebdiagnostik. Test-Band. (Third Ed.) Bern, Hans Huber, 1972.

23. Walters, A.: Psychiatric considerations of pain. In Youmans, J. R. (Ed.): Neurological Surgery. Philadelphia, W. B. Saunders Co., 1973, pp. 1615–1645.

CHAPTER 19

Rehabilitation of the Spinal Cord Injured Patient

THOMAS A. KELLEY, JR., M.D.
University of Louisville

The treatment of a patient with a traumatic spinal cord injury should ideally begin at the scene of the accident. Unfortunately, this ideal at the present is neither practical nor feasible in most parts of the world. For all practical purposes, case identification and treatment begins in the emergency room. Here in the emergency room the ultimate rehabilitation potential of the patient is determined by the avoidance of several mistakes which commonly occur during the period of emergency and acute medical and nursing care.

The prime rule in the early care of the spinal cord injured patient is to avoid any motion of the vertebral skeletal axis. This rule is commonly broken when a patient is brought to an emergency room and transferred from the stretcher to an examining table without adequate stabilization of the bony axis. There is no valid reason for transferring the patient to an examining table until early evaluation has been completed with the patient still on the stretcher. The patient with a suspected cord lesion should, in fact, have the clothing cut off so that movement is avoided; a rapid history can be obtained while the patient's clothing is being removed.

HISTORY

The mechanism of the patient's injury is of academic interest but adds little information toward guiding the plan of treatment. History should be elicited of any previous major surgical or medical illnesses, particularly endocrine problems such as diabetes. The history of allergy should be obtained, particularly that relating to medications. The history of the neurological level of the paralysis and the onset of sensory disturbance is particularly important. The patient must also be closely questioned as to whether there has been either progression or regression of the neurological involvement in the intervening period.

PHYSICAL EXAMINATION

The examination does not follow the routine pattern but should be adapted to cover the most critical systems first.

Respiratory System

Most patients will be in a state of neurogenic spinal shock, with absolute atonicity below the level of their lesion. The patient with either a cervical or a high dorsal cord lesion will present with a "paradoxical respiratory pattern." The patient will have at least a partially intact diaphragmatic excursion. However, the absence of the thoracic musculature allows chest retraction during an attempted inspiration with invagination of the intercostal musculature. Concomitantly, during attempted expiration there will be relative rebounding of the thoracic cage with evagination of the intercostal musculature. This unusual type of paradoxical respiration is best viewed at an oblique angle to the chest with good lighting. The pathomechanics which produce this respiratory pattern allow for little respiratory reserve. The patient's tidal volume and oxygen perfusion are diminished, while there is a relative increase in the dead space. If the patient's condition leads to a question of respiratory assistance, nasal oxygen or intermittent positive pressure breathing through a mask is of little help. In this case, a tracheotomy should be performed immediately. Although the tracheotomy can produce further complications, it eases the carrying out of tracheal toileting and avoids some of the problems of intubation. The posturing required for endotracheal intubation makes it a difficult and hazardous procedure in the face of an unstable cervical fracture.

Cardiovascular System

Neurogenic spinal shock produces not only atonicity of the striated musculature but also generalized atonicity of the vascular bed. Hypotension and tachycardia will mirror this anatomical configuration, with a systolic blood pressure often ranging between 60 and 80 mm of mercury. These patients, considering their age and general physical condition, will have a fairly adequate cardiac reserve. However, an indwelling venous catheter should be maintained since pressor agents may be required. The intravenous fluid of choice is a "keep vein open" (K.V.O.) drip of 5 per cent dextrose and water. An excess of fluid, especially electrolyte solutions, can overload the cardiovascular reserve, producing congestive failure which is extremely difficult to treat.

Concomitant, Non-Spinal Problems

A rapid evaluation should be performed to assess the possibility of non-vertebral fracture, intracranial lesions or significant intra-abdominal lesions. The presence of a ruptured viscus or evidence of intraperitoneal or retroperitoneal hemorrhage requires quick, tempo-rary immobilization of the spinal fracture and early surgical intervention. However, as has been mentioned earlier, the presence of rather profound hypotension and tachycardia does not necessarily signal the presence of a closed cavity lesion. A concomitant non-spinal abdominal lesion worsens the prognosis in a geometric rather than an arithmetic fashion, and the presence of significant intracranial lesions produces a rather dim prognosis.

Motor System Evaluation

The presence of a paradoxical respiratory pattern points to a lesion of the high dorsal or cervical neuraxis. In this case, the motor power of the lower extremities can be grossly assessed by asking the patient to move any portion of the leg, and observing any active motion. If no movement is elicited, one should move to the upper extremity in order to ascertain a neurological level. There is overlap of the root innervation in most of the musculature. Also, the root which exits from the foramina at the fracture level may be incompletely injured. Both of these facts lead to slight inaccuracies. However, most of the confusion of neurological level is due to the interposition of peripheral nerve terminology and ascribing it to a root distribution. A simple outline can be constructed to provide an evaluation of the functional motor level without moving the patient.

MUSCLE GRADING. During the evaluation, the joint movement initiated by the tests of muscle should be observed and if the limb can be brought through full range, the manual resistance should be given in order to provide strength grading. The muscle and tendon should also be palpated to avoid confusion caused by muscle substitution. The muscles can be graded from Zero (0) to Normal (N) with intermediate grades of Trace (TR), Poor (P), Fair (F), Good (G). The muscle grades have the following significance; 0, no observable or palpable movement of a muscle; TR, palpable movement of the muscle without any movement of the joint involved; P, active contraction which carries the joint through one half of its range of motion against gravity; F, the joint carries through full range of motion against gravity; G, the joint can be carried through full range against moderate resistance and N, the muscle can be carried through full range against maximal resistance.

TABLE 19–1.

Root Level	Muscle	Muscle Action	Palpation
C7–C8	First dorsal interosseous	Abduction of the second digit from the midline	Over radial border of the second metacarpal
C6–C7	Flexor carpi ulnaris	Wrist flexion	Tendon over volar wrist crease— ulnar aspect
C(5)–C6	Extensor carpi radialis	Wrist exten- sion with radial devia- tion	Tendon over dorsal wrist crease— radial aspect
*C5–C(6)	Biceps	Elbow flexion with full forearm supination	Anterior midarm
C(3)–C4	Deltoid	Abduction of the shoulder	Over the shoulder mantle
C3	Trapezius	Shoulder shrug	Over medial shoulder mantle

*The most common traumatic cervical spinal cord lesion is at a C5–C6 level. The patient will present active movement of shoulder abduction, elbow flexion, pseudopronation and supination provided by the brachioradialis and a TR to F extensor carpi radialis longus which produces wrist extension with radial deviation.

Motor Evaluation of Lower Extremities

If a paradoxical respiratory pattern is not present and one suspects a lower dorsal or lumbar lesion, a careful assessment of the lower extremities should be carried out before evaluating the upper extremities.

Sensory Evaluation

Rapid and accurate sensory evaluation and determination of sensory level in a patient with spinal cord injury is usually rather difficult. The patient's anxiety interferes with quick response for sensory comparison. In addition, there is frequently pain in a radicular distribution secondary to root compression at the fracture site. Despite these difficulties, a careful sensory evaluation should be performed to provide a confirmatory comparison to the motor examination. Sensation should be tested by employing a sharp pin and moving both from the suspected insensate to the sensate areas and the reverse. One should also test individually in each of the suspected der-

matomic distributions. Even with a suspected cervical lesion a full sensory evaluation should be carried out, beginning with the sacral segments in order to facilitate later comparative examinations. A simple body diagram should be employed, with differential markings for areas of relative hypalgesia and analgesia.

Urological Evaluation

The urinary bladder is atonic or markedly hypotonic in the presence of "spinal shock," and many of these patients have recently consumed copious quantities of ethanolic liquids. However, except in the presence of profound hypotension, renal function is not particularly impaired. The urinary bladder can rapidly become overdistended, resulting in multiple mucosal tears which later provide excellent avenues for the formation of multiple bladder diverticuli.

A small (no. 16 F.) silastic indwelling urinary catheter should be inserted under sterile conditions and connected to free drainage into a closed system. A constant intake

TABLE 19–2.

Root	Muscle	Muscle Action	Palpation
S2–S4	Gluteus maximus Gluteus medius	Hip extension and abduction	Superior and lateral to ischial tuberosity
L5,S1	Triceps surae	Plantar flexion of ankle	Posterior leg
L4–L5	Anterior tibial	Dorsiflexion and inversion of ankle	Tendon over medial ante- rior aspect of ankle joint
L(3)–L4	Quadriceps	Knee extension	Over anterior thigh or pa- tellar tendon
L1–L3	Iliopsoas*	Hip flexion	Tendon below inguinal ligament
D8–L1	Rectus abdominis**	Elevation of trunk	Over medial aspect of abdomen

*If a fracture of the lower dorsal or upper lumbar region is suspected, active contraction of the iliopsoas should be avoided. Vigorous contraction of this muscle provides a significant distractive force to the level of possible fracture.
**A similar distractive force can be provided by active contraction of the abdominal musculature. In addition, because of gross overlap of root levels, isolation of a particular root is far from perfect when testing the abdominal musculature.

TABLE 19-3.

Dermatomic Distribution	Areas To Be Tested
S2-S4*	Onion-skin layering in perianal region
S1	Medial aspect of ankle
L5	Anterolateral aspect of ankle
L4	Lower anterior thigh
L2-L3	Upper anterior thigh
D12,L1	Region of inguinal ligament
D10	Umbilicus
D7-D8	Epigastrium
D5**	Nipple line
C8	Fifth digit distal palmar aspect
C7	Third digit distal palmar aspect
C6	Second digit distal palmar aspect
C5	Base of first metacarpal on radial aspect
C4	Shoulder mantle

*It is necessary to have two other people gently abduct the thighs in order to adequately test the S2-S4 dermatomic segments. However, careful assessment is particularly important, since partial preservation of sensation is found in a "central cord lesion."

**A common mistake is to check sensation from distal to proximal in the thorax, and when a level near the nipple line is found it is listed as dorsal 5. Because the cervical and upper thoracic dermatomic patterns layer across the anterior chest wall in thin segments, one must check the upper extremity as soon as a level is found to be near the nipple line.

and output record should be started and kept with the patient at all times. In all patients the catheter should be securely taped to the anterior superior spine of the ilium in order to lessen the chances of accidental removal with the bag inflated. In the male patient, if the catheter is allowed to cross below the thigh, the natural curve of the penile urethra is disrupted at the level of the symphysis pubis and pressure is applied to the posterior portion of the urethra. This pressure can be indicated in the later formation of penoscrotal abscesses.

General Medical Review

At this point, with the institution of necessary respiratory and urinary care and with the hemodynamic situation under control, it is well to quickly assess the general medical status of the patient and also to quickly review those systems which have not been evaluated until this time. The patient may also complain of lancinating pain in a radicular pattern which conforms to the apparent fracture site. There would appear to be an apparent need for analgesia. However, analgesic-sedative class drugs can cause: 1) respiratory depression in a patient with a poor respiratory reserve; 2) emesis, with movement of the neuraxis and the possibility of aspiration; 3) iatrogenic addiction—this type of patient, with long term medical problems, is particularly subject to this problem; and 4), of most importance, the release of the protective spasm of the paraspinal musculature and produce worsening of the neurological picture. Radicular irritation produces reflex muscular spasm, which has the side effect of splinting the cervical spine. If the reflex is broken, the protective spasm is released. After reviewing the histories of several cases which were converted from incomplete to complete lesions after the use of analgesic or sedative drugs it is now felt that the use of these agents is contraindicated until good vertebral skeletal stabilization has been achieved.

X-Ray

With a clinical neurological level determined, x-rays should be obtained to localize the level and extent of the fracture or fracture-subluxation. Although portable x-rays may not provide the ultimate in detailed delineation, they are necessary to avoid moving the patient. It is agreed that in many situations a series of A-P, lateral and bilateral oblique views are desirable. However, with a suspected spinal cord injured patient the desired goal is to obtain the minimum number of views with the minimum of patient movement that will establish the level of bony instability. Multiple segmental fractures are possible, but are the exception to the rule. Therefore, the x-ray approach can be divided into three major categories, compatible with the three major segmental areas of fracture: 1) cervical; 2) dorsal; 3) lumbar.

CERVICAL

A trans-table lateral will in most cases provide the necessary information. Other views which require elevation or rotation of the body will in most cases produce little added information. If a low cervical lesion is suspected and/or muscle spasm has effectively foreshortened the neck, the shoulders may well obscure a lesion. Firm but gentle manual traction on the upper extremities will allow a better view of the cervical spine below the fifth cervical vertebra. If partial phrenic nerve involvement is suspected, a small plate can be slid under the lower dorsal area and a double exposure film will often demonstrate non-movement of the diaphragm.

DORSAL

The supraimposition of several structures interferes with the clear demarcation of the upper and mid-dorsal bony architecture. However, if the arms are maintained in an elevated position the trans-table lateral view will in most cases pinpoint the lesion. The intact dorsal cage provides relative protection to the upper dorsal spine. The relative infrequency of fractures in this region would confirm this fact. A review of a series of spinal cord injured patients revealed that relatively few had significant disruption of the bony structures between D1 and D6. Of the patients who did have significant fractures in this region, all had compromised the integrity of the dorsal cage either through fracture-subluxation of the sternum or through displaced fractures of the majority of the ribs. With patients who have sustained fractures between D1 and D6, a trans-table view of the sternum and a view of the rib cage should be obtained in order to avoid later complications produced by the instability in these cases.

LUMBAR

In addition to anterior wedge fracture and anterior-posterior subluxation, the lumbar spine is more prone to lateral displacement, especially with severe vehicular and defenestration trauma. Therefore, A-P as well as lateral views are desirable. A significant percentage of these cases will have concomitant pelvic fractures which can be demonstrated by using a large X-ray cassette.

TREATMENT

Early Fracture Stabilization

With the confirmed neurological diagnosis, the rule of avoiding movement of the patient is still of prime importance. A cervical fracture cannot be adequately immobilized with sandbags. They are essentially window dressing. Non-skeletal traction provides only slightly better results. The head weighs approximately twelve pounds. The coefficient of friction from the bed sheet significantly increases the effective weight of the head. Therefore, the use of five to 10 pounds of halter traction produces neither a reductive nor a distractive force. The major result of this type of treatment is the production of submandibular ulcerations and pain in the temporomandibular joint.

In the presence of a significant cervical fracture, adequate immediate stabilization can be provided only with skeletal traction. Halo-pelvic traction provides excellent stabilization, but is not at this time used as commonly as tong skeletal attachment. After implacement of a set of serial adjustable tongs, it is obvious that weights of 20 lbs or greater are required if any distractive force is to be transmitted to the spine. After application of this amount of weight, repeat trans-table lateral x-rays can be obtained to assess any change, and the amount of weight can be adjusted as necessary. It is often noted that the patient's radicular pain begins to diminish as adequate reduction is approached. A slight angle of flexion of the cervical spine will increase the effective traction. Conversely, as an increasing angle of extension is employed, the efficiency ratio of the traction is diminished and the possibility of deep decubitus ulceration of the occiput is increased.

Bed Care

The medical, surgical and nursing care of the patient can be facilitated and expedited if the patient is transferred to a turning frame prior to the application of tong skeletal traction. The transfer should be carried out with a four-man lift to the supine positioned frame. One person is responsible for each of the following segments: 1) Head and neck; 2) upper thoracic region and upper extremities; 3) lower thoracic region and pelvis; and 4) lower extremities.

One popular type of turning frame is the "circle bed." After reviewing the experience of some general hospitals in using this type of frame, we feel that its use is contraindicated in the care of acute spinal cord injured patients. This frame has a high incidence of mechanical failure, and it permits nursing mistakes with disastrous consequences. The frame presents problems with maintaining constant traction while the patient is being turned. If there is a malfunction while the patient is being turned and the frame should open, the patient is left in an extremely precarious position. And, in addition, if the frame should malfunction when the patient is in the erect position, postural hypotension can rapidly ensue and produce severe cardiac decompensation.

Of the prone-supine types of turning frames, the wedge Stryker is the safest and easiest to operate when used with two safety belts. The patient can be turned quickly and easily by one person. The traction force is undisturbed because the traction axis remains perpendicular to the head, and the possibility of postural hypotension is avoided since the movement is prone-supine. Patient injuries from frame malfunction are also greatly decreased with this type of turning mechanism. The patient can be transported while locked in the frame and can in fact be surgically prepared and treated without transfer.

Surgical Treatment

There has been widespread controversy over the applicability of early surgical intervention in the care of the spinal cord injured patient. One of the arguments against surgical intervention has been the cited mortality and morbidity, especially in those patients with cervical lesions. Another argument against surgical intervention has been the cited possibility of producing further injury to the root at the inferior portion of the fracture site in cervical spinal injuries, especially with the critical difference in functional capabilities that a single root level differential does make in this type of patient. Proponents of early surgical intervention have often cited the case which demonstrates worsening of the neurological condition, especially with a rising level of paralytic involvement, as a definite indication for intervention. In most cases, the controversy has led to endless debate without any particular solution. It can be agreed that early mobilization without compromise of the neural structures lends itself to a definite decrease in non-spinal complications of the skin, urinary system, skeletal system and psyche. Early mobilization lends itself to speeding up the training to bring the patient to his highest level of functional independence within the framework of the neurological injury. Perhaps the contro-

versy would be best approached with a definition of the goal of the surgical procedure; that is, whether it is designed as a "decompressive laminectomy" or whether it is designed to provide skeletal stabilization. In most cases, it would appear that the goal orientation in cervical and thoracic lesions should be toward *stabilization;* whereas in the lumbar region the goal of *decompression and stabilization* is perhaps more pertinent.

If the schemata of variable treatment for different levels of injury is to be followed, the lesions, of necessity, must be divided into the segmental components of 1) lumbar, 2) thoracic and 3) cervical.

LUMBAR. It is obvious that any lesion below the conus medullaris produces a lower motor neuron involvement with regenerative capabilities, somewhat comparable to those of a peripheral nerve injury. Early and adequate surgical decompression, with removal of extraneous material from the neural canal, in the absence of gross root avulsion, would appear to definitely improve the prognosis in this group of patients. Maintenance of general body functioning and prevention of skeletal and non-skeletal complications is most easily provided in this group and, therefore, immediate stabilization is of secondary concern.

THORACIC. As was noted previously, investigation should be carried out early, especially in the upper thoracic injury, to discern whether there may not well be concomitant rib or sternal fractures which have reduced the stability or integrity of the thoracic cage. In those cases in which it is evident, repair of the sternal fracture-subluxation may well increase the structural integrity. Vertebral rod fixation procedures allow early mobilization of the patient. In addition, a hinged, total contact, rigid polypropethylene jacket closely fitted to the thoracic cage and the iliac crest affords a good deal of protection for the spines of these patients. This type of jacket is easily removable to facilitate skin and nursing care.

CERVICAL. Severe wedge fracturing or comminution of the vertebral body does not provide a situation that is amenable to an anterior exploration approach with circular plug replacement. A posterior approach with articular and extra-articular fixation has been used in this type of case. However, more recently, the anterior approach with cervical corporectomy and intrabody fusion would appear to facilitate early mobilization of the patient, even with the presently inadequate orthoses to provide extraskeletal stabilization. This approach appears to have eliminated the problem of anterior resubluxation with slippage at the fracture site.

POSTSURGICAL CARE

The major requirement during the early period of postsurgical care is the prevention, through simple procedures, of the major complications which can prolong the period of hospitalization or prevent the patient's return to the highest functional capability.

Urological Care

The problem of urinary system ossification, related to diet in part, is primarily due to exorbitant calcium mobilization through the metabolism of nonstressed bone. The increased excretion of protein, calcium and phosphorus in the face of the inevitable presence of bacteria in the urinary tract presents a major problem for medical management. The problem of bacterial infection, especially organisms of the urea-splitting variety, can be lessened but not eliminated with judicious use of antimicrobial agents. A diminution of bacterial count decreases the amount of particulate material which is present for nidus formation; however, the basic problem of excess excretion of protein and electrolytes is not solved. Part of the answer to the problem appears to lie in the adage "Moss does not grow in a rapidly flowing stream." Since renal function is intact, a major part of the solution to the problem is to provide the maximum amount of solvent to dissolve the particulate matter which is being excreted. This can be accomplished by demanding a urine output of at least five liters a day. A urinometer can be used to observe the urinary specific gravity in the morning and evening. This procedure provides a double check of the daily calculated urinary output. As a general rule, the patient will not have major problems if the urinary specific gravity constantly remains less than 1.005.

Most of the patients in this phase of care are maintained on open drainage with an indwelling silastic catheter. As previously mentioned, the catheter must be securely attached to the anterior-superior pelvic brim to lessen the chances of accidental removal, with the catastrophic occurrence of pelvic thrombophlebitis, and also diminish the occurrence of penoscrotal abscess formation.

The catheter-urethra interface should be carefully cleansed three times per day with soap and a bacteriostatic solution, and the bladder irrigated with 1 liter of $\frac{1}{4}$ per cent acetic acid solution. This procedure also checks the patency of the catheter. Patients with a propensity to put out heavy crystalline material can be irrigated once a day with Renacidin.

The urine should be kept as bacteria-free as possible. The patient can be followed by obtaining routine urinalysis on a weekly basis. If there are a significant number of WBC's and bacteria, a culture and sensitivity is performed. In the presence of over 100,000 colonies per ml, appropriate antibiotic therapy is instituted. When the urine is relatively noncontaminated, an intermittent catheter clamping program is instituted and rapidly increased to $2\frac{1}{2}$ hours clamped and $\frac{1}{2}$ hour open. The catheter is then removed and a modified form of intermittent catheterization is performed. The patient is asked to attempt to void and Credé every four hours, and a catheterized residual urine is obtained. If the residual urine remains at less than 100 ml, the time between catheterizations is gradually increased to six, eight, and then 12 hours. Patients who are infection free continue to gradually increase the interval until they recheck every two weeks. Even male patients who have successful timevoiding programs will often continue to employ an external urinary collecting device in order to avoid any instances of incontinence. Female patients who are socially active often opt for prolonged catheterization in order to avoid the possibility of accidental voiding. When the patient can be moved without concern for the stability of the vertebral axis, a baseline intravenous pyelogram is performed. This is repeated on a regular basis and a cystometrogram is performed if hydronephrosis or hydroureter is suspected.

Decubitus Ulceration

The prime cause of decubitus ulceration is the presence of external pressure which exceeds the subcutaneous vascular system's ability to oxygenate the tissue. The end-arteriolar pressure of approximately 29 mm Hg provides a reference point to the critical amount of pressure the body can withstand. The time required to produce tissue necrosis is inversely related to the amount of pressure applied to the cutaneous and subcutaneous tissues. With the presence of significant pressure most spinal cord injured patients will develop critical changes in approximately two hours. Two other factors to be considered are the presence of exogenous macerating liquid and the ability of the body to disperse the pressure over a larger area. In the case of superficial bony prominences, the second factor is markedly diminished. Considering the above, one can easily establish the prime areas for the occurrence of decubitus ulceration.

1. Patient supine:
   a. sacral alae
   b. posterior calcaneus
   c. lateral malleolus
   d. occiput
2. Patient prone:
   a. anterior superior iliac spine
   b. patellae
3. Side lying:
   a. greater trochanter
   b. lateral malleolus
4. Sitting position:
   a. ischial tuberosities

Except in cases in which the care must be compromised due to extenuating circumstances, the only reason for a patient to develop a decubitus ulcer is poor nursing care. Turning frames, water mattresses, alternating air mattresses and gel pads provide an aid to, but should not be substituted for, good nursing care. No matter what type of bed the patient is placed upon, the major areas of pressure must be relieved by turning and positioning the patient at least every two hours, and more frequently if skin changes occur. Each time the patient is turned a meticulous check should be made of problem areas. With adequate lighting, the skin should be checked for erythema. Note should be made if with digital pressure there is not rapid blanching of any erythematous area, and rapid capillary filling when the pressure is removed. The check should be repeated before the patient is turned the next time. As long as non-blanching rubor persists, the area should not be used for weight bearing. In most cases it is necessary to provide extra protection to the posterior calcaneus and the lateral malleolus by using foam rubber boots. When the patient is sitting in a wheelchair, a gel pad can be employed; however, it is still necessary to carry out a wheelchair pushup every 20 to 30 minutes to relieve pressure under the ischial tuberosity.

The hydra-headed approach to the management of decubitus ulceration would lead one to question its efficacy. Treatment regimens which employ salt, sugar, dirt, lyophilized human albumin, Karaya gum powder, among others, appear to have two things in common: 1) marked increase in the amount of nursing care to the skin, and 2) universal partial success. Since pressure, maceration and shear forces are the primary causative factors of decubitus it is obvious that these factors must be eliminated no matter what the remainder of the regimen includes. Vigorous surgical debridement without elimination of recurrent pressure is tantamount to a creeping corporectomy. A large decubitus can also produce, through the transudation of protein and hemorrhagic diathesis, a severe protein depletion state with a negative nitrogen balance and anemia, both of which must be reversed.

The occurrence of a significant decubitus ulceration does not delay functional retraining by days but rather by weeks or months. The best treatment of decubiti is their prevention. If one must treat an ulceration, the foremost considerations are meticulous cleaning followed by the elimination of body depletion states and pressure.

Deep Venous Thrombosis

Pulmonary embolization is one of the major early complications in the care of these cases. The clinical and subclinical (autopsy) incidence appears to be approximately 40 per cent in these patients. The major sources of the thrombi are the deep pelvic veins and the deep venous system of the lower extremities. Although occurrence of pulmonary emboli cannot be completely eliminated, the incidence from pelvic sources can be markedly diminished by: 1) meticulous urinary catheter care, especially the prevention of excess pressure and traction on the bladder; and 2) extreme care in the nontraumatic use of rectal tubes.

Thrombus formation in the lower extremities is difficult to avoid, in view of the hematological pooling and diminished vascular flow. At the end of an operative procedure the vascular bed in the lower extremities should be carefully drained by elevating and emptying each leg. Thereafter, precise wrapping of the extremities should be carried out three times per day. An overlapping figure-of-eight technique should be used, starting at the metatarsophalangeal joints and ending at the groin. Custom fitted, long leg elastic hose, with open toe and closed heel, and 30 mm Hg pressure at the ankle appear to be of definite benefit. The use of anticoagulant medication after the development of deep thrombophlebitis can produce a major risk in view of the significant incidence of gastrointestinal stress ulcers in these patients.

Pulmonary Embolus

Pneumonia is a fairly common complication in the early course of the spinal cord injured patient. These patients, with limited respiratory capacity and reserve, are unable to fully aerate basal lung segments or produce an adequate cough for tracheobronchial cleansing. The tracheostomy patient makes obvious the need for frequent tracheal toileting; however, the need for careful respiratory care is also mandatory in the remainder of cases. The benefit of moisturized assisted intermittent positive pressure breathing is recognized in the care of many postoperative patients; however, it is often overlooked as a long-term measure in the care of the spinal cord injured patient. In addition to the use of IPPB, the patient can be assisted in producing increased aeration and tracheal toileting by manually stabilizing the chest and abdomen and demanding repeated efforts for a cough. This procedure can easily be carried out by nursing personnel each time the patient is to be turned.

Bowel Program

There is general hypomotility of the gastrointestinal tract, with a marked tendency toward constipation and impaction. One approach to the care of this problem has been the use of extremely low residue formula. However, these diets are generally intolerable, expensive and difficult to control. Another more practical approach is the use of a high residue diet plus bulk-forming medications or "stool softeners," with a consistently high fluid intake, as is required for the care of the renal system. Glycerin suppositories, or at times a more astringent medication, should be used at approximately the same time every 48 hours

to develop inherent rhythmicity of the bowel. It is important to place the suppository against the rectal mucosa and avoid burying it in the fecal mass. Most paraplegic patients can replace the suppositories with digital stimulation. However, strict adherence to a time schedule is necessary to provide cyclic evacuation. A low level enema may be used if no results are obtained after three days. But enema dependence is quickly acquired, and is difficult to change. Most patients prefer to cycle evacuation for the evening so that they have fewer problems after returning to work. This approach provides an early and practical beginning for a bowel retraining program which allows evacuation with the least number of unexpected bowel movements.

Stress Ulcer

Stress ulceration of the gastrointestinal tract occurs in approximately 25 per cent of patients with spinal cord injuries. This complication is most difficult to deal with, since pinpoint symptomatology is rarely present. The patient's basic neurological problem produces a diminution or absence of visceral awareness which is often coupled with the late appearance of blood, secondary to hypoactivity of the gastrointestinal tract. The treatment, if ulcers develop, is also difficult because the standard medication and diet regimen used in most patients with gastrointestinal ulceration can, in spinal cord patients, create early and serious renal complications. Prevention coupled with expectant awareness is the course of choice. The use of mild appropriate sedative medication, firm, gentle guidance from the physician, and good nursing care with frequent doses of TLC (tender loving care) appear to be the most beneficial regimen. If the patient does require anticoagulant medication because of thrombophlebitis or pulmonary embolus, the physician must be quite aware of the possible development of massive bleeding from stress ulcer.

Hypertension

Autonomic hyperreflexia can present a vexing problem in patients with upper dorsal or cervical cord lesions. It is present in these patients because the prime cause is interruption of the sympathetic feedback system. Afferent input produces generalized vasoconstriction below the patient's neurological level. There is an immediate elevation of blood pressure which stimulates the baroreceptors of the aortic arch and carotid sinus. This produces a vagal response, with resultant bradycardia. However, this change is not adequate to significantly alter the hypertensive state. The commonest direct cause is distention of the bladder, although distention of any viscus will produce the syndrome. Clinically the patient presents with headache, hyperhidrosis, cutis anserinus, facial erythema and dilation of the conjunctival vasculature. On physical examination the patient will have marked hypertension and a marked bradycardia. If the syndrome is not controlled it can produce intracerebral hemorrhagic diathesis or fatal cardiac arrhythmias, or both.

The syndrome may be reversed when the distended viscus is deflated; however, the viscus should not be deflated rapidly. For instance, if the urinary bladder contains 1200 ml the patient should be catheterized and approximately 200 ml removed at a time. If the viscus is rapidly deflated the syndrome may be accentuated. Patients having a surgical procedure on a viscus may require medicinal control. Likewise, patients who are postoperative from procedures which may have irritated the trigone may require medication for several days to effect control of the syndrome. The drug of choice would appear to be pentolinium tartrate, 20 mg orally three times a day.

Heterotrophic Ossification

Approximately 25 per cent of patients with spinal cord injury develop significant amounts of myositis ossificans, with calcification of soft tissue structures. The theories of causation are multiple (e.g., microtrauma, partial avulsion of muscle, post-hemorrhagic), as are the avenues of treatment (e.g., absolute rest, aggressive range of motion, surgical intervention). Although ossification can occur anywhere, the more common sites are about the elbow flexors, the hip flexors and knees. The involvement can be insidiously progressive and can immobilize multiple joints and vastly interfere with functional performance. Presently, the most promising approach appears to be passive maintenance of range of motion. Future hope lies in a medication which is presently undergoing double-blind evaluation, and which will possibly prevent this nonskeletal ossification.

Diet

The patient with spinal cord injury has a major problem with excess protein release and depletion at a time when his body is in negative protein balance. Also present is the problem of abundant calcium release. Although there is some excretion of the calcium through the gastrointestinal system, the major amount is excreted via the renal system. The dual problem of excessive protein and calcium mobilization has in the past been treated with normal diet and high calcium intake, in an attempt to provide replacement. This approach is based upon a false assumption. Although the negative nitrogen balance can, to a certain extent, be offset with a high caloric, high protein intake, the addition of exogenous calcium does not remedy the problem of calcium mobilization, but rather increases the load which must be excreted. This leads to the formulation of a diet which has a high caloric count, generally 2000 calories or above, with at least 100 gm of protein and a low calcium component (400 mg). The diet should have very little spice but a fair amount of fiber content to provide bulk.

Sexual and Reproductive Functions

After even initial conscious awareness, if not acceptance, of their neurological status these patients begin to demonstrate symptomatology of reactive depression. Because of the age grouping of the majority of these patients, a major, but often overlooked, problem is the question of sexual and reproductive function. The patient may be reticent to discuss the question until it becomes an overwhelming part of the depressive reaction. In this situation, the problem is often brought to the fore when the persons present are not knowledgeably equipped to deal with the situation. As part of the general care of the patient, explanation can be provided to avert ensuing problems.

Logically, the explanation must be divided into the problems of female and male but, in addition, the problem of the male must be considered in the light of either an upper or lower motor neuron lesion and in light of the effect on potency or fertility.

In the male with an upper motor neuron lesion, after spinal shock has abated, reflex erection without cerebral control is elicited by stimulation of the genital structures. The tumescent state will persist as long as reflex stimulation is provided. If there is a problem, in most cases it is not the initiation of erection but rather the occurrence of priapism. A male with a traumatic lower motor neuron lesion with interruption of the parasympathetic reflex pathways will be impotent.

Conversely, a large percentage (approximately 95 per cent) of patients with an upper motor neuron lesion will be sterile and later develop testicular atrophy. The reason is not clear; loss of temperature control below the level of the lesion, urethral reflux, and recurrent infections have all been proposed as causative agents. In dealing with these patients, the fact of potency is stressed, and in early discussions the possibility of fertility is dealt with by advising the patient to take precautions if he does not wish to take a chance of impregnating. There is a high incidence of normal testicular function in the male with a lower motor neuron lesion. If spermatozoa can be mechanically recovered, impregnation is theoretically possible.

The problems of the female patient with either an upper or a lower motor neuron lesion are somewhat comparable. Studies are presently underway in an attempt to elucidate the phenomenon of amenorrhea after spinal cord injury which appears to last until spinal shock subsides. The first superficial reasoning of a Selye stress syndrome as the cause does not fit the clinical picture in these cases. There is some slight evidence that, although amenorrheic, these patients might not necessarily be anovulatory. After return of the ovarian cycle, the fertility potential of these patients is not altered. If anything, they may stand at greater risk. This, in and of itself, presents a problem because of the increased proclivity to the development of deep vein thrombophlebitis and the problem of adequate protection of the urinary system during gestation. Pregnancy is highly inadvisable for at least two years after the onset of the neurological lesion. A secondary problem is the provision of prophylactic measures for this group of females, the majority of whom are nulliparous. Cervical diaphragms are not well retained or easily placed. Intrauterine devices appear to be more easily expelled and, since the patient is prone to phlebitis, oral anovulatory preparations present a definite risk. If the patient does become pregnant this should not be an unusual obstetrical problem except in the patient with severe spasticity. This can present bodily risk to the obstetrician during attempted examination if he is unprepared. Labor and vaginal delivery in both types of cases present no particular problems; if anything, the problem of soft tissue outlet obstruction is eliminated. For unknown reasons, even the severe spasticity of the upper motor neuron patient appears to lessen or disappear during labor and delivery.

In summary, the male with an upper motor neuron lesion is generally potent but sterile; the reverse is true in the lower motor neuron lesion. In the female patient, the ability to procreate and deliver is essentially unaltered.

REHABILITATION

Range of Motion and Positioning

Extra-articular soft tissue contractures can develop quite rapidly and insidiously if active preventive measures are not followed. The theory of very frequent range of motion exercises to increase neurological return is a common fallacy and should not be fostered. ("If a little will help, a lot will cure.") Joint contractures can be avoided if full range of motion to each joint which the patient cannot actively control in full is carried out twice a day. The contractures which develop most readily produce loss of shoulder abduction and elbow extension, forearm supination and pronation and wrist and digit flexion, and produce an intrinsic minus hand. In the lower extremity, contractures produce the loss of internal rotation of the hip, flexion of the knee and dorsiflexion of the ankle. Considering the joints which are most commonly involved, one can also correctly position the patient in bed to avoid some of the problems. The upper extremities should be positioned with the hand above the elbow and the elbow above the shoulder, when the patient is supine. The lower extremities can be held in internal rotation with rolled bath blankets. A footboard or similar device should be employed to keep the sheets from being tucked tightly and forcing the ankles into fixed equinus. Once contractures are allowed to develop, the care required by the patient will be unnecessarily prolonged and functional return, despite neurological return, may be prevented.

Hypotension

When the patient has a stable neuraxis, mobilization can begin. However, the patient has had a long period of enforced bed rest and has persistent absence of vascular control below the neurological level. These factors produce acute hypotension with possible cardiac decompensation when the patient is brought to the erect position. The use of lower extremity Ace bandage wrapping and abdominal binders will partially correct the problem. However, the patient's body must reaccommodate to the upright position. To effect accommodation, the patient can be placed on a tilt table and the angle of incline and time of elevation gradually increased. In patients who have difficulty adapting, 5 per cent CO_2 by face mask will provide central vasodilation and peripheral vasoconstriction. As soon as the patient is able to passively stand for approximately 10 minutes he can progress to a reclining wheelchair.

Mobilization

These patients are of necessity placed in a dependent position during their early care. Yet, one of the aims of the treatment program is to produce independence. The patient can begin moving himself about even before sitting is allowed. A well padded, self-propelled, prone stretcher allows him to get out of his room and adopt a feeling of freedom. After the patient is accommodated to the upright position he should be provided with his own wheelchair. The wheelchair should be of sturdy construction but easily collapsible. The arm rests should be removable desk-type and well padded, to facilitate transfer activities and to allow the patient to more closely approach a table or desk. Swingaway, elevated, removable leg rests with heel loops allow better control of dependent edema and facilitate removal of the device for transfer activities; the heel loops tend to better position the legs. Solid rubber tires, toggle brakes, and 8-inch front casters with caster and reverse locks provide safer travel. The addition of wheel projections aids the quadriparetic patient in propelling the chair. If narrow dorways are en-

countered, a Narrow-matic device can diminish the width of the chair without disturbing the patient. A motorized model with proportional control is available for patients with severe impairment. Although the initial outlay is rather substantial, a well engineered and constructed chair will save money and prevent trouble.

Splints and Devices

The tenodesis action of the wrist and digits is a normal function produced by the differential flexor-extensor tendon lengths. A neurologically intact person who is at complete rest will produce finger flexion when the wrist is passively extended. This phenomenon is reinforced to produce grasp in the quadriparetic patient. If the fingers are allowed to develop slight flexion contracture of the interphalangeal joints the grasp is enhanced and becomes more functional. A patient with a functional extensor carpi radialis longus, to produce wrist extension, can be fitted with a flexor hinge driven tenodesis splint. With this splint the second and third digits are flexed toward the fixed first digit when the wrist is extended (i.e., wrist extension is converted mechanically into finger flexion). A patient who lacks active wrist extension can be equipped with an externally powered tenodesis splint; the orthosis is activated when a switch is activated by another movement of the body.

For patients with cervical injuries a most useful device is the universal cuff. This is an elasticized cuff which fits over the hand and has a pouch along its palmar axis. It will accept eating utensils, pencils or typing sticks and can be donned by the patients themselves. As a general rule, a patient will reject gimmick devices; however, there are numerous self-help devices (i.e., long-handled shoehorn, plate guard) which will increase the patient's functional capability if he is trained to use them well.

Exercise

In the spinal cord injury patient the upper extremities, for all practical purposes, must replace the function of the lower extremities. The quadriparetic patient must have excellent strength for transfer activities and wheelchair pushups; the paraparetic patient must have strength and endurance for ambulation activities. Most patients can be started on an exercise program while still bedbound. The weights can then be increased as tolerated, and disuse atrophy be prevented. When the patient's spinal fracture is stabilized, the amount of weight and the time of exercise should be quickly increased. Despite patient recognition of the need for muscular development, repetition produces boredom. This can be avoided by the judicious use of occupational therapy which produces a task oriented exercise program. A patient will work for a prolonged period on a weighted sanding project, if at the end of a period of time a finished product is produced. Paraplegics will often have contests to see who can loom the most material, despite the fact that a resistance of 30 pounds is included.

Mat activities are introduced to teach the patient passive control and positioning of the lower extremities. In addition, the patient must be trained in body balancing exercises so that he can use his upper extremities for activities other than maintaining the sitting position. The patient then progresses to transfer activities. In most instances, a side-sliding transfer technique is employed by removing the arm of the wheelchair and if necessary using a transfer board.

Bracing

Numerous types of braces are used on the cervical spine without much success in absolute control of motion. In fact, either the patient is able to voluntarily control abnormal movement or a cervical-pelvic halo traction is required. Some support to increase sitting balance can be provided by a Hoke corset with duralumin paravertebral and axillary stays. Somewhat greater support can be produced for the patient with a dorsal lesion by using a Knight–Taylor brace. However the dorsal spine can be truly protected only by employing a molded total contact hinged jacket constructed of rigid, easily cleaned material. This type of jacket has advantages over a plaster Minerva jacket in the production of a skintight fit without excessive focal pressure. Also, it can be easily removed, one half shell at a time, for skin inspection and care.

A back brace, if required, can be incorporated into the braces for the lower extremities. The braces should be considered from the shoes up. The shoe is the foundation of the brace and is not to be lightly regarded. It should be a well-fitted oxford with an 8/8 rubber heel, 12 iron leather sole, solid steel shank with long medial counter, and a blucher closure. Attachment to the brace by a split flat caliper attachment with drop rivets will allow the patient to change shoes. Most patients can use a 105 degree Klenzak ankle joint. Steel or duralumin uprights may be used, depending on the patient's weight and the presence of spasticity. A medial or lateral drop box lock with spring bullet can be used on one clevis knee joint, and a bail lock used on the contralateral side. Drop box hip locks with spring bullets can be used if the brace is to be connected to a pelvic band. As a general rule, patients with lesions above D4 cannot become functional ambulators with braces; they have neither the balance nor, more importantly, the cardiorespiratory reserve. The exceptions to this rule are usually heavily muscled, thin, young male patients. Patients with lesions below D4 without intercurrent problems (i.e., obesity, pulmonary disease, fractures) can be taught to ambulate with braces and crutches. Much has been made of the fact that many patients do not continue to use their braces after a period of time, leading some to question their utility—this is a very shortsighted view. The patient, while it is still feasible, should be given a trial at ambulation so that he does not later report, "If only I had been given a chance, things would be different." A second, more important, reason for bracing a patient is the increased strength and endurance of the upper extremities that ambulation produces. The repetitive lifting of the body weight provides an exercise which cannot be otherwise duplicated. The resultant musculature may not, in the long run, be used for ambulation but it is of great help in carrying out the activities of daily living, especially wheelchair transfer activities. Most patients use adjustable aluminum forearm crutches during ambulation; they are lightweight and easily stored and provide a platform when resting. The forearm band should be hinged to turn completely around in order to avoid a forearm fracture during the inevitable fall.

Activities of Daily Living

The average person prepares for his daily activities without conscious effort. Bathing, grooming and dressing are almost automatic activities. However, in the patient with residual paresis a systematic approach to these activities must be adopted. Dressing then becomes an act which is a total of many subsystems. Techniques must be adapted for placing trousers over extremities which do not cooperate and for pulling up trousers while in the supine position. Each of the patient's activities must be evaluated. Then, either with assistive devices or substitute movements, the patient must be taught to perform the tasks. Both the patient with braces and the patient confined to a wheelchair must be able to function as independently as possible. A patient who cannot perform a wheelchair transfer to bed, toilet or automobile is a prisoner in the wheelchair. Likewise, the person who is not taught to drive an automobile with hand controls is being deprived of a major avenue of independence. Over 300 activities of daily living must be evaluated and the patient must be trained to perform the tasks. This portion of the rehabilitative process, while not as obvious as exercise or gait training, is just as important.

Spasticity

Spasticity appears in the majority of patients with spinal cord injuries as the effects of spinal shock abate. In some patients it is hardly bothersome, while in others it grossly interferes with function. Spasticity may limit ambulation activities or even wheelchair independence and can lead to skin breakdown because of the shearing forces and difficulty in positioning. The involuntary movements can be medically dampened in many patients through the use of diazepam or dantrolene. However, the patient with significant spasticity usually requires ablative surgery, and most patients will reject this type of surgery until there is little alternative. At times, a simple peripheral neurectomy or tenotomy will bias the tonicity enough to allow increased function. Other procedures which can be employed are anterior or posterior rhizotomy, cordotomy, myelotomy, or intrathecal introduction of absolute alcohol. The procedure for an "alcohol wash" is quick, is easily performed, and requires only a lumbar puncture. However, a side effect is ablation of potency in the male patient. This side effect can usually be avoided with a Bischoff type myelo-

tomy; however, this procedure does require a laminectomy. To decrease the occurrence of psychological side effects, any of the above procedures must be fully explained to the patient, and the patient must decide if the spasticity interferes enough with his activities to warrant the contemplated procedure.

Phantom Phenomenon

Phantom sensation and pain are well recognized and appreciated in amputation patients. These phenomena are also present in peripheral nerve injuries, brachial plexus lesions, hemiparesis and spinal cord injuries. Therefore, it would perhaps be better to consider the process to be the result of denervation rather than amputation. Several theories have been propounded to explain the occurrence. The most commonly accepted theory relates to the concept of "body image" which is considered to be a stable cognitive feature refined from past sensory experience. The phantom would therefore be the persistence of the fixed body image beyond the time of denervation. The phantom extremities usually do not conform to the position of the patient's extremities.

The patient with a spinal cord injury may also, in addition to phantom extremities, have a phantom bladder, penis, or rectum. There is no treatment per se; however, the phenomenon should be fully discussed with the patient. In doing so, one can avoid the costly traps produced when a patient 1) feels that he is becoming non compos mentis; 2) accepts the phantom as evidence of neurological return and passively awaits further return; or 3) becomes iatrogenically addicted while being treated for phantom pain.

Functional Versus Neurological Level

The goal of treatment for the patient is greatly influenced by the residual neurological function. A patient without motor power cannot be retrained to carry out highly functional activities. Likewise, the goal must be limited if there is little cardiorespiratory reserve. Complete cervical lesions above C4 have shoulder shrug but no movement of the extremities which can be harnessed; the respiratory reserve is greatly compromised as well. Neurological function at C4-C5 produces enough movement of the extremity so that, with assistive splinting and external motor assist, limited wheelchair activities can be performed. In many cases a motorized wheelchair will be employed. C5-C6 is the commonest cervical level of injury: the patient can use a self-powered tenodesis splint to produce grasp and is able to propel a wheelchair for short distances. The lack of full sensation in the hand interferes with fine coordinate activities and the patient will require assistance for wheelchair transfer activities.

At C6-C7, the patient has wrist flexors and extensors and triceps. The patient's wheelchair endurance is increased; he is better able to transfer; and he can drive an automobile with hand controls. C8-D1 patients have complete motor and sensory function of the upper extremities for the provision of fine coordinate hand skills, while a strong latissimus dorsi allows transfer activities with more ease. These patients are completely independent from a wheelchair. D4-D12 patients have increasing repiratory reserve; sitting balance should be adequate especially in the lower lesions; they are completely independent from a wheelchair and, in the absence of complicating factors, should be independent in ambulation with braces and crutches.

With L1 to L3 levels of injury, patients should be completely independent with long leg braces and canes. L4-L5 patients are independent with short leg braces to merely control the ankle joint. S1-S5 patients require no bracing but will have an abnormal gait and difficulty with bowel and bladder control. So, while there are many similarities in patients with spinal cord injuries at various levels there is a variance in the treatment approach and the goal depending upon the neurological level.

SUMMARY

Just a few years ago, the life of the patient with spinal cord injury was quite short. Today, the life span has been markedly increased through the use of modern medical care. Therefore, both from a humanistic and an economic viewpoint, these patients must receive excellent, not just adequate, care from the onset. The avoidance of the complications which have been outlined represents a cost saving of several thousands of dollars per patient. Excellent care also produces a human being who can be reintegrated into society. The patient must be discharged from an institutional setting as quickly as feasible; however, ongoing followup care is mandatory. Medically, the patient must have urological evaluation at six months after discharge and yearly thereafter. Of equal importance is the psychological support and educational retraining necessary to allow the individual to be highly productive within his functional capability; that is, accepting the disability but reducing the handicap. In cooperation with vocational rehabilitation, the patient enters the next phase of rehabilitation, becoming a productive member of society.

References

1. Abramson, A. S.: Modern concepts of management of the patient with spinal cord injury. Arch. Phys. Med. 48:113–121, 1967.
2. Bell, E., Elliott, R. M., and Von Werssowetz, O. F.: Muscle strength and resultant function in cervical cord lesions. Amer. J. Occup. Ther. 15:106–109, 1961.
3. Campbell, E. W., Jr.: Bladder dysfunction related to lesions of the spinal cord. South. Med. J. 60:364–366, 1967.
4. Cate, J. ten, Boeles, J. T., and Visser, P.: Contributions to the physiology of spinal shock. Acta. Physiol. Pharmacol. Neerl. 8:315–325, 1959.
5. Chesire, D. J.: The complete and centralised treatment of paraplegia. Paraplegia 6:59–73, 1968.
6. Comarr, A. E.: Sexual function among patients with spinal cord injury. Urol. Int. 25:134–168, 1970.
7. Comarr, A. E., Kawaichi, G. K., and Bors, E.: Renal calculosis of patients with traumatic cord lesions. J. Urol. 87:647–656, 1962.
8. Cox, F.: Staffing of nursing personnel spinal cord injury service. Proc. Ann. Clin. Spinal Cord Inj. Conf. 17:111–112, 1967.
9. Damanski, M.: The care of tetraplegic patients after discharge from hospital. Practitioner 185:780–792, 1960.
10. Davenport, L. F.: The use of drugs in the care of spinal cord injury patients. Proc. Ann. Clin. Spinal Cord Inj. Conf. 16:69, 1967.
11. Druckman, R., et al.: Central pain of spinal cord origin: Pathogenesis and surgical relief in one patient. Neurology (Minneap) 15:518–522, 1965.
12. Fällstrom, C. E.: A study on working capacity of persons physically disabled by neurologic disease or injury. Effect of rehabilitation. Acta Neurol. Scand. 40:(Suppl 6):1–112, 1963.
13. Freed, M. M., et al.: Life expectancy, survival rates, and causes of death in civilian patients with spinal cord trauma. Arch. Phys. Med. 47:457–463, 1966.
14. Gregg, R. A., et al.: Spinal cord lesions and rehabilitation: Review of cases discharged from the Duke Medical Center, Neurosurgical Division. South. Med. J. 61:589–597, 1968.
15. Gucker, T.: Rehabilitation in injuries of the spinal cord. J. Occup. Med. 4:61–64, 1962.

16. Jackson, R. W.: Sexual rehabilitation after cord injury. Paraplegia *10*:50–55, 1972.
17. Jousse, A. T., et al.: The management of the spastic contracted bladder in spinal cord dysfunction. Proc. Ann. Clin. Spinal Cord Inj. Conf. *15*:140–151, 1966.
18. Kaplan, L. I., et al.: A reappraisal of braces and other mechanical aids in patients with spinal cord dysfunction: results of a followup study. Arch. Phys. Med. *47*:393–405, 1966.
19. Klein, S. J., et al.: Urinary tract disease in spinal cord injury patients, I. A brief outline of the problem. Paraplegia *7*:6–9, 1969.
20. Knapp, M. E.: Practical physical medicine and rehabilitation. 11. Spinal cord injury. Postgrad. Med. *42A*:111–116, 1967.
21. Knorr, N. J., et al.: Spinal cord injury: psychiatric considerations. Maryland Med. J. *19*:105–108, 1970.
22. LaBan, M. M., et al.: Blood volume following spinal cord injury. Arch. Phys. Med. *50*:439–441, 1969.
23. Morales, P.: Neurogenic bladder in traumatic paraplegia. New York J. Med. *68*:2031–2037, 1968.
24. Moulton, A., et al.: Chest movements in patients with traumatic injuries of the cervical cord. Clin. Sci. *39*:407–422, 1970.
25. Munro, D.: The role of fusion or wiring in the treatment of acute traumatic instability of the spine. Paraplegia *3*:97–111, 1965.
26. Nieder, R. M., et al.: Autonomic hyperreflexia in urologic surgery. J.A.M.A. *213*:867–869, 1970.
27. Remvig, O.: Rehabilitation of patients with spinal cord injuries. Acta Psychiat. Scand. *36*(suppl 150):282–294, 1961.
28. Rosenthal, A. M.: A rational therapeutic program for patients with spinal cord transsection. Med. Times *90*:407–413, 1962.
29. Rossier, A.: The organization and function of the spinal cord injury service of the Veterans Administration Hospital, Long Beach, California. J. Int. Coll. Surg. *39*:225–237, 1963.
30. Runge, M.: Self-dressing techniques for patients with spinal cord injury. Amer. J. Occup. Ther. *21*:367–375, 1967.
31. Shul, J. R., et al.: Pulmonary embolism in patients with spinal cord injuries. Arch. Phys. Med. *47*:444–449, 1966.
32. Silver, J. R.: The oxygen cost of breathing in tetraplegic patients. Paraplegic *1*:204–214, 1963.
33. Suwanwela, C., Alexander, E., Jr., and Davis, C. H., Jr.: Prognosis in spinal cord injury, with special reference to patients with motor paralysis and sensory preservation. J. Neurosurg. *19*:220–227, 1962.
34. Trigiano, L. L., et al.: Physical rehabilitation of quadriplegic patients. Arch. Phys. Med. Rehab. *51*:592–594, 1970.
35. Tudor, L. L.: Bladder and bowel retraining. Amer. J. Nurs. *70*:2391–2393, 1970.
36. Webb, J.: Decubitus ulcers. Proc. Ann. Clin. Spinal Cord Inj. Conf. *17*:113–114, 1967.
37. Weber, D. K., et al.: A review of sexual function following spinal cord trauma. Phys. Ther. *51*:290–295, 1971.
38. Wilcox, N. E., et al.: A statistical analysis of 423 consecutive patients admitted to the Spinal Cord Injury Center, Ranchos Los Amigos Hospital, 1 January 1964 through 31 December 1967. Paraplegia *8*:27–35, 1970.
39. Wilcox, N. E., and Stauffer, E. S.: Follow-up of 423 consecutive patients admitted to the Spinal Cord Center, Ranchos Los Amigos Hospital 1 January to 31 December 1967. Paraplegia *10*:115–122, 1972.

INDEX

Note: In this index, page numbers in *italics* refer to illustrations; page numbers followed by (t) refer to tables.

Ankylosing spondylitis (*continued*)
  bilateral sacroiliitis in, 737, 738
  calcification and spur formation in, 733, *736*
  cardiovascular disease in, 729
  cauda equina syndrome in, 728
  cervical spine in, 727–729
  cervicodorsal kyphosis in, 727, *727*
  chin on chest deformity in, 792–796
  clinical features of, 725–728
  clinical laboratory studies in, 730
  course of, 725, 734–737
  diagnosis of, 737
    pain in, 725
    stiffness in, 725
  differential diagnosis of, 737–743
    acro-osteolysis in, 742
    adult rheumatoid arthritis in, 738
    ankylosing hyperostosis in, 786
    colitic spondylitis in, 739
    diseases with "ossifying diathesis" in, 741
    fluorosis in, 741
    heredofamilial vascular and articular cal-
      cification in, 742
    hypoparathyroidism in, 741
    hypophosphatemic rickets in, 741
    infections in, 740
    juvenile rheumatoid arthritis in, 738
    lumbosacral strain in, 737
    myositis ossificans progressiva in, 741
    neoplasia in, 740
    osteitis condensans ilii in, 739, *739*
    Paget's disease in, 742, *742*
    psoriatic spondylitis in, 739
    Reiter's spondylitis in, 739
    sacroiliac disease in paraplegia in, 738
    sarcoidosis in, 743
    spondylolisthesis in, 737
    spondylolysis in, 738
  dislocation of atlantoaxial joint in, 728, 733
  dorsal spine in, 726–727
  erythrocyte sedimentation rate in, 730
  extra-articular bone lesions in, 729
  extra-spinal arthritis in, 728
  flexion deformity in, *727, 728*
  fuzzy new bone formation in, 734, *737*
  hip joint disease in, 733, *736*
  HL-A antigens and, 722
  incidence of, 721
  in differential diagnosis of ochronosis, 788
  in differential diagnosis of Reiter's spondylitis,
    756
  interspinous ligaments in, 733
  lumbar spine in, 726
  meningeal involvement in, 728
  neurological involvement in, 728
  onset of, 721, 725
  ossification in, 723, *723, 724, 724*
  osteitis in, 723
  osteophytes in, *735*
  osteoporosis in, 723, *734*
  paraplegia in, 728
  paraspinal muscle atrophy in, 727, *727*
  pathologic changes preceding, 724
  pathology of, 722–725
    at lumbar vertebrae, 723, *724*
    in manubriosternal joint, 723, *723*
    schematic representation of, *724*

Ankylosing spondylitis (*continued*)
  progression of spinal deformity in, 734
  pulmonary disease in, 729
  pulmonary fibrosis in, 729
  radiographic findings in, 730
  recurrent iritis in, 729
  referred pain in, 727
  rheumatoid factor in, 730
  rib cage in, 726–727
  sacroiliac joints in, 725, 730, 731, *731*
  sacroiliitis in, *731*
  sclerosis in, 723, *723, 724*
  severe hip disease in, 736
  sphincter disturbances in, 728
  squaring of lumbar vertebrae in, 732, *732*
  symptoms of, 725
  syndesmophyte formation in, 724, *724*
  syndesmophytes in, 732, 734, *734, 735*
  synonyms of, 721
  synovitis in, 730
  thoracic spine in, 726
  trauma and, 728
  treatment of, 743–745
    anti-rheumatic agents in, 744
    aspirin in, 744
    corticosteroids in, 744
    corticotropin in, 744
    hyperextension exercises in, 803
    indomethacin in, 744
    osteotomy in, 803
    phenylbutazone in, 744
    prognosis in, 743
    radiation therapy in 744
    rest-exercise program in, 743
    stages in, 803
    therapeutic exercise in, 743
    "trolley track" configuration in, 733, *735*
  ulcerative colitis in, 748
  widening of joint spaces in, 730
Ansa hypoglossi, 86
Anterior horn cell degeneration, 62
Antidepressants, for spinal pain, 848
Anti-rheumatic drugs, in treatment of psoriatic
  arthritis, 751
Anulus fibrosus, 80, *80*
  development of, 9
  elastic properties of, 50
  structure of, 32
Apical ligament, 25
Aplasia, odontoid, 173
Apophyseal joint, subluxation of facets of, *397*
Arachnoid cyst, following lumbar disc surgery,
  499
Arch, cervical, ossification of, *8*
  lumbar, ossification of, *8*
  neural, *8*
  thoracic, ossification of, *8*
  malformation of, 161, *168*
Arnold-Chiari syndrome, 55
Arterial hypoxemia, 285
Arteriosclerosis, and atlantoaxial instability, 163
Arteriovenous malformation, 55
  and back pain, 57
  and radicular pain, 58
Artery(ies), basilar, 85
  carotid, 87
  cervical, deep, 43